MASTER TECHNIQUES IN ORTHOPAEDIC SURGERY
■
THE FOOT AND ANKLE

MASTER TECHNIQUES IN ORTHOPAEDIC SURGERY

Series Editor
Roby C. Thompson, Jr., M.D.

Volume Editors

THE FOOT AND ANKLE
Kenneth A. Johnson, M.D.

RECONSTRUCTIVE KNEE SURGERY
Douglas W. Jackson, M.D.

KNEE ARTHROPLASTY
Paul A. Lotke, M.D.

THE HIP
Clement B. Sledge, M.D.

THE SPINE
David S. Bradford, M.D.

THE SHOULDER
Edward V. Craig, M.D.

THE ELBOW
Bernard F. Morrey, M.D.

THE WRIST
Richard H. Gelberman, M.D.

THE HAND
James W. Strickland, M.D.

THE FOOT AND ANKLE

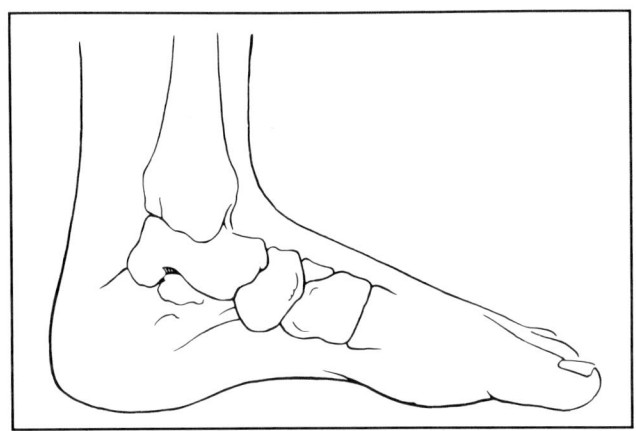

Editor

KENNETH A. JOHNSON, M.D.
Chairman
Division of Foot and Ankle Surgery
Mayo Clinic Scottsdale
Scottsdale, Arizona
Professor of Orthopaedics
Mayo Medical School
Rochester, Minnesota

Illustrator
Deborah Ravin
Phoenix, Arizona

Raven Press ● New York

Raven Press, Ltd., 1185 Avenue of the Americas, New York, New York 10036

© 1994 Raven Press, Ltd. All rights reserved. This book is protected by copyright. No part of it may be reproduced, stored in a retrieval system, or transmitted, in any form or by any means, electronic, mechanical, photocopying, or recording, or otherwise, without the written permission of the publisher.

Made in the United States of America

Library of Congress Cataloging-in-Publication Data

The Foot and ankle / editor, Kenneth A. Johnson ; illustrator, Deborah Ravin.
    p. cm.—(Master techniques in orthopaedic surgery)
  Includes bibliographical references and index.
  ISBN 0-7817-0030-2
  1. Foot—Surgery. 2. Ankle—Surgery. I. Johnson, Kenneth A., 1940– . II. Series.
  [DNLM: 1. Foot—surgery. 2. Ankle—surgery. WE 168 F687 1994 v. 2]
RD781.F572 1994
617.5'85059—dc20
DNLM/DLC
for Library of Congress   93-20598

    The material contained in this volume was submitted as previously unpublished material, except in the instances in which credit has been given to the source from which some of the illustrative material was derived.
    Great care has been taken to maintain the accuracy of the information contained in the volume. However, neither Raven Press nor the editor can be held responsible for errors or for any consequences arising from the use of the information contained herein.
    Materials appearing in this book prepared by individuals as part of their official duties as U.S. Government employees are not covered by the above-mentioned copyright.

9 8 7 6 5 4 3 2 1

To the Fellows in foot and ankle surgery for whom I have the opportunity to be a teacher. They are all unique, friends, and contributed to a joint experience in the care of foot and ankle pain and deformity. With appreciation:

Charles E. Graham, M.D.
Michael J. Shereff, M.D.
Paul V. Spiegl, M.D.
W. Grant Braly, M.D.
Richard J. Claridge, M.D.
Barry W. Liechty, M.D.
Ian J. Alexander, M.D.
David E. Strom, M.D.
David A. Friscia, M.D.
Charles L. Saltzman, M.D.
Robert D. Teasdall, M.D.
Jon C. Gehrke, M.D.
Todd A. Kile, M.D.

■

CONTENTS

Contributors xi

Acknowledgments xiii

Foreword xv

Preface xvii

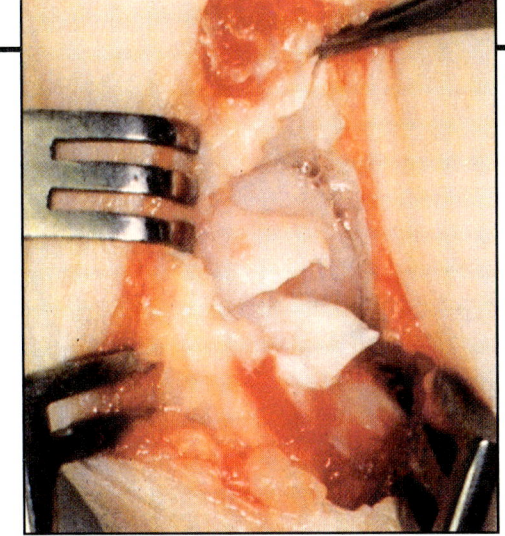

PART I   PHALANGES

Chapter 1
  Marginal Toenail Ablation   3
  Melanie Sanders

Chapter 2
  Phenol Matrixectomy   15
  Irwin L. Bliss

Chapter 3
  Hallux Interphalangeal Arthrodesis   21
  Ian J. Alexander

PART II   METATARSOPHALANGEAL JOINTS

Chapter 4
  Chevron Osteotomy   31
  Kenneth A. Johnson

Chapter 5
  Hallux Metatarsophalangeal Arthrodesis   49
  Ian J. Alexander

Chapter 6
  **Hallux Proximal Phalanx Osteotomy:
      The Akin Procedure   65**
  Carol Frey

Chapter 7
  Michell Osteotomy   73
  Kent K. Wu

Chapter 8
  Proximal First Metatarsal Osteotomy   85
  Michael J. Coughlin

Chapter 9
  Cuneiform-Metatarsal Arthrodesis 107
  Mark S. Myerson

Chapter 10
  Cheilectomy 119
  Glenn B. Pfeffer

Chapter 11
  Realignment of the Overlapping Second Toe 135
  E. Greer Richardson

Chapter 12
  Resection Arthroplasty of the Second and Third Toes 149
  Robert D. Teasdall

PART III METATARSALS

Chapter 13
  Primary Interdigital Neuroma Resection 163
  James A. Amis

Chapter 14
  Secondary Interdigital Neuroma Resection 179
  Jeffrey E. Johnson

Chapter 15
  Osteotomy of the Fifth Metatarsal 189
  Harold B. Kitaoka

Chapter 16
  Rheumatoid Forefoot Reconstruction 197
  Charles L. Saltzman

Chapter 17
  Transmetatarsal Amputation 213
  James W. Brodsky

PART IV CUNEIFORM-METATARSAL JOINTS

Chapter 18
  Cuneiform-Metatarsal Arthrodesis (Lisfranc) 231
  Bruce J. Sangeorzan and Sigvard T. Hansen, Jr.

PART V MIDTARSAL

Chapter 19
  Talonavicular Arthrodesis 249
  G. James Sammarco

CONTRIBUTORS

Ian J. Alexander, M.D., F.R.C.S.(C)
Associate Professor, Department of Orthopaedic Surgery, Northeast Ohio Universities College of Medicine, Rootstown, Ohio; Department of Orthopaedics, Crystal Clinic, Suite 102, 3975 Embassy Parkway, Akron, Ohio 44313

James A. Amis, M.D.
Volunteer Assistant Professor, Department of Orthopaedics, University of Cincinnati Medical College, 3219 Clinton Avenue, Suite 300, Cincinnati, Ohio 45220

Donald E. Baxter, M.D.
Clinical Professor, Department of Orthopaedic Surgery, Baylor College of Medicine, 7500 Beechnut, Suite 175, Houston, Texas 77074

Irwin L. Bliss, M.D.
Assistant Clinical Professor of Orthopaedic Surgery, Department of Orthopaedics, University of California–Los Angeles, Los Angeles, California; and 2080 Century Park East, Suite 1500, Los Angeles, California 90067

Walther H. O. Bohne, M.D.
Associate Professor of Orthopaedic Surgery, New York Hospital-Cornell University Medical Center, New York, New York; Department of Orthopaedic Surgery, The Hospital of Special Surgery, 535 East 70th Street, New York, New York 10021

R. Luke Bordelon, M.D.
Clinical Professor of Orthopaedics, Department of Orthopaedics, Louisiana State University School of Medicine, 5069 Highway I-49 South, Opelousas, Louisiana 70570

W. Grant Braly, M.D.
Assistant Clinical Professor, Section of Foot and Ankle Surgery, Department of Orthopaedic Surgery, Baylor College of Medicine, Houston, Texas; and Scurlock Tower, 6560 Fannin, Suite 2100, Houston, Texas 77030-2727

James W. Brodsky, M.D.
Associate Clinical Professor, Department of Orthopaedic Surgery, University of Texas Southwestern Medical School Dallas, Texas; Department of Orthopaedic Surgery, Baylor University Medical Center, 3500 Gaston Avenue, Dallas, Texas; Orthopaedic Associates of Dallas, 411 N. Washington #7000, Dallas, Texas 75246

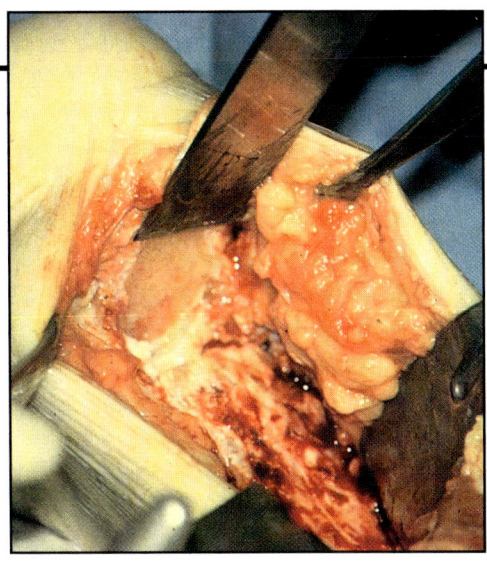

Jason H. Calhoun, M.D., M.Eng.
Associate Professor, Chief, Orthopaedic Surgery, Department of Orthopaedic Surgery, University of Texas Medical Branch, 6.136 McCullough Building, Galveston, Texas 77555-0792

Michael J. Coughlin, M.D.
Private practice, Orthopaedic Surgery, 901 North Curtis Road, Boise, Idaho 83706; Clinical Associate Professor of Surgery, Division of Orthopaedic Surgery and Rehabilitation, Department of Surgery, Oregon Health Sciences University, Portland, Oregon 97201

Carol Frey, M.D.
Associate Clinical Professor, Department of Orthopaedic Surgery, University of Southern California; Director, Orthopaedic Foot & Ankle Center, 2300 South Hope Street, Suite 700, Los Angeles, California 90007

William G. Hamilton, M.D.
Assistant Clinical Professor of Orthopaedic Surgery, Columbia University College of Physicians and Surgeons, New York, New York; Senior Attending Orthopaedic Surgeon, St. Luke's-Roosevelt Hospital Center, New York, New York; and 343 West 58th Street, New York, NY 10019

Sigvard T. Hansen, Jr., M.D.
Professor, Department of Orthopaedics, University of Washington, Harborview Medical Center, 325 Ninth Avenue ZA-48, Seattle, Washington 98104

Marion C. Harper, M.D.
Clinical Professor, Department of Orthopaedic Surgery and Rehabilitation, Vanderbilt University, Nashville, Tennessee; Centennial Medical Center, The Atrium, Suite 204, 250 25th Avenue North, Nashville, Tennessee 37203

Jeffrey E. Johnson, M.D.
Associate Professor, Department of Orthopaedic Surgery, Medical College of Wisconsin, 8700 West Wisconsin Avenue, Milwaukee, Wisconsin 53226

Kenneth A. Johnson, M.D.
Chairman, Division of Foot and Ankle Surgery, Mayo Clinic Scottsdale, 13400 East Shea Boulevard, Scottsdale, Arizona 85259; Professor of Orthopaedics, Mayo Medical School, Rochester, Minnesota

Harold B. Kitaoka, M.D.
Consultant, Department of Orthopaedics, Mayo Clinic and Mayo Foundation, Assistant Professor of Orthopaedics, Mayo Medical School, 200 First Street SW, Rochester, Minnesota 55905

Arthur Manoli II, M.D.
Professor of Orthopaedic Surgery, Wayne State University, Detroit, Michigan; Department of Orthopaedic Surgery, Hutzel Hospital, Suite 1-South, 4707 St. Antoine, Detroit, Michigan 48201

Mark S. Myerson, M.D.
Director, Foot & Ankle Center, Department of Orthopaedic Surgery, Union Memorial Hospital, 3333 North Calvert Street, Baltimore, Maryland 21218

Glenn B. Pfeffer, M.D.
Assistant Clinical Professor, Department of Orthopaedics, University of California-San Francisco, San Francisco, California; Chief, Orthopaedic Foot and Ankle Surgery, California Pacific Medical Center, Pacific Campus, 2100 Webster Street, Suite 115, San Francisco, California 94115

E. Greer Richardson, M.D.
Associate Professor, Department of Orthopaedics, University of Tennessee, College of Medicine, 66 North Pauline Street, Memphis, Tennessee; The Campbell Clinic, 869 Madison Avenue, Memphis, Tennessee 38103

Michael M. Romash, M.D.
Associate Clinical Professor, Department of Surgery, Uniform Services University of Health Sciences, Bethesda, Maryland; and 700 North Battlefield Boulevard, Suite D, Chesapeake, Virginia 23320

Charles L. Saltzman, M.D.
Assistant Professor, Department of Orthopaedic Surgery, University of Iowa, RCP-1067, UIHC, Iowa City, Iowa 55242

G. James Sammarco, M.D.
Volunteer Professor of Orthopaedic Surgery, University of Cincinnati, Cincinnati, Ohio; The Center for Orthopaedic Care, Inc., 2123 Auburn Avenue, Suite 235, Cincinnati, Ohio 45219

Melanie Sanders, M.D.
Orthopaedic Foot & Ankle Surgery, Suite 300, 3850 Shore Drive, Indianapolis, Indiana 46254

Bruce J. Sangeorzan, M.D.
Associate Professor, Department of Orthopaedics, University of Washington/Harborview Medical Center, 325 Ninth Avenue, ZA-48/6S21 Seattle, Washington 98104

Michael J. Shereff, M.D.
Associate Professor, Department of Orthopaedic Surgery, Director, Division of Foot and Ankle Surgery, Medical College of Wisconsin, 8700 West Wisconsin Avenue, Milwaukee, Wisconsin 53226

Ronald W. Smith, M.D.
Associate Clinical Professor, Division of Orthopaedic Surgery, University of California at Los Angeles School of Medicine, Los Angeles, California; and 2651 Elm Avenue, Long Beach, California 90806

Mark Sobel, M.D.
Director, Orthopaedic Foot and Ankle Service, Beth Israel Medical Center, North Division, New York, New York; Beth Israel Medical Center Petrie Campus, First Avenue and 17th Street, New York, New York; private practice: 755 Park Avenue, New York, New York 10021

Robert D. Teasdall, M.D.
Assistant Professor, Department of Orthopaedics, The Bowman Gray School of Medicine, Medical Center Boulevard, Winston-Salem, North Carolina 27157

Keith L. Wapner, M.D.
Associate Professor of Orthopaedic Surgery, Director, Division Foot and Ankle Surgery, Thomas Jefferson University, 838 Walnut Street, Philadelphia, Pennsylvania; Chief, Orthopaedic Surgery, Thomas Jefferson Ford Road Campus, 3900 Ford Road, Philadelphia, Pennsylvania 19107

Kent K. Wu, M.D.
Senior Orthopaedic Surgeon, Bone and Joint Center, Henry Ford Hospital, 2799 West Grand Boulevard, Detroit, Michigan 48202

ACKNOWLEDGMENTS

The illustrator, Deborah Ravin, is gratefully acknowledged for her talent and expertise in illustrating. I thank Nancy Gray for her excellence in secretarial assistance during the preparation of the manuscripts. And Raven editors, Kathey Alexander and Danette Knopp, are thanked for their patience and support in the final assembling of this book.

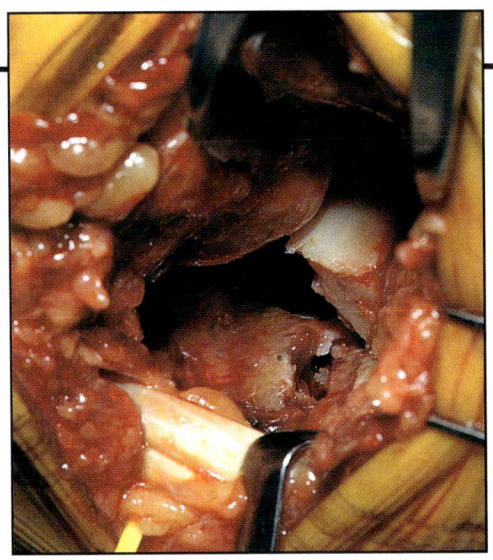

SERIES PREFACE

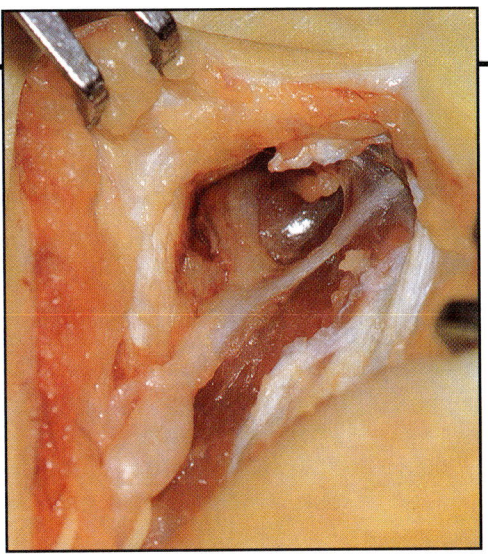

Master Techniques in Orthopaedic Surgery is a series of nine volumes designed to provide direct, detailed access to techniques preferred by orthopaedic surgeons who are recognized by their colleagues as "masters" in their specialty. The volume editors are leaders who, through their research and educational efforts, have earned the respect of their peers. The chapter authors, selected for their experience and skills, present the techniques in a personal manner, bringing their unique perspectives and observations to the reader.

These atlases are designed to help the practitioner deal with the difficult but common problems encountered in daily practice. Experimental techniques and technology that are so sophisticated that most cases are referred to a treatment center are avoided, as are straightforward surgical techniques that seldom cause difficulty.

These books take you into the operating room and let you peer over the shoulder of the surgeon at work. The color photographs and accompanying drawings guide you step-by-step through a procedure. The commentary, organized in a standardized format throughout the series, offers you specific technical advice, as well as tips and pearls gained through the surgeons' years of experience.

The shared knowledge and expertise found in these pages are presented to enable the surgeon to undertake surgical procedures with greater confidence and improved proficiency.

Roby C. Thompson, Jr., M.D.
Series Editor

PREFACE

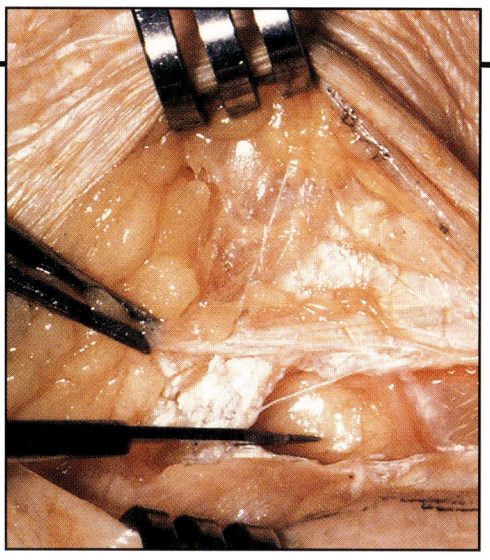

Every surgeon has a *way* of doing a surgical procedure. This book contains the ways a group of orthopaedic surgeons approach an array of foot and ankle procedures.

The authors of this volume are young and old, male and female, nonacademic and academic. Their common bond is that they are all surgeons with a specific practice interest in the foot and ankle, and they have demonstrated a master's quality by sharing their experience with their peers through the written or spoken word. They have done the procedures, looked at the results, worried about the complications, and tried to technically improve their performance. "Masters" does not imply omnipotence or infallibility. It does suggest honesty, experience, and thoughtfulness.

The procedures selected range from toenail ablation to involved multiple arthrodesis. They are the surgical challenges that face the general orthopaedic surgeon. It is not expected that another surgeon will try to replicate the technique as described. But, it is expected that incorporating some of the authors' thoughts with your own will facilitate an improved surgical procedure and result.

Not only does the surgeon instruct by word but also by illustrations and intraoperative photographs. A single illustrator, Deborah Ravin, provided all of the artwork in the clarifying style.

I agreed to edit this volume because Roby C. Thompson unambiguously suggested I would. More importantly, the foot and ankle is an integral part of orthopaedic surgery. About one of every five patients in the general orthopaedic office will be seen for a foot and ankle problem. We need to be informed about newer methods of ankle ligament repair, changes in thought about hallux valgus procedures, nerve entrapment causing heel pain and so on. The collective experience of 31 surgeons is presented in 37 chapters with approximately 180 illustrations and more than 400 photographs/radiographs. Bring this book with you to the operating room, dog-ear the pages, write in the margins, drip coffee on the illustrations, and get betadine stains on the binding. It is a friendly book, to be used.

Kenneth A. Johnson, M.D.

MASTER TECHNIQUES IN ORTHOPAEDIC SURGERY
■
THE FOOT AND ANKLE

PART I

Phalanges

1

Marginal Toenail Ablation

Melanie Sanders

INDICATIONS/CONTRAINDICATIONS

The surgical management of ingrown toenails is generally reserved for those cases where optimum conservation management has failed (1–3,5). There are cases where my threshold for treatment is much lower, such as in the diabetic patient or in patients with total joint replacements. In those instances, I feel it is better to prevent recurrent infections and the possibility of sepsis, and I recommend surgery much sooner. Additional indications for surgical management include extremely deformed fungal nails where pressure from the surface of the shoe causes significant pain for the patient. Chronic suppurative lesions with granulation tissue may require surgical decompression in order to facilitate healing so that definitive surgical treatment can be performed. The major contraindication for surgery is embarrassed vascular supply to the great toe. Chronic infections may carry a relative contraindication for procedures that involve matricectomy because of the concern of transfer of infection to deep tissues.

PREOPERATIVE PLANNING

Evaluation of the patient before the surgical procedure should include a history of the frequency of recurrence of infections and how recalcitrant they may be to treatment. If there is concern about deep infection, anteroposterior (AP) and oblique radiographs of the great toe should be taken and examined for evidence of periosteal elevation or bone erosion. Plain radiographs are generally sufficient to reveal underlying unusual bony shapes, such as enchondromas, which are occasional causes of nail deformity or infection. In the majority of cases, more involved and costly studies are not necessary as a part of preoperative planning. Patients are

---

M. Sanders, M.D.: Orthopaedic Foot & Ankle Surgery, Suite 300, 3850 Shore Drive, Indianapolis, IN 46254.

encouraged to improve their general foot hygiene before surgery and specifically to clean the area at least daily with a good antiseptic for 3 days before surgery.

SURGERY

This procedure can be performed under any number of anesthetics. Digital or ankle blocks both work well. Some patients will request general or spinal anesthetic because of anxiety. Regardless of the anesthetic used, I feel it is desirable to perform a digital block with Marcaine at the end of the case to provide prolonged pain relief for the patient postoperatively. With the patient supine, the foot should be prepped to the level of the ankle. If a procedure is to be done with gross infection present, I do not exsanguinate the toe. My preference at that point is to use either an ankle or thigh tourniquet. In cases that are performed for onychogryphosis or tubular nail where there is no infection, using a large Penrose as an Esmarch bandage works quite well (Fig. 1). It is important to use a hemostat to secure the Penrose to avoid the disaster of leaving the Penrose in place at the end of the case when the dressing is applied.

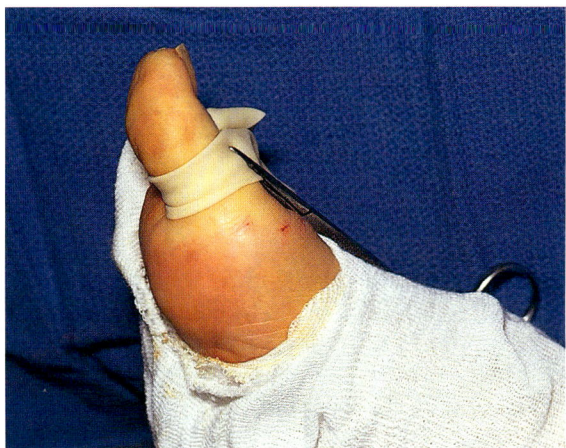

Figure 1. Large Penrose drain is used to exsanguinate the toe initially, and then is secured with a hemostat to act as a tourniquet.

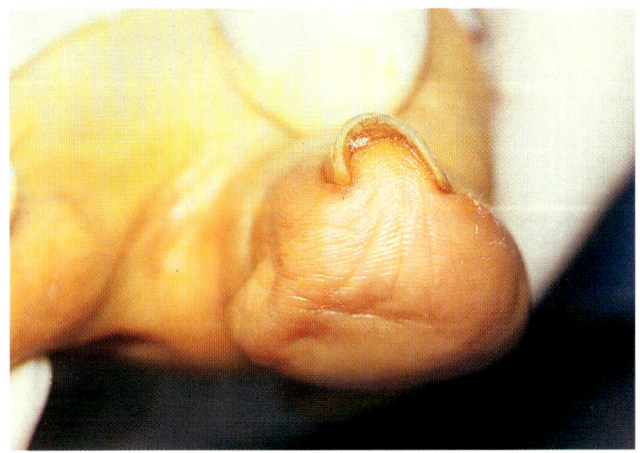 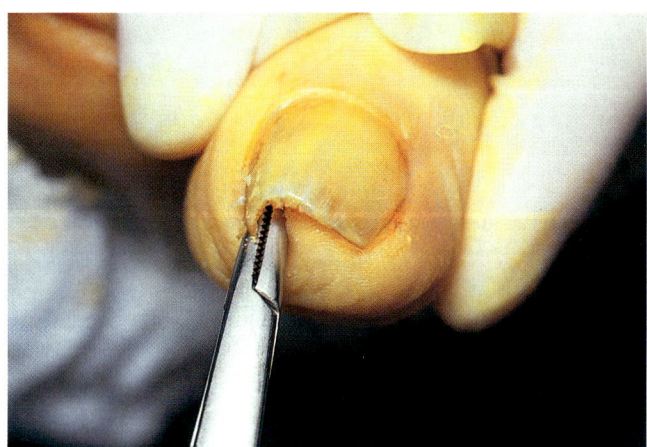

Figure 2. A: Tubular nail. **B:** A small curved hemostat is used to bluntly elevate the nail from the nail bed.

Figure 3. Nail splitter introduced to cut the nail longitudinally.

Technique. Once a bloodless field is established, the toenail is approached from its distal end. I generally find a small curved hemostat works well to separate the nail from the underlying nail bed. If the entire nail is to be removed, this can be accomplished with gentle and persistent blunt dissection toward the base of the nail (Fig. 2). This technique is carried out in a more limited fashion on either the medial or lateral margins or both in cases where only partial nail ablation is to be performed. In the case of partial nail ablation, a nail splitter is then used to separate the margin of the nail from the central portion. This is carried up under the edge of the ungual fold (Fig. 3). The nail is then removed from the operative field (Fig. 4).

For the next stage of the operation, I find loupe magnification to be extremely helpful. Oblique incisions are made at the proximal corners of the ungual fold (Fig. 5). These incisions are carried only to a depth of the fatty tissue underlying the dermis, their purpose being facilitation of exposure of the underlying matrix. There is matrix surface that can form nail under the edge of the ungual fold, curving around the base of the toenail and in the nail bed distal to the lunula. It is necessary to excise this inferior surface of the ungual fold (Fig. 6). The knife is inserted parallel to the overlying ungual fold, sharply separating it from the

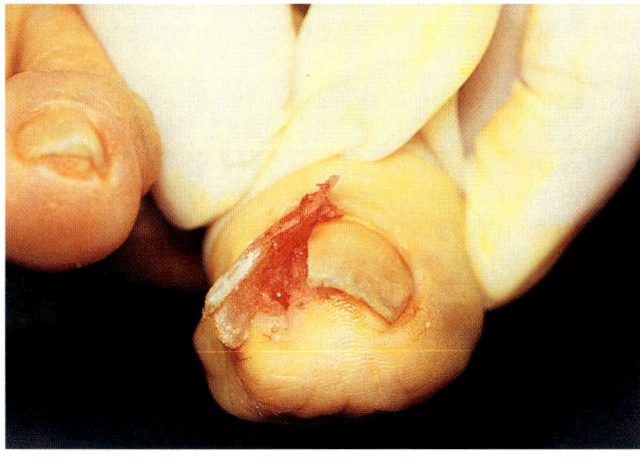
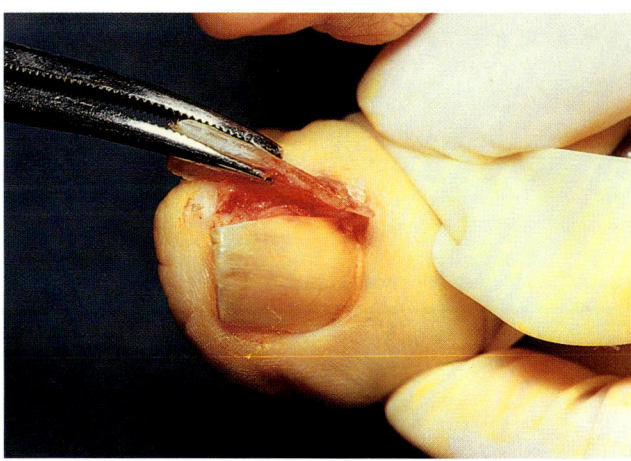

Figure 4. A: Lateral nail lifted away from the underlying nail bed. **B:** Completion of avulsion of the nail.

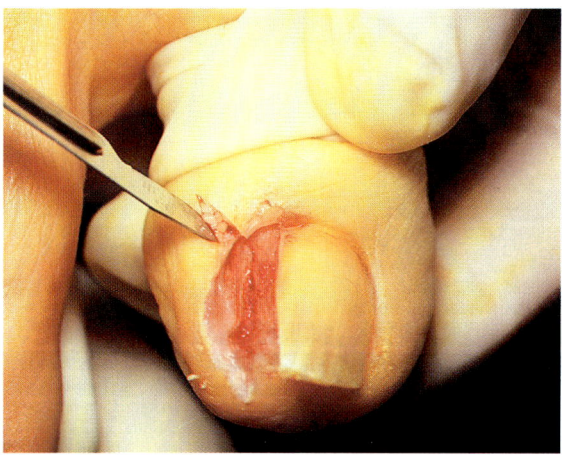

Figure 5. Oblique proximal incision.

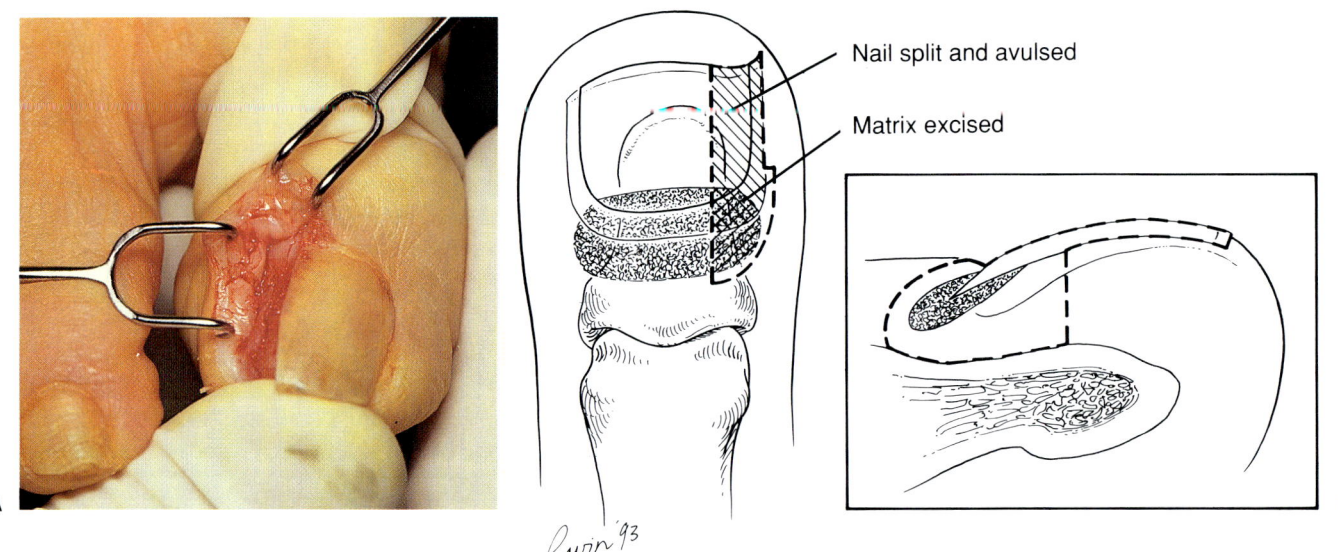

Figure 6. A: Completed exposure of the matrix. Notice the change in color between the nail bed and the matrix. **B:** Extent of tissue resection for marginal nail ablation procedure.

underlying matrix. This technique is carried out along the lateral ungual fold as well. The nail bed is then cut horizontally at a level slightly distal to the lunula. In some, but not all patients, a change in coloration can be noted where the matrix darkens at its junction from a pale color to the normal pink or red of the nail bed. This transverse incision in the nail bed and matrix surface is carried down to the level of the bone. At this stage, the corner of the matrix is grasped gently with forceps and a sharp instrument (either a #15 scalpel blade or a beaver blade) is used to separate the matrix from the surrounding and underlying fat tissue (Fig. 7).

Partial matricectomy generally yields a piece of tissue that is approximately 0.75 cm × 0.75 cm (Fig. 8). This should be carefully examined to note whether there are any holes or rents present in the specimen. If these are perceived, a careful search for this tissue should be undertaken, although this is sometimes fruitless. If there is concern as to whether the matrix was incompletely removed,

1 MARGINAL TOENAIL ABLATION

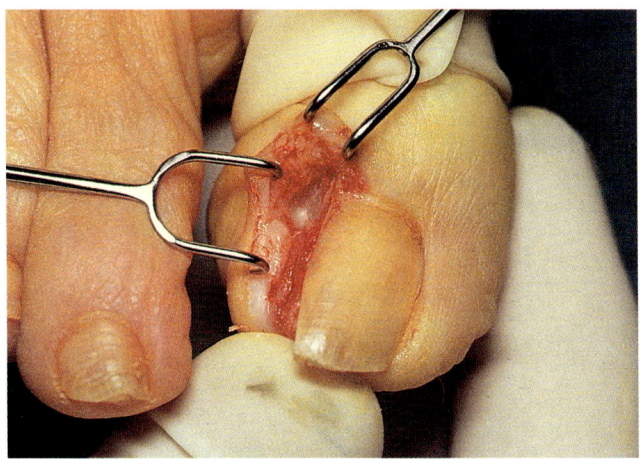

Figure 7. Removal of matrix. Surface of the proximal phalanx is visible in the wound.

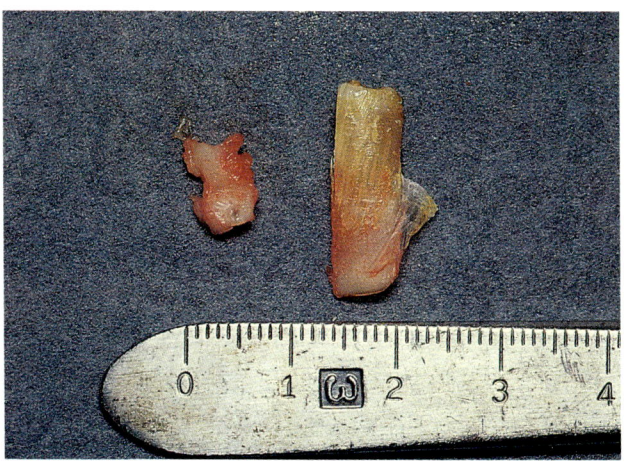

Figure 8. Specimens from partial matricectomy and nail.

I generally will use a small curette to elevate the periosteum on the phalanx and to remove any fibrous tissue that might represent matrix. Some patients have an extremely deep shape to the matrix on either corner. In these cases, it is sometimes helpful to use a small skin hook to help elevate the matrix from the underlying tissue. I find it is also helpful in those cases when this is recognized as a problem during the case, to extend the oblique incision slightly. The danger here is that the matrix will be transected leaving a corner of the matrix behind.

A complete matricectomy requires excision of the matrix across the entire base of the nail bed (Fig. 9). Generally this is carried out at a level slightly distal to the distal edge of the lunula. Resection of this tissue causes a significant defect to be present, but this is necessary in order to remove all of the germinal tissue. At this stage, standard irrigation is generally performed. I often use cautery in an attempt to minimize bleeding. It is also possible to use small pieces of Gelfoam packed particularly in the medial and lateral gutters of the area of resection (Fig. 10). The oblique incisions at the corner are generally closed with a nonabsorbable nylon suture with a mattress stitch. In some cases of partial nail ablation, I will make a small hole in the lateral nail edge using a large needle and place one suture

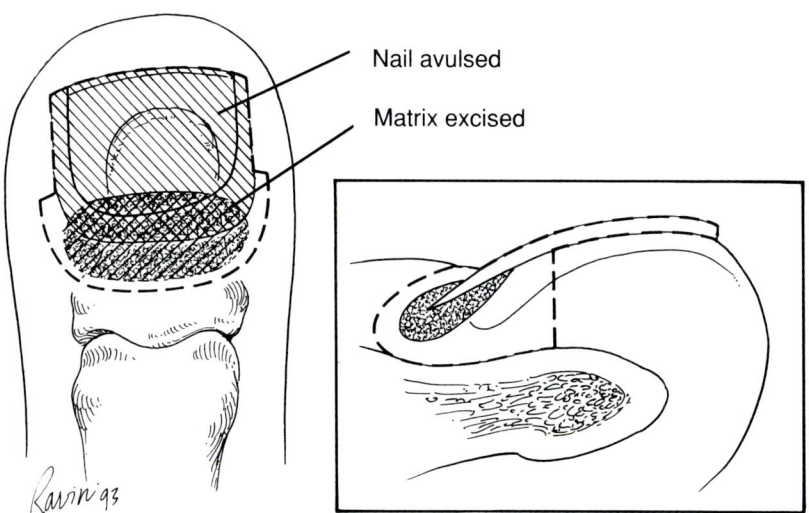

Figure 9. Extent of tissue resection for total nail matrix ablation.

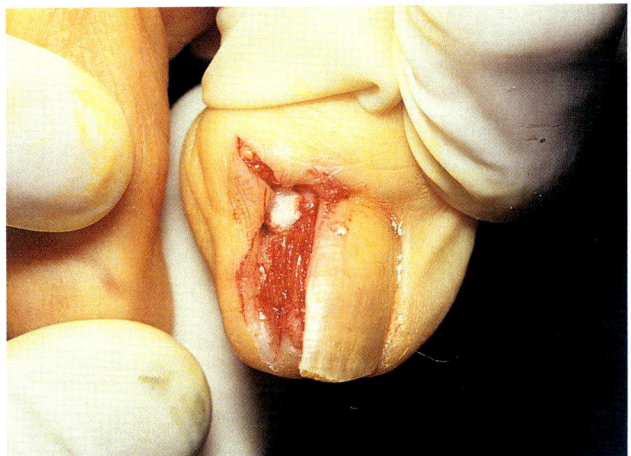

Figure 10. Gelfoam packed in wound.

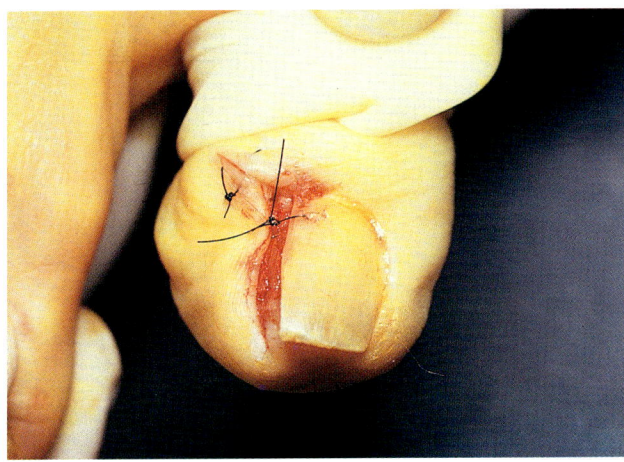

Figure 11. Closure of the wound with nonabsorbable nylon suture.

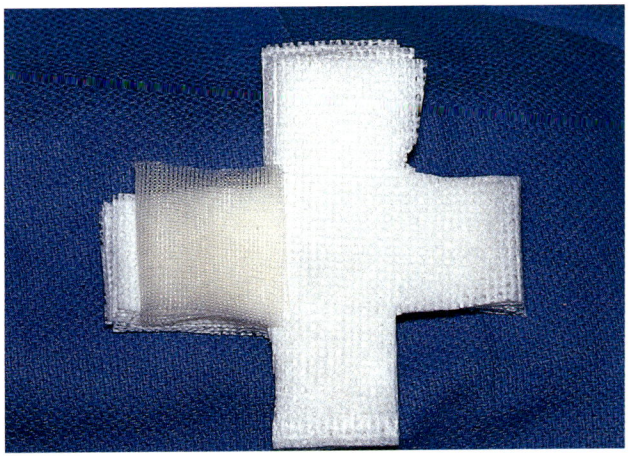

Figure 12. Dressing.

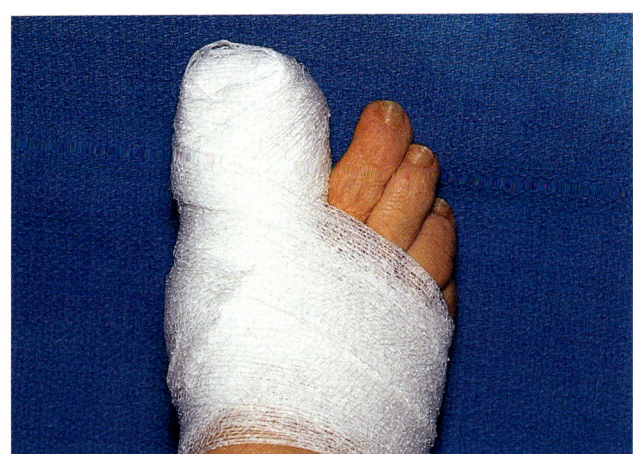

Figure 13. Completed dressing.

through the lateral ungual fold and the nail to encourage healing of the tissue in better position (Fig. 11). At this point the dressing is ready to be applied. Any nonadherent material can be used underlying a bulky dressing. I will generally place a pile of 4 × 4s that have been cut in the shape of a cross over the end of the toe, as this allows a dressing that form-fits quite nicely (Fig. 12). A 2-inch Kling is necessary to get a good firm dressing, and the dressing generally also is brought up onto the forefoot (Fig. 13). The digital block with Marcaine can be performed before or after the dressing is applied.

POSTOPERATIVE MANAGEMENT

Patients are allowed to go home the same day of surgery in any shoe that is comfortable and does not cause any pressure on the dorsum of the great toe. Patients are often most comfortable in an old shoe with an area cut to accommodate the dressing or in a sandal, although some do opt for the use of a wooden-soled shoe. Generally this type of accommodation is necessary for a period of 2 to 4 days after surgery. Patients are sent home from the surgical procedure with a page of instructions, including specific instructions which state to expect bleeding. Bleeding can often be quite profuse and will at times saturate the dressing by the

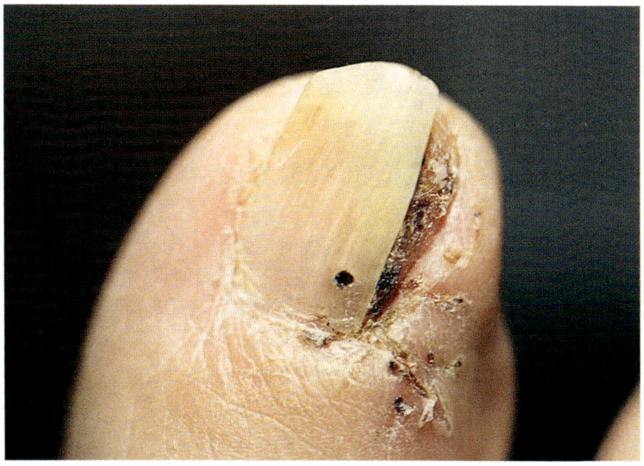

Figure 14. Appearance of toe after suture removal, 14 days postoperative.

time the patient has reached the recovery area. Patients are instructed to change their dressing approximately 36 or 48 hours after surgery. I suggest that they use saline or sterile water to saturate the dressing so that it can be removed as painlessly as possible. Generally bleeding has subsided by the second postoperative day, and the patient can put a smaller nonadherent dressing over the toe. Patients are cautioned against any kind of soaking or immersion of the foot, and are asked to keep the surgical area clean and dry. Additional instructions include ice and elevation, particularly for the first 3 to 4 days. The use of the digital block generally lessens the postoperative pain significantly and patients are often able to discontinue pain medications after 1 or 2 days. If a surgical procedure is done in the face of infection, I will consider the use of prophylactic oral antibiotics at home. Most patients receive one dose of prophylactic antibiotic in the surgical suite intravenously.

Patients return to the office at 10 days after surgery for suture removal and at that time any necessary changes in care of the surgical site are implemented. Many patients come to the first postoperative follow-up visit wearing enclosed shoes and hose (Fig. 14). Any deviation from steady improvement would make me suspect a postoperative infection. The second follow-up visit is scheduled 2 to 3 months postoperative.

COMPLICATIONS

The most common complication from the procedure is the persistence of nail horns or spikes after ablation of the nail and matrix. These occur because of remnants or islands of germinal matrix that still form nail. In some instances these are not particularly troublesome to the patient and are managed by periodic trimming or removal by the patient. At other times they are quite problematic and can result in the need for further surgery. Sometimes adequate removal of the nail spike can be performed with an en bloc type of excision; however, at times it is necessary to manage the problem with a more extensive procedure such as a terminal Syme amputation (4). Some patients do form a cornified layer of tissue overlying the nail bed, which can appear to be toenail but is not adherent to the nail bed and can be removed easily.

The second problem that may be considered a complication by both the patient and the physician is formation of what may appear to be nail tissue over the nail bed. This most commonly occurs when this procedure is performed for fungal infection in the toenail and may be the result of fungal infection still within the skin of the great toe. I have found that this generally responds well to the use of topical antifungal medications.

ILLUSTRATIVE CASE FOR TECHNIQUE

This 53-year-old diabetic patient had experienced several episodes of redness, erythema, and drainage from very mild toenail deformities and requested surgical management because of recurring pain (Fig. 15). Complete ablation of the nail and matrix was recommended for this patient. The procedure was performed as an outpatient (which required special management due to her diabetes). The toenail was elevated off of the underlying nail bed with a curved hemostat (Fig. 16). After avulsion of the nail, it was removed from the surgical field (Fig. 17). Two oblique incisions were then made at the corners of the ungual folds and a #15 blade was used to separate the matrix from the overlying skin fold (Fig. 18). A transverse incision was then made through the nail bed down to the bone from the medial to the lateral extent of the great toenail surface (Fig. 19). The matrix was then removed sharply with careful dissection under loupe magnification. The

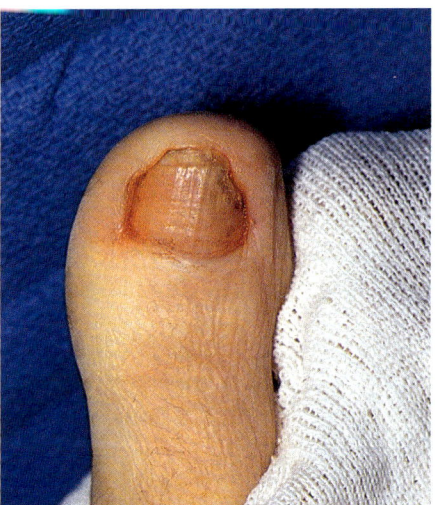

Figure 15. Preoperative view. Note incorrect nail trimming, which had contributed to recurrent acute inflammatory episodes.

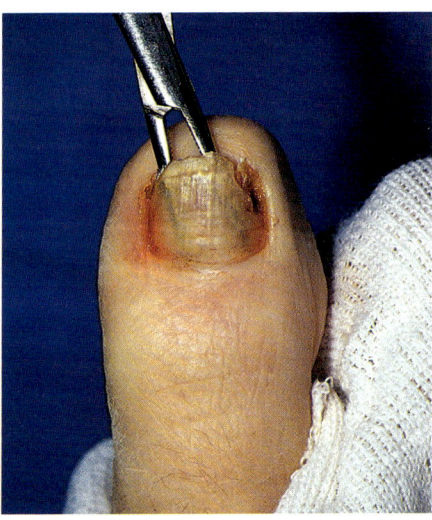

Figure 16. Blunt dissection with hemostat.

1 MARGINAL TOENAIL ABLATION

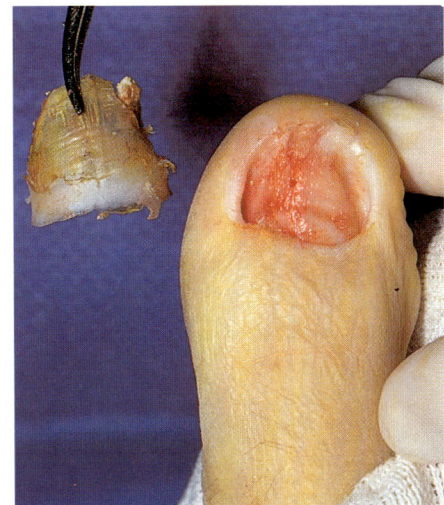

Figure 17. Complete avulsion of nail.

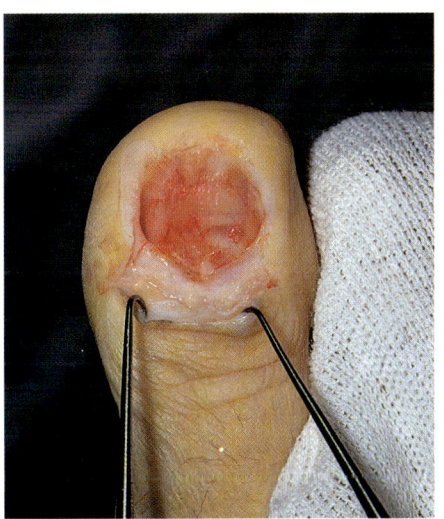

Figure 18. Matrix dissected free from overlying skin and subcutaneous tissue.

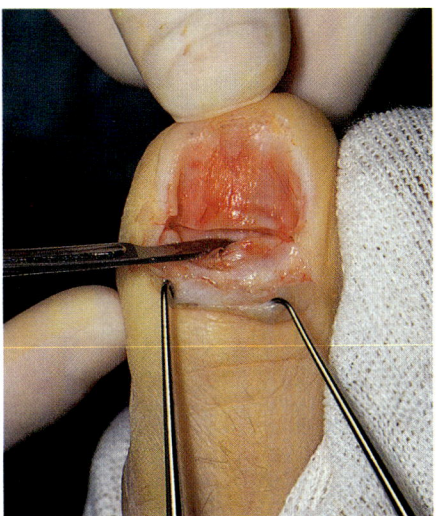

Figure 19. Transverse nail bed incision.

matrix was carefully examined for any evidence of tears or loss of tissue during the procedure (Fig. 20). Irrigation of the wound was performed and cautery was used along with gentle curettage. The matrix bed was packed with Gelfoam and thrombin, and the lateral incisions closed with Ethilon. Long-term follow-up healing of the toe is demonstrated in Fig. 21.

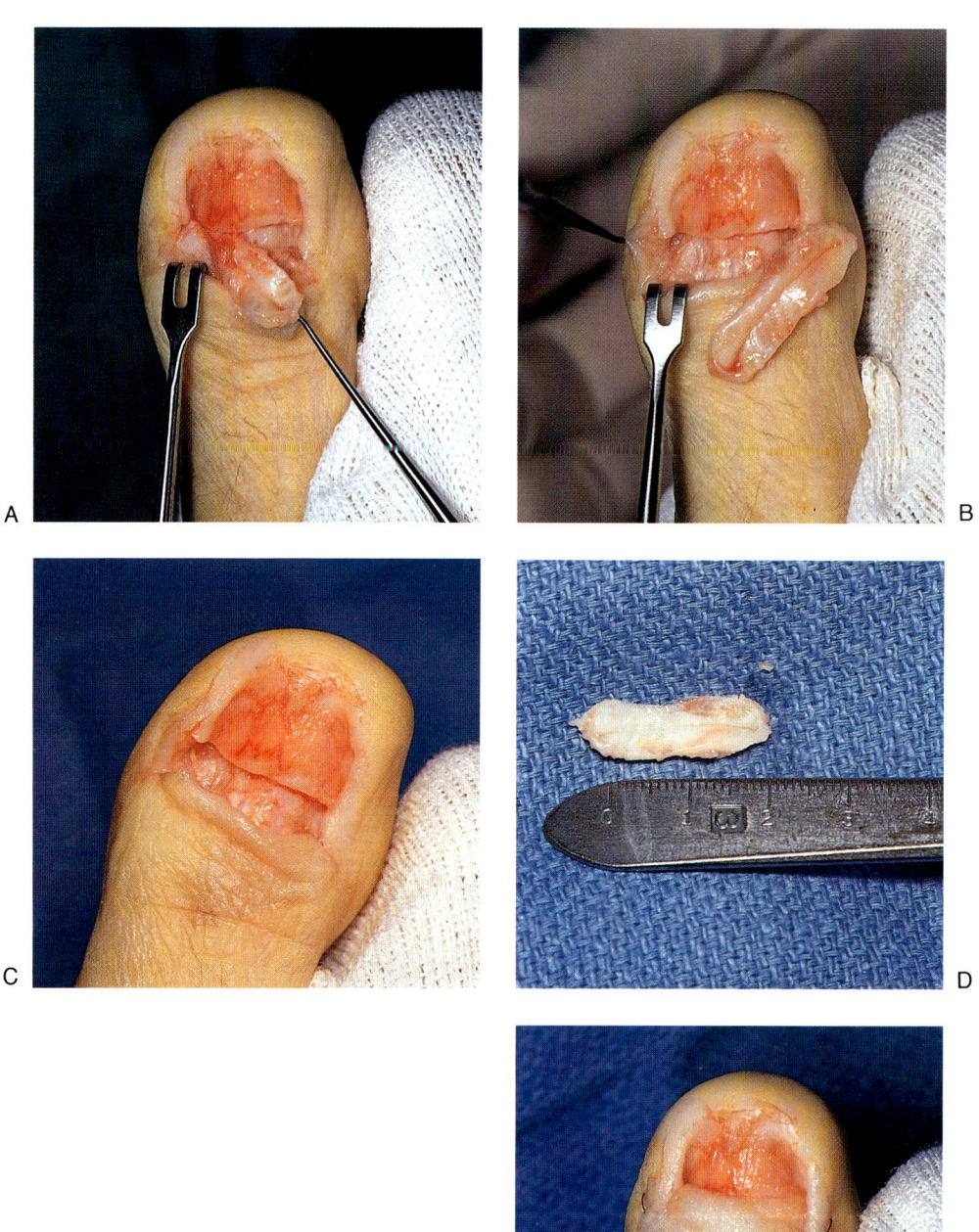

Figure 20. A: Dissection of matrix from underlying bone, incomplete. **B:** Complete matrix removal. **C:** Defect created after total matrix excision. **D:** Specimen from matrix excision. **E:** Packing with Gelfoam and thrombin in place.

1 MARGINAL TOENAIL ABLATION

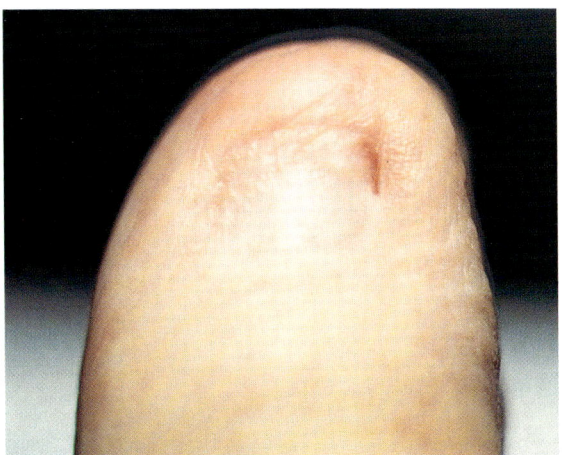

Figure 21. Example of clinical appearance 6 months postoperatively.

RECOMMENDED READING

1. Dixon, G. L.: Treatment of ingrown toenail. *Foot Ankle*, 3(5): 254–260, 1983.
2. Heifetz, C. J.: Ingrown toenail: a clinical study. *Am. J. Surg.*, 38(2): 298–315, 1937.
3. Johnson, K. A.: *Surgery of the Foot and Ankle,* pp. 91–96. New York: Raven Press, 1989.
4. Thompson, T. C., and Terwilliger, C.: The terminal Syme operation for ingrown toenail. *Surg. Clin. North Am.*, 31: 575–584, 1951.
5. Zadik, F. R.: Obliteration of the nail bed of the great toe without shortening the terminal phalanx. *J. Bone Joint Surg.*, 32B(1): 66–667, 1950.

2

Phenol Matrixectomy

Irwin L. Bliss

INDICATIONS/CONTRAINDICATIONS

Recurrent ingrown toenails in the younger patient or painful calluses in the nail groove (due to chronic deformation of the nail bed and nail plate) in the older patient are the primary indications for partial nail ablation. Approximately 85% of the geriatric population have at least one toe with a symptomatic incurving nail due to pressure in the offended nail groove (Fig. 1). Diabetic patients with deformed nails are at risk for infection and this concern can be obviated safely if the border ablation is carried out before vascular insufficiency is an issue.

Multiple approaches to the problem of partial nail ablation have been described. Some include soft tissue correction involving a variety of surgical procedures; all include removal of the involved portion of the matrix with the surrounding portion of the lateral skinfold. Other techniques have included the use of electrocautery and thermal ablation with laser.

Phenol ablation offers several advantages. The procedure does not require an incision and therefore avoids all the risks and complications of a surgical procedures. No special equipment is required. The procedure can be completed easily in the office.

The normal nail plate and nail bed are flat. In a young patient with an ingrown nail, the edge of the nail turns in (incurvation) but the nail bed remains flat. In the older patient, both the nail plate and nail bed deform almost symmetrically. Incurvation of the nail may be thought of as part of a continuum with the end of the spectrum being a tubular nail. The amount of nail removed should leave no residual incurving corners. If the degree of incurving is so severe that removing all the incurving corners leaves nothing but a narrow central portion, it is more reasonable to do a total nail ablation.

I. L. Bliss, M.D.: Department of Orthopaedics, University of California, Los Angeles, Los Angeles, CA 90024-1783; and *private practice*, Suite 1500, 2080 Century Park East, Los Angeles, CA 90067.

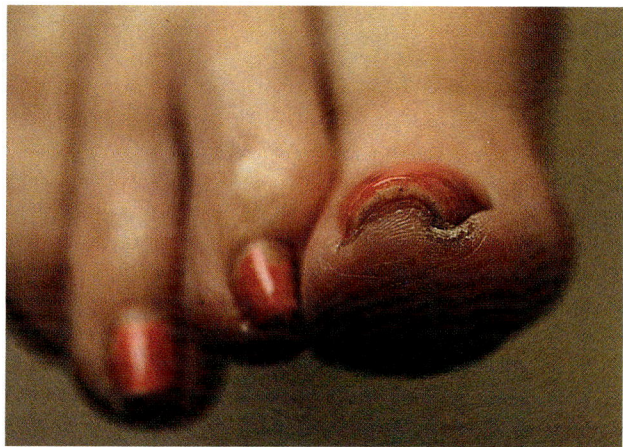

Figure 1. Painful callus in nail groove.

Total matrixectomy can be accomplished with this technique. In this instance the entire nail plate is avulsed and the entire undersurface of the eponychium is scraped as well as the dorsal portion of the proximal phalanx on which the matrix rests.

PREOPERATIVE PLANNING

If the deformity of the nail is suggestive, obtain radiographs of the hallux to rule out a subungual exostosis (Figs. 2 and 3).

Fungal infection in conjunction with or as a cause of a nail defect is not a contraindication to phenol matrixectomy; however, it would alter the postoperative treatment. Therefore, it is important to make a definitive diagnosis and this cannot be done by clinical appearance (Fig. 4). Either a culture on Sabourand's agar or a microscopic evaluation of a KOH preparation will indicate if a fungal infection is present.

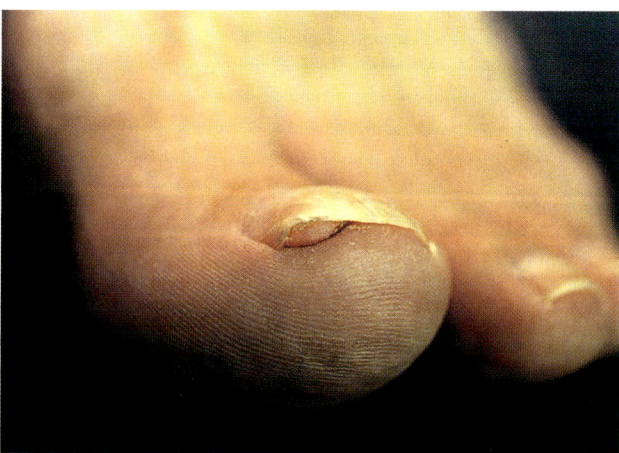

Figure 2. Subungual prominence from exostosis.

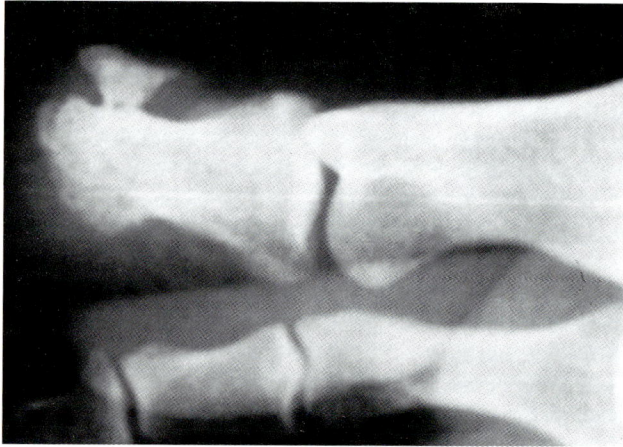

Figure 3. Radiograph of toe in Fig. 2.

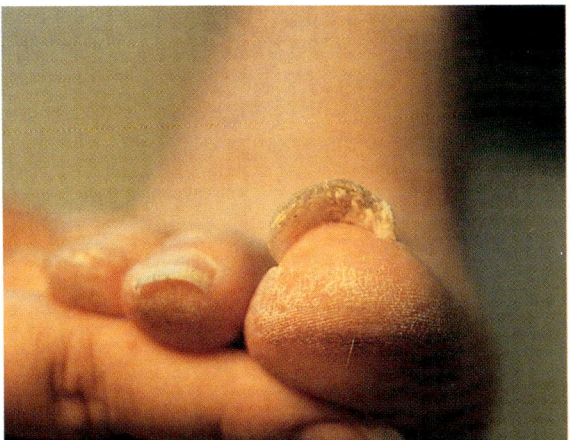

Figure 4. Subungual material can be debris or fungus.

SURGERY

The patient is placed supine on the table with the hip and knee flexed so that the foot is plantigrade. The nails are cleaned of subungual debris and trimmed. The foot is then scrubbed and a Betadine prep is used on the involved toe. The remainder of the foot is draped out.

A digital block is completed with lidocaine or bupivacaine and when satisfactory anesthesia is obtained, the toe is exsanguinated by circumferential pressure. A ¼-inch Penrose drain is wrapped around the base of the toe over a gauze sponge (Fig. 5).

Technique. The incurved border of the nail (Fig. 6) is elevated with a spatula (Fig. 7) and is then cut with a nail clipper (Fig. 8). The cut portion of the nail is removed.

The matrix, including that portion that is on the undersurface of the eponychium, is removed with a curette as is the exposed portion of nail bed under the removed segment of nail plate (Fig. 9). To facilitate access to the epinychial undersurface, apply digital pressure to the dorsum of the toe, proximal to the matrix, in a distal direction as this often brings additional, inaccessible matrix into the field.

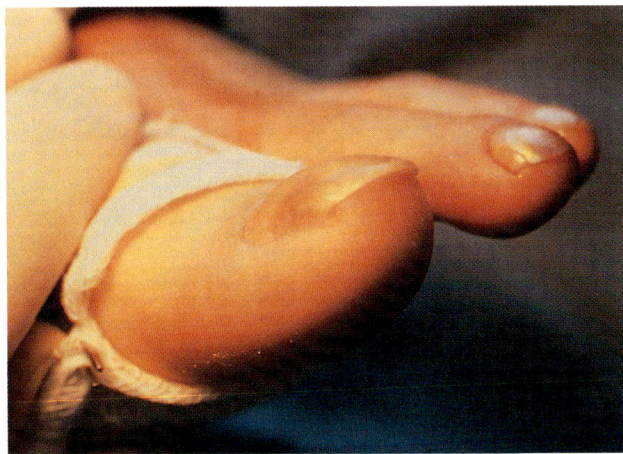

Figure 5. Toe is exsanguinated and a Penrose drain is applied over gauze sponge at base of toe.

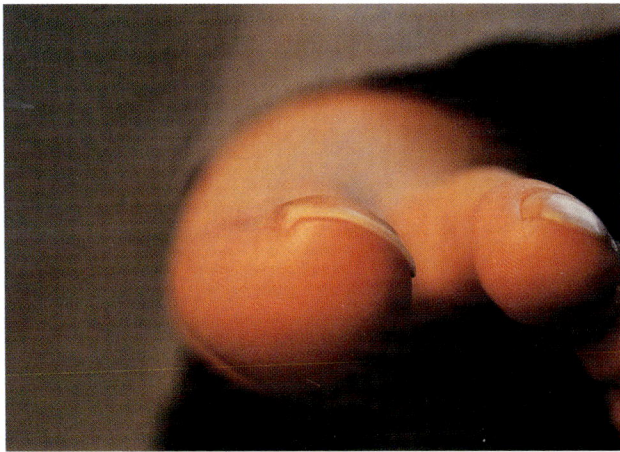

Figure 6. The 90° downward turn of medial border of hallux nail plate.

A cotton swab with approximately 50% of its bulk removed is dipped into 89% phenol (avoid excessive saturation of the swab) and then introduced under the eponychium into the area of the matrix. There it is rotated for approximately 30 seconds and removed (Fig. 10). This step is repeated. A third cotton swab, similarly debulked, is dipped into isopropyl alcohol and introduced into the depths of

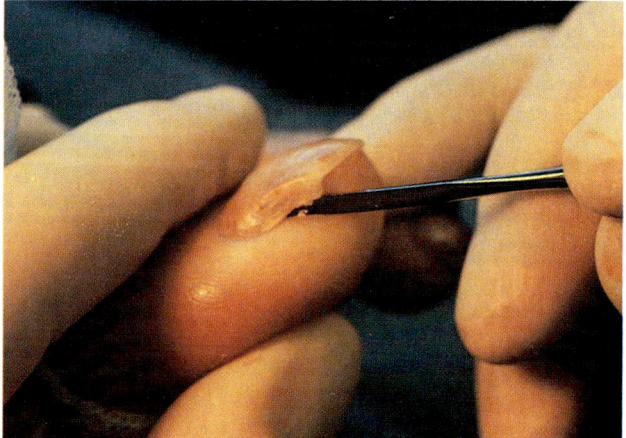

Figure 7. Incurved border of nail is elevated with spatula.

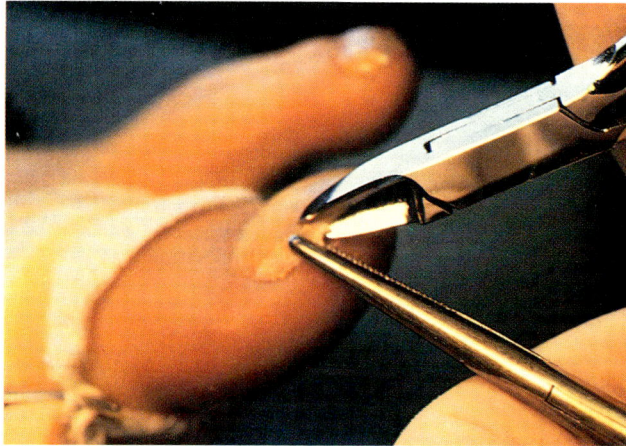

Figure 8. Nail cut with clipper.

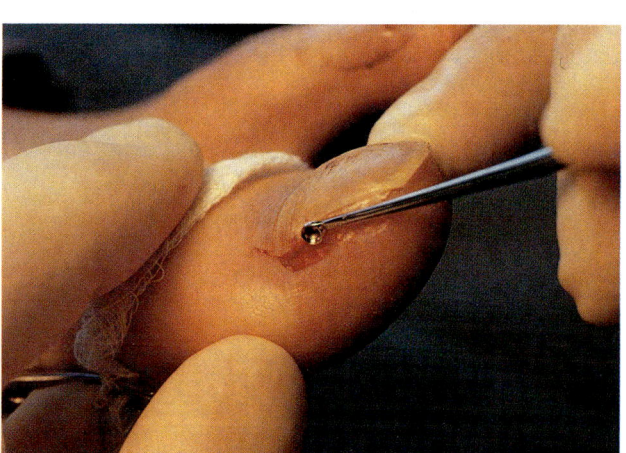

Figure 9. Matrix and nail bed removed with curette.

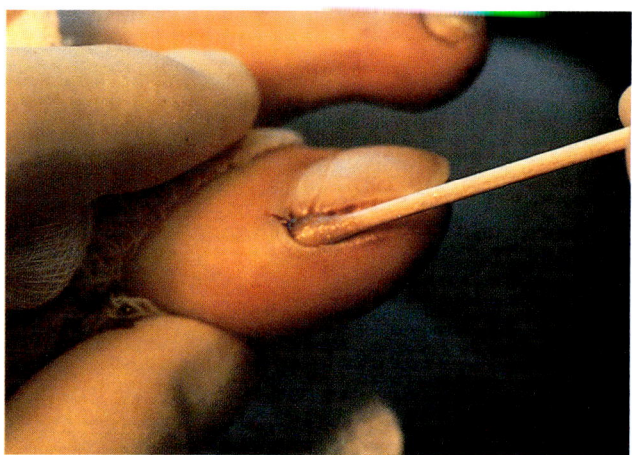

Figure 10. Debulked cotton swab used to introduce phenol and then isopropyl alcohol.

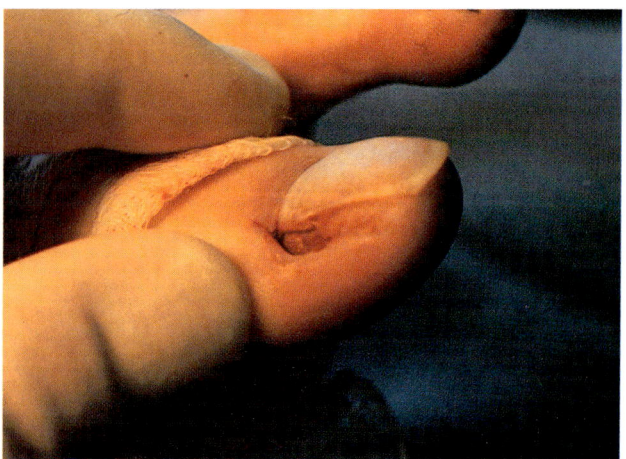

Figure 11. Appearance at end of procedure.

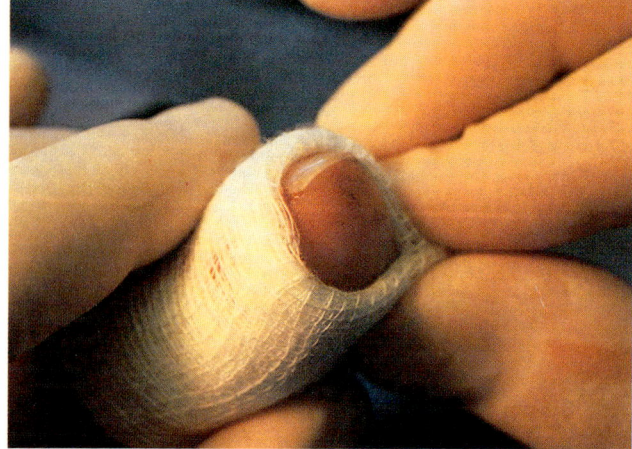

Figure 12. Bandage applied and covered with Coban.

the wound in the area of the matrix as were the first two swabs and is kept there for approximately 30 seconds. The isopropyl alcohol neutralizes the necrotizing effect of the phenol. (Fig. 11).

The raw areas are then covered with Neosporin cream and a small compression bandage is applied after which the Penrose drain tourniquet is removed (Fig. 12).

POSTOPERATIVE MANAGEMENT

Patients are advised to expect some serous drainage (days to weeks) representing the chemical burn induced by the phenol. The duration and the amount of drainage can be limited significantly with the use of nonsteroidal anti-inflammatory medications. In addition, patients are advised to soak the foot in lukewarm saline 10 to 15 minutes t.i.d. Prolonged drainage might suggest a low-grade superficial infection and, for this reason, application of Neosporin or Betadine following the soaks is helpful.

Patients may wear sandals for a day or two and then regular shoes as tolerated. Patients return in 3 days for removal of clot and debris. They are also encouraged to clean the surgical area with a sponge or cloth as a means of ongoing debridement.

COMPLICATIONS

Aside from the possibilities of prolonged serous drainage and occasional mild pain, the main complication would be partial recurrence or spicule formation.

It should be noted that the matrix is formed embryologically from an epidermal invagination and therefore the underside of the eponychium has growth cells as well as the dorsum of the phalanx (Fig. 13) and failure to remove this segment will result in regrowth of nail or spicule formation.

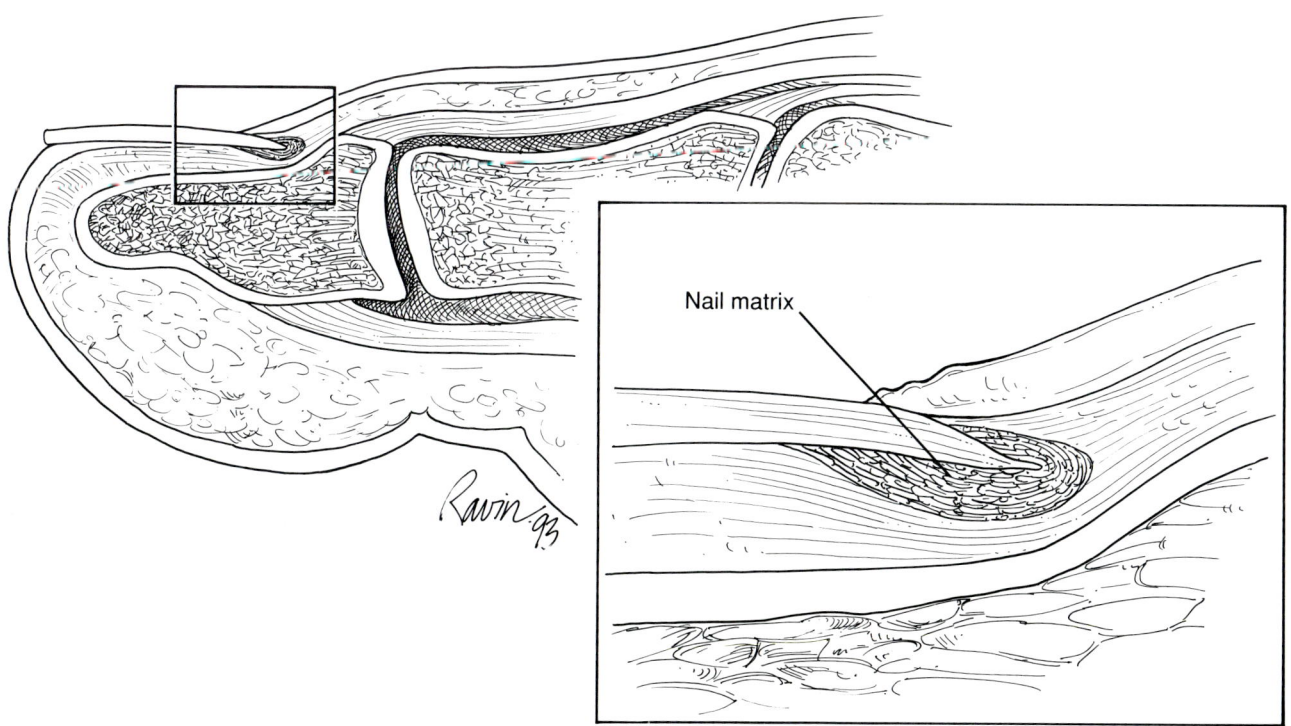

Figure 13. Lateral view of distal phalanx showing germinal cells under eponychium and at base of nail bed.

Phenol must be kept in a cool dark area and changed on a regular basis because it will deteriorate rather quickly after exposure to air.

The surgical field must be dry because phenol mixed with blood alters the pH, compromising the effectiveness of the phenol and turning the area black. The phenol technique will fail if old phenol is used, if the phenol is not applied to all the appropriate areas, or if an insufficient amount of nail is removed at the primary procedure.

ILLUSTRATIVE CASE FOR TECHNIQUE

This 40-year-old man had multiple episodes of pain along the lateral margin of his great toe. Soaking and occasional antibiotics were necessary to control his acute pain symptoms. Because of the chronic difficulty, a phenol nail margin ablation was done. Figure 14 shows his great toenail appearance 1 year later with no recurrence of symptoms.

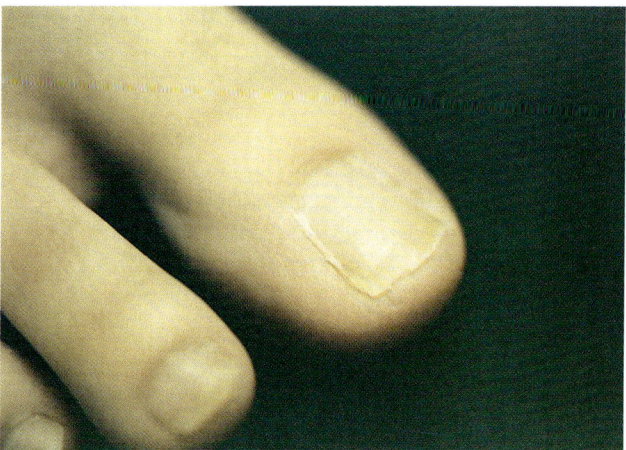

Figure 14. Appearance 1 year after procedure.

RECOMMENDED READING

1. McGlamry, E. D.: *Comprehensive Textbook of Foot Surgery.* Williams & Wilkins, Baltimore, 1987, p. 21.
2. Yale, J.: Phenol-alcohol technique for correction of infected ingrown toenail. *J. Am. Podiatr. Med. Assoc.,* 64: 46–53, 1974.

3
Hallux Interphalangeal Arthrodesis

Ian J. Alexander

INDICATIONS/CONTRAINDICATIONS

Arthrodesis of the hallux interphalangeal (IP) joint is primarily indicated for deformity and arthritis of the IP joint. In certain instances it is used independently or as an adjunct to tendon transfers when the IP and metatarsophalangeal (MP) joints are unstable or malaligned due to soft tissue deficiency or muscular imbalances. Examples of this include a claw hallux secondary to intrinsic muscle denervation (e.g., Charcot-Marie-Tooth disease), flexor hallucis brevis detachment after sesamoidectomy, and hallux varus deformity after bunionectomy. The IP arthrodesis serves to stabilize the joint when the extensor hallucis longus is transferred to the metatarsal neck in the Jones procedure or to the lateral aspect of the phalangeal base in the correction of hallux varus. When short flexor deficiency is the indication for IP fusion, arthrodesis of the IP joint eliminates the flexion deformity at the IP joint and allows the flexor hallucis longus to flex the hallux at the MP joint restoring great toe function.

PREOPERATIVE PLANNING

Preoperative examination of the foot should include a careful assessment of the circulatory status of the foot and the integrity of the skin in the area of the proposed surgery. Range of motion of the first MP joint must be assessed, particularly in patients with a claw deformity of the hallux. If the hallux cannot be passively

---

I. J. Alexander, MD: Department of Orthopedic Surgery, Northeast Ohio Universities College of Medicine, Rootstown, Ohio 44272; and Department of Orthopaedics, Crystal Clinic, Suite 102, Akron, Ohio 44313.

flexed to at least the neutral (sagittal) position, surgery on the MTP joint at the time of the IP fusion may be necessary to ensure good postoperative position of the hallux. In cases involving transfer of the extensor hallucis longus, care must be taken to assess function of the extensor hallucis brevis. Absence of the extensor hallucis brevis will result in a drop hallux if the longus is transferred.

Weight-bearing anterior, posterior, and lateral radiographs of the foot are obtained. The degree of deformity present at the IP joint of the great toe is assessed. With loss of articular surface from one side or the other such as following trauma, the amount of bone to be removed from the head of the proximal phalanx can be assessed and the degree of great toe shortening estimated. The goal is to place the IP joint in neutral flexion and extension in the sagittal plane as well as neutral varus and valgus in the transverse (axial) plane.

The length of screw to be used at the time of surgery can be estimated by measuring the combined length of the proximal and distal phalanges and then planning for bone resection of about 4 mm. When combined with the intraoperative measurement, this will ensure that the longitudinal screw will not penetrate the MP joint.

SURGERY

IP joint shape limits surface preparation for arthrodesis of this joint to either straight cutting or simply denuding the articular surfaces.

Technique. This procedure is best accomplished through a dorsal transverse incision across the joint with terminal curves or an L-shaped incision (Figs. 1–3). The dorsal capsule and medial and lateral ligaments are divided to allow adequate visualization of the joint surfaces (Fig. 4). A saw can be used to prepare the fusion site (Figs. 5–9), or the surfaces are prepared by removing only the articular

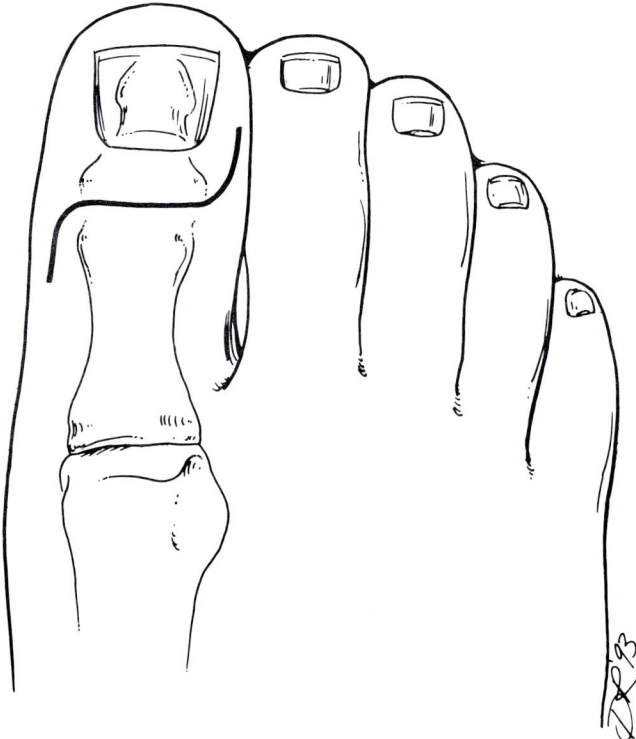

Figure 1. Incision for hallux interphalangeal (IP) arthrodesis.

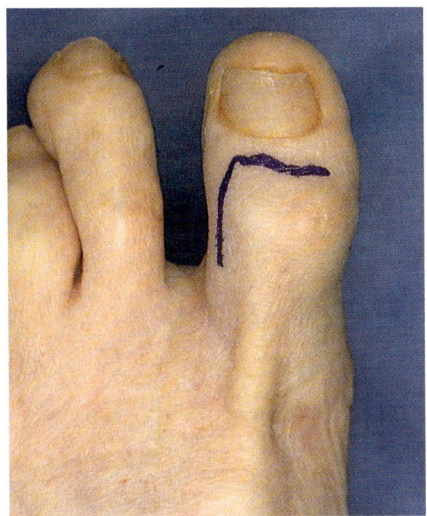

Figure 2. Marking for an L-shaped incision across the IP joint and down the lateral aspect is seen.

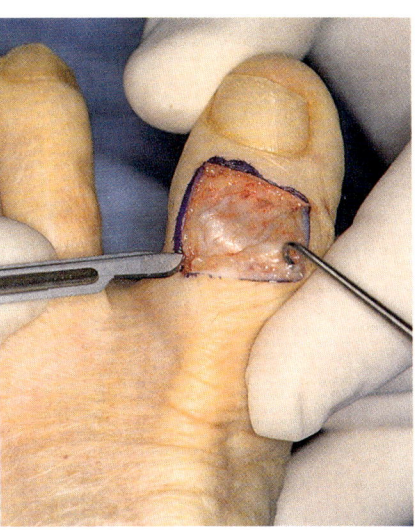

Figure 3. This incision is deepened with special care being taken to protect the full-thickness flap. Note that the incision is just proximal to the growth matrix of the nail and the extensor hallucis longus tendon is seen in the depths of the wound.

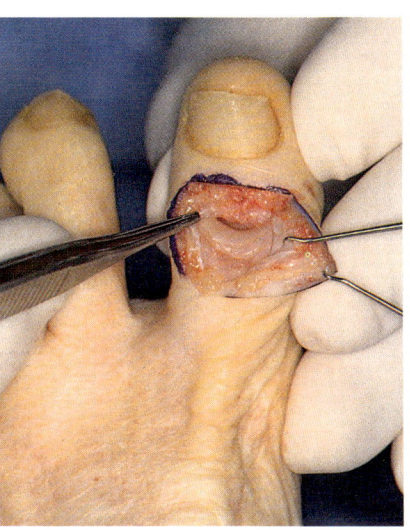

Figure 4. The joint is exposed by cutting the collateral ligaments of the joint and transection of about two-thirds of the width of the extensor hallucis longus tendon. The medial one-third of the tendon is kept intact on the medial side of the joint. Note the thumb forceps pointing to the collateral ligament on the lateral side of the IP joint.

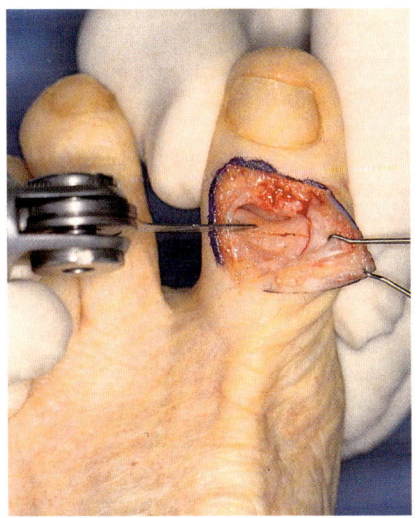

Figure 5. First the distal aspect of the proximal phalanx is removed. This is only about 2 mm in width.

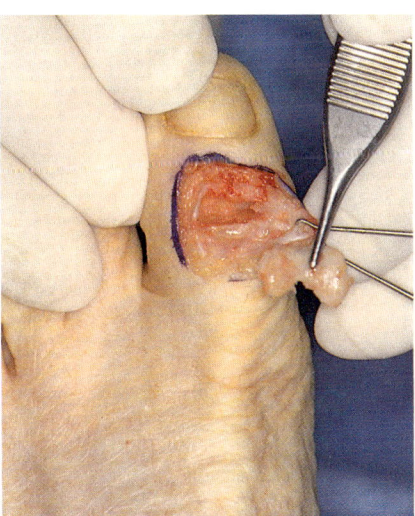

Figure 6. A resected bone from the distal end of the proximal phalanx in the thumb forceps.

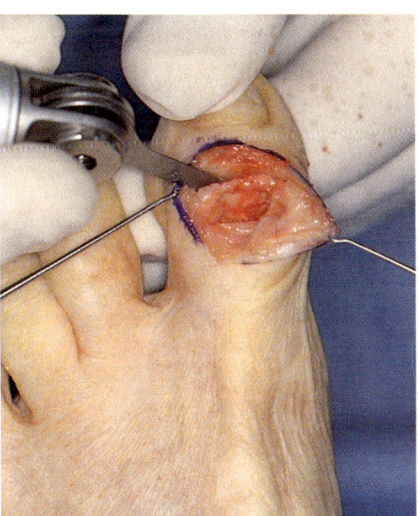

Figure 7. The proximal aspect of the distal phalanx is removed using a sagittal saw.

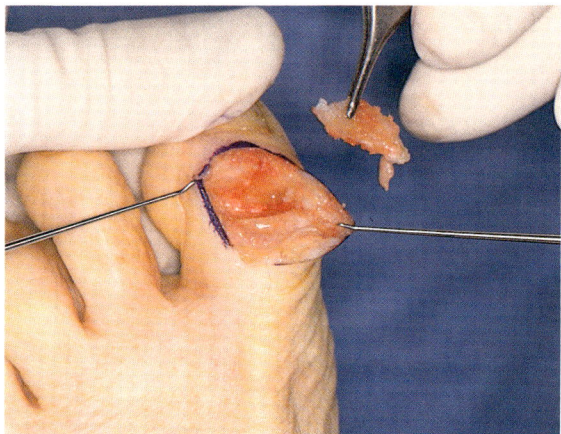

Figure 8. Only about 2 mm in width of this slightly concave joint is removed and the surface is held in the thumb forceps.

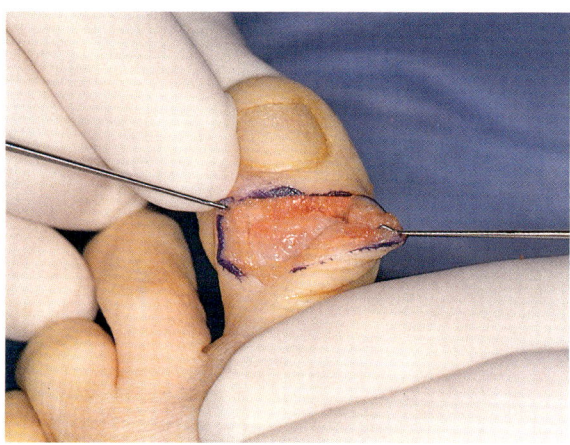

Figure 9. The two surfaces are opposed. The dorsal cortex of the proximal phalanx and the dorsal cortex of the distal phalanx should align themselves in a flush manner.

cartilage and dense subchondral bone following the contours of the joint line. After removing the articular surfaces the distal phalanx is drilled retrograde, exiting the toe tip just below the nail (Figs. 10 and 11). The joint surfaces are then apposed and position and contact are checked. Then with the drill bit entering the terminal phalanx distally through the previously drilled tract, the proximal phalanx is drilled (Figs. 12 and 13). Fixation is achieved with a 4.0 mm cancellous lag screw that compresses the fusion site, a technique described by Shives and Johnson (1) (Figs. 14–17). Lack of rotational control provided by the screw alone has led to nonunion in a few of our patients despite excellent initial screw fixation. To prevent this rotation, an obliquely placed 0.045 or smaller K-wire is currently utilized to transfix the joint (Fig. 18). Intraoperative radiographs in two planes are advisable to assess bone contact at the fusion site and screw and pin position.

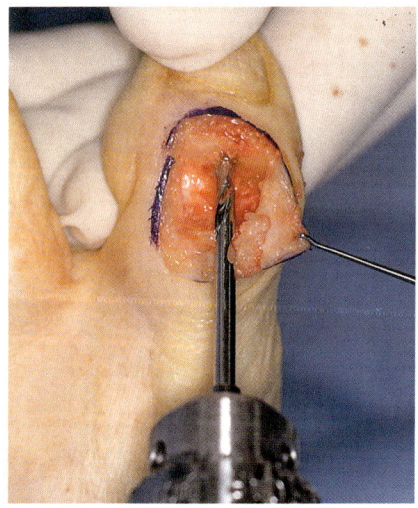

Figure 10. A 4-mm drill bit is used to drill the distal phalanx starting from its proximal aspect through the wound.

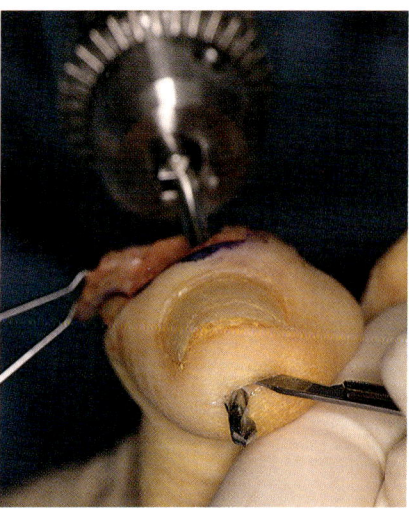

Figure 11. The skin on the tip of the toe is incised where the drill bit tents the skin.

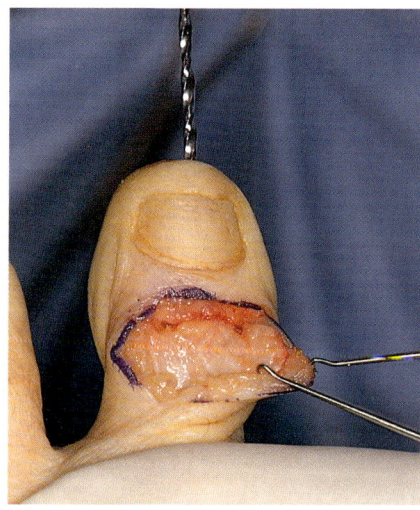

Figure 12. A 2.0-mm drill bit is placed down the drill pathway in the distal phalanx while the arthrodesis site is held in the proper position.

3 HALLUX INTERPHALANGEAL ARTHRODESIS

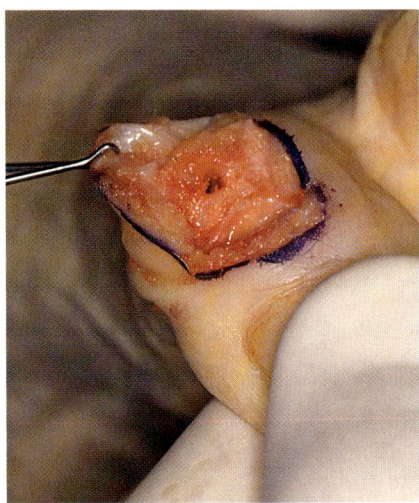

Figure 13. This drill bit should enter the resected end of the proximal phalanx in its midportion, which is seen here.

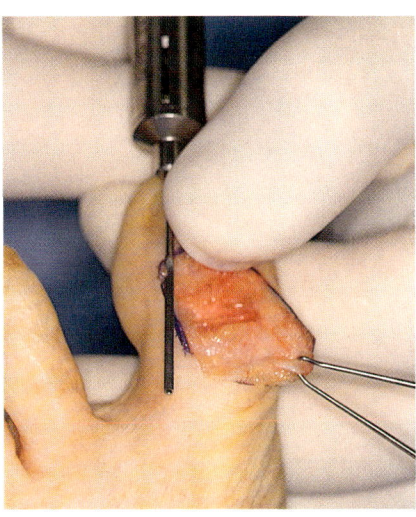

Figure 14. The length of screw to be used is measured directly on the toe and compared with an estimate made from the preoperative radiograph.

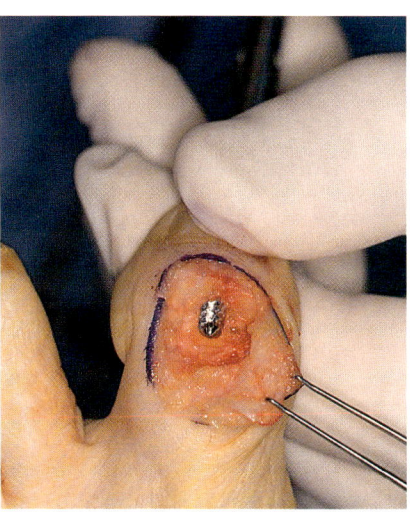

Figure 15. The appropriate 4.0 cancellous bone screw is advanced through the tip of the toe and out the proximal surface of the distal phalanx.

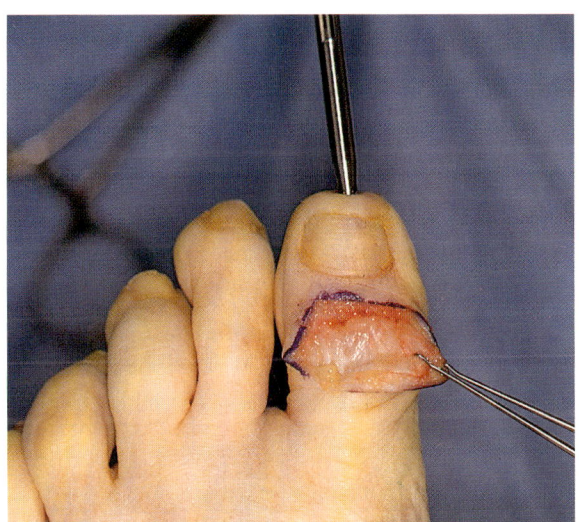

Figure 16. The screw is then tightened bringing the two surfaces of the arthrodesis site closely opposed.

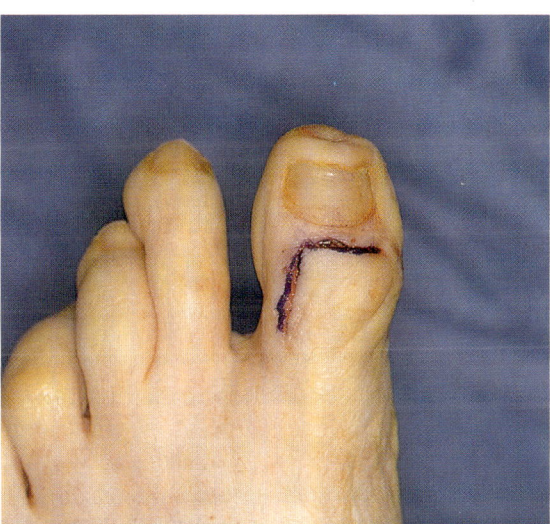

Figure 17. The skin is closed with the surgeon's suture of choice.

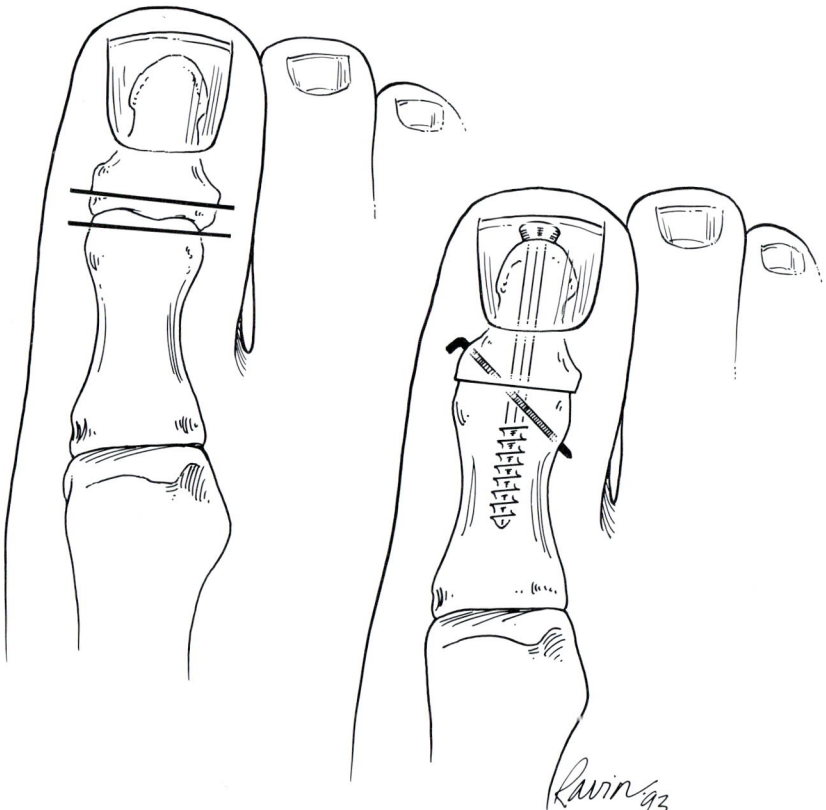

Figure 18. To control rotation, a Kirschner wire may be placed obliquely across the arthrodesis site.

POSTOPERATIVE MANAGEMENT

Six weeks in a wooden postoperative shoe is usually sufficient immobilization, but it is also advisable to recommend limited activity and total avoidance of weight bearing on the hallux until solid union is apparent radiographically. The screw and wire are removed under toe block anesthesia in the office at 3 months if healing is complete. Lacking back-cutting threads, the 4.0 lag screw can be difficult to remove, particularly if more than 3 months have elapsed since insertion. With the supplemental oblique K-wire, success rate and patient satisfaction with the outcome of this procedure has been excellent.

COMPLICATIONS

Less than optional outcomes are usually the result of nonunion, which may be related to inadequate fixation, failure to achieve adequate bony apposition, or premature loading of the digit. Salvage is with a repeat arthrodesis. Postoperatively, a non–weight-bearing cast is applied that extends over the hallux and is maintained until union is confirmed clinically and radiographically. Although conceivable, malposition is rarely a problem. Screw removal is advisable, particularly if the head is prominent. This was reinforced by my own experience with an immunosuppressed woman with rheumatoid arthritis who stubbed her toe, dehisced over the screw head, and subsequently developed osteomyelitis.

3 HALLUX INTERPHALANGEAL ARTHRODESIS

ILLUSTRATIVE CASE FOR TECHNIQUE

An active 14-year-old boy presents with a painful deformity of the IP joint of the hallux subsequent to a stroke. The deformity consisted of a flexion contracture and associated valgus deviation (35°) at the IP joint of the hallux (Fig. 19A).

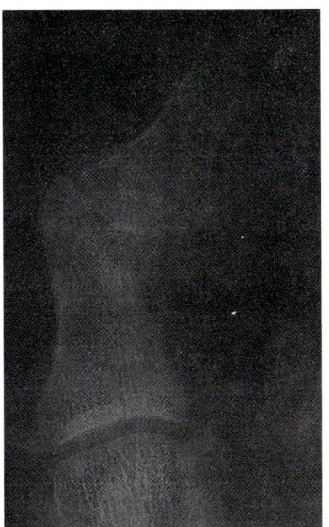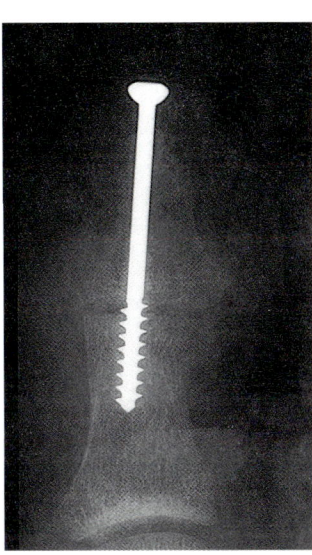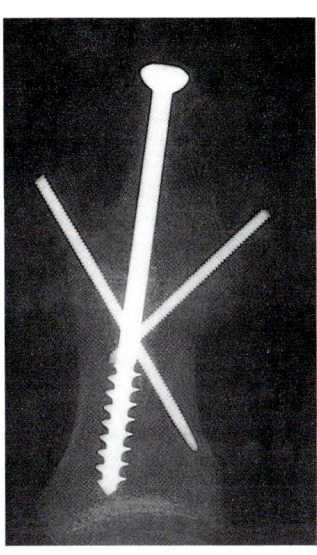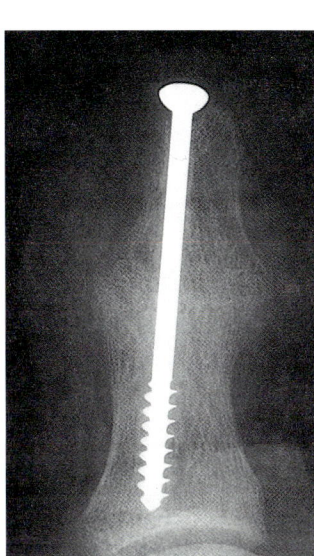

Figure 19. A: Anteroposterior radiograph shows the posttraumatic deformity of the IP joint of the great toe. **B:** Postoperatively the patient was extremely active, the screw backed out and a painful nonunion ensued. **C:** Repeat arthrodesis involved "freshening" the surfaces, reinsertion of a longitudinal screw and supplemental fixation with crossed K-wires. Usually a single oblique wire will suffice. **D:** A solid arthrodesis occurred and the K-wires were removed.

An IP arthrodesis was performed by straight cutting the articular surface to correct the alignment. Excellent fixation was obtained in the dense bone with a single 4.0 lag screw and surface apposition was checked with intraoperative films.

Postoperatively, the patient remained active, even marching with his school band. By 4 weeks, radiolucency was apparent at the fusion site and the screw had started to back out (Fig. 19B).

Repeat arthrodesis was performed with a combination of a single screw and crossed K-wires (Fig. 19C). The patient was placed in a short leg walking cast as an additional precaution. Solid union was achieved (Fig. 19D).

RECOMMENDED READING

1. Shives, T. C., and Johnson, K. A.: Arthrodesis of the interphalangeal joint of the great toe—an improved technique. *Foot Ankle,* 1:26–29, 1980.

PART II

Metatarsophalangeal Joints

4

Chevron Osteotomy

Kenneth A. Johnson

INDICATIONS/CONTRAINDICATIONS

Pain is the primary indication for a chevron osteotomy. The pain is located over the medial eminence and is related to the use of enclosed shoes. How much pain with shoewear should be present before a chevron osteotomy is suggested is a nebulous clinical decision. Suggesting a hallux valgus procedure such as a chevron osteotomy (Fig. 1) in anticipation of difficulty at some uncertain time in the future does not seem reasonable. A procedure solely for cosmetic reasons is questionable.

A hallux valgus deformity with an intermetatarsal 1–2 angle of 16° or less is considered an indication for chevron osteotomy. This figure of 16° was determined from both an empiric and scientific basis. Empirically, when the intermetatarsal angle was more than 16°, patient satisfaction was not as consistent as for those with the lesser deformity. On a scientific basis, the width of the first metatarsal head in essence determines how much the intermetatarsal angle can be narrowed. Each millimeter of lateral shift of the metatarsal head will decrease the intermetatarsal angle approximately 1°. Since the width of the metatarsal head at the level of osteotomy allows only about 6 mm of lateral shift, the maximum correction is about 6°. Because the normal intermetatarsal 1–2 angle is 10° or less, the reduction to a normal intermetatarsal 1–2 angle can only occur when the preoperative deformity is 16° or less.

The patient's age is also a factor in selecting the chevron osteotomy. Patients over 60 years of age do not seem to do as well as younger patients. The reasons for this are unclear. Perhaps stiffer tissues, increased expectations, or shoe-wear demands could be implicated. It is granted, however, that an older person with a hallux valgus may have a very supple deformity and be appropriate for a chevron osteotomy.

K. A. Johnson, M.D.: Division of Foot and Ankle Surgery, Mayo Clinic Scottsdale, Scottsdale, AZ 85259.

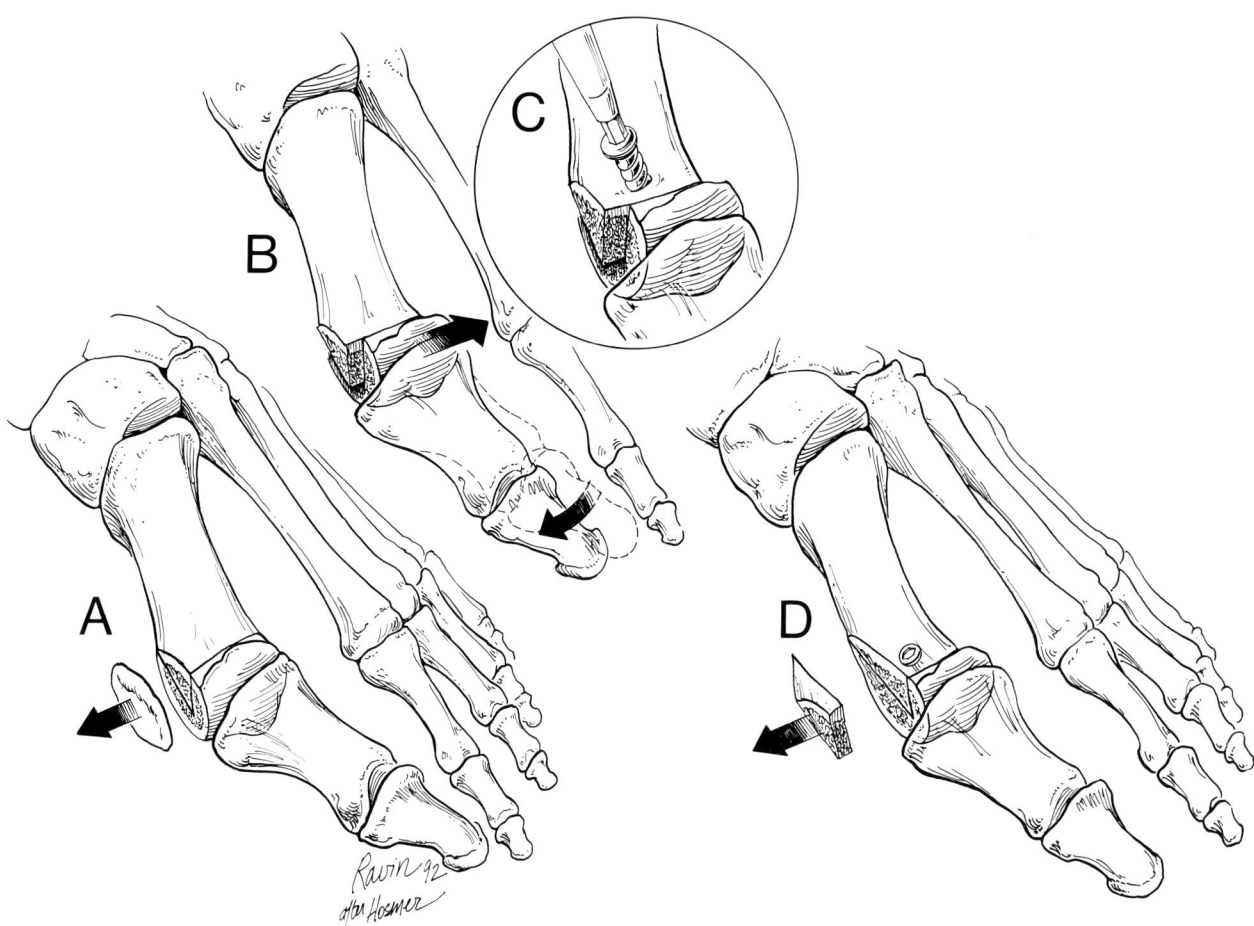

Figure 1. A: Removal of the medial eminence. The location for the modified chevron osteotomy is shown. **B:** With osteotomy completion, the metatarsal head is displaced lateralward about 5 to 7 mm. Relaxation of the adductor hallucis allows some realignment at the metatarsophalangeal joint. **C:** A 2.7-mm screw provides osteotomy fixation and compression. **D:** The uncovered portion of the metaphysis is removed completing the bone aspects of the chevron procedure.

A mobile and smooth metatarsophalangeal joint as indicated with varus-valgus stress is also a necessary precondition for a chevron osteotomy. This can be tested clinically by moving the great toe manually from a valgus to a varus position. Supple and smooth motion is a further indication that the chevron procedure is appropriate.

Absence of pain, an intermetatarsal 1–2 angle of more than 16°, a physiologically older person, and a stiff metatarsophalangeal joint are all considered contraindications for a chevron osteotomy. Degenerative arthritis of the metatarsophalangeal joint is usually not a concomitant finding with a mild hallux valgus. Some peripheral osteophyte formation and joint narrowing is acceptable as long as the varus-

TABLE 1. *Chevron osteotomy indications and contraindications*

	Indications	Contraindications
Symptoms	Pain	No pain
Intermetatarsal 1–2 angle	16° or less	>16°
Age	Younger	Older
Joint mobility	Supple-smooth	Rigid-rough
Previous hallux valgus surgery	No	Yes

valgus stress testing is mobile and smooth. More severe degenerative arthritis suggestive of hallux rigidus is a contraindication for a chevron osteotomy.

Prior hallux valgus surgery usually eliminates the chevron procedure from consideration. The chevron procedure is not a salvage procedure, and therefore is infrequently utilized after another procedure has been inadequate (Table 1).

PREOPERATIVE PLANNING

Planning for a chevron osteotomy includes a detailed discussion of symptoms and expectations, examination of the foot, general health evaluation, radiologic interpretation, and anesthetic discussion.

An ideal patient for a chevron osteotomy describes the symptoms in realistic terms and has appropriate expectations. When the pain is excruciating, involves the whole foot as well as the leg, and is present with or without shoes, a chevron osteotomy may not be the answer. Likewise, beware if the procedure is expected to make the patient run faster and leap higher as well as allow greater dexterity.

Besides noting the presence of the hallux valgus deformity, the foot examination should include the mobility of the metatarsophalangeal joint in flexion-extension and varus-valgus planes. Check that the neurovascular status of the foot is normal and look for any difficulties with lesser toe position or callus formation beneath the lesser metatarsal heads. An adjunctive procedure to the lesser metatarsal heads is rarely indicated with a chevron osteotomy. In fact, placing the great toe metatarsal head in an improved weight-bearing position with the chevron osteotomy may decrease lesser metatarsal callus formation and pain.

A general health evaluation is important mainly to anticipate difficulties that may occur. Diabetes mellitus, peripheral vascular disease, medications such as prednisone or methotrexate, and allergies all have specific implications.

Radiologic evaluation should include full weight-bearing anteroposterior and lateral views. The intermetatarsal 1–2 angle is measured as the angle between lines drawn from the center of the head to the center of the base for the first and second metatarsals. The hallux valgus angle measured between the line down the first metatarsal and line drawn down the shaft of the proximal phalanx is of lesser importance. Degenerative arthritis at the metatarsophalangeal joint can be evaluated on both the anteroposterior and lateral radiographs. The presence of metatarsus adduction with a normal intermetatarsal 1–2 angle should be noted. In such a situation, there is no "space" into which the metatarsal head can be translocated.

A chevron osteotomy can be done under local or general anesthesia as either outpatient or inpatient status. If both feet are to be treated surgically, the amount of local anesthesia necessary to provide adequate anesthesia to both feet may exceed safety limits. In such a situation, general anesthesia is preferred. Also, if the patient is "needle shy" or particularly anxious, a general anesthesia may be easier on both the patient and the surgeon.

Most often chevron osteotomy will be done on an outpatient basis in an outpatient surgical facility. Occasionally, because of general health difficulties or an absence of family support, it will be necessary to admit the patient to the hospital one night postoperative. The availability of home infusion services and nursing care has made the necessity of inpatient care infrequent.

This modification of the chevron osteotomy changed the configuration of the osteotomy and screw fixation. The conventional chevron osteotomy had the potential to slip back into its original position and lose correction. Although it is not known exactly in what percentage of cases this occurred, there is no doubt it did occur. Changes in radiograph projection and quality make postoperative comparisons with preoperative films difficult. Screw fixation insures the metatarsal head will stay in the proper position. Additionally, screw fixation allows early weight bearing without osteotomy displacement. With the conventional chevron osteotomy cast immobilization was utilized for 3 weeks. When screw fixation is used, it is not necessary to immobilize the foot. As is described in "Postoperative Management" later in this chapter, a 1-week period of cast immobilization is used. This period of casting, however, is done primarily for pain relief and not to protect the osteotomy site.

A variety of osteotomy configurations were considered before adopting the modification described. This particular configuration is stable particularly against distal fragment dorsiflexion and is easily adaptable to screw fixation. Other types of mechanical fixation were also considered—Kirschner wire, absorbable pin, compression Herbert screw, staples, bone pegs—but when the degree of fixation and cost were considered, the 2.7-mm screw was felt to be preferable.

SURGERY

The patient is positioned supine on the surgical table. A thigh tourniquet or a rubber Esmarch bandage around the ankle may be used for bleeding control. If local ankle block anesthesia is used, the ankle compression bandage is necessary. Padding the ankle with a surgical towel before applying the tourniquet along with intravenous sedation increases patient acceptance of the compression at the ankle.

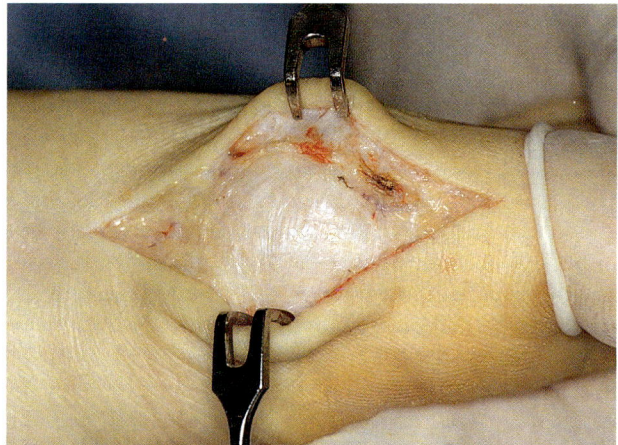

Figure 2. Medial exposure of metatarsophalangeal joint capsule.

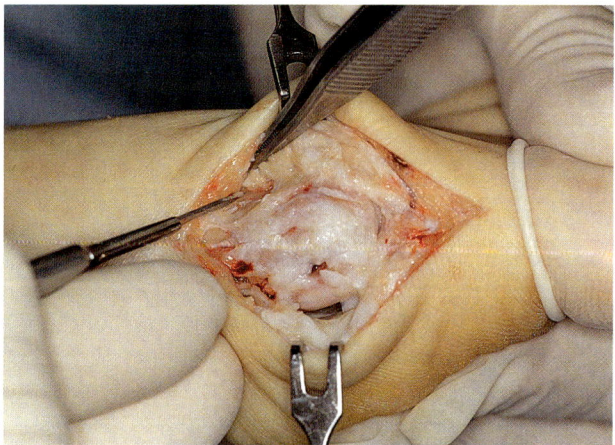

Figure 3. Elevation of the medial capsule and ligament structures.

The surgeon sits at the end of the table with an assistant on the side of the table closest to the foot. For a right-handed surgeon, a right-foot chevron procedure is a bit less difficult since it will be easier to position the dominant hand toward the medial eminence of the foot.

The skin incision is dorsomedial, about 7 cm in length, and centered over the medial eminence (Fig. 2). The subcutaneous tissue is elevated from the capsule over the medial eminence, taking care to protect not only the dorsomedial nerve branch of the superficial peroneal nerve, but also the plantar medial nerve to the great toe from the medial plantar nerve. If the plantar medial nerve is surgically injured, it is a significant problem since the subsequent end-bulb neuroma will be repetitively irritated with weight bearing.

Technique. When the medial capsule has been exposed, a midline longitudinal medial incision in the capsule is made and the capsular structure dissected off the medial eminence (Fig. 3). Avoid injury to the dorsomedial and plantar medial nerves to the great toe. This can be done by making the initial skin incision only about 2 mm dorsal to the medial midline of the medial eminence. Dissection through the subcutaneous tissue is made to the capsule over the medial eminence and then the subcutaneous tissues dorsalward and plantarward are swept off the capsule, which elevates the nerves away from injury. The dorsomedial aspect of the metatarsal metaphysis is also exposed in preparation for later screw fixation of the osteotomy.

Stripping of capsule from the lateral aspect of the metatarsal head may deprive the metatarsal head of its blood supply and is not indicated. For placement of the screw the capsule is elevated from the dorsomedial aspect of the metaphysis but not from the lateral side of the metatarsal head. Whether or not a perforation of the lateral joint capsule and release of the adductor hallucis at the joint line should be done is controversial. Advocates point out such surgical manipulations are distal to the vascular supply to metatarsal head and feel that the correction of the valgus angulation of the great toe may be improved. Opponents of lateral capsular release feel that it complicates the procedure and is not necessary, that it is not possible to get a true adductor hallucis release without extensive dissection, and that the possibility of the subsequent avascular necrosis is enhanced when such a release is done. In fact, just translocating the metatarsal head along with the phalanges laterally brings the insertion of the adductor hallucis closer to its origin and is in effect a physiologic release.

The metatarsophalangeal joint is opened only enough to allow visualization of the sagittal groove of the medial eminence. Starting at the sagittal groove, the medial eminence is removed parallel to the medial border of the foot (Fig. 4). The

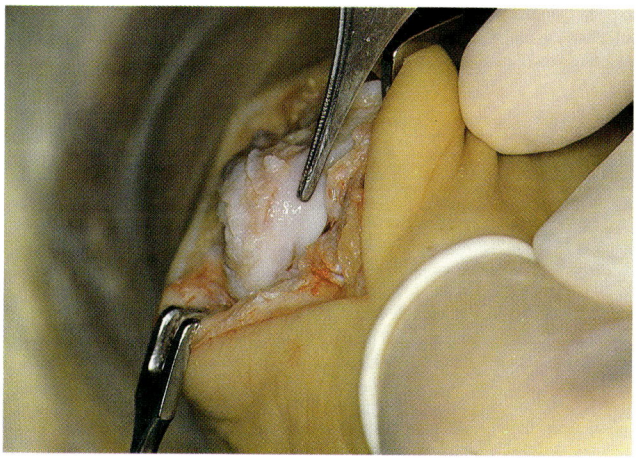
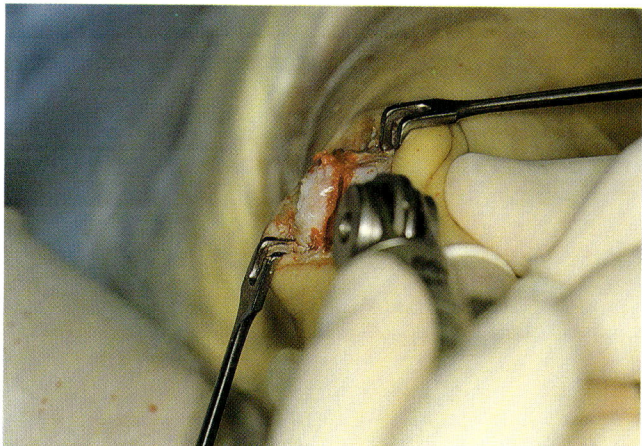

Figure 4. A: Location of the sagittal groove is shown at the tip of the thumb forceps. **B:** Medial eminence removed parallel to medial foot border.

Hall-Micro-Saw 100 sagittal with a 5053-232 blade (Zimmer Co., Warsaw, Indiana) is ideal for medial eminence removal, subsequent osteotomy, and metaphysis realignment.

Removal of the medial eminence along the medial border of the foot is done to present a smooth flat surface for shoe-wear. If medial eminence resection is done along the shaft of the first metatarsal, there is a tendency to leave the distal medial aspect of the metatarsal head prominent and cause pain later. An area of cancellous bone approximately the size of a teardrop-shaped nickel will be exposed with removal of the medial eminence (Fig. 5).

The metatarsal is now ready for the osteotomy. The chevron osteotomy has been modified to facilitate its stabilization with a screw (Fig. 6). The inferior arm of the osteotomy is made parallel to the plantar surface of the foot, starting from a point just a few millimeters proximal to the resected surface of the medial eminence and midway between the superior and inferior margins of the first metatarsal head (Fig. 7A). This provides an elongated plantar extension tongue of the osteotomized metatarsal head. The second arm of the chevron osteotomy is from the apex of the inferior osteotomy arm, directed dorsally about 70° from the plane of the plantar surface of the foot. The superior context of the metatarsal is broached with this arm of the osteotomy just proximal to the articular surface of the metatarsal head.

The modified chevron osteotomy itself has some potential pitfalls. The apex of the osteotomy should be within a few millimeters of the distal cut edge of the medial eminence resection in the wide portion of the metaphysis. If not placed far enough distalward, the width of metatarsal is insufficient to allow enough lateral displacement. Also, the plantarward arm of the osteotomy should be parallel to the plane of the sole of the foot. If instead the natural tendency to angulate the plantarward arm downward toward the heel of the foot is done, there will be a shortened plantar tongue extension of the capital fragment and screw fixation will be difficult. Probably the most difficult site of the chevron osteotomy is where the plantarward arm leaves the metatarsal shaft proximally. This is cortical bone that needs to be cut obliquely. If the osteotomy is not completed in this site, however, the metatarsal head will tend to rotate during translocation and give an improper head alignment as well as poor osteotomy apposition.

The metatarsal shaft is now grasped with a large towel clip and the capital fragment manually displaced laterally 5 to 7 mm (Figs. 7B and 8). Particular attention is given to translocating the capital fragment lateralward without any tilting or angulation. This is best observed by looking at the inferior osteotomy edges

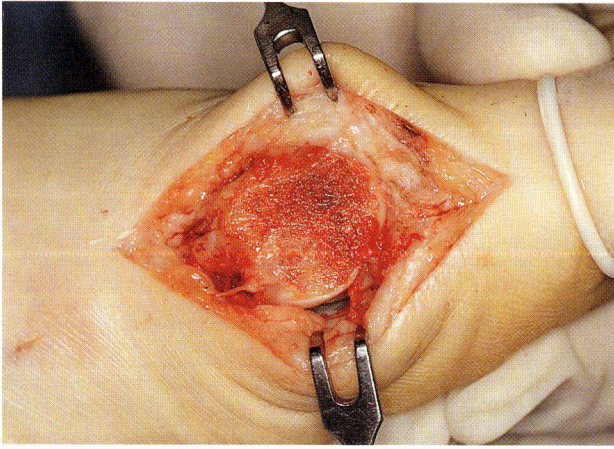

Figure 5. Appearance of the metatarsal head after medial eminence removal.

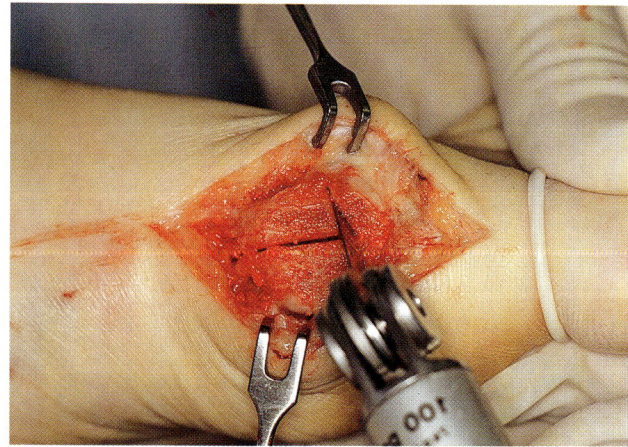

Figure 6. The inferior arm of the chevron osteotomy has been completed and short superior arm is being cut with the saw blade.

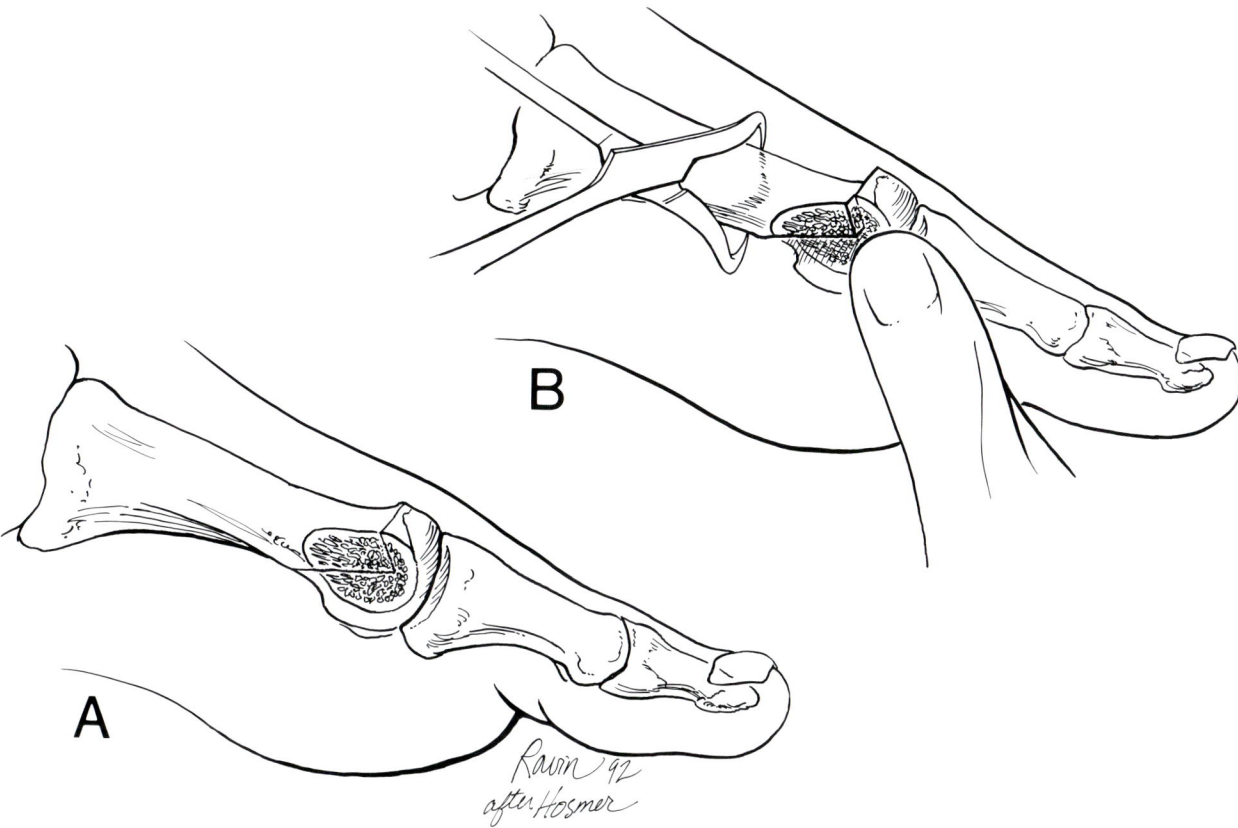

Figure 7. A: Correct location for the modified osteotomy arms of the chevron osteotomy. **B:** Utilizing a small towel clip for countertraction, the metatarsal head is displaced laterally.

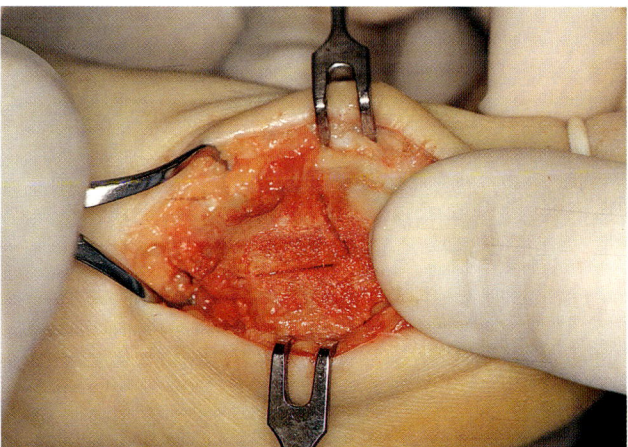

Figure 8. Pressure with the thumb over the capital fragment allows shifting of the metatarsal head.

and being certain they are still parallel after translocation. Longitudinal compression on the great toe will coapt the osteotomy; it should be inherently stable and not "spring" back to the original position (Figs. 9 and 10).

Attention is now given to the dorsal aspect of the metaphysis just behind the upper arm of the osteotomy. The drill bit is the 2.0-mm size for the 2.7-mm screw. Entrance on the superior metaphysis is about 3 mm proximal to the superior arm of the chevron osteotomy and about 3 mm lateral to the edge of the capital portion that was osteotomized with removal of the medial eminence (Fig. 11). The 2.0-mm drill bit is directed about 10° distalward from a perpendicular line to the first metatarsal shaft and about 10° to 15° lateralward from a plane perpendicular to the surface of the foot. (Fig. 12). This orientation of the drill will engage the laterally displaced tongue of the capital fragment. The reason for the distalward orientation of the drill bit is to provide compression to the superior limb of the modified chevron osteotomy, as well as the inferior limb. This orientation will also place the tip of the screw behind the plantarward articular surface of the metatarsal head and militate against the possibility of sesamoid impingement on

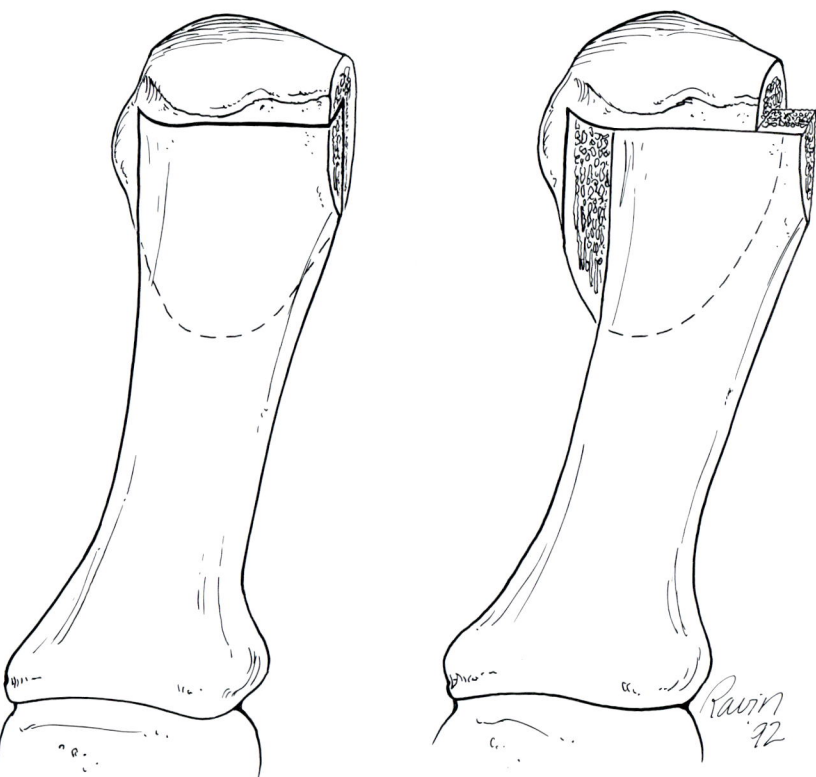

Figure 9. The metatarsal head is displaced from its original position *(left)* to the corrected position *(right)*.

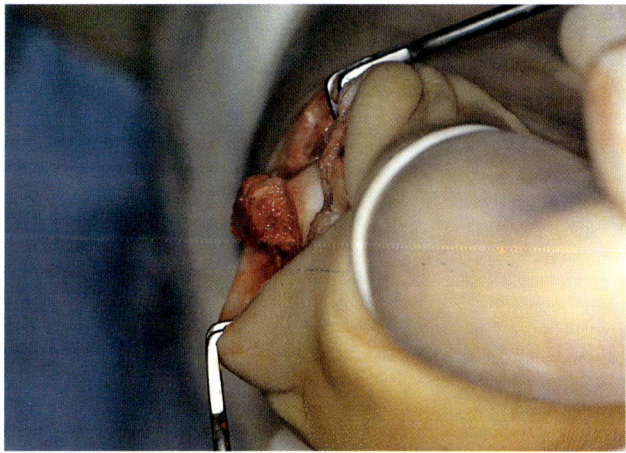

Figure 10. This end view shows the metatarsal head displaced lateralward about 6 mm.

the screw tip. Following the 2.0-mm drill, a 2.7-mm tap of the drill hole is made and a countersink used to the dorsal aspect of the metaphysis. A 2.7-mm drill is then run through the dorsal cortex to provide a lag effect on the osteotomy. A depth gauge is utilized to measure for the screw length, which is almost always 16 or 18 mm in length (Fig. 13). As the screw is inserted and is tightened the osteotomy will close and should be very stable (Figs. 14 and 15).

The placement of the screw for fixation of the osteotomy should not be difficult. Only a few pitfalls seem to be present. It is important that the drill hole not be started in the dorsal metaphysis too far medial. Otherwise, when the step for

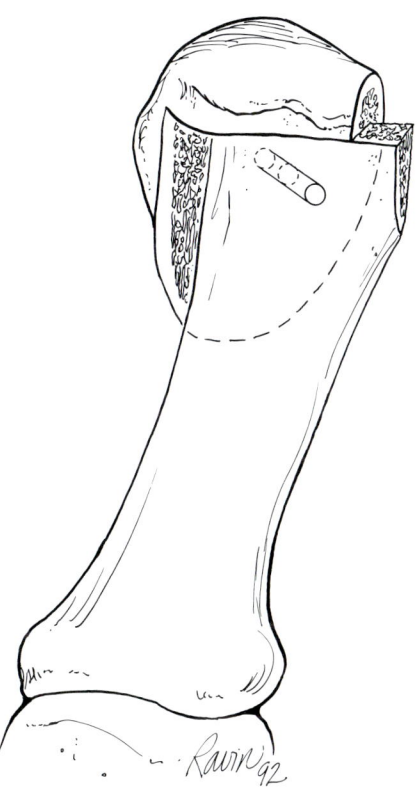

Figure 11. Diagrammatic representation of drill hole position.

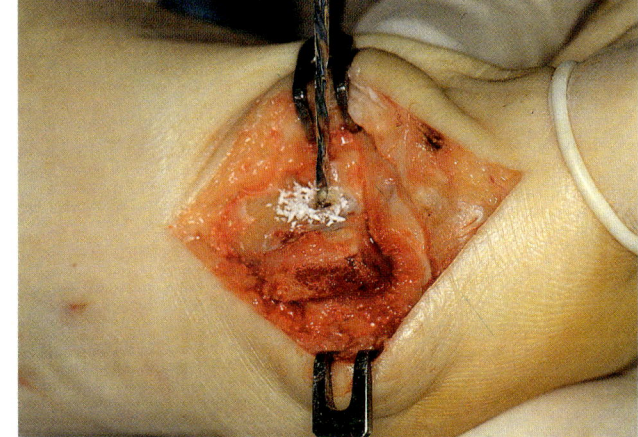

Figure 12. The 2.0-mm drill bit starting in the dorsal metaphysis.

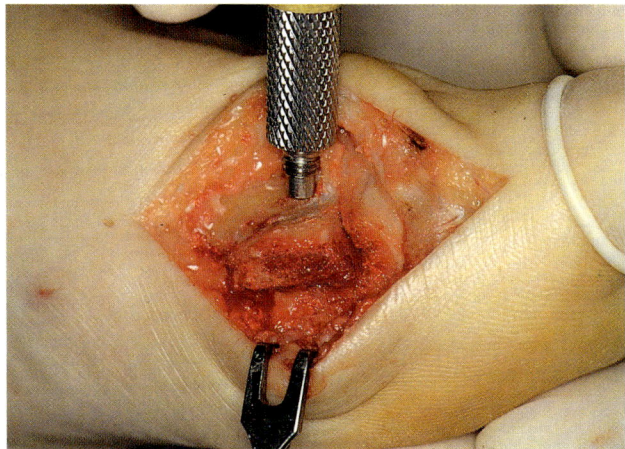

Figure 13. A depth gauge indicates proper length of screw.

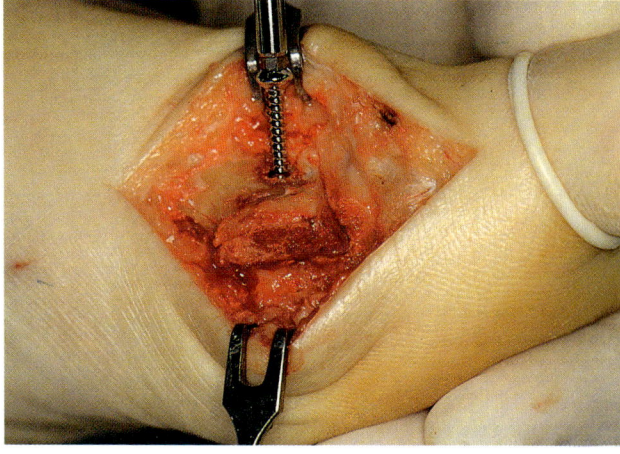

Figure 14. Insertion of the 2.7-mm screw.

Figure 15. A: Angulation of the screw slightly distalward and lateralward is shown. **B:** Compression *(arrows)* is present across the osteotomy.

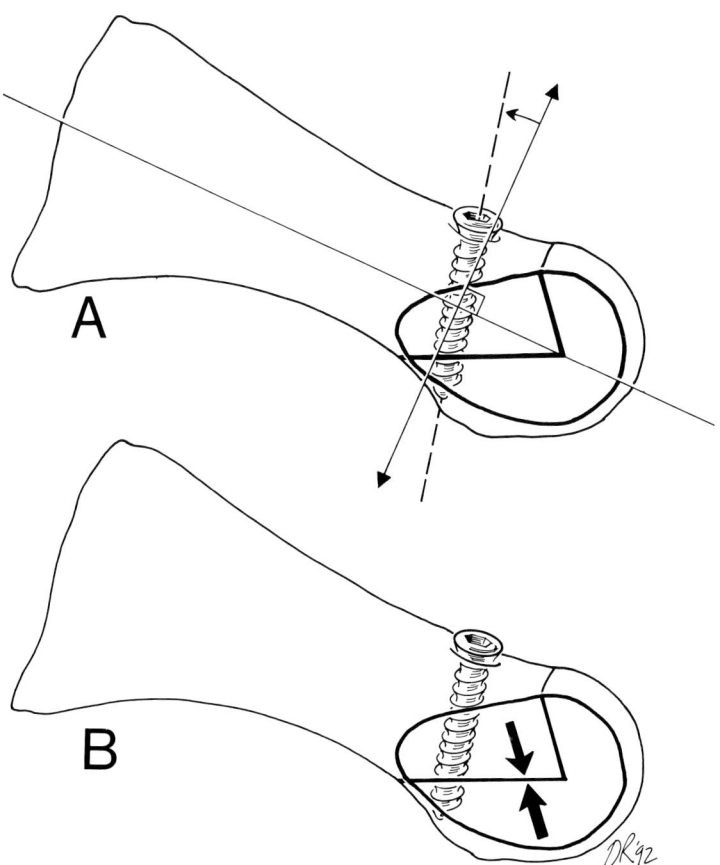

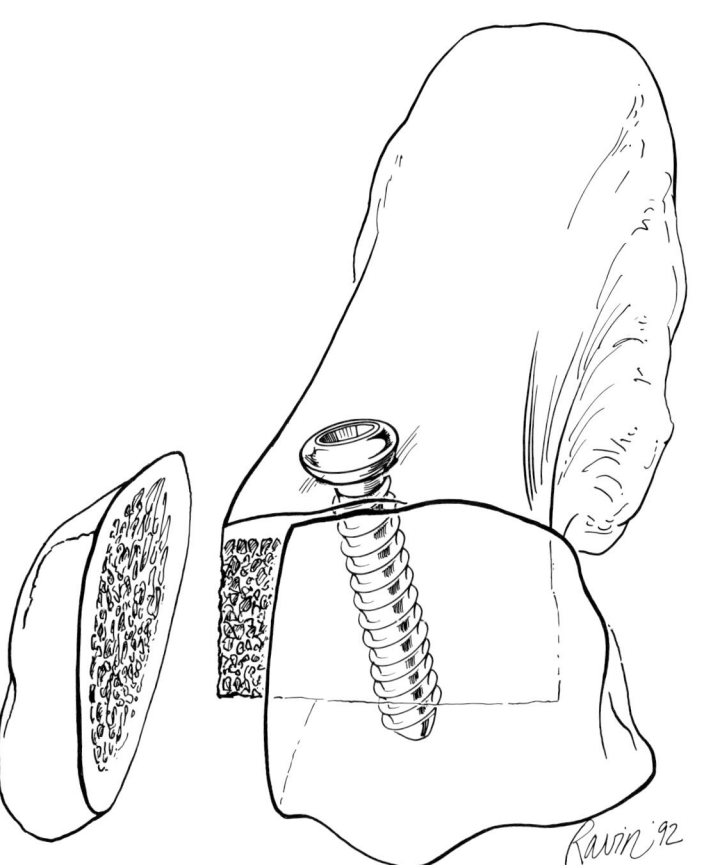

Figure 16. This illustration shows the relative amounts of medial eminence removed and lateral capital fragment displacement.

resection of the uncovered exposed portion of the metaphysis is done the screw head will be in the way or the amount of bone around the screw will be too weak. Another potential problem with screw fixation is not directing the screw plantar lateral so as to engage the plantar tongue of the capital fragment. If the screw is not measured correctly, protuberance of the screw into the sesamoid path may occur. Remembering that the proper length of the screw will only be about 16 to 18 mm should help avoid such a pitfall (Fig. 16).

Resection of the uncovered portion of metaphysis is now performed parallel to the medial border of the foot (Fig. 17). Directing the saw blade from the dorsal aspect of the metatarsal facilitates a smooth straight resection along the medial border of the foot (Fig. 18). Finally, a small needle-nosed bone rongeur is used

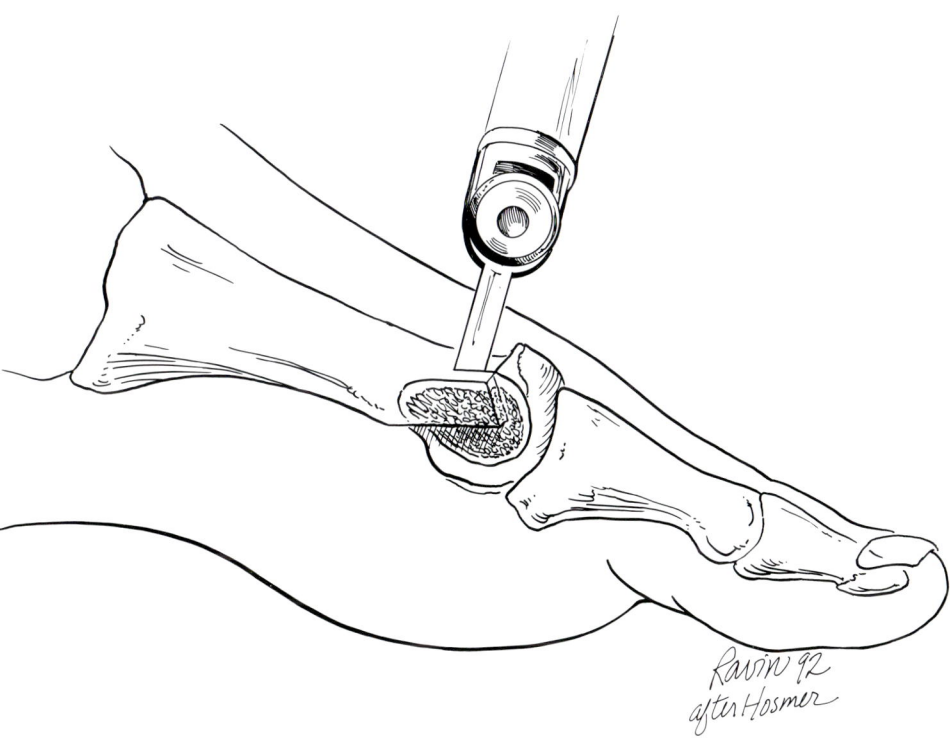

Figure 17. The uncovered position of the metaphysis is removed.

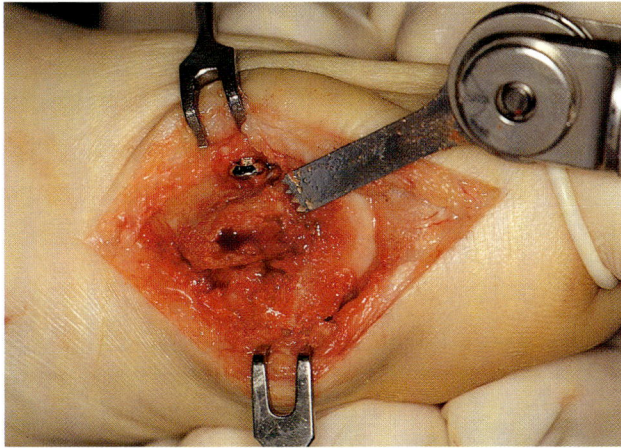

Figure 18. The saw blade is directed along the capital fragment cut surface as a template to remove the uncovered metaphysis.

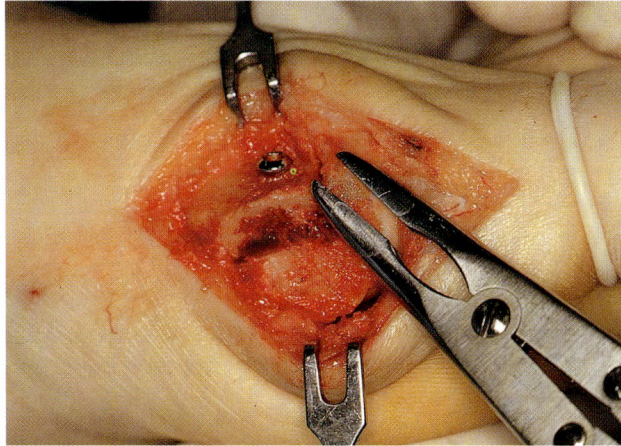

Figure 19. The dorsomedial aspect of the metatarsal head is smoothed.

to smooth off the dorsomedial aspect of the metatarsal head so it will not be prominent with shoe-wear (Fig. 19). The osteotomy is complete (Figs. 20 and 21).

Soft tissue reconstruction after completion of the osteotomy is very important. With the longitudinal incision in the medial capsule followed by removal of the medial eminence and osteotomy, excess capsule tissue will be available. An ellipse of capsule tissue is removed prior to capsular closure. The amount to be removed is determined by having an assistant hold the foot and great toe in neutral flexion-extension and in an overcorrected position of about 10° varus. Using a thumb forceps or skin hook on each capsular flap, the capsule is overlapped and an estimate made of the width of capsule to be resected (Fig. 22). This is usually taken from the inferior capsular flap and measures about 3 to 5 mm in width. With the great toe again held in the overcorrected position of about 10° varus, the medial capsular closure is made with 2-0 nonabsorbable buried knot sutures (Fig. 23). After the first two or three sutures have been placed, the tension on the medial capsule is checked by releasing the toe and observing it in a resting position; it should rest unsupported at about a neutral position in the plane of varus-valgus while at neutral position in the plane of flexion-extension. If at this point the great toe position is in valgus, succeeding capsular sutures are placed to imbricate more of the capsule. By repetitively testing and taking large tissue bites if the toe goes into valgus, or lesser tissue bites if the toe remains in varus, the final unsupported position of the great toe should be neutral when the medial capsule is tightly closed

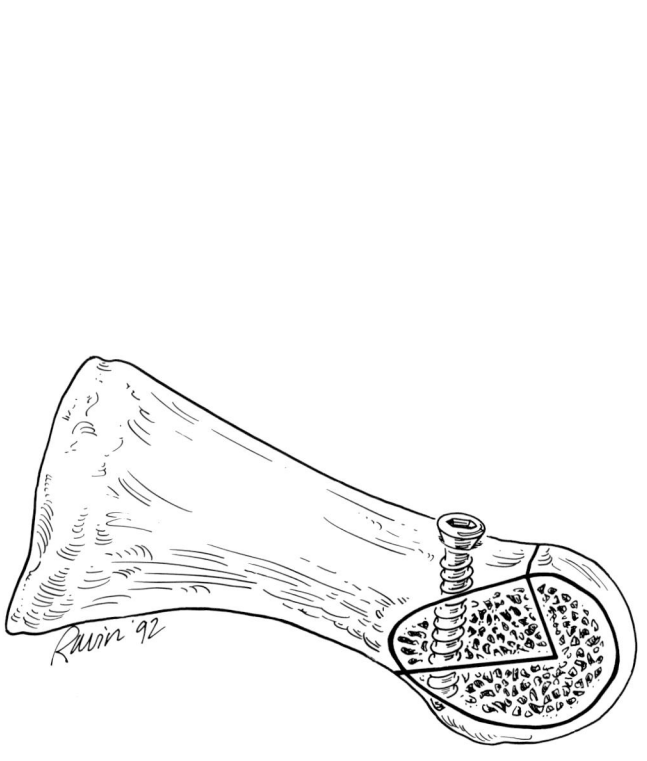

Figure 20. This side view shows the completed osteotomy and screw fixation.

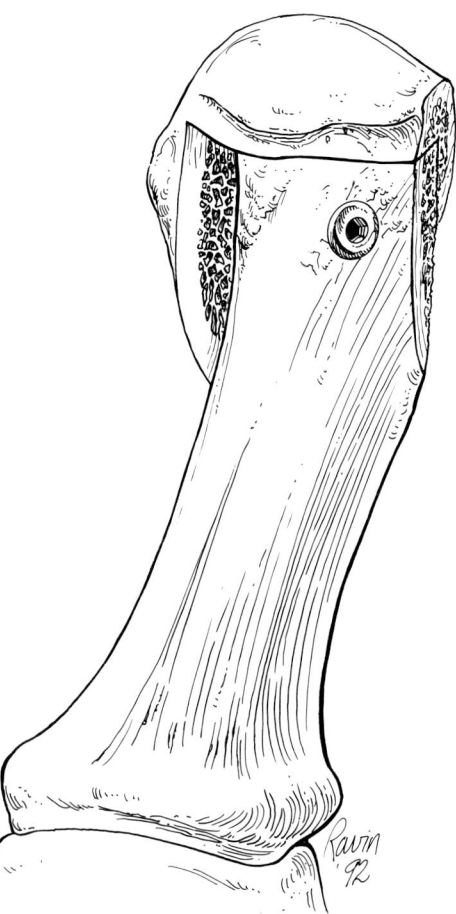

Figure 21. A top view of the completed modified chevron osteotomy.

(Fig. 24). That is, the phalanges will be in line with the longitudinal axis of the first metatarsal. Closing the capsule tightly in this manner keeps the sesamoids beneath the metatarsal head. Skin closure is usually made with absorbable subcuticular sutures and Steri-strips.

The wound is dressed with a 4" × 4" sponge folded once and placed over the wound. A 2" Kling bandage is applied in a spica weave–type pattern to hold the toe in the proper neutral position as well as provide medial-lateral compression to the metatarsal heads (Fig. 25). Anteroposterior and lateral radiographs are taken in the recovery room.

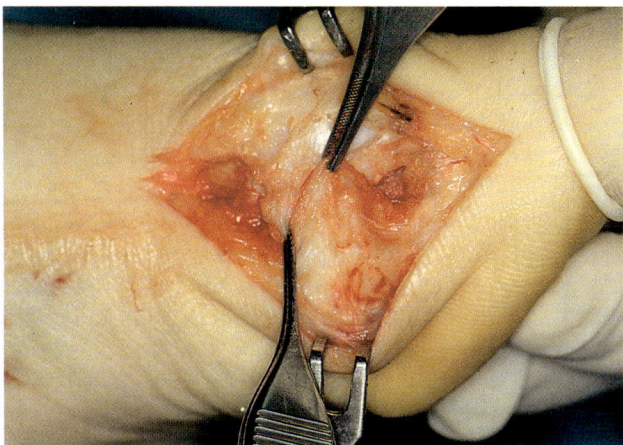

Figure 22. Estimating the width of redundant capsule after completion of chevron osteotomy and fixation.

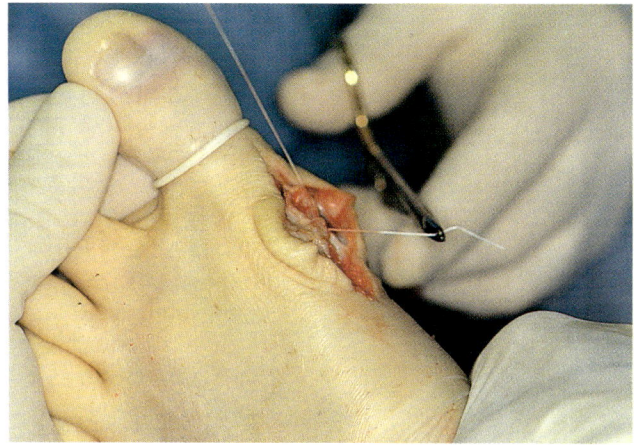

Figure 23. Closure of the medial capsule with the great toe in an overcorrected position.

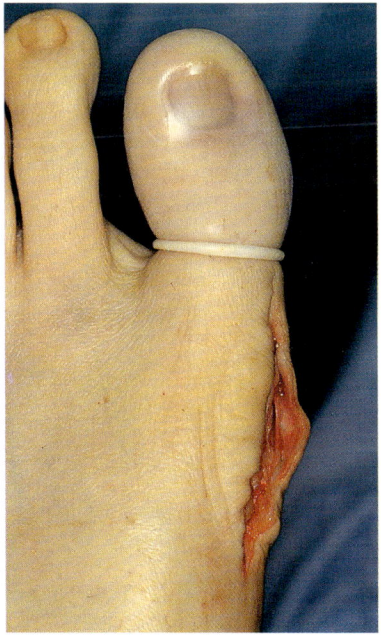

Figure 24. The great toe will rest passively in a proper position after medial capsule closure.

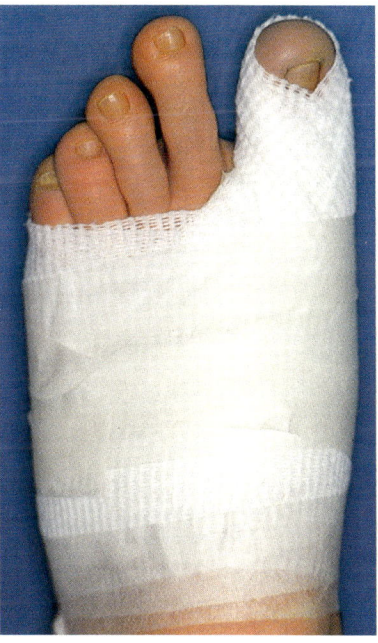

Figure 25. Soft tissue dressing helps maintain great toe position.

POSTOPERATIVE MANAGEMENT

After completion of the modified chevron osteotomy the previously described spica type of soft tissue dressing is applied (Table 2). This is followed by a compression dressing with plaster splinting. Such a dressing provides immobilization, compression without constriction, and comfort. The patient can bear weight on the dressing. Crutches are usually used for balance as well as limiting pressure on the foot while it is still tender initially.

After 1 to 3 days, the compression dressing is removed, a new spica splint dressing applied to the great toe, and a short leg walking cast applied. The forward edge of the cast should protrude beyond the great toe and gently support it on the superior, inferior, and medial sides. A heel is applied in line with the tibia. Such a heel position decreases the pressures placed on the great toe with walking and makes full weight bearing reasonable as well as comfortable.

The cast is removed about 8 to 10 days after surgery, and the patient is instructed in flexion-extension active exercises for the great toe. Trying to increase movement at the extremes of the range of motion is emphasized. No formal physical therapy is felt to be necessary. At this 8th- to 10th-day visit, the patient is provided with a hallux valgus night splint. Such a splint protects the medial capsular suture line as the scar matures over the first month postoperative. A stiff-soled postoperative type shoe is provided for use during the following 3 weeks.

At 3 weeks postoperative, the patient returns and anteroposterior and lateral radiographs of the foot are taken to be compared with the immediate postoperative radiographs. At this visit, an expected range of motion at the metatarsophalangeal joint should be from about 10° of plantar flexion to 30° of dorsiflexion. The patient is advised that this motion should gradually increase over the next several weeks to a normal range. Also at this visit, the patient is instructed to gradually work back toward normal footwear starting initially with a soft and wide lace-up type of shoe. The perils of high-heeled shoes are proffered at this time, but rarely heeded.

If at the 3-week visit the great toe is in a good alignment, radiographs are satisfactory. If the wound is well healed and motion is returning, the patient is dismissed. Otherwise the patient will be seen again at about 6 weeks after surgery for a final recheck usually without repeat of the radiographs.

The surgeon's expectations for patient satisfaction after the modified chevron osteotomy depend to a large degree on proper patient selection. If the procedure is done for the patient group already described, the satisfaction rate will be about 90% to 95% after several months. Relief of pain from pressure over the medial eminence is quite consistent. Improved comfort with shoe-wear is also to be ex-

TABLE 2. *Postoperative care for chevron osteotomy*

Time postoperative	Care
Immediate	Soft spica splinting
	Compressive dressing with plaster
	Radiographs
1–3 days	Soft spica splinting
	Short leg walking cast with great toe extension
7–10 days	Cast removal
	Stiff-soled postoperative shoe
	Great toe motion exercises
3 weeks	Radiographs
	Gradually resume normal footwear
	Check motion, wound
	Possible dismissal
6 weeks	Recheck
	Probable dismissal

pected. Not infrequently the person will try to use increasingly narrow and stylish pumps and may complain of pain in the foot. It needs to be pointed out to these patients that preoperatively such shoes were not comfortable and that even women with no foot problems can have pain with such a shoe. Cosmesis is usually not much of a problem either before or after a chevron osteotomy. If cosmesis seems to be an important aspect of the hallux valgus deformity during preoperative discussion, caution should be exercised in suggesting surgical care.

The perceived length of recuperation from any foot surgical procedure is variable from patient to patient. When the question arises regarding how long it will take to recover, an answer of several months to complete recovery seems generically reasonable. It is a gradual recovery with symptoms abating asymptomatically to normal. Some patients feel they are normal at 3 weeks while others, fortunately few, feel it takes forever. As estimate of several months seems to be a practical but unscientific answer.

COMPLICATIONS

Complications unique to the modified chevron osteotomy can occur. Some are real such as recurrent valgus at the metatarsophalangeal joint, insufficient narrowing of the forefoot, and unfulfilled patient expectations. Some are potential but have not been encountered, such as avascular necrosis of the metatarsal head and incongruity at the metatarsophalangeal joint. Complications include the following:

1. *Recurrent metatarsophalangeal valgus.* This problem is usually due to inadequate plication of the medial joint capsule at the time of the surgical procedure or dehiscence of the capsular suture line. Inadequate plication can be avoided by close attention to this aspect of the technique. If the capsular suture line separates the valgus deformity return will be precipitous and usually occur within the first several weeks after surgery.

    If the metatarsophalangeal valgus is a significant problem, then plication and resuturing of the capsule with a longer period of immobilization can be done.

2. *Insufficient narrowing of the forefoot.* This usually occurs when there is an associated metatarsus adductus. In such a situation there simply is no "place" to put the metatarsal head and the forefoot is not narrowed sufficiently. It does not seem reasonable to do osteotomies of all the lesser metatarsals in addition to the modified chevron osteotomy for metatarsus adductus. Avoidance of the complication is by proper preoperative assessment and selection of the patient for the modified chevron osteotomy.

3. *Unfulfilled patient expectations.* Preoperative discussion should include the expectations of the patient. When cosmetic concerns or the desire to wear fashionable pumps is the main patient drive to have surgical care, a cautious approach by the surgeon is suggested. Trying to explain in detail appropriate expectations will avoid or at least make defensible possible conflict later.

4. *Avascular necrosis.* Ischemia with necrosis and collapse of the metatarsal head can occur after a distal metatarsal osteotomy. Preservation of the lateral blood supply to the capital fragment will avoid such a problem. A lateral capsular perforation distal to the metatarsal head along with an adductor hallucis tenotomy should not interfere with the vascular supply to the metatarsal head. Such an adjunctive procedure just has not been necessary. Stripping of soft tissue from the lateral metatarsal head and then completion of a distal osteotomy is inappropriate and may cause avascular necrosis.

5. *Incongruity at the metatarsophalangeal joint.* Rotating the metatarsal head so the articular surface faces medialward has been suggested as a variation of the chevron osteotomy that would help realign the great toe. If such a procedure is done, the metatarsal head may rotate out from under the proximal

phalanx base, resulting in an incongruous joint prone to degenerative arthritis and stiffness. Likewise, an osteotomy of the proximal phalanx to aid in realignment may rotate the base of the proximal phalanx off the metatarsal head and cause malalignment. If malalignment occurs, a period of several months of observation is suggested. Later if the joint is painful, an arthrodesis of the metatarsophalangeal joint may be performed as a salvage procedure.

ILLUSTRATIVE CASE FOR TECHNIQUE

This 32-year-old woman described pain at the medial eminence region of her right foot only. Apparently the prominence appeared during her teenage years and she felt it was enlarging (Fig. 26). Trying to fit a proper shoe for the right foot while having the mate shoe stay on the left foot was a significant problem. Cosmesis was not much of a difficulty for her, but she did not want to end up with feet like her mother's.

Her foot was essentially normal except for the great toe, which was erythematous over the prominent medial eminence. Motion of the first metatarsophalangeal joint was from 80° of dorsiflexion to 30° of plantar flexion measured from the line of the first metatarsal. The great toe was supple in varus-valgus passive motion with no indication of degenerative arthritis.

The radiographs on the anteroposterior weight-bearing view (Fig. 27A) demonstrated an intermetatarsal 1–2 angle of 12° and a metatarsophalangeal angle of 24°. The tibialward sesamoid was centered in a subluxed position under the metatarsal head. The lateral view (Fig. 27B) did not yield much information. Sometimes dorsal osteophytes indicating degenerative arthritis may be evident on a lateral view and not on the anteroposterior radiography.

A chevron osteotomy with screw fixation was performed in the outpatient surgical suite under local anesthesia. The patient went home the same day with the foot in a bulky dressing; she had a walking cast applied the following day. This cast was removed in 1 week and she then used a postoperative recuperation shoe for another 2 weeks.

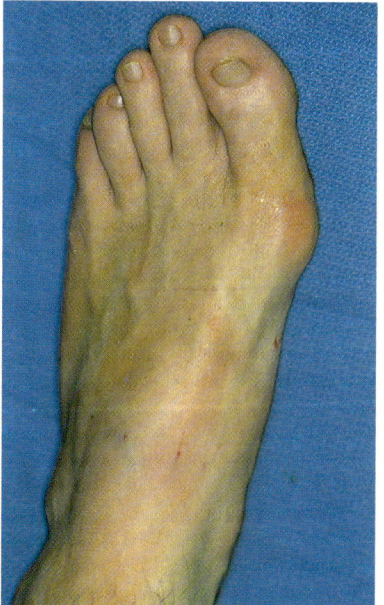

Figure 26. Photograph of metatarsophalangeal appearance before modified chevron osteotomy.

4 CHEVRON OSTEOTOMY

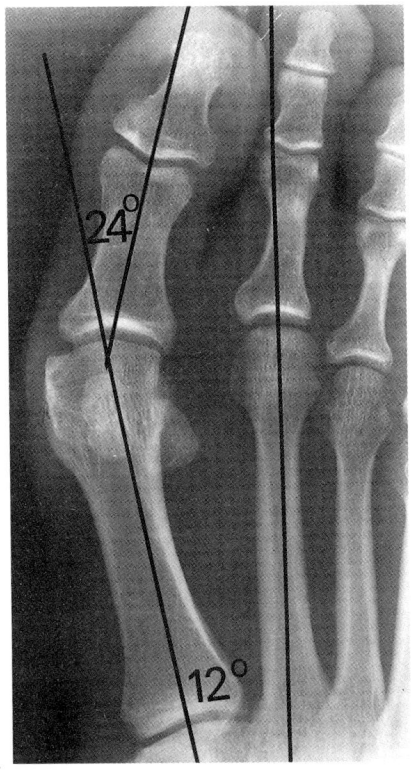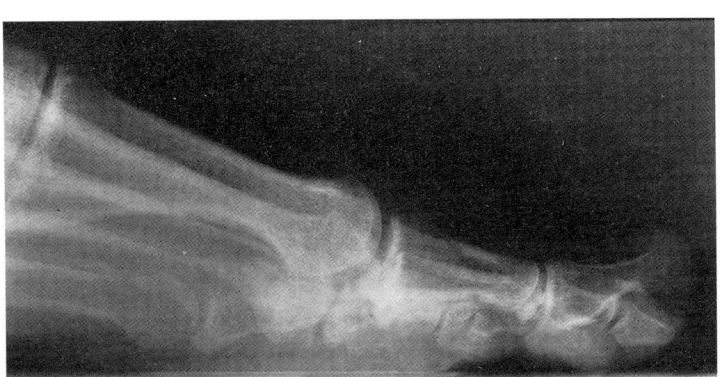

Figure 27. A: AP radiograph of patient's foot. **B:** Lateral radiograph.

The radiographs 4 weeks postoperative (Fig. 28) show the lateral translocation of the metatarsal head to be 7 mm. The intermetatarsal 1–2 angle decreased to 5° while without any lateral adductor release the metatarsophalangeal angle decreased to 14°. The sesamoid position has improved to normal. Although the screw

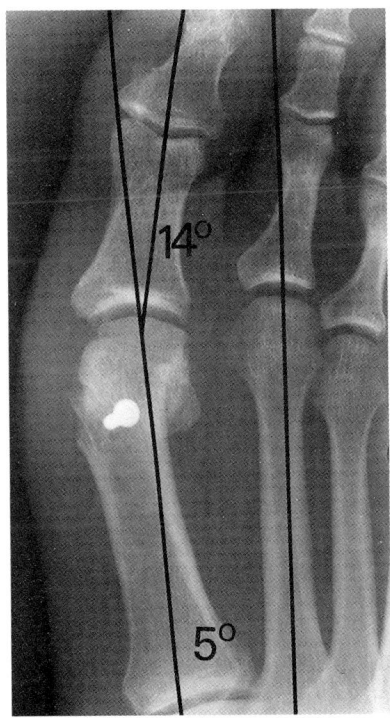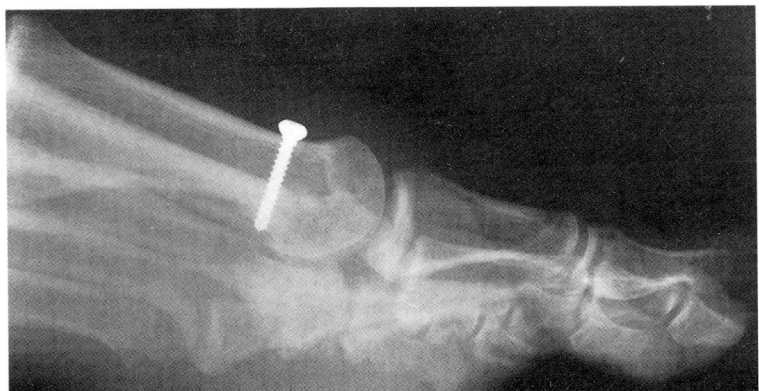

Figure 28. A: Postoperative radiographs show the realigned metatarsal after chevron osteotomy. AP view. **B:** Lateral view.

head could have been countersunk a bit more, prominence of the screw head was not a problem probably because it is situated in a concavity just behind the dorsal articular surface rim.

At follow-up 18 months later, she described no pain, limited joint motion, or difficulty with shoe selection, and overall she was satisfied.

RECOMMENDED READING

1. Austin, D., and Leventen, E.: A new osteotomy for hallux valgus. *Clin. Orthop.*, 157: 25–30, 1981.
2. Coughlin, M. J.: Chevron procedure. *Contemp. Orthop.*, 23: 45–49, 1991.
3. Hattrup, S., and Johnson, K.: Chevron osteotomy: analysis of factors in patients' dissatisfaction. *Foot Ankle*, 5: 327–332, 1985.
4. Johnson, K., Cofield, R., and Morrey, B.: Chevron osteotomy for hallux valgus. *Clin. Orthop.*, 142: 44–47, 1979.
5. Leventen, E.: The chevron procedure. *Orthopedics*, 13: 973–978, 1990.

5

Hallux Metatarsophalangeal Arthrodesis

Ian J. Alexander

INDICATIONS/CONTRAINDICATIONS

Although many surgeons shy away from first metatarsophalangeal (MP) arthrodesis as an option in their treatment of disorders of the MP joint, their concerns in many cases are unjustified. Unquestionably, arthrodesis of the first MP joint has an adverse effect on foot mechanics, but in situations where first MP mechanics are already abnormal, fusion of the joint to eliminate pain or severe deformity may actually improve foot function.

Indications for first MP arthrodesis include painful degenerative, inflammatory, or posttraumatic arthritis, marked deformity, and occasionally chronic instability. Arthrodesis in many cases is the optimal means of salvaging failed first MP joint surgery. When systemic disease such as rheumatoid arthritis or previous surgery has created a bony defect at the first MP joint, a solid arthrodesis with a well-positioned hallux of reasonable length may be achieved with an interposition bone graft technique.

Contraindications to first MP arthrodesis include impaired vascularity and significant neuropathy. Arthrodesis of the first MP joint should also be cautiously considered if there is coexistent arthritis of the interphalangeal (IP) joint of the hallux. Leaving the IP joint alone in these circumstances will lead to accentuation of IP joint symptoms. Fusing both joints simultaneously creates a very stiff ray that is prone to overload. Under these circumstances, combining an MP joint resection arthroplasty with an IP fusion may be a reasonable option.

Alternatives to first MP arthrodesis include resection or implant arthroplasty. Resection arthroplasty is a reasonable alternative for patients with combined mild-

---

I. J. Alexander, M.D.: Department of Orthopaedic Surgery, Northeast Ohio Universities College of Medicine, Rootstown, OH 44272; the Department of Orthopaedics, Crystal Clinic, Suite 102, 3975 Embassy Parkway, Akron, OH 44313.

to-moderate hallux valgus and arthritis who are reluctant to have an arthrodesis due to limitations placed on their shoe-wear selection. First MP joint implants should be approached with reservations. I feel there are essentially no indications for unipolar Silastic implants. The use of bipolar Silastic implants for the first MP joint in rheumatoid arthritis is probably the only defensible indication, and its use is waning. Metal/polyethylene component first MP arthroplasties are experimental and their poor track record in the past with designs similar to those currently being promoted should dampen any enthusiasm for these devices. If they fail, the bone resection associated with their insertion presents a difficult reconstructive problem.

Successful arthrodesis depends on achieving a solid fusion with a hallux in optimal position. I will focus on achieving these objectives in primary cases as well as in complex reconstructive problems of the distal first ray.

PREOPERATIVE PLANNING

The preoperative examination of the patient should ensure adequate circulation and integrity of the skin over the sight of the proposed surgical incision.

Preoperative weight bearing AP and lateral radiographs of the feet are mandatory. Angles that should be measured include: hallux valgus angle, intermetatarsal 1–2 angle, and angle of inclination of the first metatarsal. If narrowing of the IMT 1–2 angle is part of the objective of the first MPT fusion, as in severe hallux valgus, attention should be paid to the base of the first metatarsal. The presence of a facet on the lateral aspect of the first metatarsal base abutting against the second metatarsal should make the surgeon aware that normal reduction of the IM 1–2 angle (average usually 8°–9°) will not occur.

It is important that the most desirable position of the hallux in the three primary planes is determined before surgery.

Failure to position the hallux well in the sagittal (flexion-extension) plane is the positioning error. Excessive hallux extension results in dorsal toe irritation by the shoe at the IP joint. Also, reduced hallux function will predispose the patient to secondary metatarsalgia. Excessive plantar flexion may result in hallux overload and painful plantar callosities at the plantar aspect of the IP joint region. This is particularly apt to occur when a sesamoid lies in the flexor hallucis longus just proximal to its insertion. Sagittal position is optimal in most cases when the sagittal axis to the proximal phalanx is parallel to the floor when the foot is plantigrade. Because the sesamoids elevate the first metatarsal head and due to the normal sigmoid curvature of the plantar surface of the proximal phalanx, the head of a proximal phalanx that is fused parallel to the plantar aspect of the foot will clear the floor by 5 to 10 mm (Fig. 1). This clearance allows for relatively normal roll-off during walking without hallux overload, and dorsal toe irritation is rarely a problem. This position also gives women some leeway in terms of shoe heel height.

The optimal sagittal arthrodesis angle (AA) is widely quoted as 25° to 30°. This is usually correct, as in most individuals the metatarsal inclination angle (MIA) to the floor measures between 25° and 30° (Fig. 2). In the case of pes planus and pes cavus, however, routinely fusing the hallux at 25° to 30° will result in malposition. For example, if the MIA is 15° (pes planus) and the AA is 30°, the hallux will be fused at 15° of dorsiflexion and dorsal toe irritation will almost certainly result. On the other hand, if the MIA is 45° (pes cavus) and the AA is 30° the hallux will be plantar flexed 15° and overload may result. To achieve a hallux that is parallel to the floor the AA should equal the MIA. The MIA can be easily determined from the preoperative standing lateral radiograph by measuring the angle between the floor and a line intersecting the top of the head and the base of the first metatarsal (Fig. 2). To intraoperatively assess sagittal plane position, pressure is applied to the plantar aspect of the foot with a flat rigid surface (Fig. 3). With this load-bearing simulation, the head of the proximal phalanx should clear the surface by 5 to 10 mm. If the head rests against the surface, plantar flexion is excessive. If the operator's index fingertip passes easily under the phalangeal head, extension is excessive. Observation from the side should show the hallux to be parallel to the rigid surface.

Two clinical problems result from transverse (axial) plane malposition. Excessive valgus results in painful great toe–second toe impingement, and excessive varus may lead to IP joint degeneration. Again, recommending a specific hallux valgus (HV) angle of 15° to 20° as optimal for all cases is not appropriate. An example is first MP arthrodesis for hallux rigidus. In many hallux rigidus patients the hallux valgus angle is only 0° to 5° with the second toe parallel to and resting against the hallux (Fig. 4). If the hallux, in this case, is fused at 15° to 20° of valgus, painful great toe–second toe impingement and crossover will predictably occur (Fig. 5). In this instance the optimal transverse plane fusion angle is the same as the preoperative HV angle. The best rule, therefore, is to fuse the great

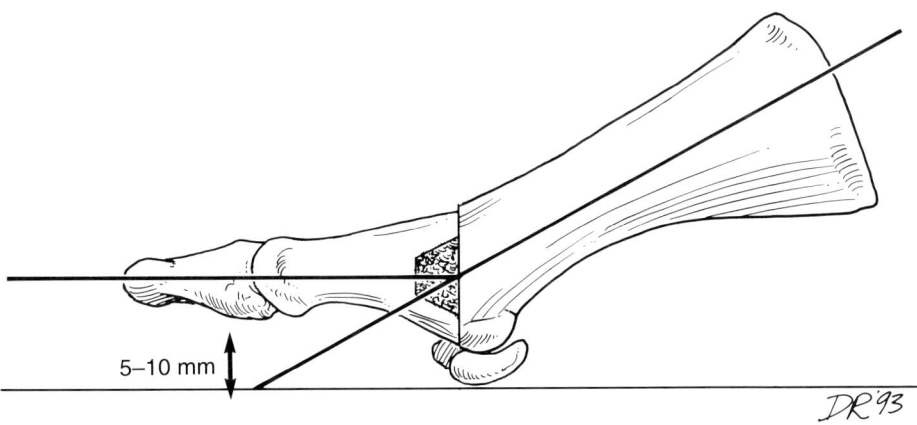

Figure 1. Proper sagittal plane position.

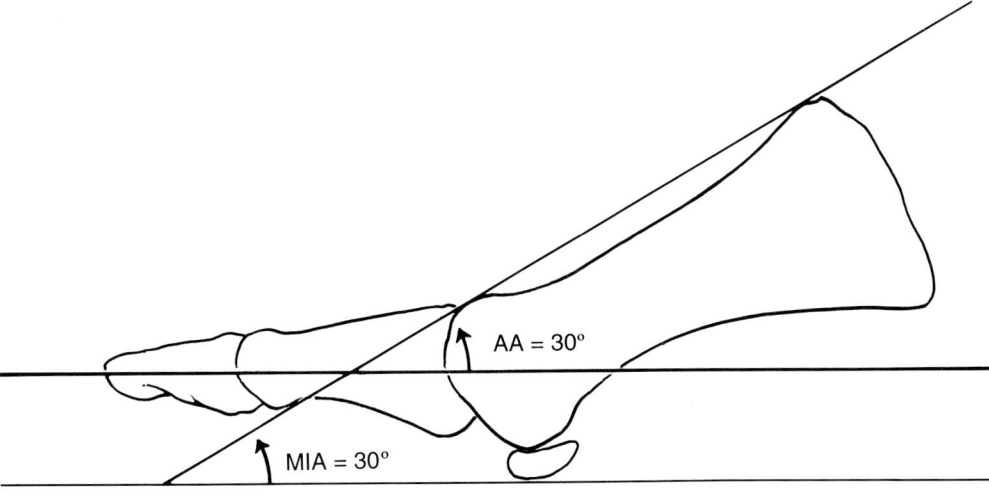

Figure 2. Measurement of metatarsal inclination angle (MIA) and arthrodesis angle (AA).

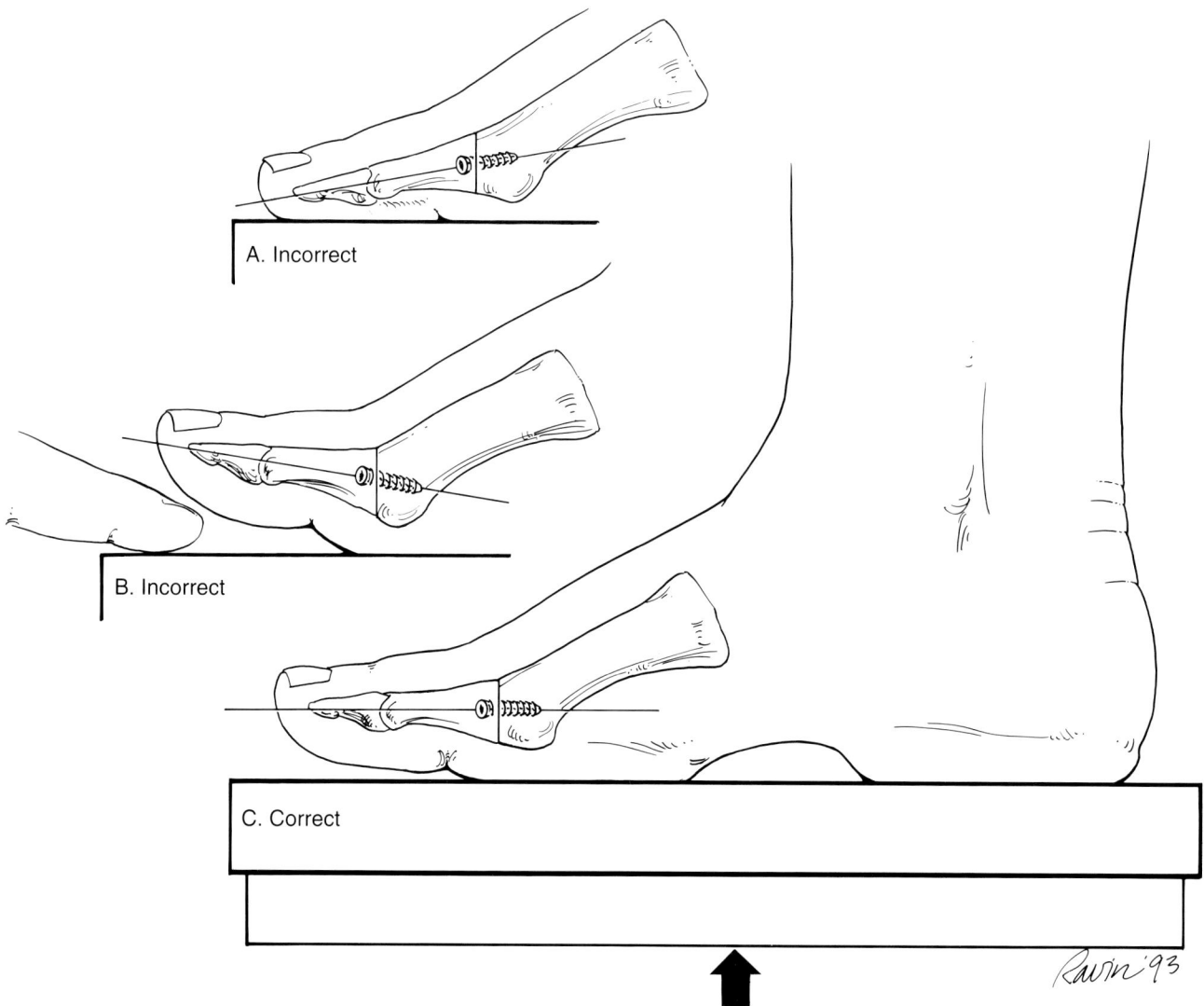

Figure 3. Intraoperatively checking sagittal plane position (A) excessive plantar flexion, (B) excessive dorsiflexion, (C) correct position.

toe in a transverse plane position that avoids second toe impingement if the preoperative HV angle is less than 15°. If the preoperative HV angle exceeds 15°, the hallux is best fused at approximately 10° to 15° of valgus. Correction of a malaligned second toe may also be necessary to prevent impingement problems if preoperatively it is deviated medially.

To be sure that impingement in the second toe will not be a problem postoperatively, a small gap should be present between the great and second toe during the load-bearing simulation intraoperatively.

Coronal plane rotation, often referred to as "pronation" or "supination" of the hallux, also influences outcome but is not as critical as alignment in the other primary planes. The most frequent problem in this plane is excessive pronation, which is usually encountered when severe hallux valgus is being corrected with an arthrodesis. The lateral capsular tightness resists hallux derotation. The consequence of fusing the hallux in "pronation" is that terminal push-off occurs on the plantar medial aspect of the hallux at the IP joint rather than on the fleshy pulp of the great toe, potentially causing a painful callus at the IP joint. In addition,

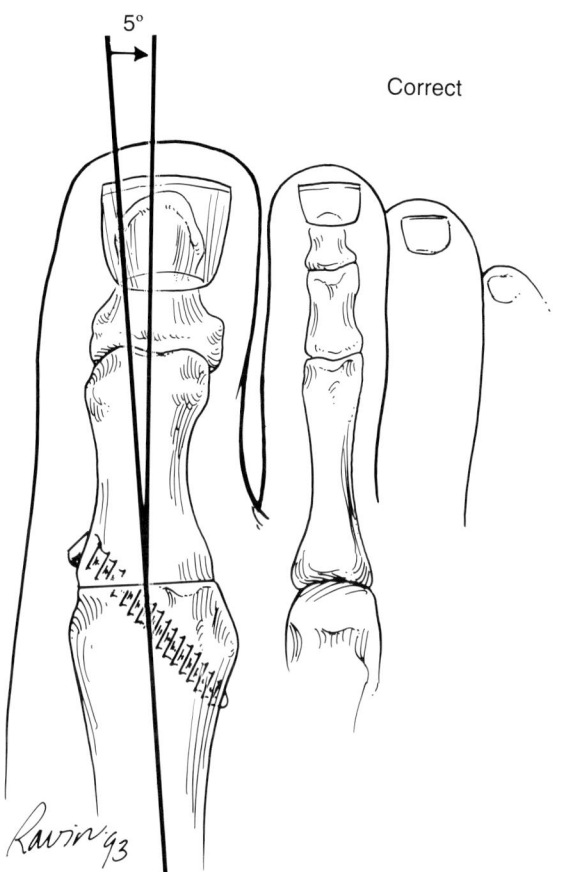
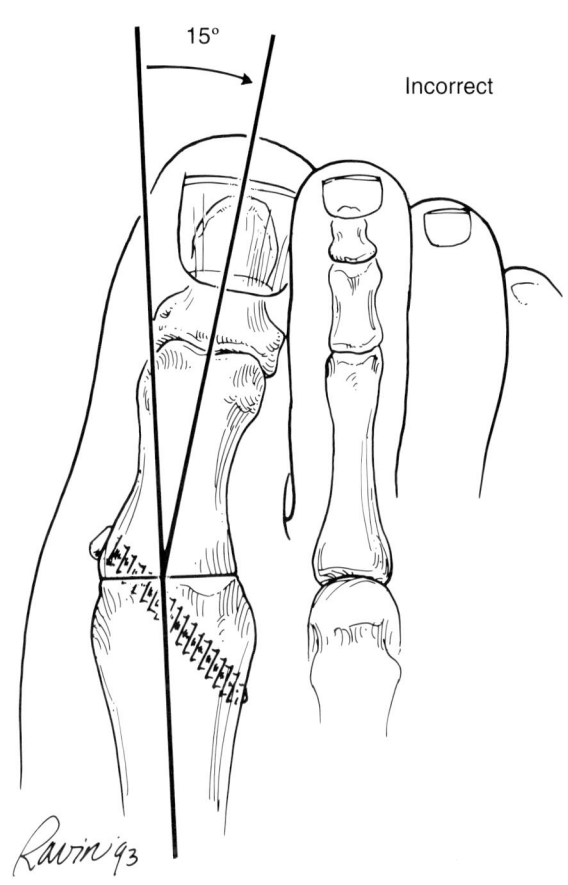

Figure 4. Transverse plane position with correct fusion alignment.

Figure 5. Transverse plane position with excessive valgus alignment.

with hallux malrotation, IP flexion/extension occurs at an angle oblique to the normal sagittal plane. Proper hallux rotation is checked intraoperatively by observing symmetry of nail plate alignment and being certain that IP flexion/extension occurs in the sagittal plan.

Besides optimizing position, obtaining a solid arthrodesis is also important in achieving a successful result. Surgical factors that contribute to reliable healing of first MP fusions include extensive cancellous bone contact, inherent stability of the fusion configuration, and rigid fixation.

An extensive cancellous bone contact and inherent stability are provided by techniques that prepare the phalangeal base and the metatarsal head into interlocking conical or truncated cone shapes. With these techniques fixation with a single small fragment screw usually provide excellent positional control (Fig. 6). Crossed screws are advisable if the bone is particularly osteoporotic (Fig. 7). Other methods of fixation have been advocated but have specific disadvantages. These other methods include longitudinal heavy threaded pins that traverse the IP joint and may contribute to late IP joint arthritis, dorsal plate and screws that are prone to mechanical failure by virtue of being located on the compression bone surface and, in addition, often have to be removed due to dorsal prominence, and multiple small K-wires that provide little compression and may require removal.

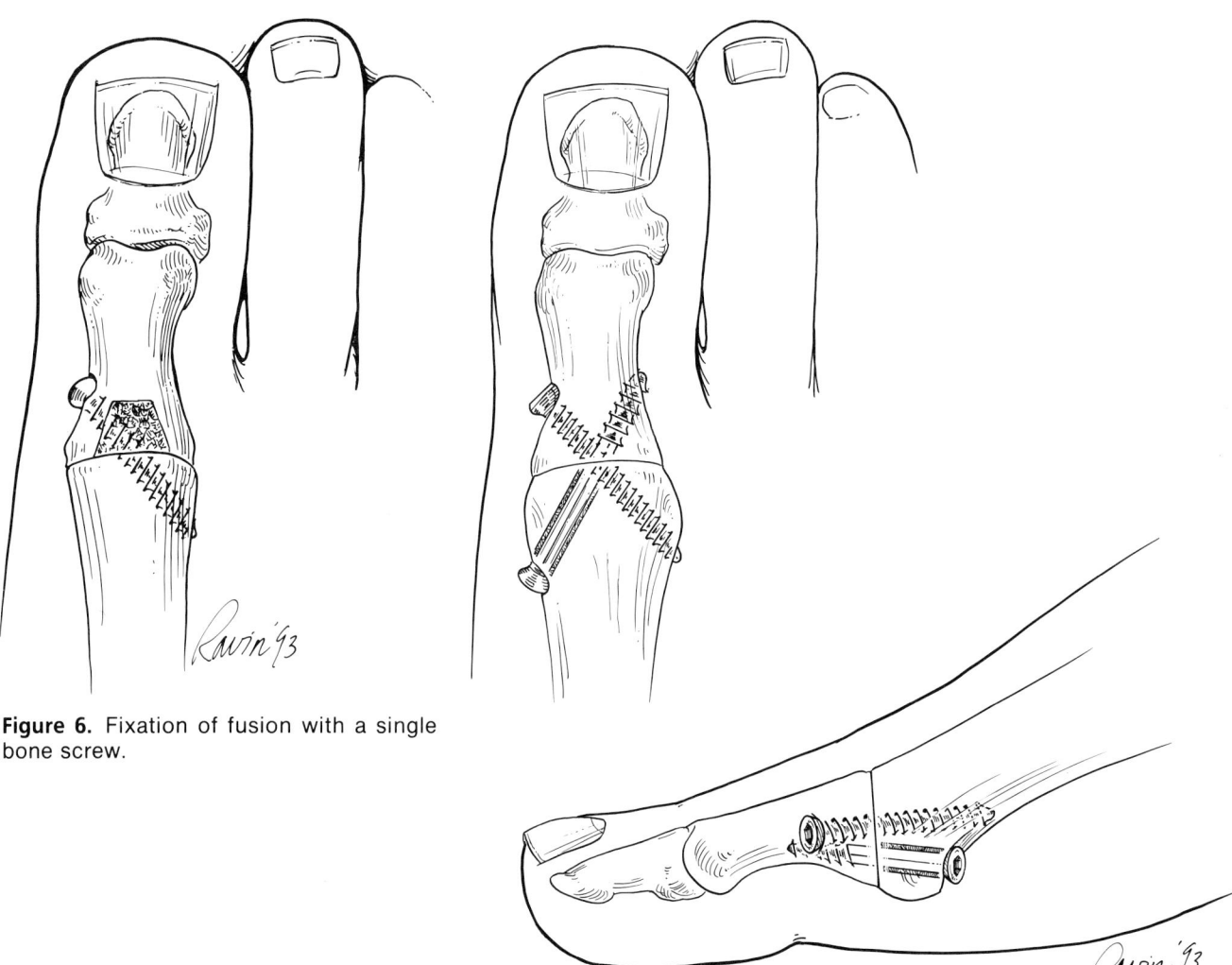

Figure 6. Fixation of fusion with a single bone screw.

Figure 7. Two-screw fixation technique.

Three methods of preparing inherently stable conical surfaces that provide extensive cancellous contact include manual surface preparation with a rongeur, the Marin reamer system (Downs, Inc., UK), and the truncated cone reamer system (Biomet Inc., Warsaw, IN).

It is possible to prepare the joint surfaces with a rongeur, but this process is tedious, and obtaining the desired position with a stable fit can be difficult. The greatest advantage of this method is that no special instrumentation is required.

The Marin reamers are manual reamers that help improve the fit provided by the rongeur technique. The Marin reamers taper the surface to a pointed cone after initial surface shaping with a rongeur. Problems encountered with this method include significant shortening of the hallux and difficult surface preparation if the bone is dense.

The truncated cone reamer system is designed to use power instrumentation to prepare the articular surface in a reproducible manner based on measurements taken from preoperative radiographs. In addition, cancellous apposition and inherent stability is maximized by the accurately machined Morse taper configuration of the prepared surfaces. Using a truncated cone versus a full cone, shortening is limited. The system consists of guides, templates, and a series of K-wire–guided reamers that facilitate accurate positioning and surface preparation (Fig. 8). In my

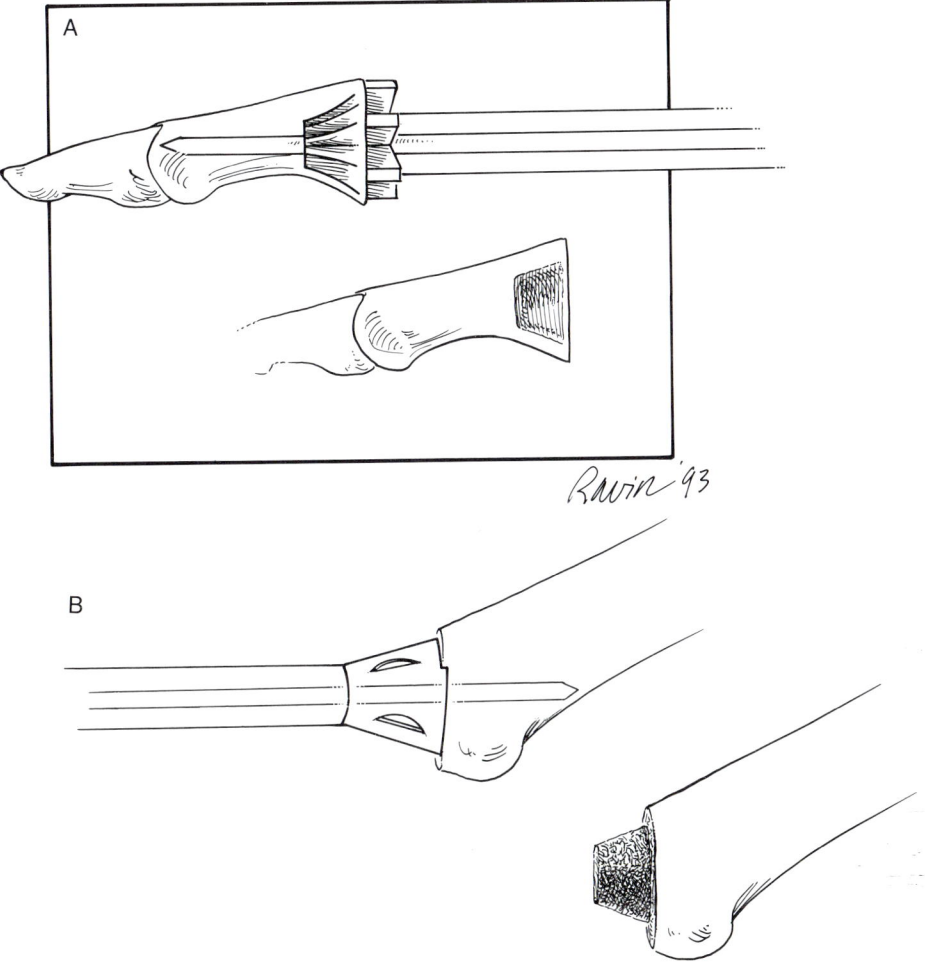

Figure 8. Overall plan for phalanx base (A) and metatarsal head (B) preparation using specialized reamers.

experience, this system has provided a reliable reproducible means of achieving a well-positioned solid arthrodesis. Fusion failures with this technique were the result of early unprotected loading of the hallux in two elderly osteoporotic females.

SURGERY

The patient is positioned supine on the operating table. Either ankle block anesthesia or general anesthesia may be utilized. If an ankle tourniquet is to be utilized, a few wraps of sterile cast padding are placed in the supramalleolar area, and subsequently, after exsanguinating the foot, the Esmarch bandage is wrapped with even tension in three to 4 layers on top of the cast padding. A thigh tourniquet can be employed in patients under general anesthesia.

Technique. A straight medial incision centered over the MP joint of the great toe is made. Flaps of tissue are not developed, but instead the incision is brought directly through the skin and subcutaneous tissue through the medial joint capsule and down to the medial cortical surface of the first metatarsal and the base of the proximal phalanx. The base of the proximal phalanx is mobilized enough to provide easy access to the proximal phalanx base with an end-on visualization. Ini-

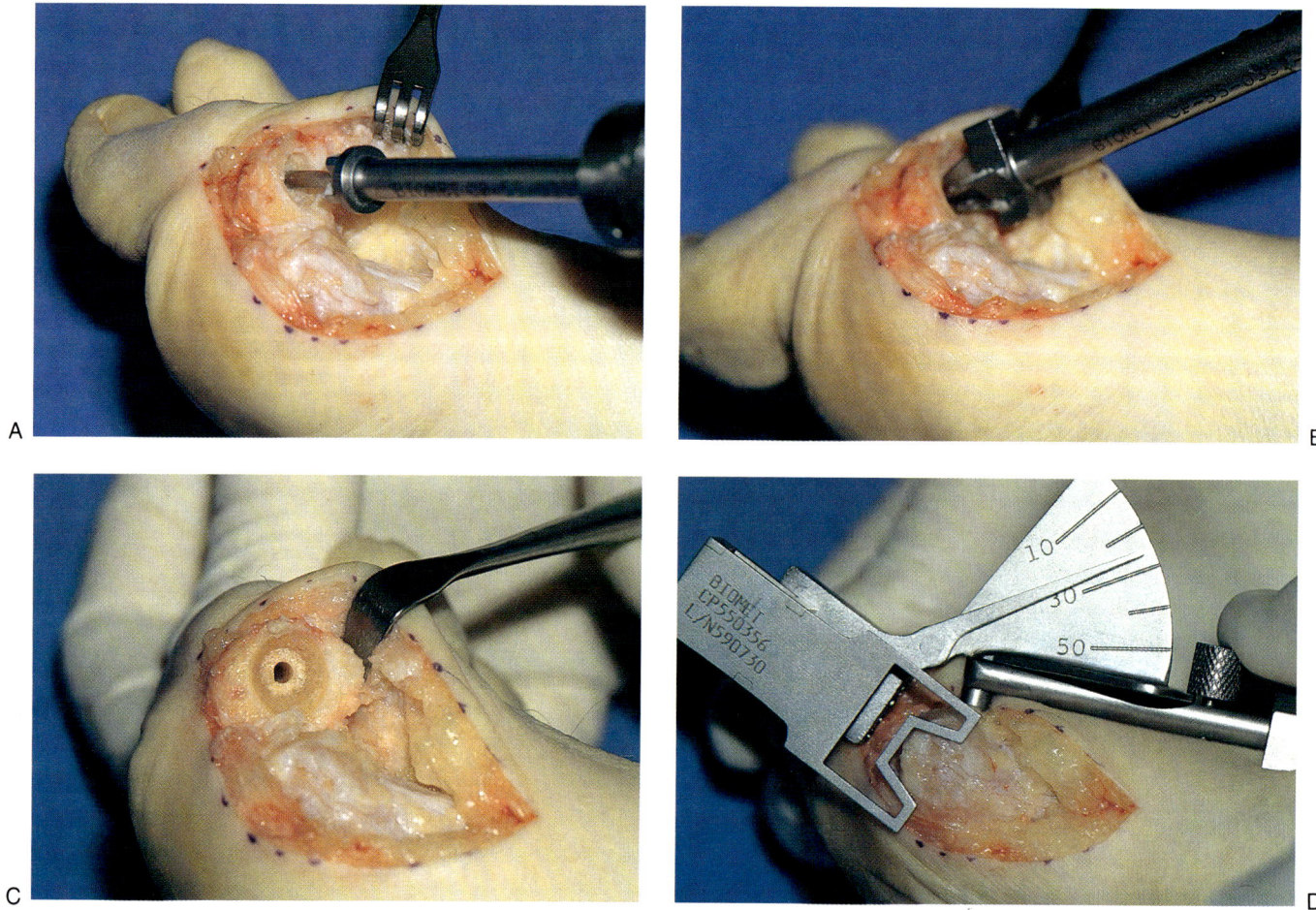

Figure 9. A: Preparing the phalangeal base with the end-cutting reamer. **B:** Cutting the truncated cone with the side-cutting reamer. **C:** Base of proximal phalanx after completion of reaming. **D:** Metatarsal guide in place to set the predetermined sagittal and transverse angles for reaming the metatarsal head.

tially a guide wire is placed down the center of the proximal phalanx. Over this guide wire, the base of the proximal phalanx is prepared with the specialized reamers (Fig. 9A–C).

The metatarsal head is then exposed and again a guide pin is inserted into the metatarsal head at the appropriate angle using the dorsal aspect of the first metatarsal as a reference (Fig. 9D). When the guide pin is properly located, the reamer system is utilized to produce a truncated cone configuration in the distal metatarsal (Fig. 9E,F).

The two surfaces are then opposed and an oblique screw is placed from the medial base of the proximal phalanx, across the arthrodesis site, and into the plantar lateral cortex of the metatarsal neck (Fig. 9G–I). Either a fully threaded 4.0 cancellous or 3.5 cortical screw is used for fixation, depending on the resistance of the bone of the far cortex to drilling. This screw should always be countersunk to avoid medial prominence of the head and cracking of the cortical shelf on the medial base of the proximal phalanx. The final position of the toe is checked in flexion-extension, varus-valgus, and rotation by simulating weight bearing on a flat rigid surface.

The wound is then closed with absorbable sutures in the capsule and the sutures of the surgeon's choice for the skin and subcutaneous tissue.

If the specialized instruments are not available, a saw, a rongeur, and a drill can be used to contour the metatarsal head and the base of the proximal phalanx

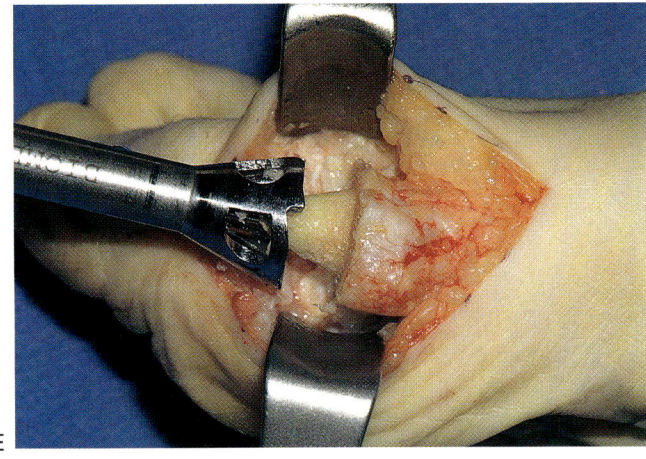
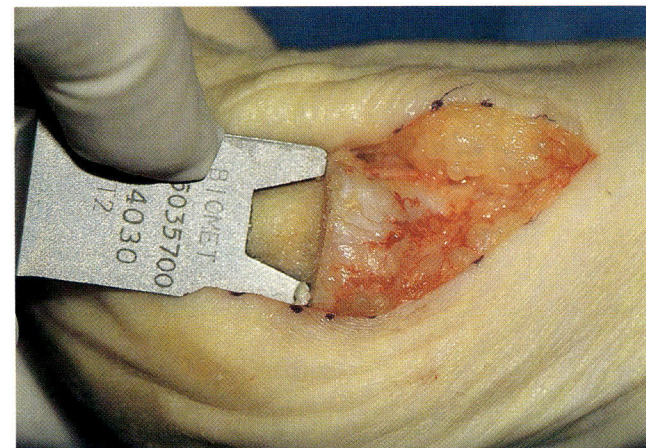
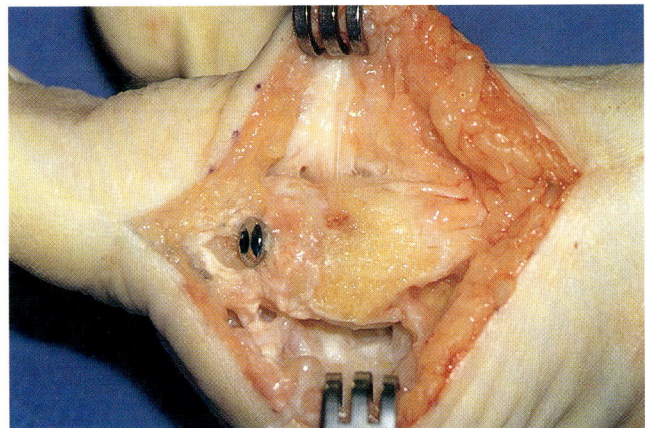
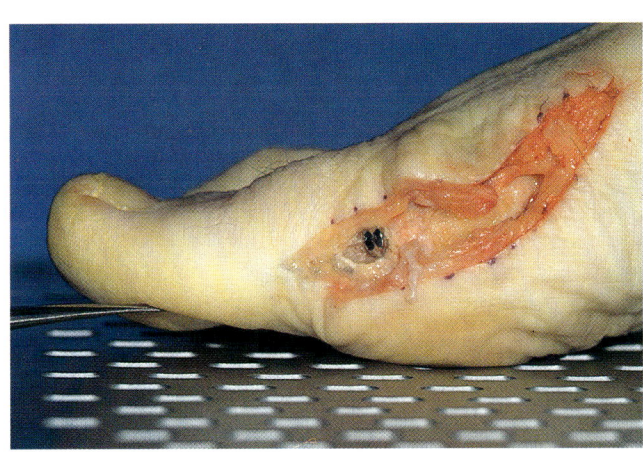
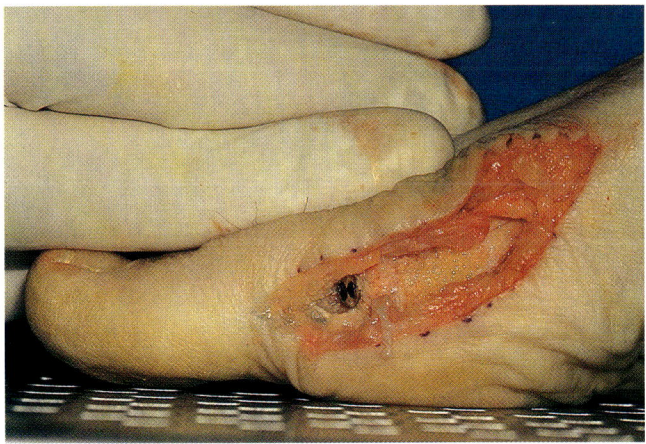

E: Metatarsal reamer and metatarsal head after reaming into a truncated cone shape. **F:** Checking the length of the metatarsal cone with the template. **G:** Male and female cones interlocked and fixed with a single oblique screw. **H:** Ensuring adequate hallux clearance under the phalangeal head. **I:** Checking the dorsal line of the first ray to be sure that the prominence of the phalangeal head is not excessive.

into a shape that provides a reasonable apposition. Regardless of the technique employed, final position of the toe is what is most critical to a successful outcome. Intraoperative evaluation of position as described in preoperative planning is essential.

When pain, deformity, or instability at the first MP joint is associated with bone deficiency due to erosive arthritis or previous surgical resection of bone, apposition of existing bone to obtain a stable, well-aligned and pain-free hallux may result in an unacceptable degree of first ray shortening. Under these circumstances, filling the defect with autogenous iliac crest bone graft will often allow one to meet the objectives of an arthrodesis while restoring first ray length and

58 PART II METATARSOPHALANGEAL JOINTS

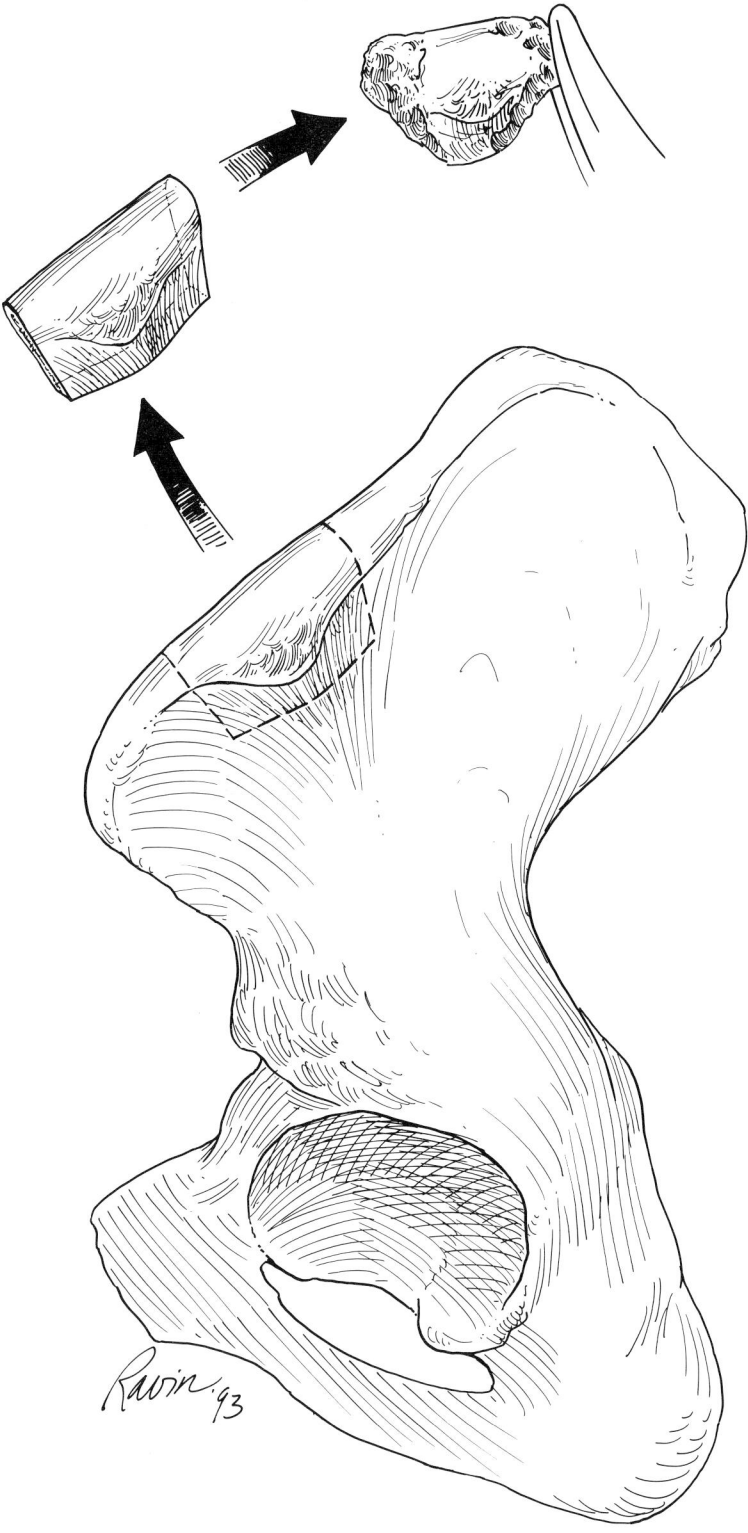

Figure 10. Harvesting and fashioning the tricortical graft.

more normal foot geometry. The basic structural component of the interposition bone graft is a tricortical block of iliac crest. This block is fashioned to fit the size, shape, and cortical deficiency of the defect to be filled (Fig. 10). The surgical approach to the joint in these individuals is usually dictated by previous surgical incisions. Frequently, there will have been multiple previous surgical approaches to the first MP joint. Neuromas of the dorsal proper digital nerve and medial plantar hallucal nerve, which would be identified on physical examination preoperatively, should be dealt with to avoid these potential sources of persistent postoperative pain.

Fibrous and other soft tissues filling the bone defects should be excised and, initially, all bone attached solidly to the metatarsal or phalanx should be left intact, even if a relatively thin cortical shell. Efforts should be made to preserve periosteal blood supply whenever possible. If the defect is asymmetric (e.g., dorsal cortical erosion with double-stem Silastic implant) it may be possible to appose the residual cortices, maintaining length. Trimming these surfaces and apposing them provides a bridge that may enhance stability and healing.

The tricortical graft is fashioned to fill the defect. Cortex should be removed from the graft to provide cancellous contact with existing bone but, whenever possible, cortex should be left on the graft surface where it will bridge cortical defects or windows. Failure to provide this cortical strut makes structural support dependent on cancellous bone, predisposing to collapse or late stress fracture.

Fixation of these fusions depends on the size and shape of the interposition graft. Crossed threaded K-wires and/or screws may provide excellent stabilization if the interposition graft is short, but fixation with a plate and screws is frequently necessary for longer segmental grafts. These plates, which are usually on the dorsal surface, are mechanically under compression and prone to failure when subjected to repetitive bending loads.

POSTOPERATIVE MANAGEMENT

Patients undergoing primary arthrodesis are routinely asked to wear a wooden postoperative shoe and to walk flat-footed, and specifically cautioned not to load the hallux. Every 2 weeks, until 6 weeks, the integrity of the fusion is checked and the bandage is changed. If any movement is present, the patient should be cast immobilized. A cast is also advisable if the patient is unreliable or osteoporotic, or if intraoperative fixation is at all questionable.

In the case of interposition graft, incorporation is a much longer process and, as a result, weight bearing is usually avoided for 3 months. After that, weight bearing is allowed in a cast with a posterior locking heel until solid healing is demonstrated on radiographs.

COMPLICATIONS

The most frequent complications of first MP arthrodesis are malposition and nonunion. A salvage of these complications consist of a redo fusion, if necessary, taking all the precautions discussed to ensure good position and to maximize the chance of solid healing. Prominent hardware may be a problem with any technique and may require removal. Damage to the dorsal proper digital nerve can cause pain and a sensitive neuroma. If desensitization fails to resolve the problem, the nerve may need to be transected and its terminal end buried into a dorsomedial drill hole in the first metatarsal.

ILLUSTRATIVE CASES FOR TECHNIQUE

A 67-year-old retired dentist presented with severe hallux valgus and painful prominence of the medial eminence. The hallux was markedly pronated and the valgus deformity was not passively correctable. After discussing possible options, the patient chose a first MP arthrodesis to obtain reliable correction without risk of recurrence. The significant decrease in the intermetatarsal 1–2 angle is easily appreciated (Fig. 11).

A woman with rheumatoid arthritis presented with pain in the first MP joint. Radiographs showed a large lytic defect in the first metatarsal head with a thin cortical shell (Fig. 12). At surgery the cyst was curetted and the articular surface and subchondral bone of the base of the phalanx and the remaining metatarsal articular surface were removed. An entirely cancellous graft was fashioned to fill the defect, and stable fixation was provided by cross screws.

Another patient had a painful MP joint after double-stem Silastic implant (Fig. 13). At surgery, almost the entire cortical rim was intact circumferentially but no cancellous bone remained in either the phalangeal base or the distal metatarsal. The bone ends were planed with a saw to provide flat apposing surfaces and a "football"-shaped totally cancellous graft was fashioned to fill the defect. Chips of cancellous bone were placed proximal and distal to the interposition graft to fill the defect and cross screws provided excellent fixation.

A woman with a painful nonfunctional great toe presented after previous bunion surgery (Fig. 14). Although the shape of the phalangeal base was unusual, this patient had apparently undergone a previous Keller resection arthroplasty. To maintain hallux length, a full tricortical graft with cancellous surfaces facing proxi-

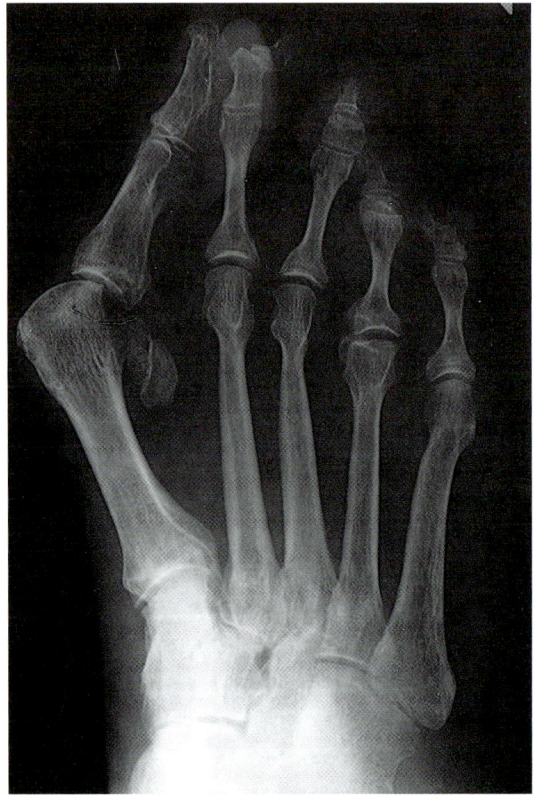 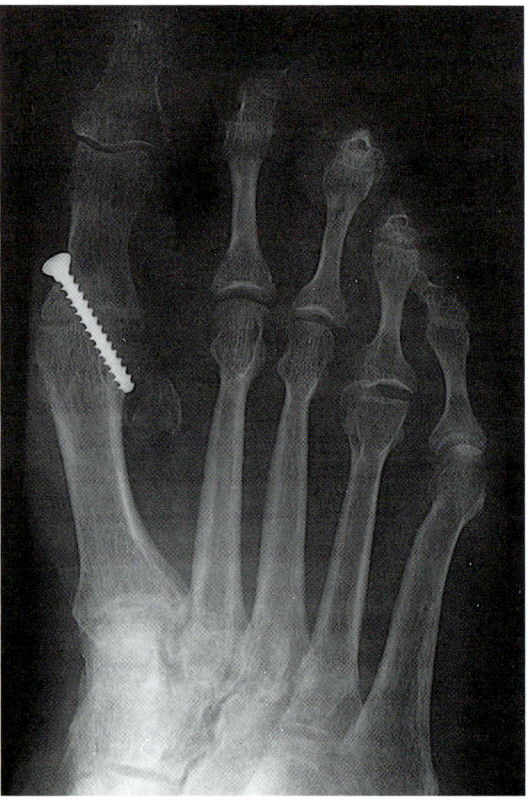

Figure 11. Case presentation. **(A)** Preoperative and **(B)** postoperative metatarsophalangeal (MP) arthrodesis.

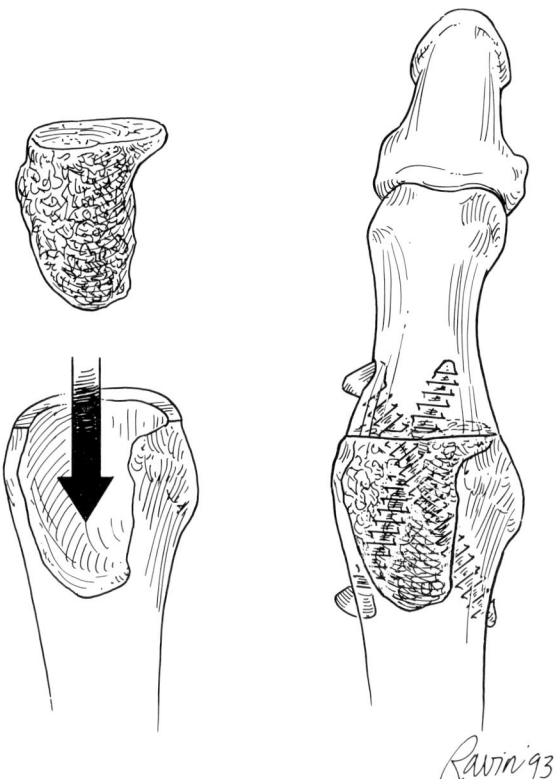

Figure 12. Bone graft preparation for irregular defect.

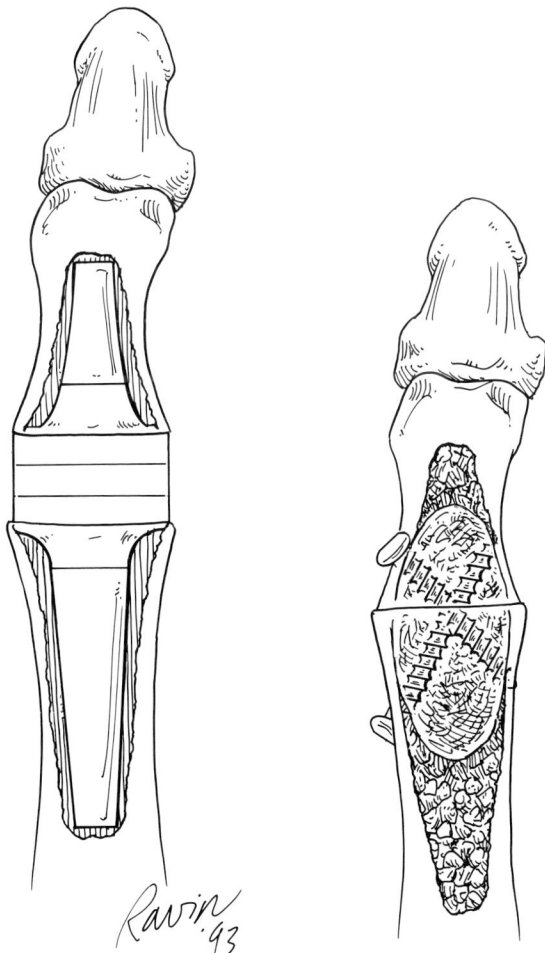

Figure 13. Combination of cortical and cancellous bone to fill extensive defect.

mally, distally, and medially was interposed and fixed with longitudinal threaded K-wires using a technique described by Coughlin and Mann.

In another case, a woman presented with a flail, malpositioned, and painful great toe after removal of a double-stem Silastic implant that had caused extensive dorsal bone destruction and perforation of the IP joint (Fig. 15). At surgery the residual phalangeal condyles surprisingly had intact articular cartilage. An extensive tricortical graft was fashioned to fill a defect and at its distal end cortical bone was removed and a dome of cancellous bone was fashioned to fit the proximal surface of the remaining phalanx. Proximal fixation was obtained with a dorsal plate and two crossed K-wires were placed distally to hold the phalanx to the interposition graft (Fig. 16).

In our follow-up of these and other interposition graft patients we found an excellent subjective outcome in terms of patient satisfaction with position, stability, and pain relief, but dynamic foot pressure analysis in almost all cases showed little or no significant hallux function.

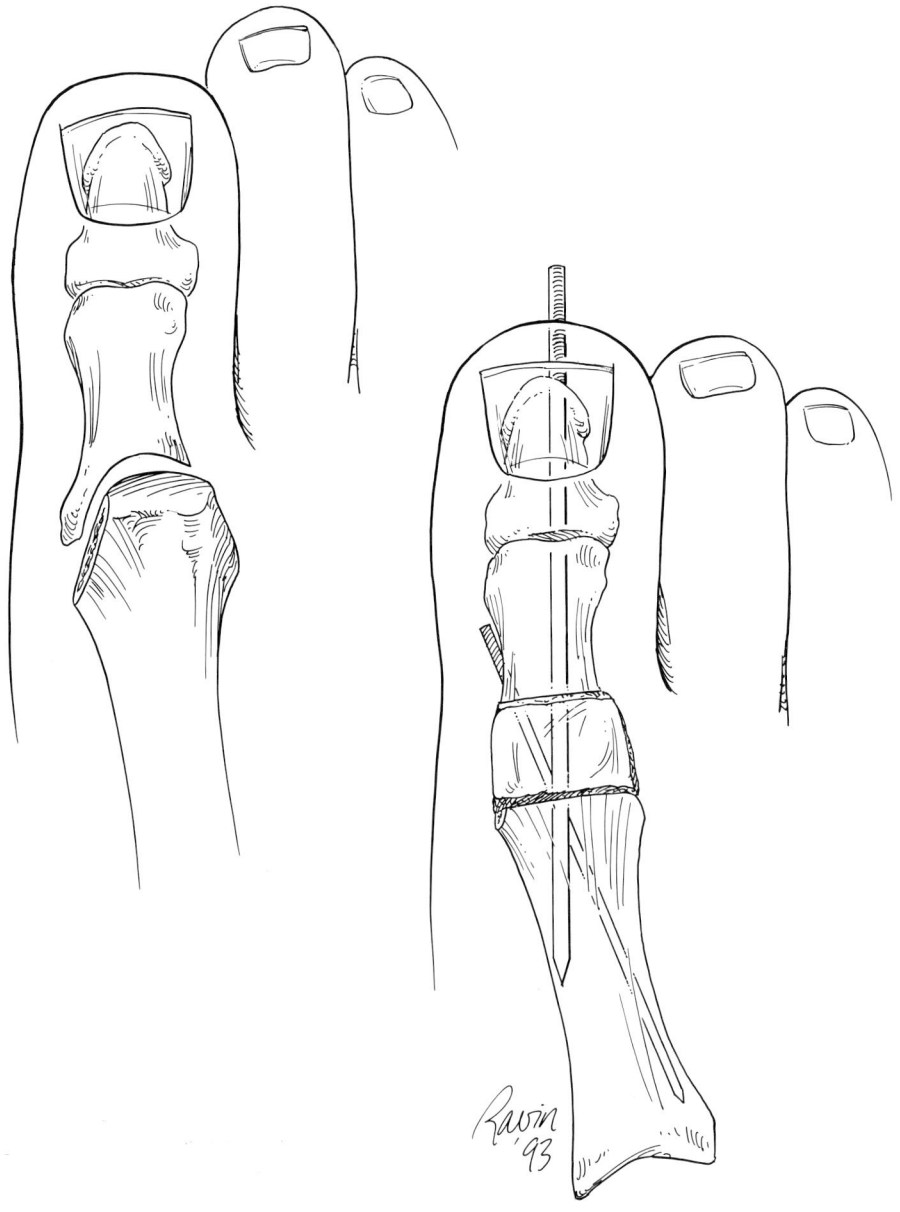

Figure 14. This block type of graft was used with K-wire fixation.

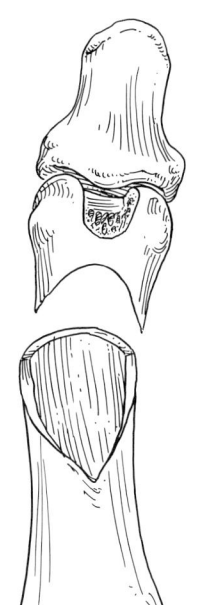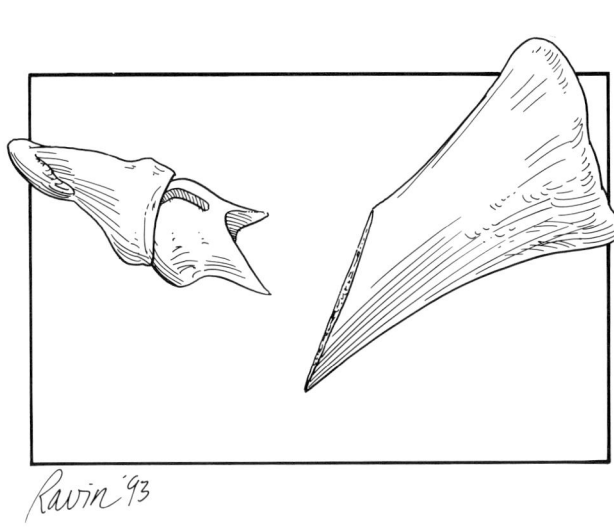

Figure 15. Extensive bone loss was present.

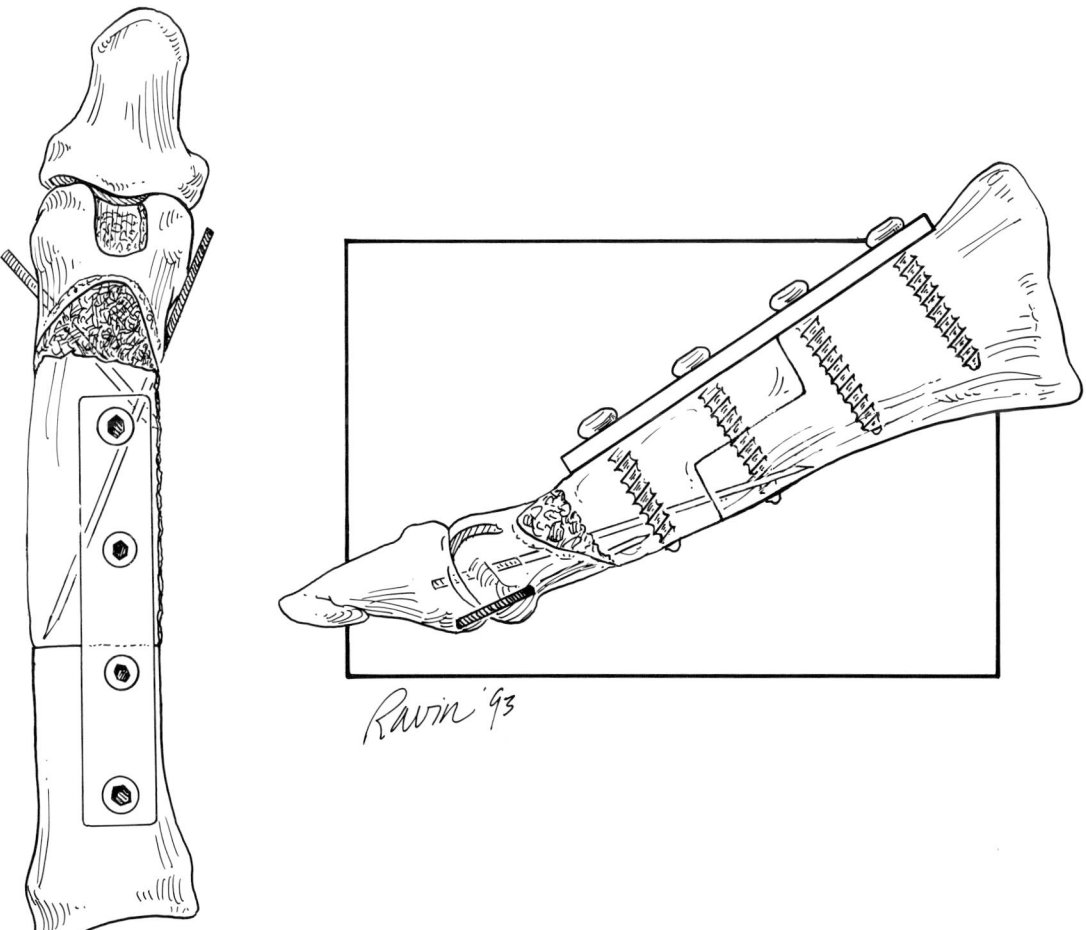

Figure 16. Cortical and cancellous bone with plate fixation was necessary.

RECOMMENDED READING

1. Coughlin, M. J., and Mann, R. A.: Arthrodesis of the first metatarsophalangeal joint as salvage for the failed Keller procedure. *J. Bone Joint Surg.*, 69A: 68–75, 1987.
2. Johnson, K. A.: *Surgery of the Foot and Ankle*. Raven Press, New York, 1989, pp. 202–208.
3. Marin, G. A.: Arthrodesis of the first metatarsophalangeal joint for hallux valgus and hallux rigidus. *Int. Surg.*, 50: 174–178, 1968.

6

Hallux Proximal Phalanx Osteotomy
The Akin Procedure

Carol Frey

INDICATIONS/CONTRAINDICATIONS

In 1925, Akin described a procedure for correction of hallux valgus that involved resection of the medial prominence of the first metatarsal head and a medial wedge osteotomy of the proximal phalanx of the great toe. Akin also described removal of the hypertrophic bone on the medial aspect of the base of the proximal phalanx of the great toe and lateral capsular release if necessary. In the following years, various modifications were added to the basic procedure described by Akin.

Indications for the Akin procedure include hallux valgus and hallux valgus interphalangeus. The procedure can also be used with success in those patients who present with a great toe valgus deformity at the metatarsophalangeal (MP) joint or the interphalangeal (IP) joint, which causes symptoms and/or deformity to develop in the second toe. The Akin procedure may also be used in cases of residual valgus deformity after previous hallux valgus surgery. Rarely, however, is an Akin procedure alone indicated for the correction of a hallux valgus deformity. In most patients the proximal phalangeal osteotomy needs to be performed in combination with some other procedure to correct all components of the hallux valgus deformity. One should avoid using the Akin procedure on the hallux deformity associated with an abnormal intermetatarsal angle, degenerative changes, or incongruity of the MP joint. In cases where a significant varus deformity of the first metatarsal is present, we feel that the Akin procedure can be combined with first metatarsal basilar osteotomy or in some cases a chevron procedure.

C. Frey, M.D.: Department of Orthopaedic Surgery, University of Southern California; and Orthopaedic Foot and Ankle Center, Los Angeles, CA 90007.

PREOPERATIVE PLANNING

The patient criterion for an Akin procedure is similar to that of other bunion procedures. Patients only become candidates for bunion surgery after they have failed an adequate course of conservative treatment, which includes a shoe with a high, wide toe box, a soft leather upper, and adequate room for all the toes to fully extend. Shoes may also be stretched with a ball-and-ring stretcher in the area of the first metatarsal prominence or when orthotics, pads, and splints have not been shown to be effective in the treatment of valgus deformities of the hallux.

On physical examination it is important to note the degree of hallux pronation associated with the bunion and valgus deformities. Only a slight degree of rotatory deformity can be corrected at the time of surgery.

The Akin procedure can be used in those patients who present with a mild hallux valgus deformity which causes symptoms and/or deformity to develop in the second toe, associated second toe deformities including hammertoes and synovitis of the MP.

Preoperatively, all patients should have anteroposterior (AP) weight bearing, lateral, and oblique radiographic views of the foot taken. Radiographic measurements include intermetatarsal angle to determine the degree of metatarsus primus varus, the first MP angle to determine the amount of hallux valgus, and the great toe IP angle to determine the amount of hallux valgus interphalangeus.

The position of the sesamoids should be measured on the AP view. Persistent lateral displacement of the sesamoids after completion of the Akin procedure can predispose to recurrence of the valgus deformity.

Arthritic changes and/or incongruity of the first MP are noted if present preoperatively and are contraindications to the Akin procedure. Radiographs should also be examined to determine the distal metatarsal articular angle (DMAA) of the metatarsal. The distal metatarsal angle is defined as the angle formed between a line that subtends the medial and lateral edges of the articular surface to a line that is transverse to the longitudinal axis of the first metatarsal. The DMAA is normally less than 10°. In patients with a DMAA of greater than 10°, the Akin procedure may be indicated to prevent resultant incongruity of the articular surfaces of the first MP joint during the correction of a valgus deformity.

One should avoid using the Akin procedure on the hallux deformity associated with an abnormal intermetatarsal 1–2 angle of over 10°, degenerative changes, or incongruity of the MP joint. The decision to incorporate the Akin proximal phalangeal osteotomy with another primary bunion procedure is usually best made at the time of surgery.

SURGERY

The Akin procedure may be performed in an outpatient setting with an ankle block anesthesia. A surgical prep to just below the knee is recommended. The patient is placed in the supine position and an ankle tourniquet may be used.

Technique. The operative technique is initiated with a longitudinal medial incision over the first MP joint and carried down through the bursa and the capsule onto the metatarsal head (Fig. 1). The flaps are elevated with a scalpel and Freer elevator. One must be careful to preserve the capsule at its attachment site at the base of the proximal phalanx. Small Homan retractors are used to protect the flexor and extensor hallucis tendons.

If prominent or symptomatic, the medial prominence of the metatarsal head is resected in line with the medial border of the foot. The same incision is extended distally to expose the basilar portion of the proximal phalanx. A ⅛-inch (3-mm) medially based wedge osteotomy is performed in the metaphyseal region of the proximal phalanx within 5 to 7 mm of the metatarsal joint using a microsagittal

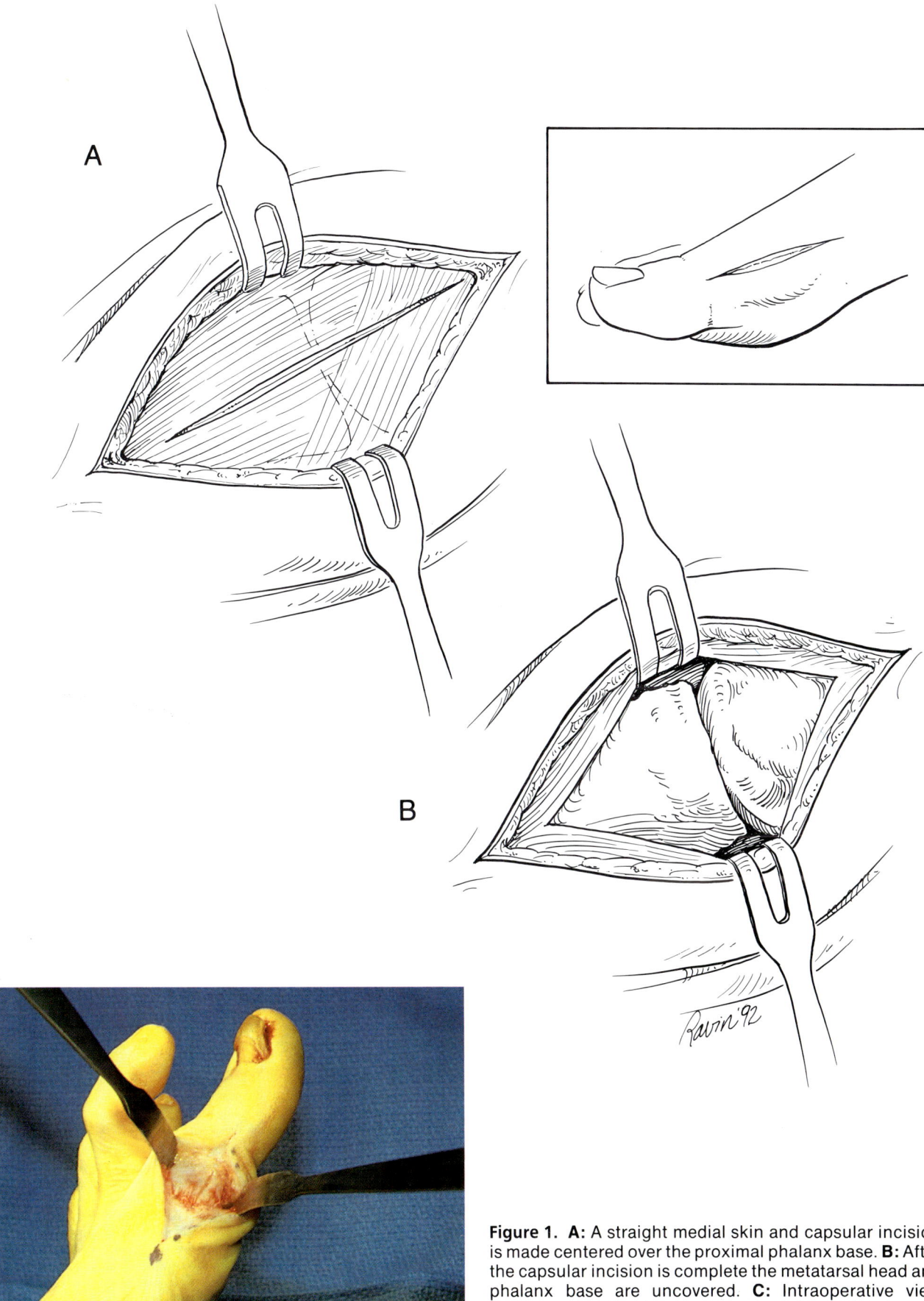

Figure 1. A: A straight medial skin and capsular incision is made centered over the proximal phalanx base. **B:** After the capsular incision is complete the metatarsal head and phalanx base are uncovered. **C:** Intraoperative view shows exposed metatarsophalangeal (MP) joint.

saw (Fig. 2). Approximately 8° of correction can be expected with this size wedge resection. Care is taken to keep the lateral periosteum intact. The wedge is closed (Fig. 3) and the corrected position maintained by two crossed K-wires placed from distal to proximal. The K-wires are then bent to 90° and left protruding through the skin (Fig. 4). Reapproximation of the capsule and the bursal incision is completed and a bunion dressing applied to maintain the corrected position.

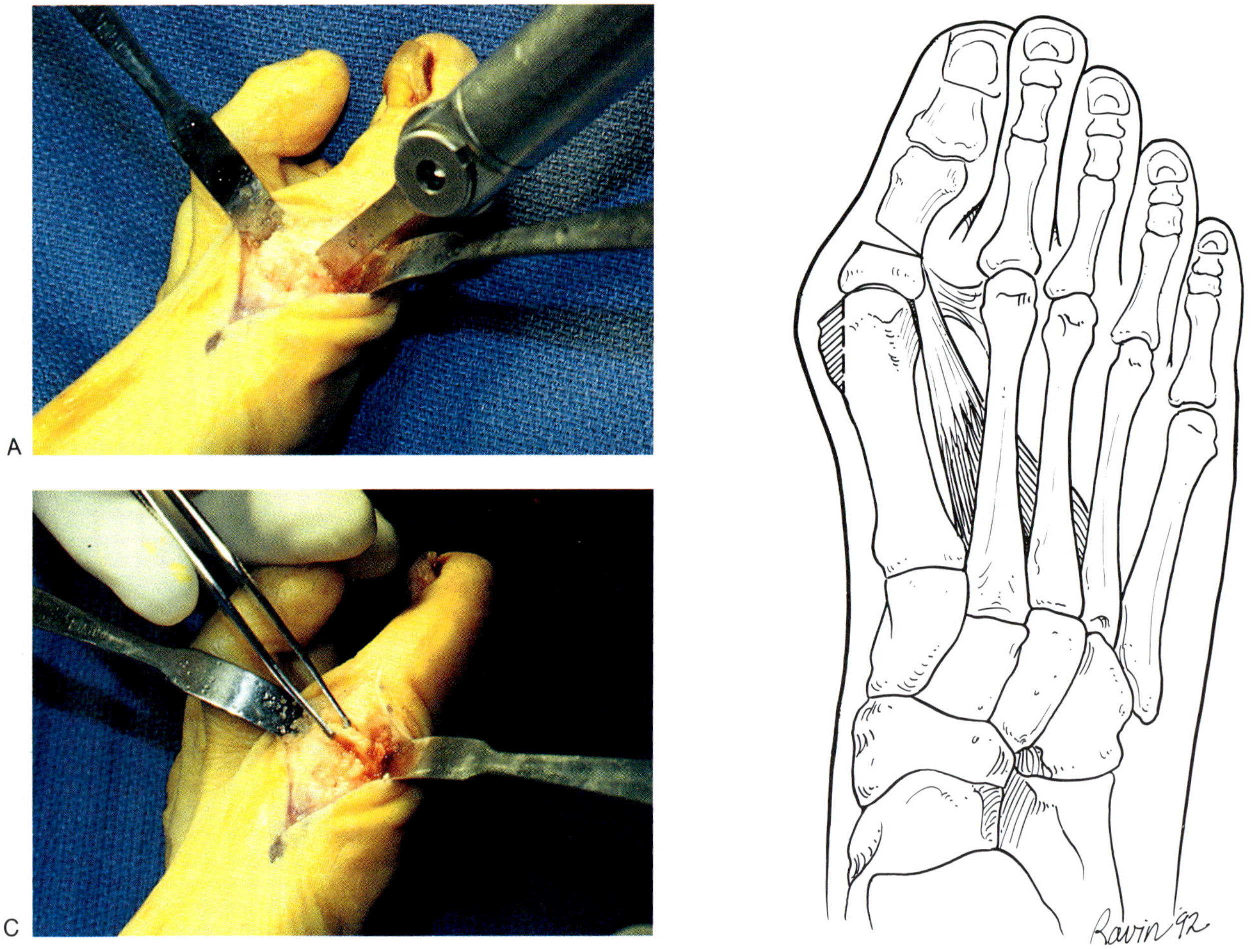

Figure 2. A: A small sagittal saw is used to make the phalanx osteotomy. **B:** Position of the osteotomy. **C:** The medial-based bone wedge is removed from the proximal phalanx.

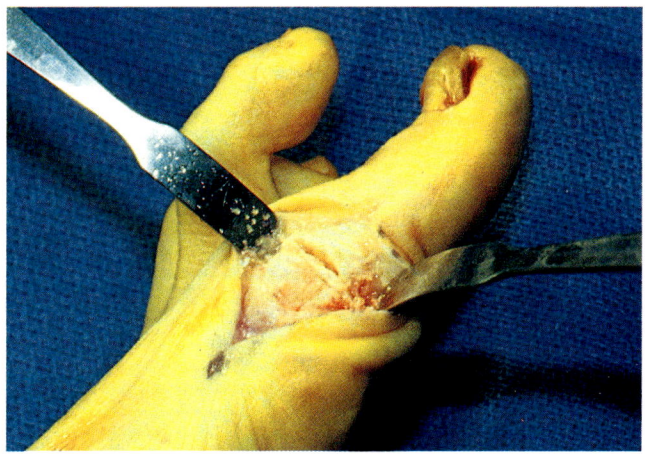

Figure 3. Closure of the phalangeal osteotomy.

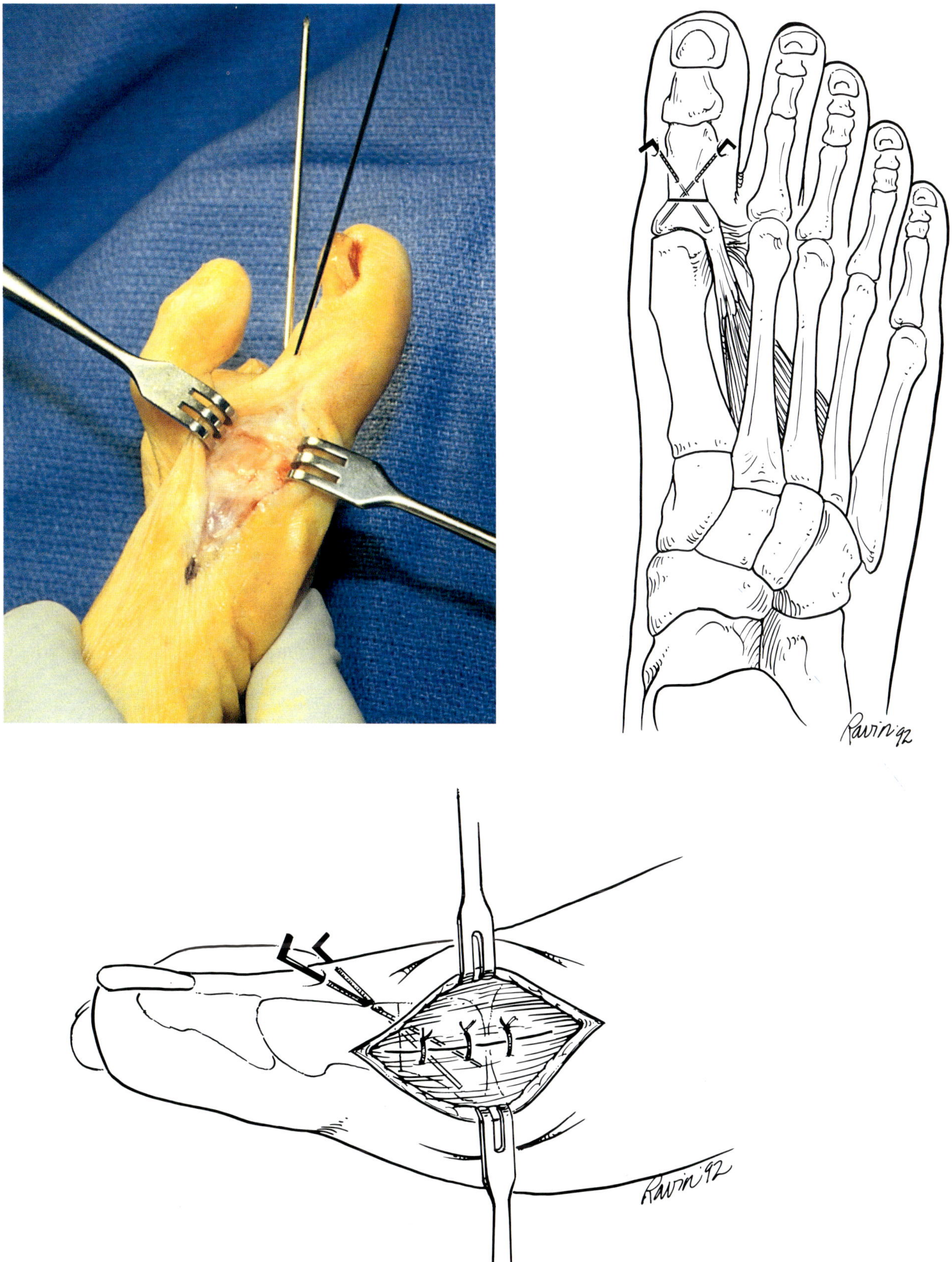

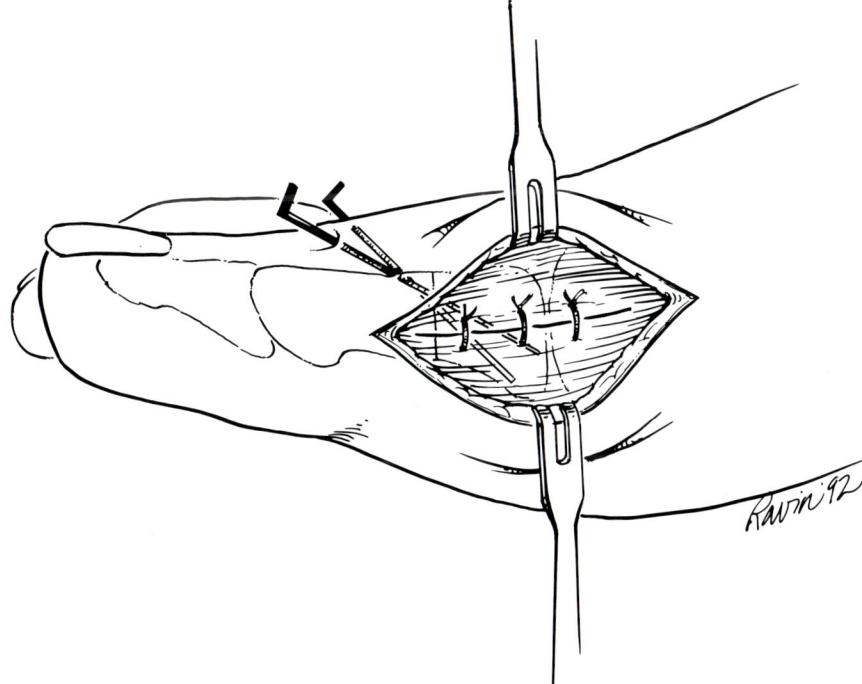

Figure 4. A: Fixation of the osteotomy with Kirschner wires. **B:** Detail view shows K-wire position. **C:** Lateral view of K-wire position.

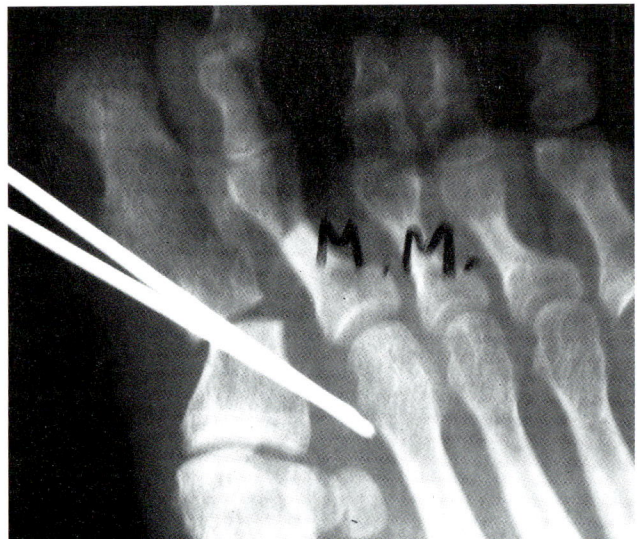 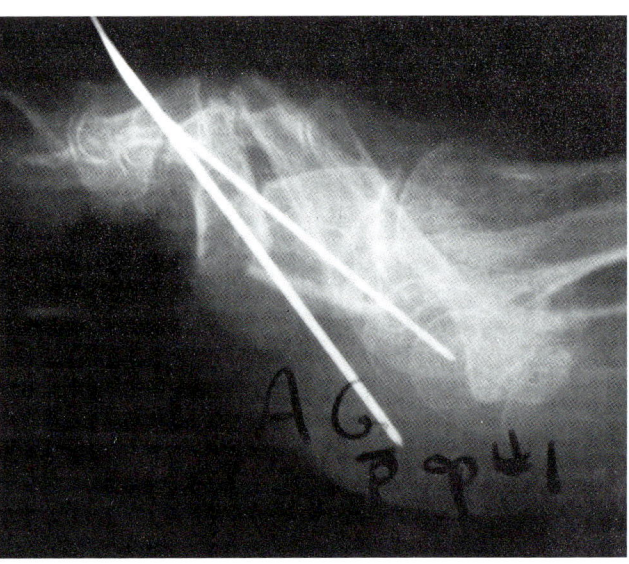

Figure 5. A: Poor bone apposition resulted in this deformed toe position. **B:** Lateral view shows apex angulation plantarward.

Technical pitfalls include fixation failure, poor bone apposition, and plantar angulation (apex plantar) at the osteotomy site (Fig. 5). Poor bone apposition can lead to the uncommon complication of nonunion. To avoid this complication, it is recommended that the surgeon obtain intraoperative radiographs to check position and apposition of bone, use some form of internal fixation, and use care in performing an accurate osteotomy.

The most common technical problem is plantar angulation at the osteotomy site. This is possibly due to the pull of the extensor hallucis longus with resultant plantar angulation across the osteotomy site or malposition of the distal fragment at the time of surgery. Intraoperative radiographs are of value to check the position of the fixation if there is any question of angulation. This problem, however, usually does not lead to any long-term complications.

POSTOPERATIVE MANAGEMENT

The patient is instructed to remain non–weight bearing with elevation of the involved extremity for the first 3 to 5 days, until the initial inflammatory phase has passed. The patient is then allowed to heel walk as tolerated in a postoperative shoe with a bunion dressing. The bunion dressing maintains the great toe in a neutral position and is changed at weekly intervals for 6 weeks allowing the osteotomy and the soft tissues to heal. The sutures are removed at 2 weeks and the pins are removed at 3 weeks in the office.

Healing is usually adequate enough to allow gentle active range of motion exercises to begin at 3 weeks. Some gentle passive range of motion exercises may be started at 4 to 6 weeks as tolerated. Radiographs are taken in the office at the first postoperative visit and at 6 weeks postoperatively. The osteotomy site is usually clinically healed at 4 to 6 weeks but radiographic healing may not occur for 3 to 6 months.

If patient selection is done correctly, the expectations for surgery include approximately an 85% chance of a good to excellent result. Most patients will be wearing a large soft shoe at 6 weeks but should not expect to fit into a fashion shoe for 3 months after surgery. As with other bunion procedures, patients should expect some postoperative swelling for up to 6 months after surgery.

COMPLICATIONS

Complications include nonunion, shortening of the toe, and recurrence of deformity. Nonunion is rare (reported in less than 1% of cases) but can occur particularly if there is poor bone apposition. Shortening of the hallux will occur in all cases and is unavoidable when performing a closing wedge osteotomy. However, shortening can be limited if a minimum of bone is removed from the proximal phalanx. Since the microsagittal saw blade will remove approximately 1 mm of bone with each cut, to make a 3-mm wedge, only 1 mm of bone actually needs to be removed. Removal of a larger wedge only suggests that the procedure was used inappropriately to correct too great a deformity at the improper level or levels. Recurrence of deformity is the most common complication and usually occurs when the indications for the procedure are being stretched. Rarely is an Akin procedure alone indicated for the correction of a hallux valgus deformity. In most patients the proximal phalangeal osteotomy needs to be performed in combination with some other procedure to correct all components of the hallux valgus deformity.

ILLUSTRATIVE CASE FOR TECHNIQUE

A 53-year-old woman presented with a 9-year history of a painful bunion and progressive deformity of the neighboring second toe. She had gotten to a point where she was symptomatic even in soft leather athletic shoes. Examination of her feet revealed a painful and prominent first metatarsal head, hallux valgus interphalangeus, and a hammertoe deformity of the second toe. There was no pronation noted of the great toe. The second toe MP joint was tender to palpation and subluxated. Radiographic examination revealed a 1–2 intermetatarsal angle of 9°, first MP angle of 17°, and a first IP joint angle of 15°. There were no radiographic arthritic changes and the DMAA was 13° (Fig. 6A).

The patient was taken to surgery where an Akin procedure that included the removal of the medial aspect of the first metatarsal head was undertaken. The second toe deformity was corrected with an extensor tenotomy and a dorsal capsulotomy. The patient followed an uneventful postoperative course (Fig. 6B).

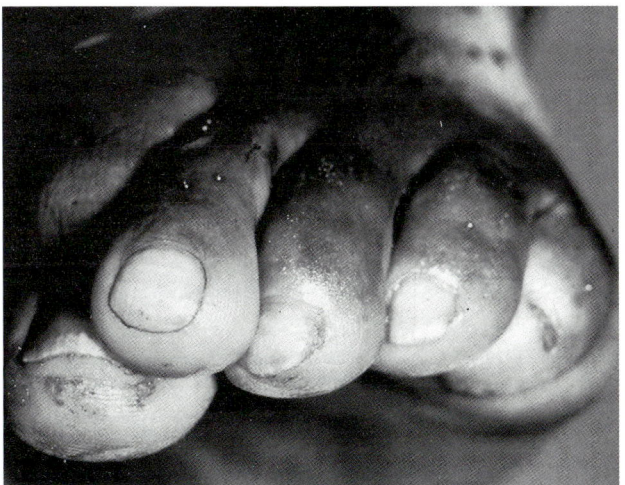
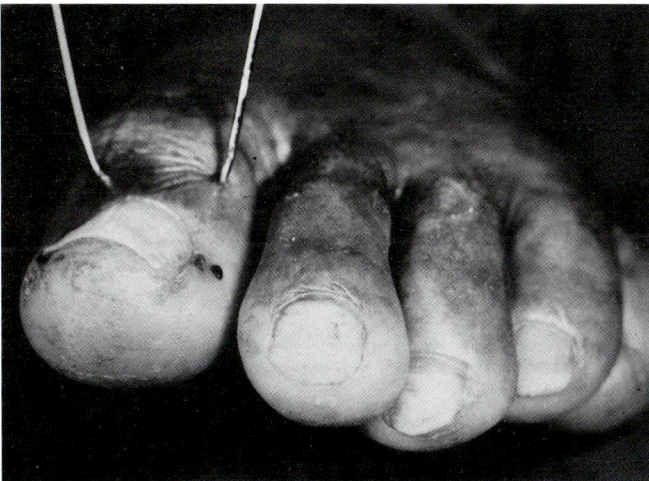

Figure 6. A: Preoperative photograph of a patient with hallux valgus interphalangeus and MP joint synovitis in the subluxated second toe. **B:** Postoperative photograph of the same patient after the Akin procedure.

Two years after surgery the patient remained asymptomatic but noted that the great toe was shortened compared to the opposite side. The great and second toe had remained in a reduced position.

RECOMMENDED READING

1. Akin, O. F.: The treatment of hallux valgus: a new operative procedure and its results. *Med. Sentinel,* 33: 678–679, 1925.
2. Colloff, B.: Proximal phalangeal osteotomy in hallux valgus, *J. Bone Joint Surg.,* 48A(7): 1442–1443, 1966.
3. Frey, C., Jahss, M., and Kummer, F. J.: The Akin procedure: an analysis of results. *Foot Ankle,* 12(1): 1–6, 1991.
4. Goldberg, I., Bahar, A., and Yosipovitch, Z.: Late results after correction of hallux valgus deformity by basilar phalangeal osteotomy. *J. Bone Joint Surg.,* 69A(1): 64–67, 1987.
5. Goldberg, I., Bahar, A., and Yosipovitch, Z.: Correspondence. *J. Bone Joint Surg.,* 69A(6): 950, 1987.
6. Seelenfruend, M.: Correction of hallux valgus deformity by basal phalanx osteotomy of the big toe. *J. Bone Joint Surg.,* 55A(7): 1411–1415, 1973.
7. Silberman, F. S.: Proximal phalangeal osteotomy for the correction of hallux valgus. *CORR,* 85: 98–100, 1972.

7

Mitchell Osteotomy

Kent K. Wu

INDICATIONS/CONTRAINDICATIONS

The Mitchell bunionectomy is used to treat mild to moderate hallux valgus and its associated deformities when the first intermetatarsal angle is up to 18° and the first metatarsophalangeal angle is up to 40°. Subluxation at the metatarsophalangeal joints may be present to a mild degree but should be easily reducible and have no significant degenerative arthritis in that joint. Patients in the older age groups of over 60 years seem to do less well than those in the younger age groups.

In addition to the usual contraindications to surgical treatment such as vascular insufficiency or infection, specific contraindications to the Mitchell osteotomy are degenerative arthritis of the metatarsophalangeal joint, marked instability of the cuneiform metatarsal articulation, a fixed valgus deformity at the metatarsophalangeal joint, and severe deformity with the intermetatarsal angle more than about 18°.

PREOPERATIVE PLANNING

The planning should include a thorough history and physical examination. The patient's complaints of pain, limitations in shoe-wear, and cosmetic concerns should be reviewed. The physical examination should focus on the severity of the prominent medial eminence and hallux valgus deformity as well as the mobility of the great toe at the metatarsophalangeal articulation in both flexion-extension and varus-valgus plane of motion.

Anteroposterior (AP) and lateral weight-bearing views of the foot along with oblique radiographs should be assessed. This allows measurement of the intermetatarsal 1–2 angle, as well the metatarsophalangeal angle. Also, presence of an acquired hammertoe deformity of the second toe should be noted, and the neces-

---

K. K. Wu, M.D.: Bone and Joint Center, Henry Ford Hospital, Detroit, MI 48202.

sity for direct surgical treatment of that portion of the foot. When a large and painful callosity is present under the first or second metatarsal head, a sesamoid view of the foot should be obtained to visualize the condition of the sesamometatarsal joint and the amount of plantar displacement of the second metatarsal head, which may be treated by a plantar condylectomy.

SURGERY

The night before the operation, the patient is instructed to scrub the feet with Phisohex or Betadine soap solution. The surgical procedure is performed on an outpatient basis under ankle block anesthesia. The patient is placed supine on the operating room table and an Esmarch bandage is used for exsanguination and as a tourniquet about the ankle.

Techniques. A 6- to 7-cm medial longitudinal midline incision extending from the basal portion of the first proximal phalanx to the distal first metatarsal shaft is made through the skin and subcutaneous tissue down to the metatarsophalangeal (MP) joint capsule and the medial eminence of the great toe (Figs. 1 and 2). The

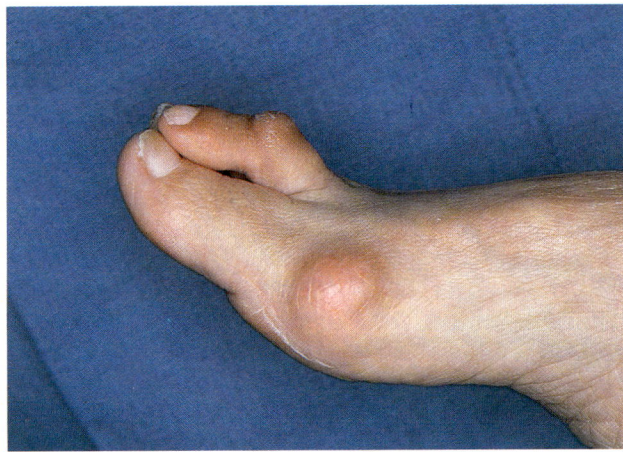

Figure 1. Lateral view of the forefoot shows a large bunion in association with a fixed crossover second hammertoe.

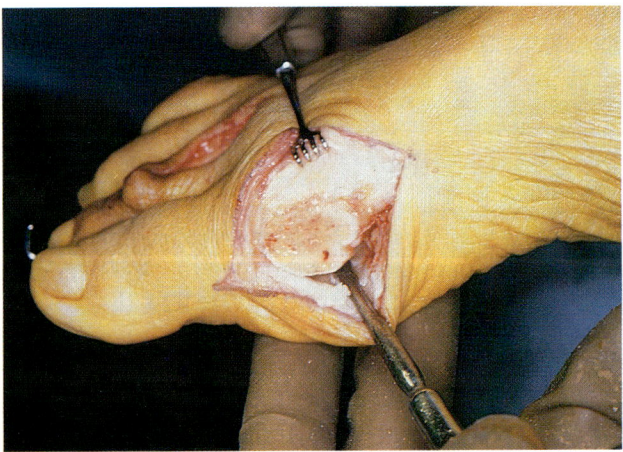

Figure 2. After correcting the second hammertoe, the bunion is removed by means of a microsaw through a medial longitudinal skin incision that also goes through the joint capsule to expose the bunion.

MP joint of the great toe is incised longitudinally and the medial eminence (bunion) is exposed by means of sharp dissection. A 1-cm strip of joint capsule is stripped from the dorsal aspect of the first metatarsal neck. A Joker retractor follows this narrowly exposed metatarsal neck and is placed on the lateral aspect of the first metatarsal neck. Protect the underlying sesamoids, by placing a second Joker retractor under the first metatarsal head. The medial eminence is removed about 1 mm medial to the sagittal groove with a microsaw (Fig. 3). Round off the sharp peripheral bone edges are rounded off with a small bone rasp.

While protecting the sesamoids with the Joker retractor, two holes are drilled through the distal portion of the first metatarsal. The distal hole emerges from the plantar side where the articular cartilage of the first metatarsal head ends. The proximal hole emerges about 1.2 to 1.8 cm proximal and 6 to 7 mm lateral to the distal hole (Figs. 4 and 5). The placement of the drill holes in relation to the osteotomy is important (Fig. 6). By inserting a straight Keith needle through the distal hole to serve as a guide, the distal partial osteotomy cut is made with a microsaw. The cut is made, 3 to 4 mm proximal to the distal hole and at a right angle to the longitudinal axis of the first metatarsal, to the desired depth (e.g., a more shallow cut for a foot with a wider first intermetatarsal angle, and a more shallow dorsal cut than its plantar cut to correct the internal rotational deformity of the great toe). The oblique proximal osteotomy should be made in a dorsoplantar direction with a 10° to 15° plantar inclination or a higher angulation when the first metatarsal is fairly short or when severe metatarsalgia is present in the lesser toes due to their excessively flexed position in a plantar direction. To minimize the unnecessary shortening of the first metatarsal, the two parallel cuts on the dorsal aspect of the first metatarsal are only 1 to 2 mm apart.

The unwanted bone is removed from the medial aspect of the osteotomy site with a small rongeur and the cut first metatarsal head is laterally and often about 2 mm plantarly displaced to engage its lateral bony ledge on the lateral aspect of the first metatarsal neck (Figs. 7 and 8). Next, two size-0 Mersilene sutures are

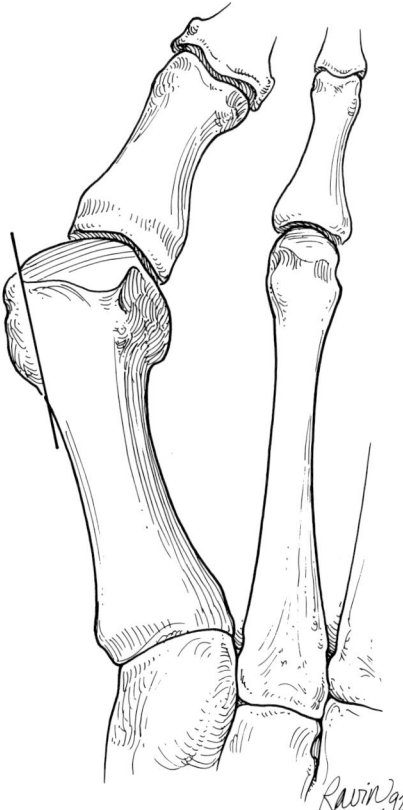

Figure 3. Plane of resection of the medial eminence, 1 mm medial to the sagittal groove.

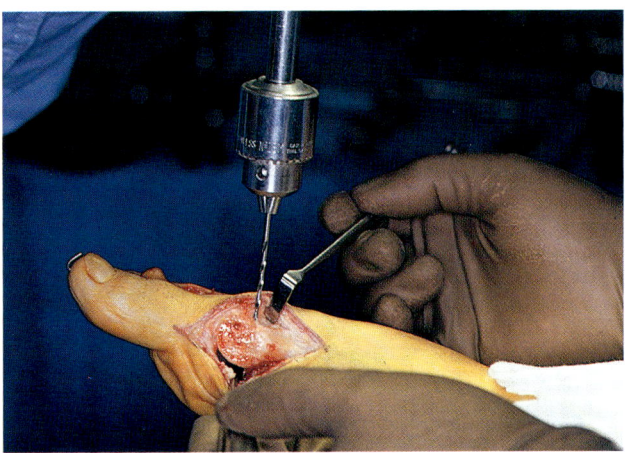

Figure 4. The distal vertical hole emerges on the plantar aspect of the first metatarsal head at the point where the articular surface ends.

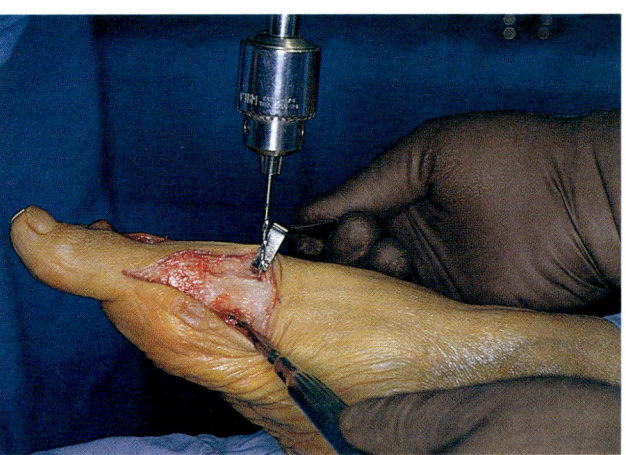

Figure 5. The proximal hole should be lateral to the distal hole. Separation between these two holes in the transverse plane determines the amount of lateral displacement of the first metatarsal head and the extent of reduction of the first intermetatarsal angle. This is because the amount of bone removed from the medial aspect of the osteotomy site is inversely proportional to the transverse distance between the two drill holes. A transverse step-out osteotomy is performed between these two drill holes. The first metatarsal head is displaced laterally and slightly plantarward.

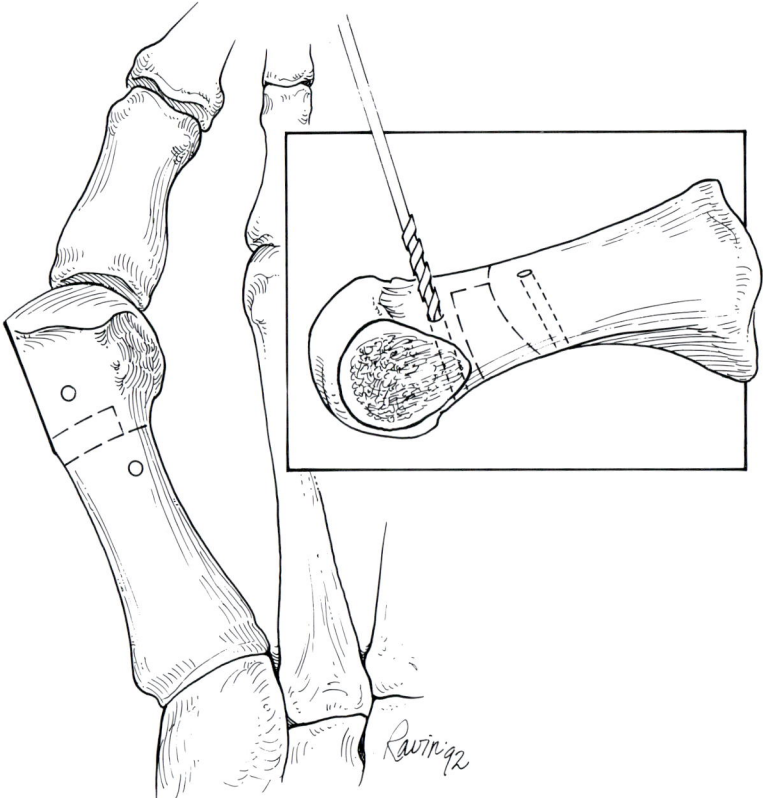

Figure 6. Relationship of the drill holes to the osteotomy cuts in the metatarsal neck.

7 MITCHELL OSTEOTOMY

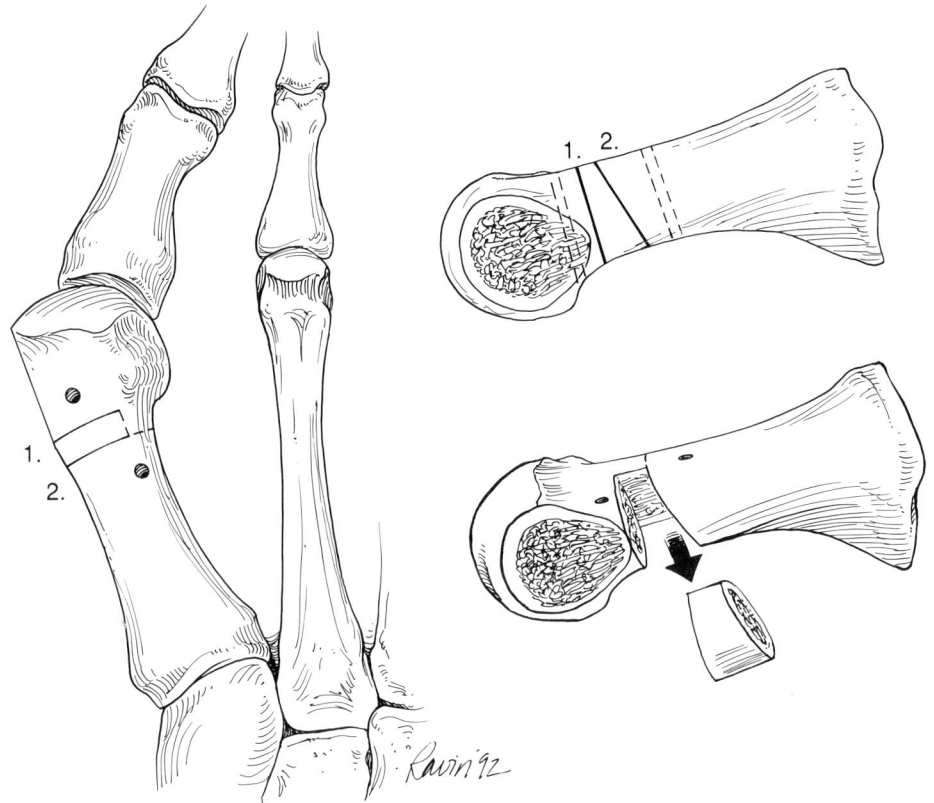

Figure 7. Bone removal is made in such a way as to plantarflex the distal metatarsal and allow lateral translocation of the metatarsal head.

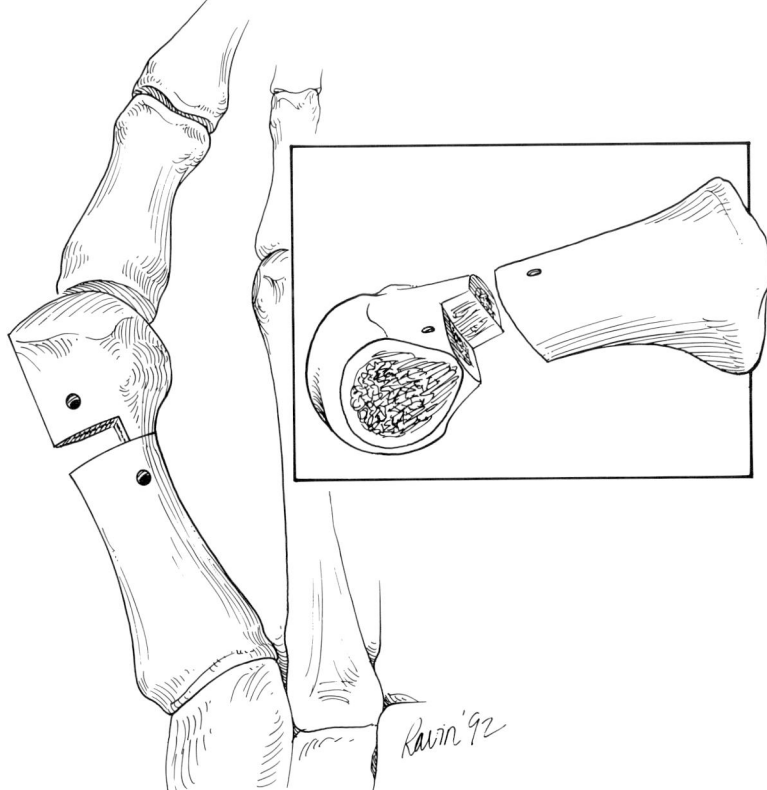

Figure 8. The lateral shelf of bone determines the lateral correction of the Mitchell osteotomy.

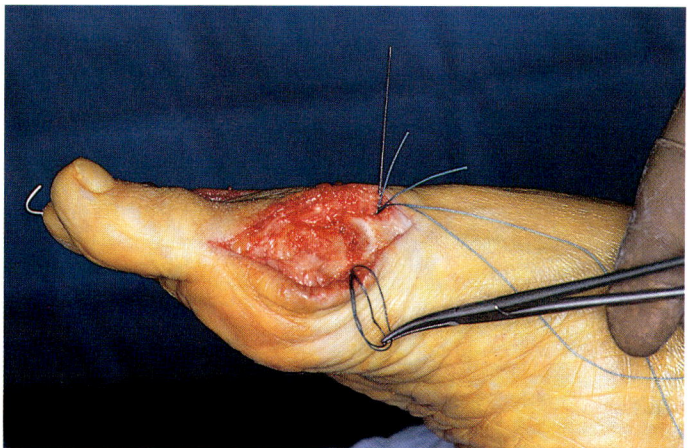

Figure 9. The two ends of two size-0 Mersilene sutures are delivered to the plantar aspect of the first metatarsal neck through the proximal drill hole with a straight Keith needle.

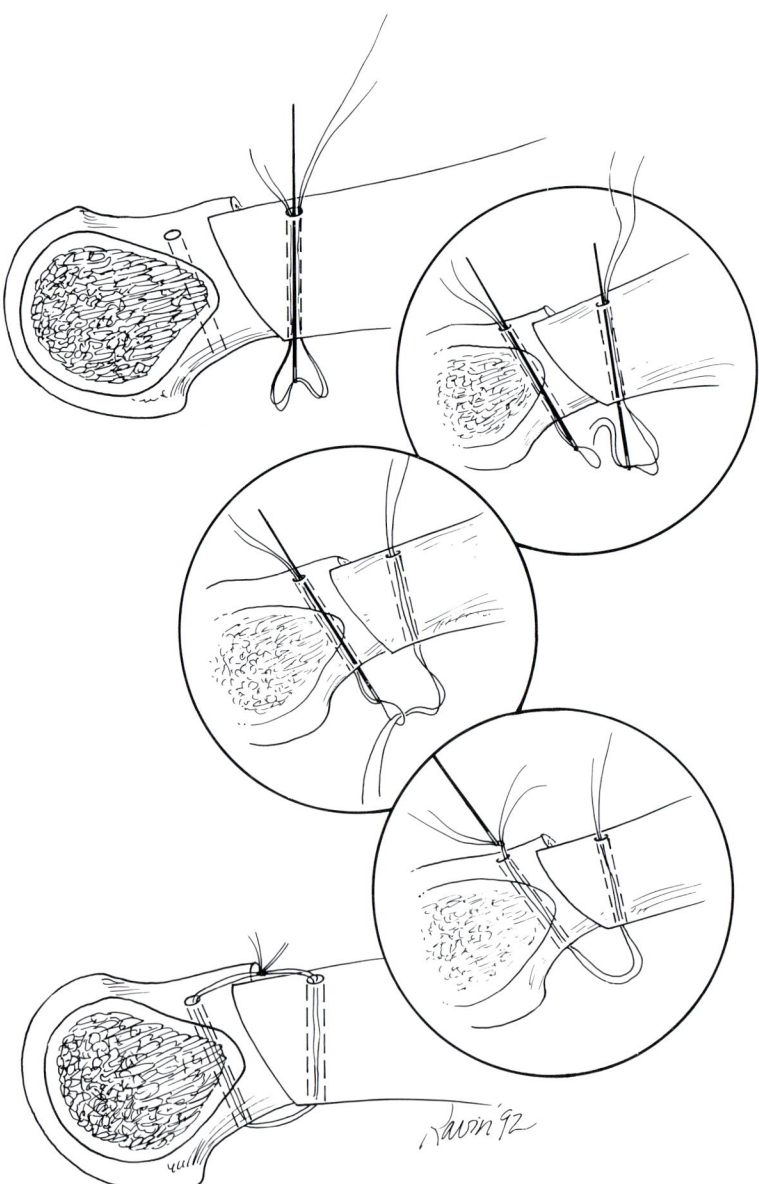

Figure 10. After the metatarsal head is displaced laterally, sutures are placed to fix the osteotomy.

passed through the proximal hole using a straight Keith needle and to pull out the two free ends with a small hemostat (Fig. 9). The two proximal hole sutures are passed through the single suture loop, which is drawn upward by pulling on the Keith needle and the two free ends of the single suture to pull the two sutures through the distal hole to the dorsal aspect of the first metatarsal head (Figs. 10 and 11). By holding the two raw bone surfaces at the osteotomy site in intimate contact, the two sutures individually are tied tightly over the dorsal aspect of the first metatarsal neck by holding the first knot down with a mosquito hemostat before the second square knot is tightened, using a total of five to six square knots to prevent slippage (Figs. 12 and 13). The bony prominence on the medial aspect of the fixed osteotomy site is removed with a microsaw (Figs. 14 and 15).

The surgical wound is washed thoroughly with a diluted Betadine solution first and followed by saline solution. To hold the great toe in a slightly overcorrected position place two 4" × 4" gauze pads folded twice in the first web space. The joint capsule is closed tightly by overlapping the MP angle of the great toe. Arthrodesis of the first MP joint with Herbert screws is indicated if a painful arthrosis of the first MP joint is associated with a hallux varus.

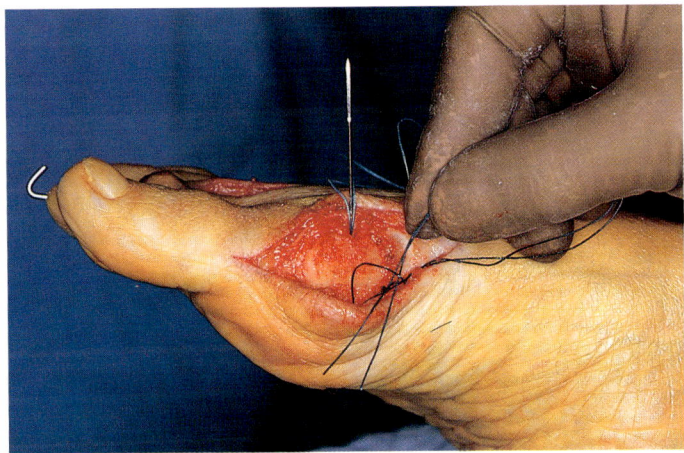

Figure 11. A single suture loop is delivered to the plantar aspect of the first metatarsal head through the distal drill hole with a straight Keith needle, and the two ends of the first two sutures are passed through the single suture loop.

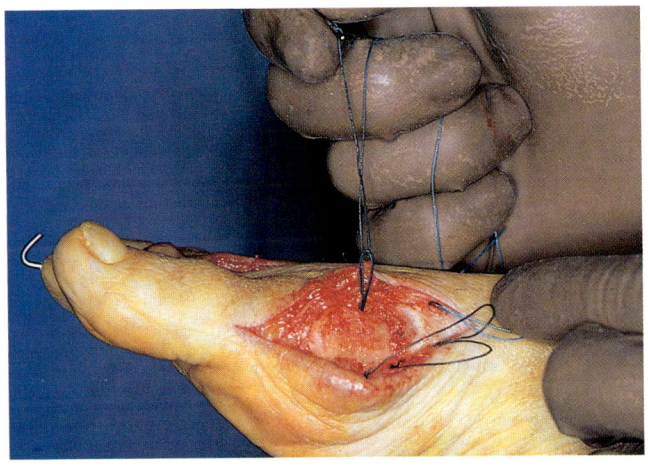 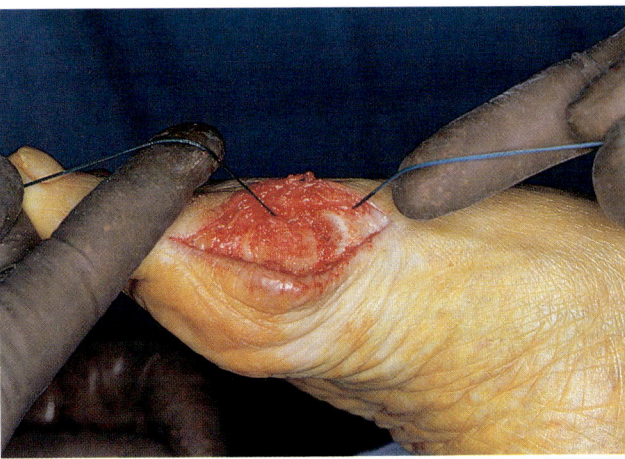

Figure 12. A, B: By pulling the two ends of the single suture upward, the two ends of the first two sutures are brought to the dorsal aspect of the first metatarsal head.

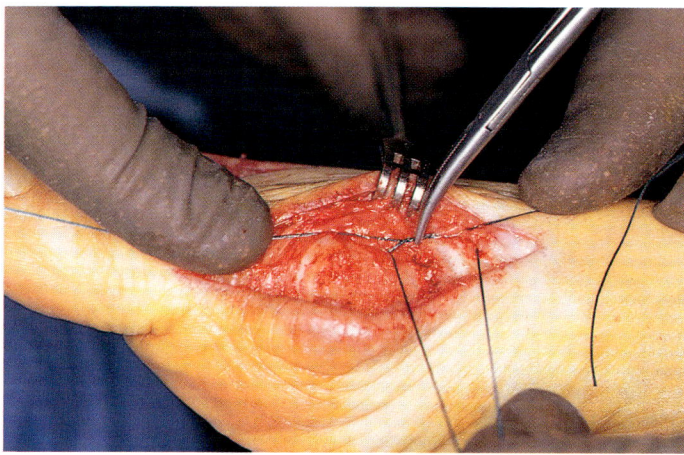

Figure 13. The two sutures are individually tied tightly across the osteotomy site. To prevent slippage of the suture knot, the first square knot should be held down tightly with a mosquito hemostat before the second square knot is tied. Four or five square knots are needed for each suture.

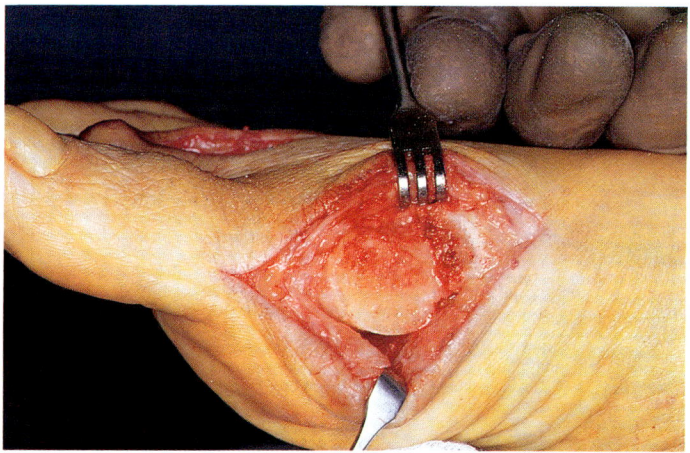

Figure 14. The protruding portion of medial aspect of the first metatarsal neck is removed with a microsaw. Note the intentional plantar displacement of the first metatarsal head.

Preoperatively, if all the lesser toes are deviated laterally, some degree of recurrence of hallux valgus can be confidently predicted because when female patients go back to their narrow, pointed high-heeled shoes, the shoe will gradually force the great toe into a valgus position to be next to the laterally deviated lesser toes. Surprisingly, the patients infrequently complain of the mild recurrence of the hallux valgus owing to the fact that their initial hallux valgus was much worse.

Pain under the second metatarsal head is a fairly common complaint and occurs in 11% of the patients with Mitchell's bunionectomy (4). Shortening (average 3.7 mm) of the first metatarsal (8) and postoperative angulations of the first metatarsal head decrease the weight-bearing function of the great toe and force the second metatarsal and to a lesser degree the third metatarsal to bear excessive amounts of the body weight, thus producing pain and plantar callosity. Needless to say, excessive shortening of the first metatarsal frequently results in metatarsalgia of the lesser toes.

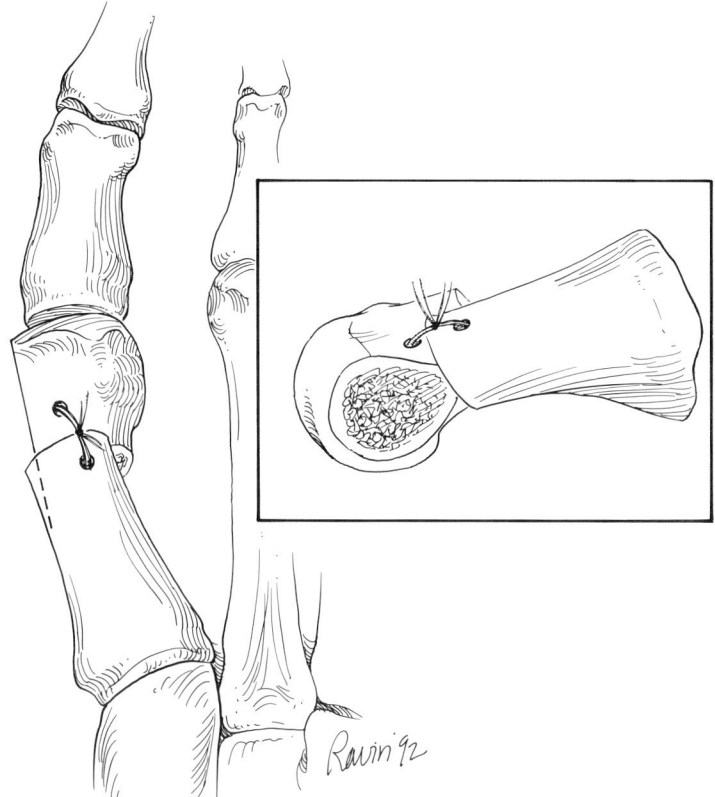

Figure 15. The completed osteotomy with suture fixation just prior to removal of the exposed bony prominence on the medial aspect of the osteotomy site.

A reliable method to minimize the incidence of developing a hallux rigidus in Mitchell's bunionectomy is to produce as little soft tissue scar around the osteotomy site as possible. This can be achieved by minimal but adequate exposure of the surgical wound to allow the removal of the bunion, and the first metatarsal neck osteotomy to be properly performed. Gentle handling of soft tissue, good hemostasis, meticulous wound closure, careful application of the compression dressing and casts, and diligent active and passive exercise of the great toe after cast removal are the important factors in preventing the development of a hallux rigidus.

The author's personal experience shows that postoperative angulations of the first metatarsal head occur in 4% of the cases of Mitchell's bunionectomy (2% dorsal angulation and 2% medial angulation) (4). If these angulations are discovered within the first 2 postoperative weeks, they usually can be reduced under local anesthesia. Under fluoroscopic guidance a small K-wire can be inserted from the tip of the great toe through the phalanges, the first metatarsal head, and the osteotomy site into the proximal part of the first metatarsal. The K-wire holds while it unites the osteotomy site in a corrected position. After 4 to 6 weeks the K-wire is removed.

When the first metatarsal head is healed in a markedly medially deviated position, a lateral displacement osteotomy with Herbert screw fixation is a good surgical option. If the healed medially deviated first metatarsal head has produced a significant amount of painful arthrosis in the first MP joint, then arthrodesis of the first MP joint becomes the surgical treatment of choice. When the first metatarsal head is healed in a moderately dorsally angulated position, only a simple cheilectomy of the protruding portion of the first metatarsal head needs to be performed.

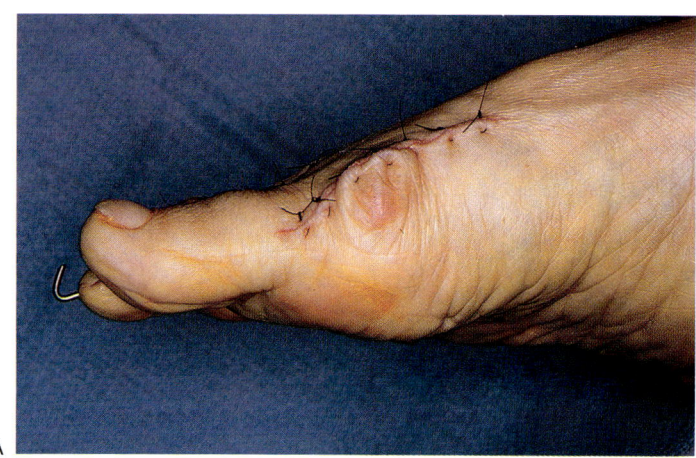 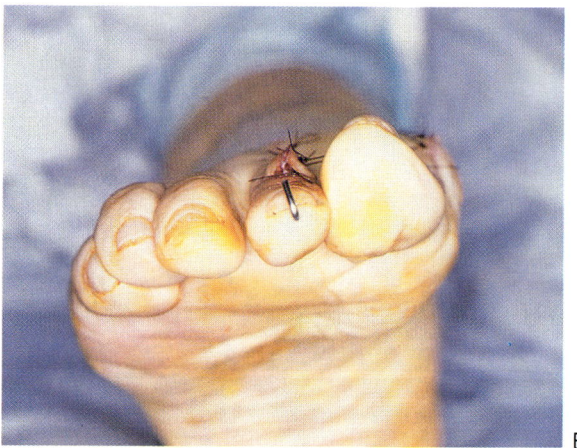

Figure 16. A,B: The joint capsule is tightly closed in an overlapping "vest over pants" manner, and the skin is closed in a regular manner. Note the correction of the hallux valgus and crossover second hammertoe deformities.

However, if the dorsal angulation is quite marked, a plantar angulation osteotomy with a double Herbert screw fixation of the new osteotomy site should be done.

When excessive bone has been removed from the medial aspect of the first metatarsal head in a lateral displacement first metatarsal neck osteotomy, the medial sesamoid can become subluxed or even dislocated medially, producing a hallux varus deformity. If the first metatarsal head still has a good articular surface, fusion of the interphalangeal (IP) joint of the great toe with transfer of the extensor hallucis longus tendon to the lateral base of the first proximal phalanx after first passing it under the first transverse metatarsal ligament as described by Johnson and Spiegl (5) can restore the normal redundant joint capsule in a "vest over pants" manner with interrupted 3-0 Vicryl sutures. The skin is closed with interrupted 4-0 nylon horizontal mattress sutures (Fig. 16). A bulky compression dressing consisting of two boxes of 4" × 4" cotton gauzes; four Klings; three presoaked and pliable tongue blades placed on the dorsal, medial, and plantar aspects of the great toe; and two 4" Ace bandages are applied over the whole foot and ankle. The Esmarch bandage is removed before the two Ace bandages are wrapped around the foot and ankle.

POSTOPERATIVE MANAGEMENT

The postoperative management consists of foot elevation on two or three pillows for 2 to 3 days, followed by dressing change and application of a bunion boot (wrapping fiberglass cast bandages over the bunionectomy dressing) 3 to 5 days postoperatively. Ten to twelve days postoperatively, the sutures are removed and a great toe spica short leg walking cast to allow full weight bearing is applied. The bunion cast is removed 6 to 8 weeks after surgery and radiographs are taken at the same time. I recommend that the patient wear a wide and comfortable shoe after cast removal and start active and passive exercises of the great toe, and gradually return to the former footwear in the ensuing weeks.

As a general rule, the Mitchell bunionectomy can be expected to yield an 85% overall good to excellent result. I have noted that the postoperative swelling tends to linger significantly longer in elderly patients than in young patients, possibly due to age-related senescence of their vascular and lymphatic systems. The reduction of metatarsus primus varus by Mitchell bunionectomy seems to be very long-lasting but the correction of hallux valgus may be lost gradually in the presence of an unstable toe, general lateral deviation of lesser toes, and wearing narrow, pointed, and high-heeled shoes.

COMPLICATIONS

The problems with Mitchell's bunionectomy are usually associated with the biplanar metatarsal neck osteotomy. If the two drilled holes are placed too close together, the osteotomy incision may extend through one of the two holes, and subsequent tying of the two sutures may cut completely through the hole and create instability. On the other hand, if the two holes are placed too far apart, much bigger suture loops have to be used to hold the osteotomy site together, and they tend to be more easily stretched out than smaller suture loops. In addition, ideally, when the first metatarsal head has been displaced laterally into its final position, the two drilled holes should form a line parallel to the longitudinal axis of the first metatarsal so that the two sutures will be tied at right angle to the osteotomy line to provide best fixation. However, if the two sutures are tied at an oblique angle with the osteotomy line, the stability of the osteotomy site may be somewhat compromised. It should also be noted that the osteotomy should simultaneously produce a lateral displacement and plantar angulation of the first metatarsal head and supination of the great toe with minimal shortening of the first metatarsal. Consequently, incorrectly performed osteotomy can produce excessive shortening, instability, undesirable angulations, and inadequate correction of the metatarsus primus varus and hallux valgus. To avoid all the above-mentioned pitfalls, the two drilled holes and the lines of cuts of the biplanar osteotomy should be carefully measured and then marked on the distal metatarsal with a surgical marking pen before carrying out the osteotomy. If the osteotomy has been incorrectly performed or the lateral bony ledge is incorrectly fashioned, correction of these mistakes commonly produces excessive shortening of the first metatarsal and/or instability of the osteotomy site. To salvage the operation, the first metatarsal head may have to be fixed in a significantly more plantarly displaced position to increase its weight-bearing function, and the osteotomy site should be held in a corrected position with K-wires or small bone screws.

ILLUSTRATIVE CASE FOR TECHNIQUE

This 52-year-old man had a chronic hallux valgus deformity with prominence of the medial eminence. Varus-valgus stress of the metatarsal phalangeal joint demonstrated smooth motion without crepitus. His preoperative intermetatarsal 1–2 angle was 18°, with a hallux-valgus angle of 40°. This is the upper limit that can be expected to be treated by a Mitchell osteotomy (Fig. 17A).

A Mitchell osteotomy was done, and it relieved the preoperative symptoms. The postoperative radiograph (image reversed) shows the intermetatarsal angle has been decreased to 5° and the valgus deformity at the metatarsophalangeal joint was 11° (Fig. 17B); 2.5-mm shortening of the first metatarsal had occurred.

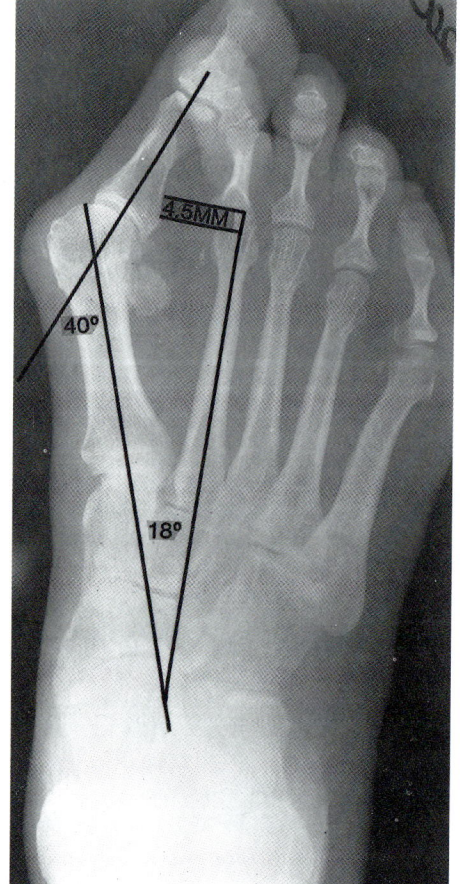
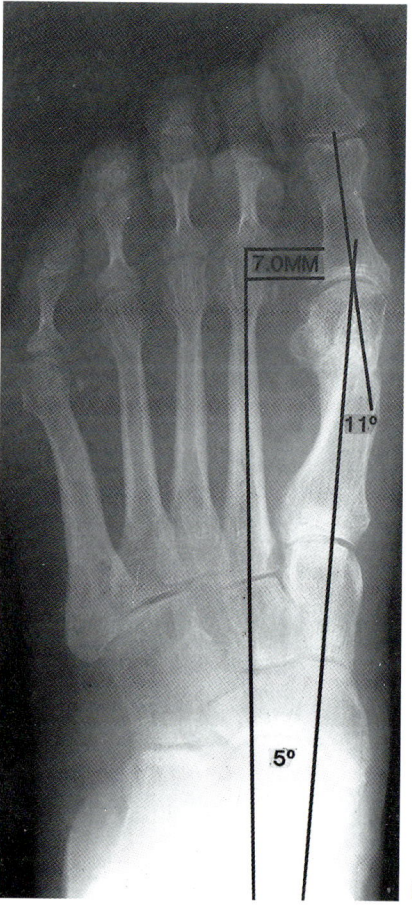

Figure 17. A: Preoperative AP foot radiograph shows first metatarsophalangeal angle of 40° and first intermetatarsal angle of 18°. **B:** Postoperative AP foot radiograph (image reversed) shows first metatarsophalangeal angle reduced to 11° and first intermetatarsal angle reduced to 5°. Shortening of the first metatarsal occurred.

RECOMMENDED READING

1. Carr, C. R., and Boyd, B. M.: Correctional osteotomy for metatarsus primus varus and hallux valgus. *J. Bone Joint Surg.,* 50A: 1353–1367, 1968.
2. Glynn, M. K., Dunlop, J. B., and Fitzpatrick, D.: The Mitchell distal metatarsal osteotomy for hallux valgus. *J. Bone Joint Surg.,* 62B: 188–191, 1980.
3. Hammond, G.: Mitchell osteotomy—bunionectomy for metatarsus primus varus and hallux valgus. In: *Instructional Course Lectures, American Academy of Orthopaedic Surgeons,* vol 21. St. Louis: C.V. Mosby, 1972; p. 246.
4. Hawkins, F. B., Mitchell, E. L., and Hedrick, D. W.: Correction of hallux valgus by metatarsal osteotomy. *J. Bone Joint Surg.,* 37A: 387–394, 1945.
5. Johnson, K. A., and Spiegl, P.: Extensor hallucis longus transfer for hallux varus deformity. *J. Bone Joint Surg.,* 66: 681, 1984.
6. Miller, J. W.: Distal first metatarsal displacement osteotomy. *J. Bone Joint Surg.,* 56A: 923–931, 1974.
7. Shapiro, F., and Heller, L.: The Mitchell distal metatarsal osteotomy in the treatment of hallux valgus. *Clin. Orthop.,* 107: 225–231, 1975.
8. Wu, K. K.: Mitchell bunionectomy: an analysis of 430 personal cases plus a review of the literature. *J. Foot Surg.,* 26: 277–292, 1987.

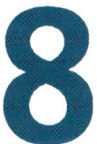

8

Proximal First Metatarsal Osteotomy

Michael J. Coughlin

INDICATIONS/CONTRAINDICATIONS

The primary indication for a distal soft tissue realignment (DSTR) with a proximal first metatarsal osteotomy (PMO) is a symptomatic hallux valgus deformity of a moderate or severe nature.

Initially, McBride described a technique involving a lateral metatarsophalangeal joint capsular release, an adductor tendon transfer into the lateral metatarsal head, a lateral sesamoid excision, medial eminence resection, and a medial capsulorrhaphy. Over the years, this technique was modified significantly, and thus, the term "distal soft tissue realignment" is preferred. Likewise, the limitations of this procedure were defined by further experience. A DSTR procedure alone achieves an average correction of the hallux-valgus angle of 17° and an average correction of the 1–2 intermetatarsal (IM) angle of 5.2° (4). The addition of a proximal metatarsal osteotomy allows a greater diminution of the 1–2 IM angle (average of 8°) and hallux valgus angle (average of 30° for severe deformity) as well. This correction is achieved without a lateral sesamoid excision, which thus decreases the incidence of a postoperative hallux varus deformity. For a mild and low moderate deformity (1–2 IM angle, <15°, hallux valgus angle <25°), a DSTR alone may be sufficient to attain a complete correction; for more severe deformities (1–2 IM angle >16°, hallux valgus angle >35°) a DSTR with a PMO may be used to achieve a correction of the hallux valgus angle. For intermediate deformities, the use of the osteotomy with DSTR depends upon the surgeon's preference and the ease with which an alignment is achieved.

M. J. Coughlin, M.D.: *Private practice*, Orthopaedic Surgery, Boise, ID 83706; Division of Orthopaedic Surgery and Rehabilitation, Department of Surgery, Oregon Health Sciences University, Portland, OR 97201.

Age does not seem to be a contraindication for this procedure although in a younger patient with an open epiphysis, the proximal metatarsal osteotomy should avoid the proximal first metatarsal epiphysis. In the older patient or the patient with a more severe deformity, decreased range of motion may occur postoperatively; however, this does not appear to influence patient satisfaction.

A subluxated or noncongruent metatarsophalangeal joint is a necessary precondition for performing a DSTR with a PMO. Radiographic evaluation can assist the surgeon in determining the congruency of the joint. A varus-valgus stress test can be used to clinically evaluate congruency as well. Manually dorsiflexing and plantar flexing the hallux metatarsophalangeal joint in varus and valgus will help to determine if the toe can be realigned with an intraarticular repair. Diminution of motion may indicate a congruent joint, which is a contraindication to this specific surgical repair.

Pain over the medial eminence is the major complaint of patients in over three-quarters of cases. Another frequent complaint is a second toe hammertoe deformity or metatarsalgia beneath the second metatarsal head.

Occasionally, a patient notes no pain, but is concerned with the cosmetic appearance of his/her foot. Surgery is ideally deferred in these patients until pain becomes a major complaint. The examiner should be aware of the patient's occupation, footwear requirements, and athletic activity as certain stressful physical activities may not be compatible with a successful surgical result. An athlete may find minor postoperative restricted range of motion much more annoying than the preoperative discomfort that led her/him to surgery. Degenerative arthritis or hallux rigidus is a relative contraindication to surgery depending upon the magnitude of the arthritic changes. Prior hallux valgus surgery is not necessarily a contraindication and this procedure may be used to salvage a previous surgical failure.

Specific contraindications for this procedure include metatarsophalangeal joint arthritis, significant metatarsus adductus, active infection, and a congruent metatarsophalangeal joint with significant distal metatarsal articular angle (DMAA) (see later discussion).

PREOPERATIVE PLANNING

Decision-making in bunion surgery starts with an in-depth history and careful physical examination. A patient's symptoms help to define the area of pain.

During the physical examination, an assessment of the neurovascular status is important to help predict healing capacity and the absence of diabetes or peripheral vascular disease. The foot is examined with the patient in a sitting and standing position and inspected for pes planus, intractable plantar keratosis, other areas of callous formation, lesser toe deformities, and the presence or absence of an interdigital neuroma. The skin overlying the medial eminence is assessed for blistering or potential skin breakdown. Range of motion of the hallux is evaluated and the magnitude of pronation of the great toe is assessed.

Weight-bearing anteroposterior radiographs, lateral radiographs, and sesamoid views are obtained. The 1–2 intermetatarsal angle is quantified (normal $\leq 9°$). The hallux valgus angle is also measured (normal $\leq 15°$) (Fig. 1).

The first MPT joint is inspected for evidence of degenerative arthritis. The forefoot is inspected for the presence of significant metatarsus adductus. Either is a contraindication for this procedure. A significant hallux valgus deformity may occur even if the 1–2 intermetatarsal angle is measured as normal due to significant metatarsus adductus. In this situation, a first metatarsal osteotomy cannot realign the first ray as there is insufficient room for a lateral displacement of the first metatarsal with the osteotomy.

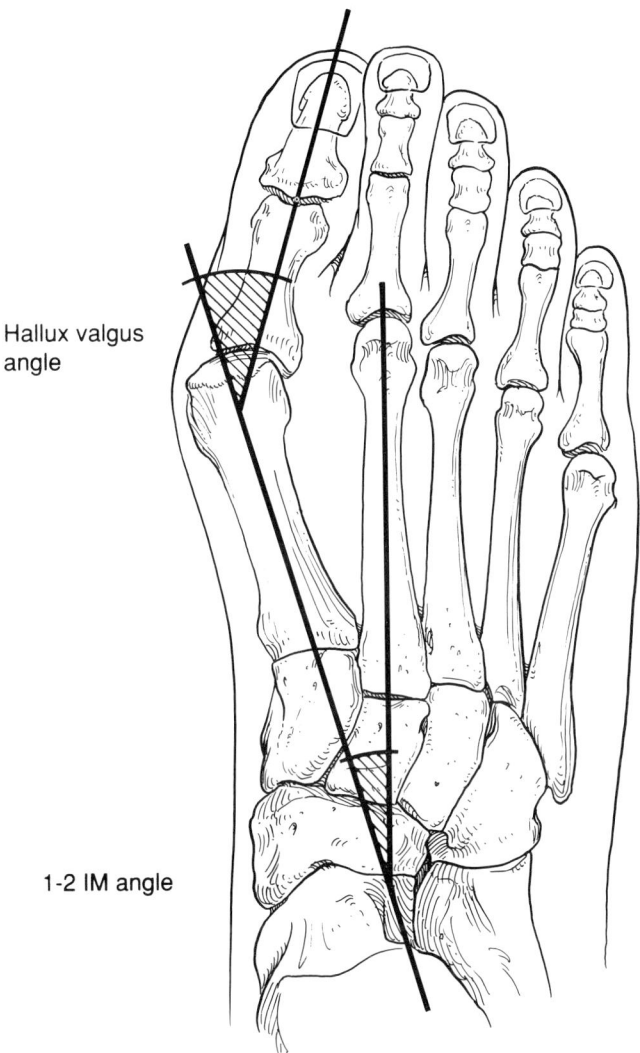

Figure 1. The hallux valgus angle describes the magnitude of the angular deformity at the first metatarsophalangeal (MP) joint. The 1–2 intermetatarsal (IM) angle describes the magnitude of divergence of the first and second metatarsals.

The congruency of the first metatarsophalangeal joint is assessed. This is the relationship between the corresponding articular surfaces of the first metatarsal head and the base of the proximal phalanx. The DMAA is formed by the angle created by two lines—one line bisects the longitudinal axis of the first metatarsal and the second line connects the medial and lateral edges of the articular surfaces of the first metatarsal head. The DMAA relates the inclination of the metatarsal head articular surface to the longitudinal axis of the first metatarsal. Normally this angle varies from 0° to 8°. An examiner must assess the magnitude of the DMAA as a hallux valgus deformity may result entirely from this inclination. When a significant DMAA is present, a surgical attempt to reduce or realign the proximal phalanx on the laterally inclined metatarsal articular surface will create an abnormal articulation that may eventually result in (a) recurrence of deformity, (b) metatarsophalangeal joint stiffness, (c) degenerative arthritis of the first metatarsophalangeal joint.

The magnitude of the hallux valgus angle must be correlated with whether the first metatarsophalangeal joint is congruent or incongruent as well as the magnitude of the DMAA (1). In a congruent joint, the proximal phalangeal articular surface is centered on the articular surface of the first metatarsal head. With an incongruent joint, the proximal phalanx is subluxated or displaced in relationship to the first metatarsal articular surface (Fig. 2).

If, on the contrary, the first metatarsophalangeal joint articulation is incongruent (or subluxated), the proximal phalanx can be realigned to the metatarsal head articular surface with an intraarticular realignment such as a distal soft tissue realignment.

The size of the medial eminence is determined on the radiograph by drawing a line from the medial border of the first metatarsal shaft. The medial eminence may be small, medium, or large in size. The position of the sagittal sulcus (Fig. 3) is an unreliable reference for the medial eminence resection since it migrates lateralward with an increased hallux valgus deformity. In severe deformities, a sagittal sulcus may be located in the midportion of the metatarsal head and lead to an excessive resection if used as a landmark for the medial eminence resection.

In a normal situation, the sesamoids are located beneath the metatarsal head. With increasing deformity, the fibular sesamoid lies exposed on an AP radiograph along the lateral border of the first metatarsal head. The magnitude of this exposure depends upon the severity of the hallux valgus deformity and the amount of pronation of the great toe.

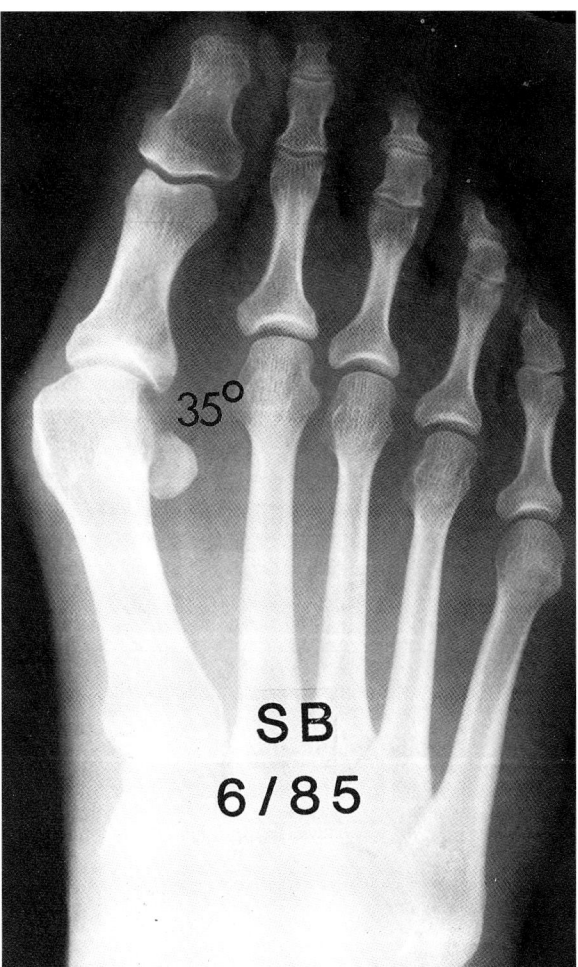

Figure 2. Subluxated metatarsophalangeal joint with hallux valgus angle of 35°, 1–2 IM angle of 18°.

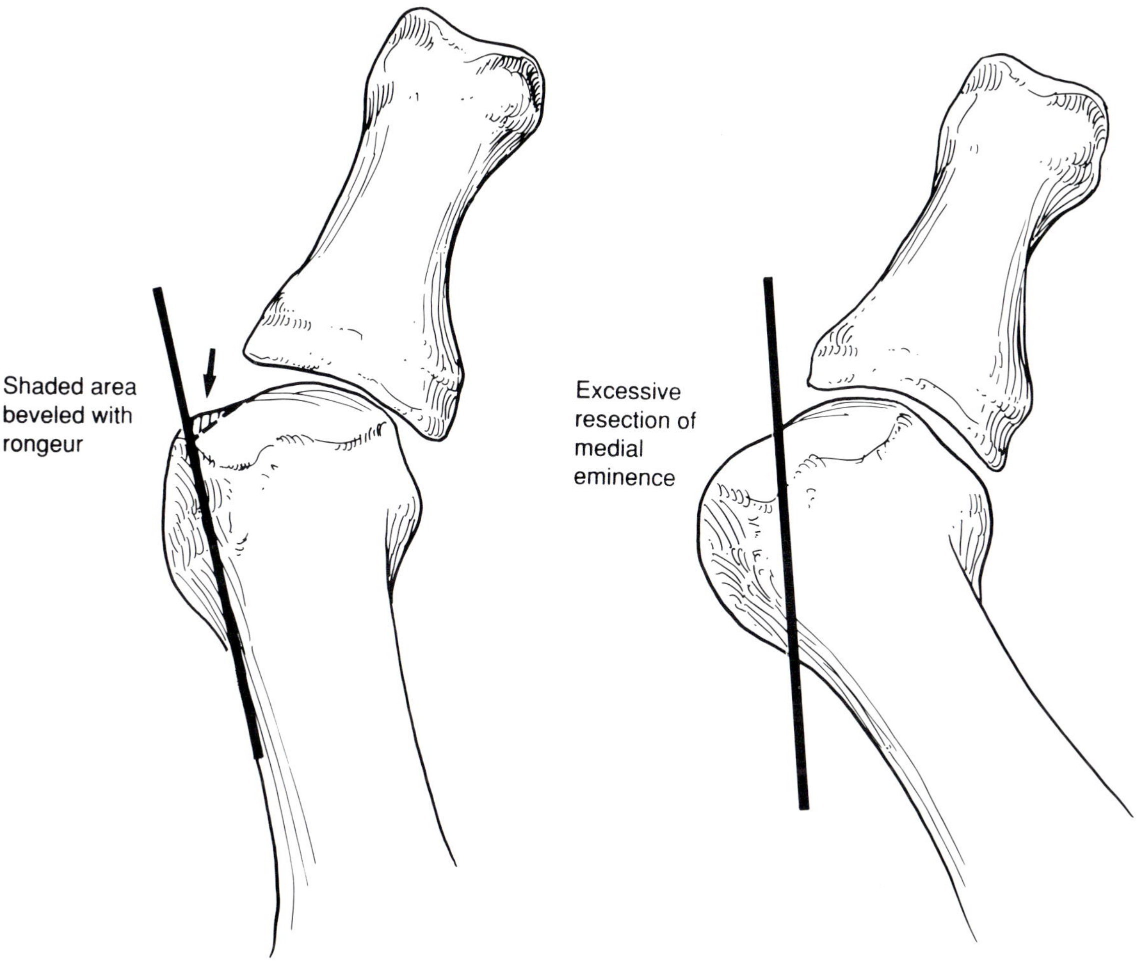

Figure 3. The sagittal sulcus is an unreliable reference for the medial eminence resection. With a small eminence, the sulcus may be the site of osteotomy. With a more severe deformity, the sulcus may be too lateral and if used will lead to an excessive resection.

In order to achieve a successful and stable correction of a hallux valgus deformity, an attempt must be made to correct all elements of the deformity present including an increased 1–2 intermetatarsal angle, an increased hallux valgus angle, a prominent medial eminence, sesamoid subluxation, and pronation of the great toe. A less than total correction of these elements may lead to recurrence of the deformity.

A DSTR with PMO may be performed on an outpatient or inpatient basis, depending on the patient's and surgeon's preference and insurance reimbursement policy. The procedure may be performed under general or regional anesthetic; however, a foot block achieves adequate anesthesia and provides long-lasting pain relief and is my preference.

SURGERY

The patient is placed in a supine position on the surgical table. The foot and lower leg are cleansed in a routine fashion. The foot is exsanguinated with an Esmarch bandage. Padding is placed around the ankle and the Esmarch bandage is used as a tourniquet. With an ankle block anesthetic, the patient is usually comfortable with an ankle tourniquet; however, on occasion, IV midazolam hydrochloride may be used to augment patient relaxation. The surgeon sits on a stool next to the contralateral leg, across the table from the operative foot. This position is used for the intermetatarsal approach. For the medial approach and the metatarsal osteotomy, the surgeon sits on the ipsilateral side looking down on the operative foot.

Technique. A 3-cm dorsal longitudinal incision is centered in the first intermetatarsal web space beginning at the distal extent of the web space and extending proximally (Fig. 4). The subcutaneous tissue is sharply incised and the first and second metatarsals are distracted with a Weitlaner retractor, exposing the conjoined adductor tendon. The tendon is dissected free from the lateral border of the sesamoid. The lateral sesamoid is completely freed up, *but is not excised*. The sesamoid is freed up on its lateral and plantar border and is released from its dorsal attachments. The metatarsal-sesamoid ligament is detached on the superior aspect of the lateral sesamoid (Fig. 5). The distal adductor tendon insertion is left attached to the base of the proximal phalanx with a stump of approximately 2 cm of tendon remaining. The tendon is released at the level of the musculotendinous junction and the adductor hallucis muscle is allowed to retract (Fig. 6). A suture is placed in the tendon stump and this is later repaired to the lateral metatarsal capsule (Fig. 7). The transverse intermetatarsal ligament is incised with care taken to avoid injury to either the common digital nerve that lies directly beneath the transverse intermetatarsal ligament, or the flexor hallucis longus tendon. The lateral metatarsophalangeal joint capsule is then perforated with several puncture wounds and the toe is angulated medially, causing a disruption of the lateral capsule. It is important to avoid an abrupt incision in the lateral capsule as this may leave a paucity of scar tissue. This tissue is needed to help provide postoperative stability on the lateral aspect of the first metatarsophalangeal joint. Also, the stump of conjoined tendon that is preserved and later sutured into the lateral metatarsophalangeal capsule helps to minimize the possibility of a postoperative

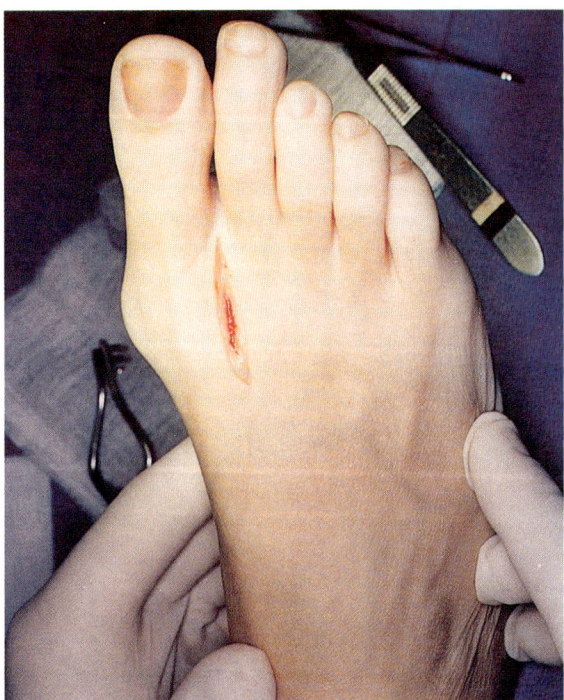

Figure 4. First intermetatarsal incision.

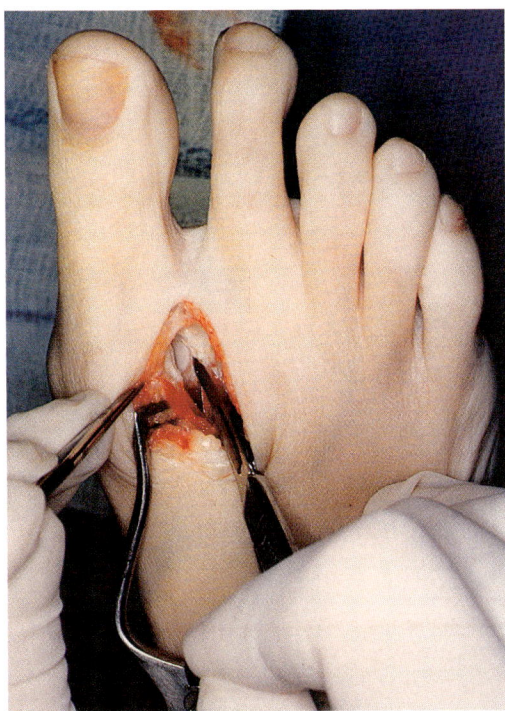

Figure 5. The sesamoid is completely freed upon on a superior aspect.

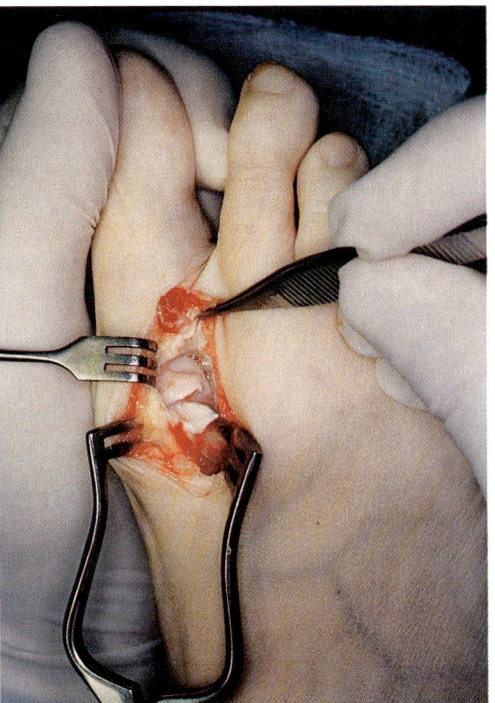

Figure 6. A lateral capsular release has been performed and a 2-cm stump of adductor tendon is retained to later repair, creating a cuff of capsule on the lateral aspect of the MP joint. (The tendon is held within the forceps.)

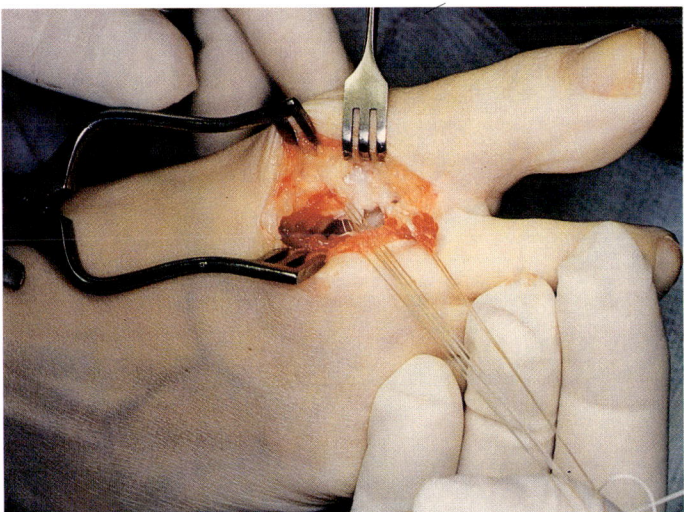

Figure 7. Three interrupted sutures are placed between the first and second MP capsule. A fourth suture is placed in the stump of adductor tendon.

hallux varus deformity. Three interrupted 2-0 absorbable sutures are placed to reef the first and second MP capsules and are later tied at the conclusion of the surgery (see Fig. 17).

A longitudinal medial incision is centered over the medial eminence beginning at the midportion of the proximal phalanx and extending 1 cm above the medial eminence. The dissection is carried directly down to the medial capsule. Care is

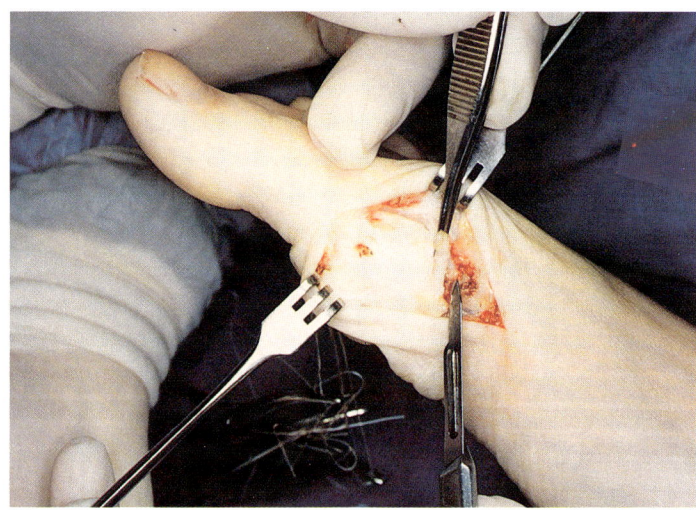

Figure 8. An L-shaped capsular release is carried out on the dorsal and proximal aspect.

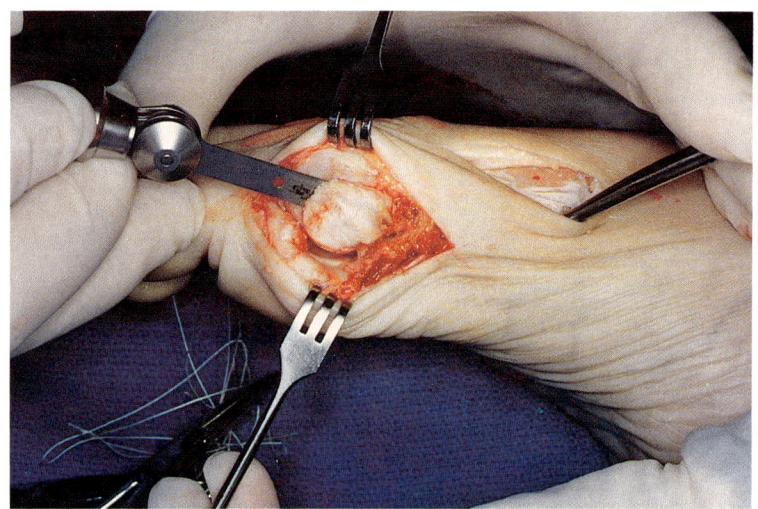

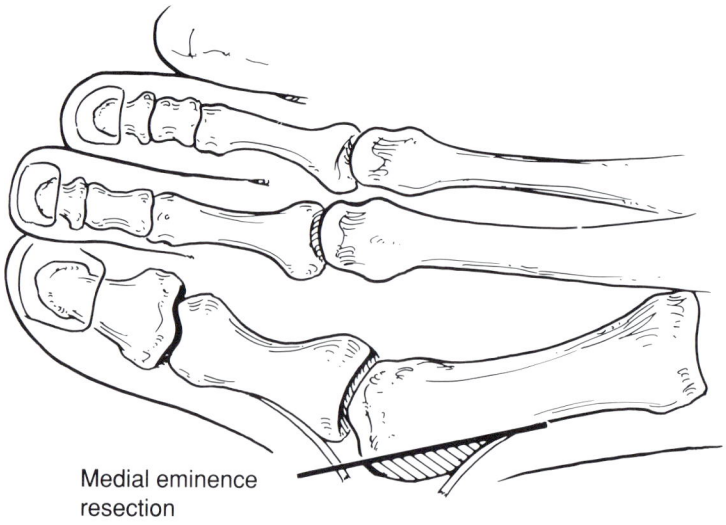

Medial eminence resection

Figure 9. A: The flap is turned downward and a sagittal saw is used to remove the medial eminence in line with the medial cortex of the first metatarsal. **B:** The medial eminence resection osteotomy is in line with the medial first metatarsal cortex.

taken to protect the medial dorsal and medial plantar digital nerves, which are swept both in a dorsal and plantar direction and protected with retractors. With a midline incision, deepened directly to the capsule, the dorsomedial sensory nerve is protected and retracted. It lies right on the capsule and may be inadvertently injured if it is not located and protected. An L-shaped distally based capsular flap is developed, releasing the capsule on the dorsal and proximal aspect (Fig. 8). The weakest attachments of the capsule are on the proximal and dorsal aspects. The strongest attachments, on the plantar and distal aspect, are preserved. This allowed excellent visualization of the first metatarsal shaft for the osteotomy of the medial eminence.

The capsule is retracted and the medial eminence is resected with an oscillating saw in a line parallel with the diaphyseal cortex of the first metatarsal (Fig. 9).

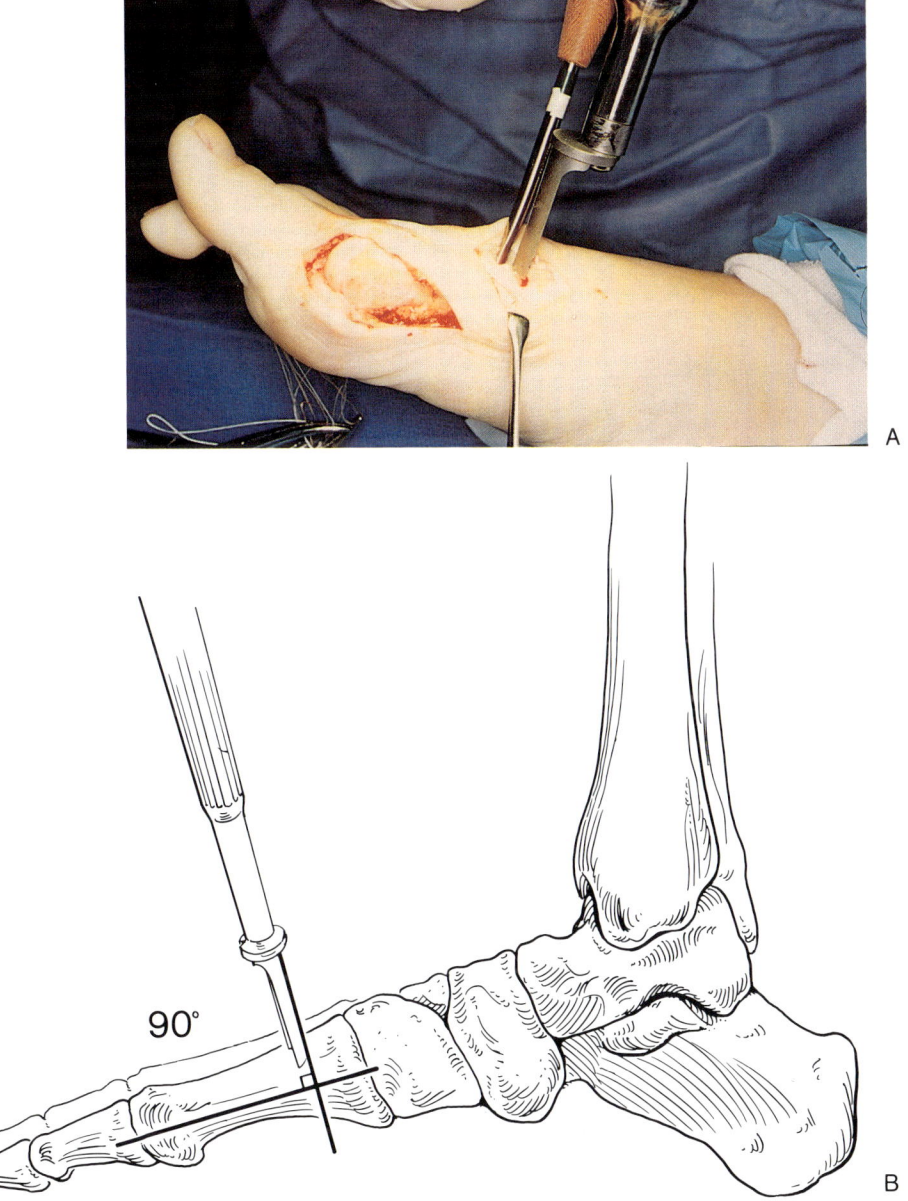

Figure 10. A: Osteotomy with excess vertical position of saw. **B:** This osteotomy is too perpendicular to the first metatarsal shaft decreasing the surface area and increasing the possibility of a dorsiflexion malunion.

Excessive resection is the most common cause of a postoperative varus deformity. The medial capsular exposure described gives a good distal view of the metatarsal shaft. A retractor can be placed in the proximal metatarsal incision and thus the proximal first metatarsal shaft can be delineated. By visualizing the first metatarsal shaft when resecting the medial eminence, an osteotomy "in-line" with the medial border of the first metatarsal shaft is performed. If the sagittal sulcus is located lateral to the medial eminence osteotomy, the prominent edge of the sulcus can be beveled with a rongeur. Use of the sagittal sulcus as a landmark for the medial eminence resection is unreliable, and in severe deformities may lead to an excessive resection.

Technique. A 3-cm dorsal longitudinal incision is centered over the dorsal proximal first metatarsal along the medial border of the extensor hallucis longus tendon.

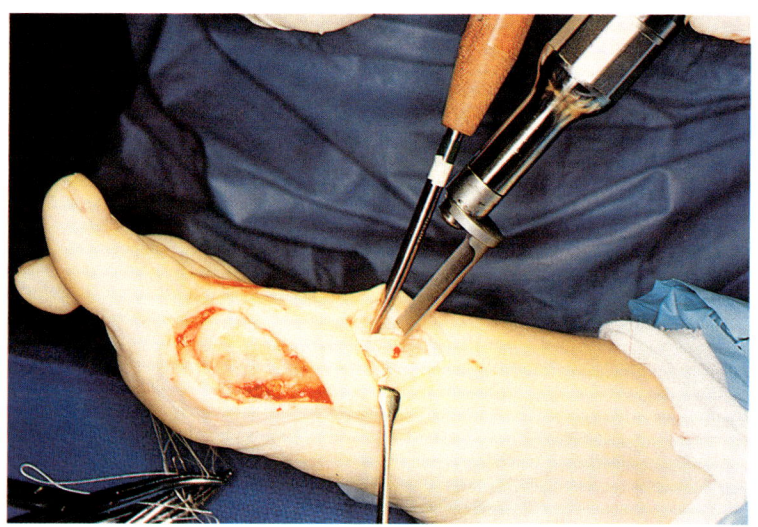

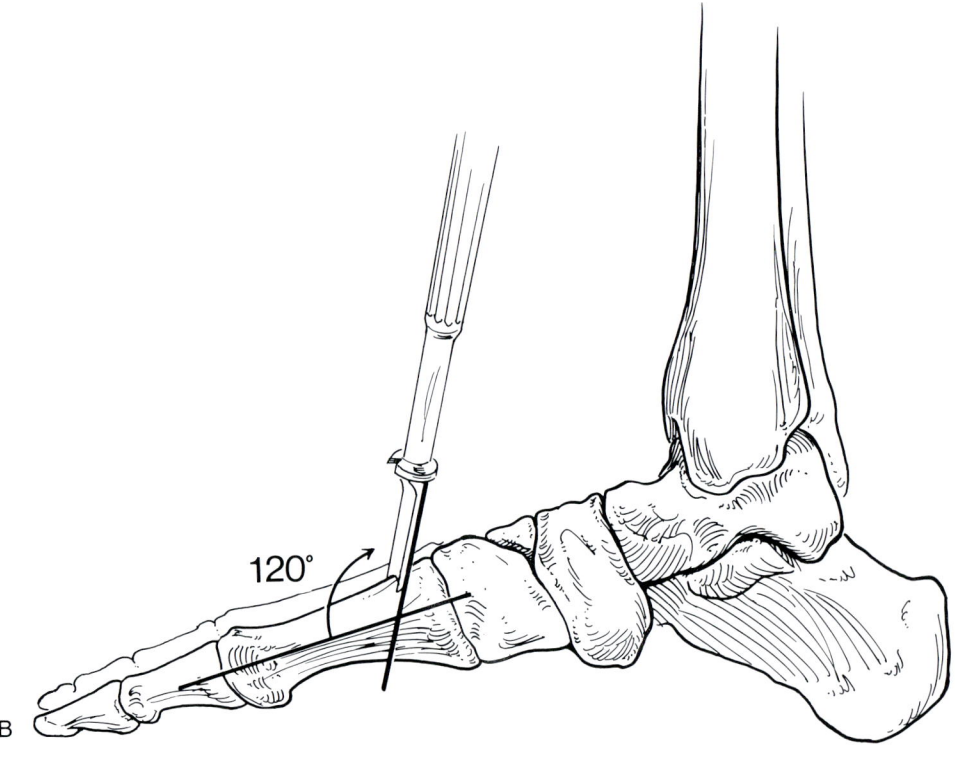

Figure 11. A: Correct angle of osteotomy. **B:** An ideal osteotomy angle at a 120° angle with the first metatarsal shaft.

The dissection is carried down to the first metatarsal shaft and the periosteum is stripped medially and laterally. The metatarsocuneiform joint is identified. A mark is placed on the first metatarsal 1 cm distal to the metatarsocuneiform joint and this is the location of the most proximal extent of the crescentic osteotomy. A Stryker microsaw provides an easily adaptable power source that can be used for the sagittal saw, curved saw, power drill, and Kirschner wire driver. A curved saw-blade (catalogue no. S5053-71A, Zimmer Co., Warsaw, IN) is used for the crescentic osteotomy. The osteotomy is oriented in a dorsal-plantar direction at a 120° angle to the metatarsal shaft. Care is taken to make the osteotomy neither perpendicular to the first metatarsal shaft nor too oblique in relationship to the first metatarsal shaft (Figs. 10, 11, and 12). The concave surface may be distal or proximal depending upon the surgeon's preference (Fig. 13).

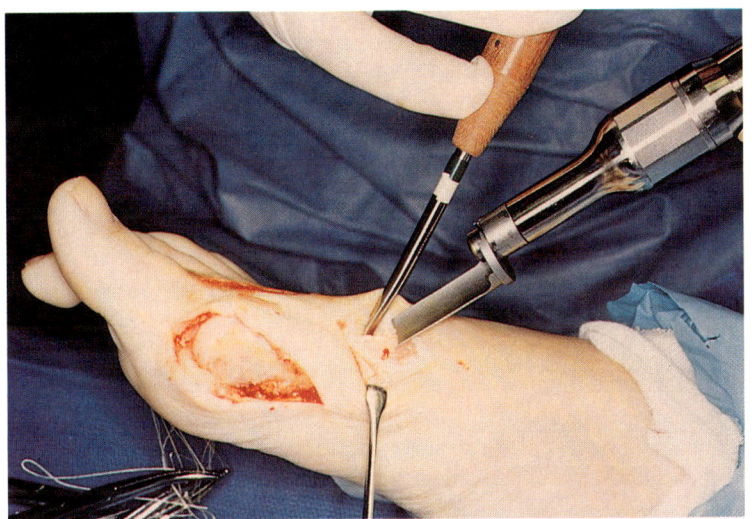

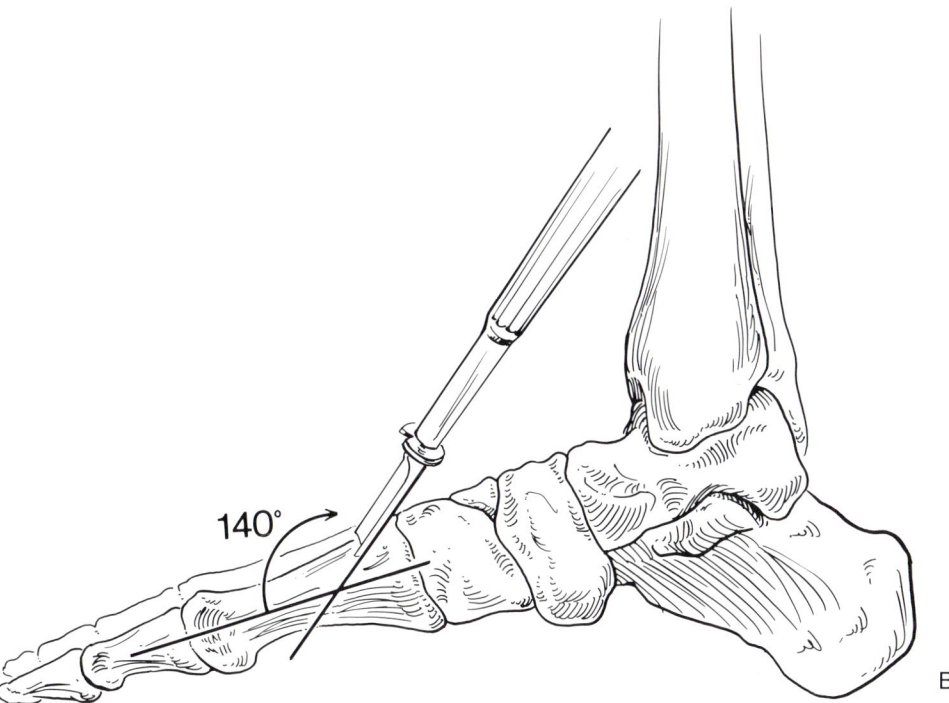

Figure 12. **A:** Excess obliquity of osteotomy saw. **B:** This osteotomy is too oblique to the first metatarsal shaft creating too long an osteotomy for the length of the saw blade.

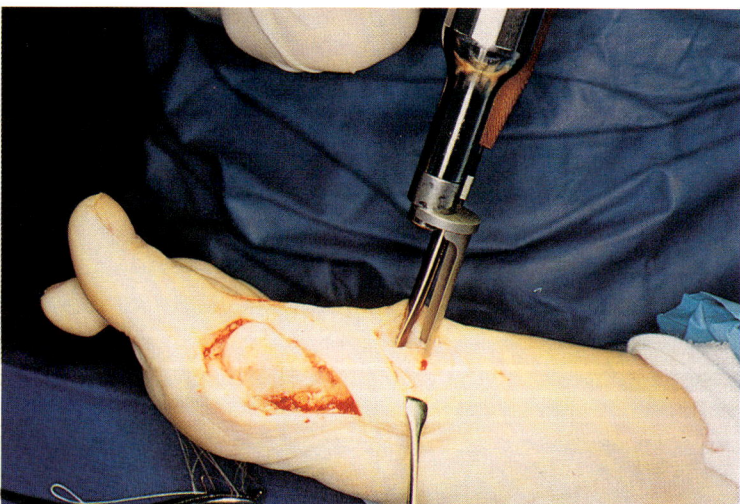

Figure 13. Technique of reverse angle, "dome distal" for proximal osteotomy.

There has been considerable debate regarding the orientation of the saw blade. It may be placed concave distal or in a concave proximal direction. Concave proximal allows the osteotomy to displace easily; however, it is easier also to overcorrect the osteotomy with this orientation. The use of intraoperative radiography enables the surgeon to assure that he is not overcorrecting the osteotomy site. A concave distal osteotomy is more difficult to displace, but does appear to to decrease the chance of overcorrection. Internal fixation with this osteotomy (concave distal) is placed approximately 8 mm distal on the metatarsal shaft, which may necessitate closer approximation of the surgical incisions.

The direction of the saw can be varied in both a distal/proximal and medial/lateral plane. Medial orientation of the saw may cause pronation of the toe and elevation of the metatarsal distally. Lateral orientation of the saw may cause supination of the toe and depression of the metatarsal head. It is desirable to maintain the saw in a neutral medial/lateral plane.

Distal/proximal inclination of the saw blade may occur as well. A distal inclination creates an osteotomy at close to a 90° angle with the metatarsal shaft and decreases the surface contact area. This may cause an increased incidence of dorsiflexion malunion at the osteotomy site. A proximal inclination creates a more oblique osteotomy (approximating 135°) and is more difficult to cut, requiring a longer osteotomy. It may also be more difficult to displace (Figs. 10 and 11).

Ideally, an osteotomy at an angle of approximately 120° is desired in relationship to the metatarsal shaft. The osteotomy is displaced by dialing the displacement. The major correction of the hallux valgus deformity occurs here. Reduction of the 1–2 intermetatarsal angle to where the first and second metatarsals are parallel helps to reduce the hallux valgus angular deformity as well. A 2 to 3 mm displacement at the osteotomy site is typically sufficient to correct the 1–2 intermetatarsal angle. Parallelism of the first and second metatarsals may be checked with intraoperative fluoroscopy. Displacement of the osteotomy site may occur due to inadequate internal fixation.

If the first metatarsal metaphysis is unusually thick, an osteotome may be needed to complete the plantar cut. The proximal fragment is displaced medially with a small elevator and the distal fragment is then rotated in a lateral direction 2 to 3 mm to reduce the 1–2 intermetatarsal angle. Care must be taken not to overcorrect the osteotomy site and create a negative 1–2 intermetatarsal angle. The osteotomy is initially fixed with a 0.062 Kirschner wire (Fig 14). The screw is not countersunk, so that it may be easily removed. A lag compression screw

8 PROXIMAL FIRST METATARSAL OSTEOTOMY

is then used to fix the osteotomy (Fig. 15). The Kirschner wire and screw fixation give rotational stability and helps to reduce the tendency for dorsiflexion at the osteotomy site. A 3.5-mm drill hole is placed in the distal fragment and a 2.5-mm drill hole is placed in the proximal fragment. The fixation hole is tapped and a compression screw fixes and compresses the osteotomy site (Fig. 16). Buried

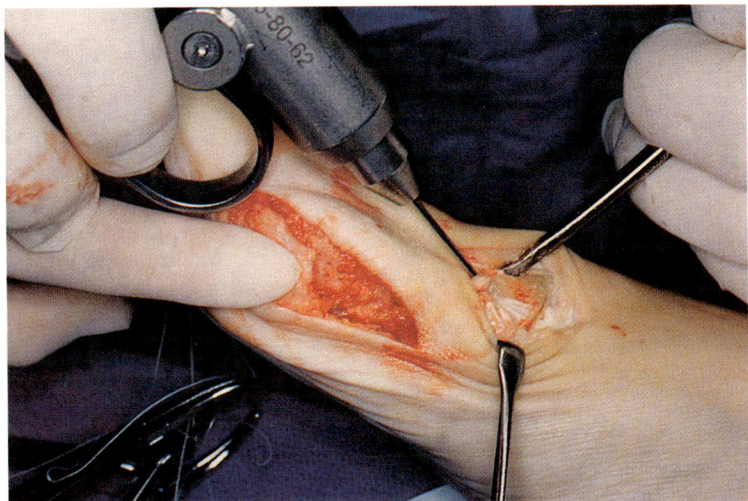

Figure 14. After the osteotomy has been displaced it is initially fixed with an 0.062 K-wire.

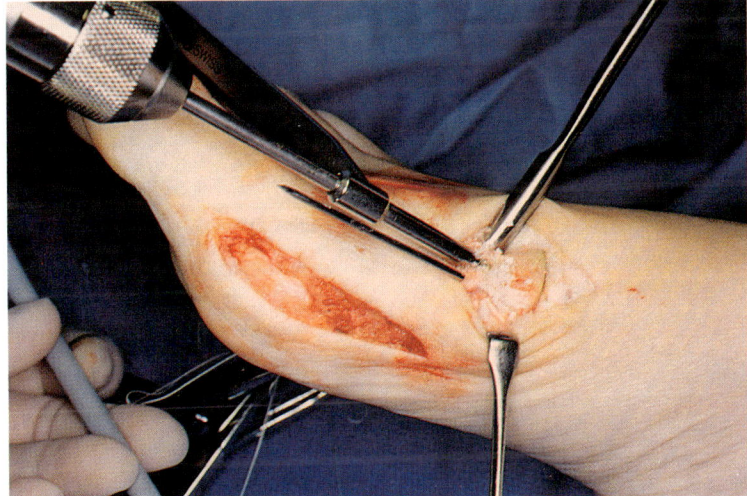

Figure 15. A lag drill hole is placed in the distal fragment.

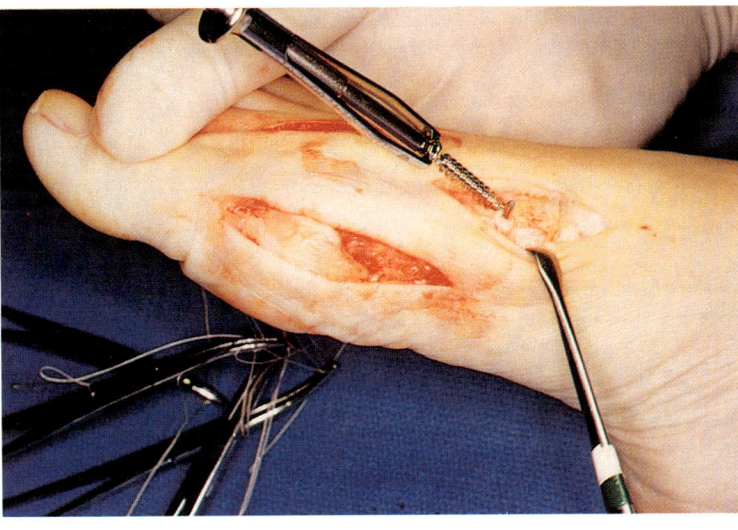

Figure 16. A lag screw is placed to secure the osteotomy. (The K-wire and pin are left in place.)

internal fixation avoids pin tract infections. The distal screw hole is placed approximately 8 to 10 mm distal to the osteotomy site. Typically, internal fixation pins are removed 6 weeks following surgery.

Following stabilization of the osteotomy, the transverse metatarsal arch is compressed and the intermetatarsal sutures are tied (Fig. 17), after which the adductor hallux tendon is sutured to the lateral metatarsal capsule (Fig. 18).

Intraoperative radiographs or fluoroscopy (Fig. 19) are beneficial in order to evaluate the correction of the 1–2 intermetatarsal angle as well as to evaluate the position of the internal fixation and the correction of the hallux valgus angle. On clinical examination during surgery, the first ray may appear to be well aligned, but the metatarsophalangeal articulation may be under- or overcorrected. Intraoperative radiographic evaluation of the alignment is helpful to decrease recurrence as well as overcorrection.

Then with the toe held in a derotated corrected position, the medial capsule is repaired with interrupted 2-0 Vicryl suture. A fixation hole may be placed in the dorsal proximal metaphysis in order to give an anchor hole for the capsular repair (Figs. 20 and 21). The L-shaped medial capsular cuff is a very strong anchor that can derotate as well as correct valgus malalignment of the great toe. The medial capsular repair is critical to the metatarsophalangeal joint realignment. A subtotal repair risks recurrence while an overcorrection may lead to a hallux varus deformity. At the completion of the procedure, the great toe rests in a corrected position without any dressing support (Fig. 22).

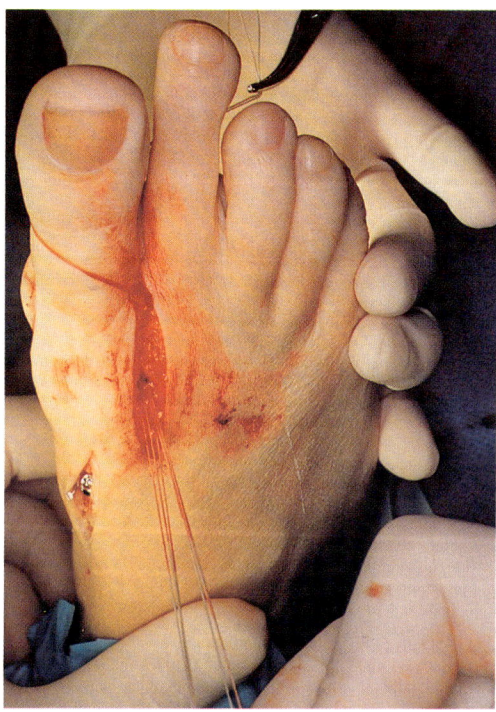

Figure 17. With the transverse metatarsal arch compressed, the intermetatarsal sutures are tied.

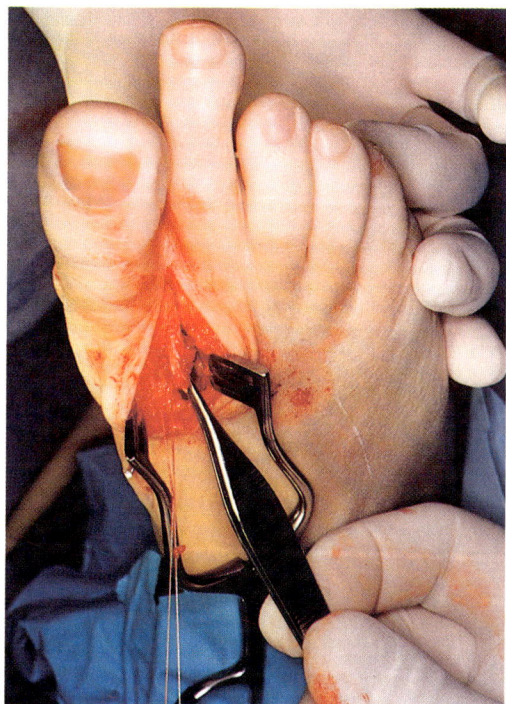

Figure 18. With tension placed on the stump of adductor tendon, it is then sutured into the lateral capsule.

8 PROXIMAL FIRST METATARSAL OSTEOTOMY

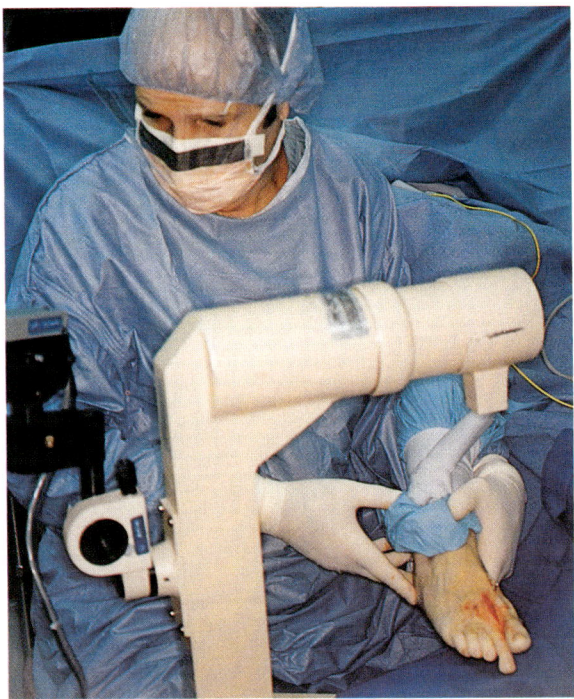

Figure 19. A mini-image intensifier is used to view the alignment of the first metatarsal and the first MP joint.

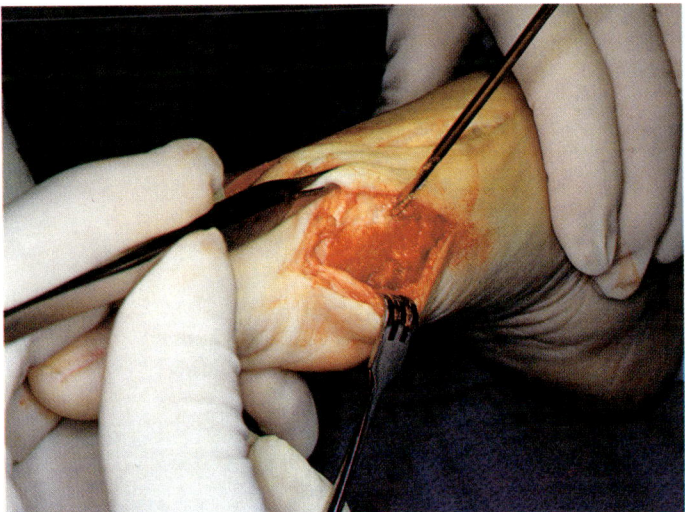

Figure 20. A drill hole is placed in the dorsal proximal first metatarsal to anchor the dorsal proximal corner of the medial capsule.

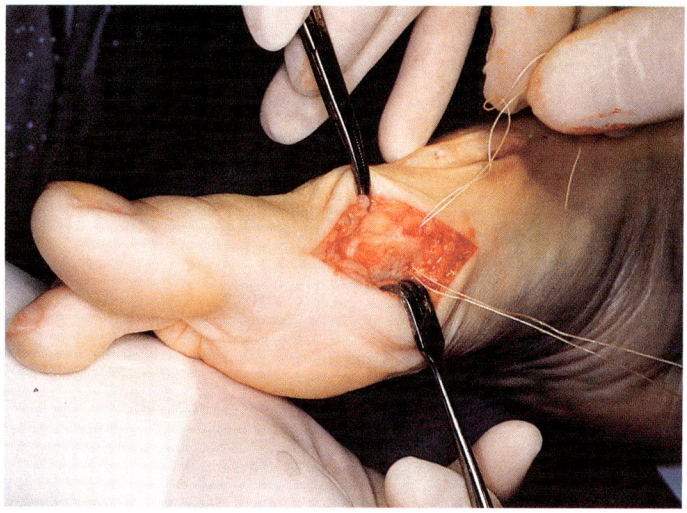

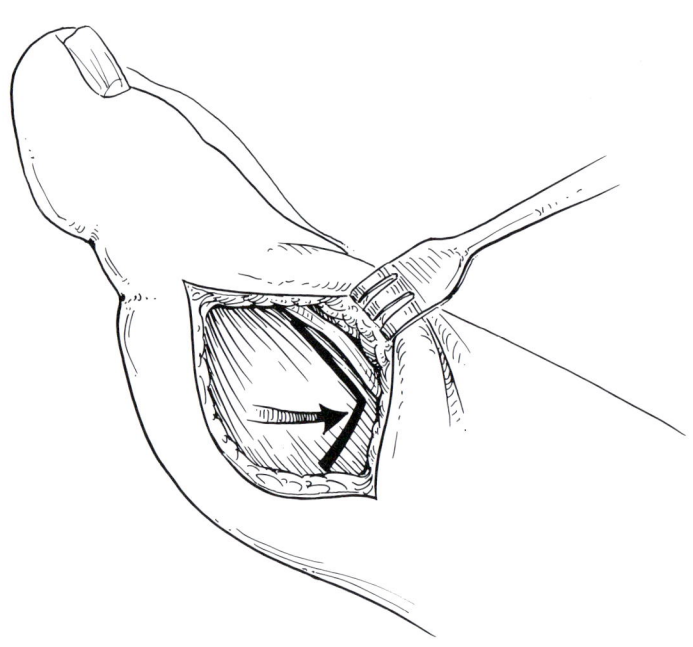

Figure 21. A: The capsule is secured with interrupted 2-0 absorbable sutures. **B:** The capsule is advanced, pulling the flap apex dorsally and proximally to help realign the great toe.

POSTOPERATIVE MANAGEMENT

After completion of the surgical procedure as described, the foot is enclosed in fluffed gauze and wrapped in a 2-inch Kling compression dressing (Fig. 23). The patient is instructed to elevate the foot on two pillows and use ice as tolerated. Crutches or a walker is used depending on a patient's preference. The patient bears weight initially on the heel and later on the outside of the foot. Six weeks following surgery, a flat-footed gait is permitted.

One to two days after surgery the dressing is changed. A gauze and tape toe spica gauze dressing is applied and changed on a weekly basis for 7 more weeks. The patient is allowed to ambulate in a postoperative shoe. At about 6 weeks, a roomy sandal is permitted. At 3 weeks following surgery, the patient is instructed

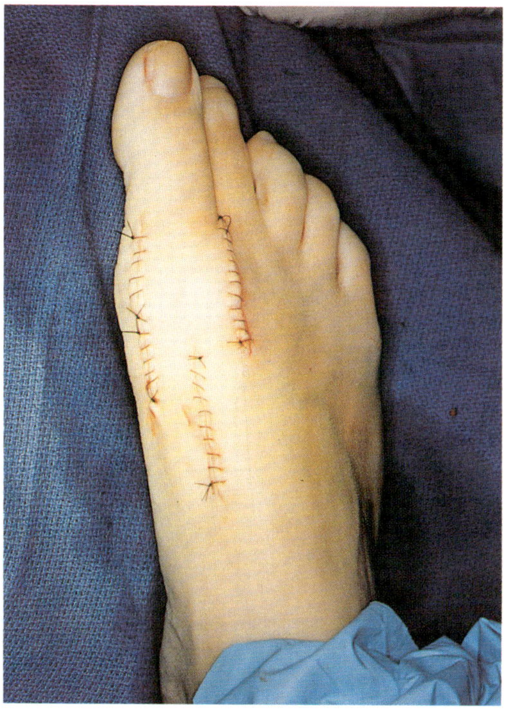

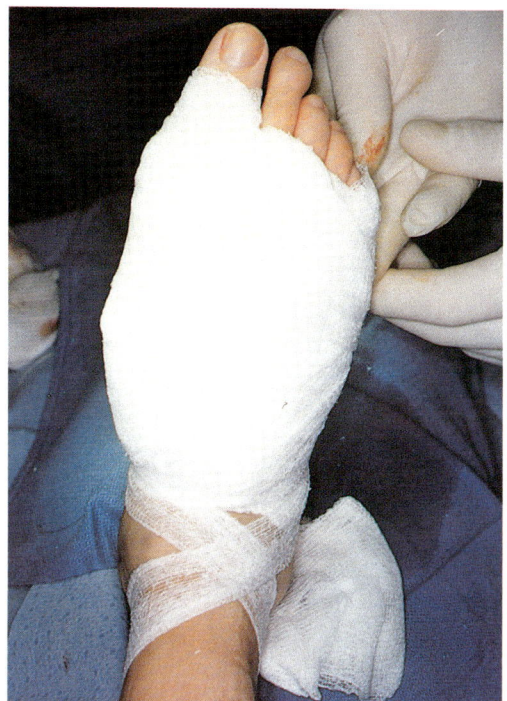

Figure 22. Foot appearance following completion of the procedure.

Figure 23. A bulky gauze and tape dressing is used postoperatively.

to start dorsal/plantar flexion stretching exercises of the toe within the confines of the tape dressing.

Following the discontinuance of dressings at 8 weeks, a more aggressive range of motion and stretching is initiated.

A frank preoperative discussion with the patient is important to cover not only patient expectations, but the surgeon's goals as well. If the procedure is selected for the patient group described, 90% to 95% patient satisfaction can be expected on a long-term basis (5).

Two-thirds of patients will be able to wear shoes that they desire (3); however, one-third of patients may still have shoe-wear restrictions. Pain relief is uniformly good and relief of associated metatarsalgia is common.

COMPLICATIONS

Complications unique to the DSTR and PMO can occur. Some of the major complications include recurrence of deformity, hallux varus or overcorrection, malalignment of the osteotomy, and delayed union. Each of these will be described separately and their prevention considered along with suggested management of the complication.

1. *Recurrent hallux valgus deformity.* This problem may result due to an insufficient lateral release, lack of reduction of the sesamoids, lack of an osteotomy, insufficient correction of the osteotomy, inadequate medial capsular plication, or inadequate correction of pronation. Complete correction at the time of surgery is the best insurance against redeformity. A redo of the procedure may be necessary if a significant redeformation occurs.

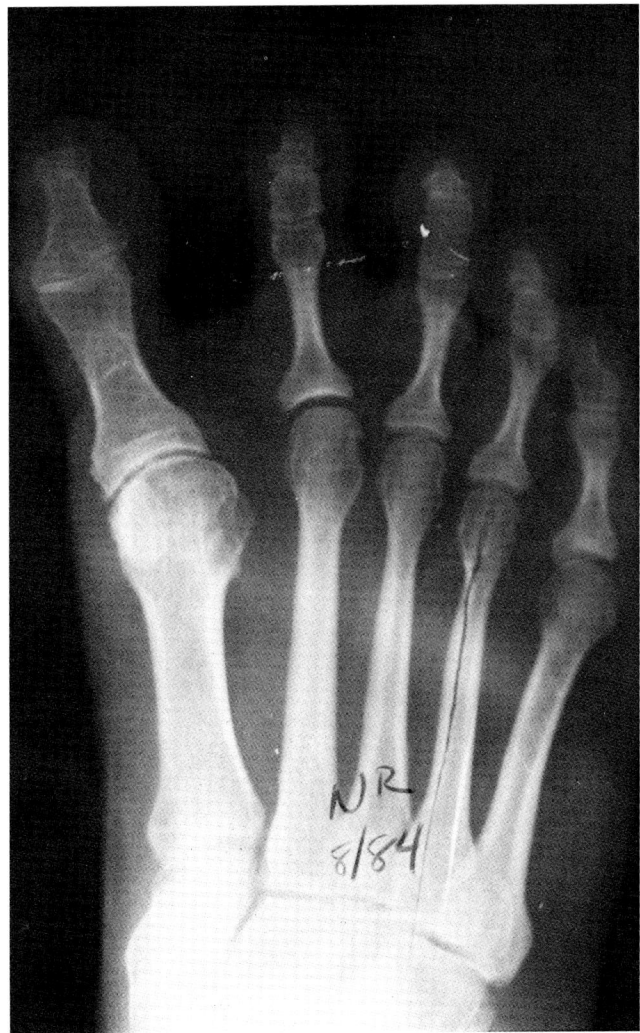

Figure 24. Following DSTR, and overcorrection has resulted. The medial sesamoid was excised. Sesamoid excision should be avoided if possible.

2. *Hallux varus.* Overcorrection or hallux varus may occur for a number of reasons (Fig. 24); overplication of the medial capsule, excessive medial eminence resection, lack of sufficient lateral capsular tissue reformation to stabilize the lateral joint, and overcorrection of the osteotomy may lead to a hallux varus deformity. Intraoperative radiography helps to insure proper alignment of the first metatarsal osteotomy and the metatarsophalangeal joint realignment. Depending upon the cause, correction of a hallux varus deformity may be achieved with a soft tissue realignment, redo osteotomy, tendon transfer (Fig. 25) (2) or metatarsophalangeal joint arthrodesis.
3. *Osteotomy delayed union.* Infrequently, one may encounter a delayed union with a first metatarsal osteotomy. The major symptoms are continued swelling and vague aching at the osteotomy site. Often the application of a below-knee walking cast will enable an expeditious healing of the osteotomy site. Excessive soft tissue stripping should be avoided at the osteotomy site.
4. *Osteotomy malunion.* Malunion of the osteotomy site can be a very difficult problem to treat. Overcorrection if severe may lead to hallux varus deformity. The surgical salvage requires a complex and extensive redo procedure with a take down of the osteotomy site and realignment, and medial capsule release

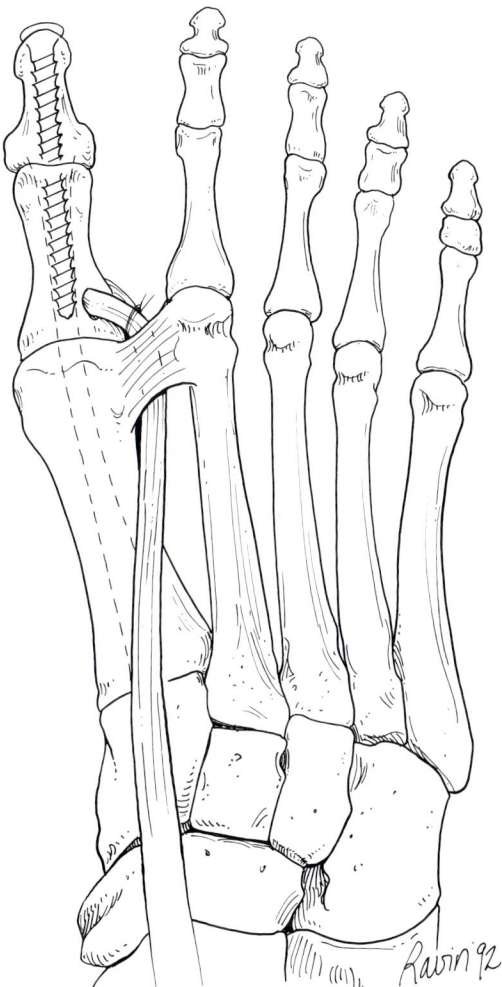

Figure 25. Diagrammatic representation of Johnson procedure (2) for hallux varus.

and realignment. A lateral capsular reefing may be necessary. The best treatment of this difficult problem is prevention. Intraoperative radiography may help to diminish the incidence of overcorrection of the osteotomy site. Dorsiflexion malunion may occur as well. Rigid internal fixation with a lag screw and Kirschner wire seems to not only prevent rotation, but gives increased stability and decreases the incidence of a dorsiflexion malunion.

ILLUSTRATIVE CASE FOR TECHNIQUE

This 43-year-old woman complained of pain over the medial eminence and increased width of her forefoot, and a symptomatic bunionette deformity. She had noticed progression of the deformity over the last 5 years and found an increased inability to wear moderately fashionable shoes. Due to continued pain she was able to wear only sneakers, which were not acceptable at work.

On physical examination, an enlarged and reddened prominence was observed over the medial eminence. Range of motion of the metatarsophalangeal joint was measured at 60° dorsiflexion, 20° plantar flexion. Range of motion remained acceptable with varus-valgus passive motion.

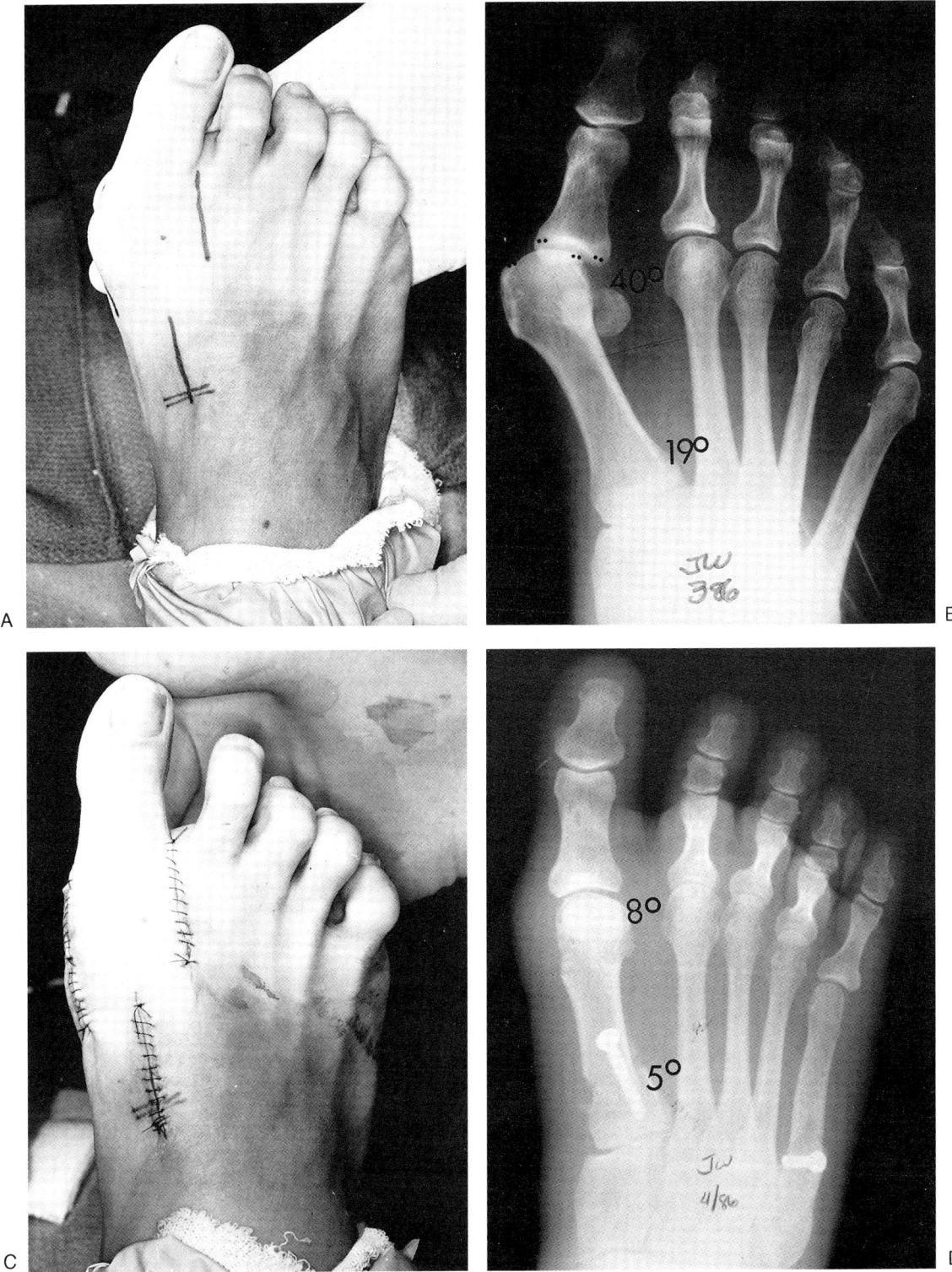

Figure 26. A: Preoperative photograph of foot. **B:** Preoperative radiograph demonstrating splay foot with 1–2 intermetatarsal angle of 19° and hallux valgus angle of 40°. The radiograph shows obvious subluxation of the first metatarsophalangeal joint. **C:** Immediately following operative correction. **D:** Following DSTR with PMO (and bunionette repair) the 1–2 intermetatarsal angle is 5° and the hallux valgus angle is 8°.

Weight-bearing radiographs of the foot demonstrated a 1–2 intermetatarsal angle of 19° and a hallux valgus angle of 40°. Sesamoid subluxation was noted with the lateral sesamoid completely subluxed into the first intermetatarsal space and the medial sesamoid laterally (Fig. 26A,B) beneath the first metatarsal head. The first metatarsophalangeal joint was incongruent or subluxated. No degenerative joint disease was demonstrated on either the AP or lateral radiograph.

A distal soft tissue realignment with proximal crescentic osteotomy was performed under a foot block (Fig. 26C). A bunionette repair was also performed. The patient was admitted as a short stay patient overnight and the dressing was changed the next day before discharge. She was discharged home, ambulating in a postoperative shoe with crutches. Dressings were changed on a weekly basis for 8 weeks following surgery. Sutures were removed 3 weeks after surgery. Radiographs were taken at 1 week postoperatively and demonstrated acceptable alignment. Six weeks following surgery, repeat radiographs demonstrated a healed (Fig. 26D) osteotomy site and the screw and Kirschner wire were removed under local anesthesia in an office setting.

The radiographs 6 weeks after surgery show the surgical correction. The 1–2 intermetatarsal angle has been decreased to 5° and the hallux valgus angle has been improved to 8°. The sesamoids have been successfully realigned. The screw head was not countersunk to aid in removal. At follow-up 2 years after surgery, the patient noted no pain or decreased range of motion and was pleased with her result.

RECOMMENDED READING

1. Coughlin, M. J.: Juvenile bunions. In: *Surgery of the Foot and Ankle*, 6th ed., edited by R. A. Mann and M. J. Coughlin, C. V. Mosby, St. Louis, 1992, pp. 297–340.
2. Johnson, K. A., and Spiegl, P. V.: Extensor hallucis longus transfer for hallux varus deformity. *J. Bone Joint Surg.*, 66A: 681–686, 1984.
3. Mann, R. A.: Decision-making in bunion surgery. In: *AAOS Instructional Course Lectures*, Vol 40. American Academy of Orthopaedic Surgeons, Chicago, IL. 1992; pp. 3–13.
4. Mann, R. A., and Coughlin, M. J.: Adult hallux valgus. In: *Surgery of the Foot and Ankle*, 6th ed., edited by R. A. Mann and M. J. Coughlin, C. V. Mosby, St. Louis, 1992, pp. 167–296.
5. Mann, R. A., Rudicel, S., and Graves, S. C.: Repair of hallux valgus with a distal soft-tissue procedure and proximal metatarsal osteotomy. *J. Bone Joint Surg.*, 74A(1): 124–129, 1992.

9

Cuneiform–Metatarsal Arthrodesis

Mark S. Myerson

INDICATIONS/CONTRAINDICATIONS

Lapidus popularized the closing wedge arthrodesis of the first metatarsocuneiform joint for the correction of hallux valgus. Over the past four decades since Lapidus last reported this work, the indications for performing this procedure as well as the operative approach have significantly changed. The goals of this operation have nevertheless remained the same: to correct and stabilize the first metatarsal at the apex of the deformity. Metatarsus primus varus is often associated with a hypermobile first ray, characterized by an increased mobility of the metatarsal in both the horizontal and sagittal planes. The presence of hypermobility associated with hallux valgus and metatarsus primus varus remains the primary indication for this procedure.

Other indications for this operation are severe metatarsus primus varus, generalized ligamentous laxity, metatarsocuneiform arthritis, the adolescent bunion with moderate to severe deformity, and selected cases of revision surgery for failed bunionectomy. Although this is a good choice of operation for correction of severe hallux valgus, it should be used only if the metatarsophalangeal (MP) joint is mobile. This operation is an excellent choice in the adolescent particularly since recurrent deformity following adolescent bunionectomy is such a common problem. However, I would recommend that this procedure be performed only if the epiphysis is closed.

The procedure is generally used in the younger age group, and I seldom use it in a patient over 60 years of age. The older patients probably fare better with other procedures with less potential morbidity, where they may be ambulatory immediately postoperatively.

M. S. Myerson, M.D.: Foot & Ankle Center, Department of Orthopaedic Surgery, Union Memorial Hospital, Baltimore, MD 21218.

The metatarsocuneiform arthrodesis is generally performed where the intermetatarsal angle is 14° or more. If generalized metatarsus adductus is present, however, the intermetatarsal angle may be less than 14°, since the position of the first metatarsal with respect to the longitudinal axis of the foot is significantly greater. Painful arthritis of the first metatarsocuneiform joint may occur in the presence of symptomatic hallux valgus, and the optimal procedure would address both these problems simultaneously.

This operation is probably contraindicated in the presence of a short first metatarsal, since further shortening is an inherent potential problem with this procedure. Also severe deformity with arthritis of the MP joint is best treated with an arthrodesis.

PREOPERATIVE PLANNING

In addition to observing parameters such as the size, shape, and function of the foot, the range of motion of the entire foot and ankle is assessed, as well as the medial longitudinal arch in weight bearing. Hypermobility of the first ray is evaluated by grasping the first metatarsal of the patient's (right) foot with the examiner's (left) hand while stabilizing the rest of the foot with the right hand. The first metatarsal is then manipulated with the right thumb and forefinger (Fig. 1). Particular attention is paid to the increased arc of motion in the dorsal direction, as this excess causes the loss of stability of the medial border of the foot in weight bearing. This excessive mobility may be associated with dorsal elevation or prominence of the first metatarsal, with weight transfer to the second metatarsal, and callosity under the second metatarsal head. This hypermobility is demonstrated radiographically as increased cortical hypertrophy along the medial border of the second metatarsal shaft (Figs. 2 and 3). Although hypermobility is usually an isolated finding in the foot, it may also be associated with generalized ligamentous laxity, and this should be evaluated.

Weight-bearing radiographs should be obtained. Measurements of the intermetatarsal 1–2 angle, the first metatarsal cuneiform and hallux valgus angles, the metatarsus adductus are then made. The lengths of the first and second metatarsals and the congruity of the hallux metatarsal phalangeal joint are noted. A laterally facing metatarsal head may be associated with a congruent MP joint, which becomes incongruent following correction of the hallux valgus. This congruity should be determined preoperatively. The range of motion of the hallux at the MP joint is measured with the hallux in the valgus position. The hallux is then straightened, and the range of motion is once again checked (Fig. 4). Although tightness of

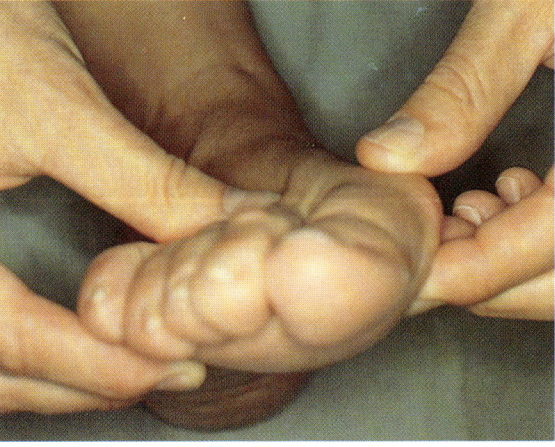

Figure 1. The evaluation for hypermobility is demonstrated.

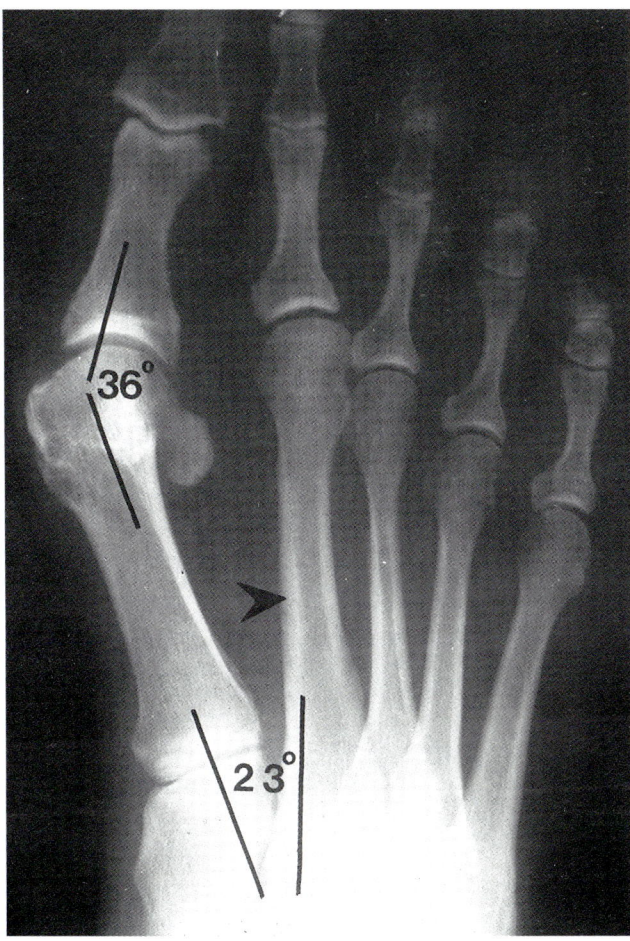

Figure 2. Hypermobility of the medial ray is demonstrated radiographically with hypertrophy of the medial border of the second metatarsal shaft.

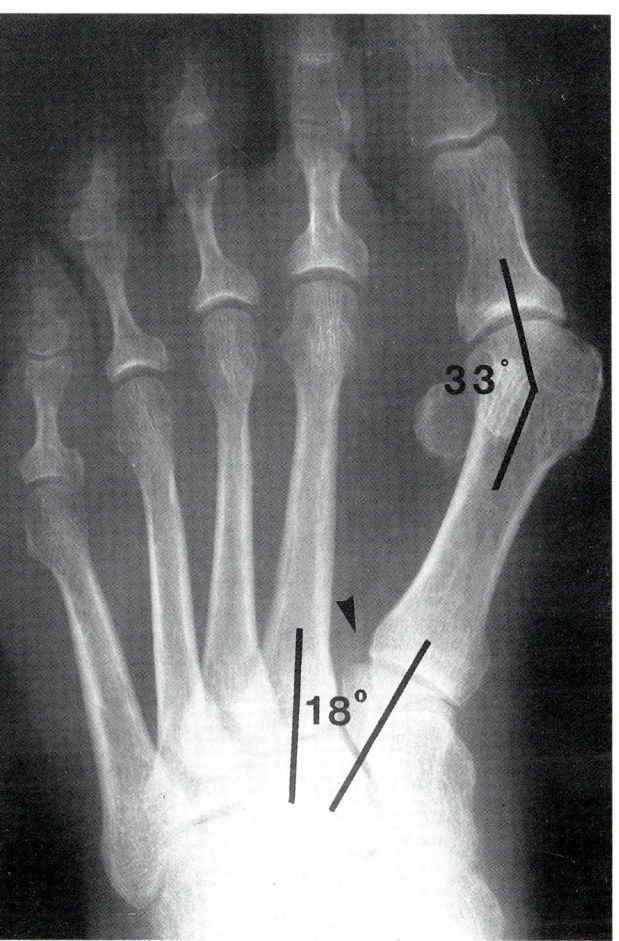

Figure 3. Hypermobility is demonstrated with instability of the base of the first metatarsal.

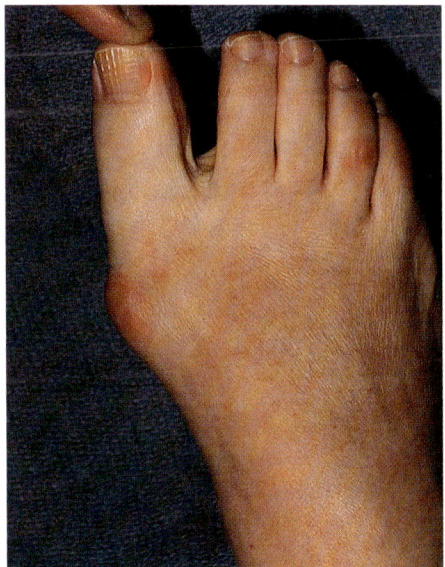

Figure 4. Motion of the hallux is checked in the valgus and the neutral position.

the lateral soft tissue structures may also contribute to this decrease in motion, incongruity of the MP joint may be present. This incongruity will cause a decrease in range of motion postoperatively. If I determine that incongruity is present, I prefer to leave the hallux in a slight valgus position, and to achieve correction with a closing wedge osteotomy at the base of the proximal phalanx (Akin). Under no circumstances, however, should this latter procedure be relied upon to correct the alignment of significant hallux valgus.

I go to great lengths to ensure patient understanding of bunion surgery. The nature of this operation as well as the various alternatives to conservative but particularly surgical treatment should be well explained. This operation involves potential problems that are unique to the arthrodesis. Patients need to be aware of the potential for complications including prolonged recovery time, pseudoarthrosis, and malunion.

Following arthrodesis, patients will experience more discomfort and swelling when compared with other similar procedures for severe hallux valgus. Problems with wound healing, incisional neuromas, and hardware removal are otherwise the same for any other bunion operation.

SURGERY

The patient is positioned supine on the operating table. Bilateral procedures are not performed simultaneously. Surgery is performed under regional ankle block anesthesia using 20 cc of 0.5% bupivacaine without admixed epinephrine. No tourniquet is used and hemostasis is controlled and bleeding minimized with the use of small hemostat clamps.

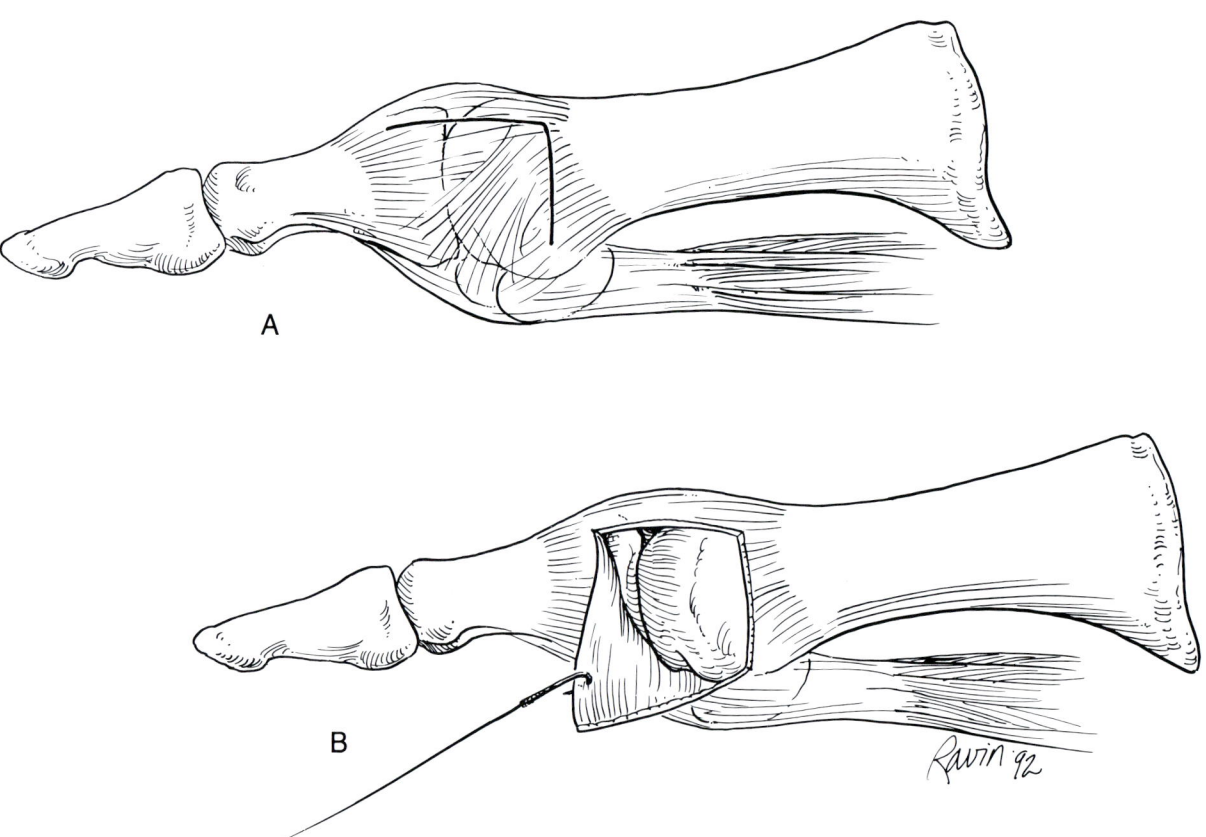

Figure 5. The capsular incision is demonstrated **(A)**, and the capsule reflected to expose the medial eminence **(B)**.

9 CUNEIFORM–METATARSAL ARTHRODESIS

Technique. A medial longitudinal incision is made over the hallux MP joint at the junction of the dorsal and plantar skin. I use an L-shaped capsular incision, with the apex dorsal and proximal (Fig. 5A). The capsule is dissected subperiosteally off the metatarsal neck exposing the entire medial eminence (Fig. 5B). The advantage of this flap is the broad exposure of the medial eminence, and later ease of capsular closure under the appropriate amount of tension, simultaneously controlling pronation of the hallux. If there is little soft tissue along the dorsomedial aspect of the metatarsal neck to reattach the capsule, then a small hole is made with an 0.062 Kirschner wire to attach the capsule.

A soft tissue release including an adductor tenotomy with partial lateral capsulotomy is performed through a separate dorsal incision over the distal intermetatarsal 1–2 space. In some adolescents with marked hypermobility of the first ray, the adductor release may not be necessary. This may be assessed by squeezing the forefoot and noting the change in position of the hallux. If the hallux assumes a corrected position without pushing it into varus, then a soft tissue release is probably unnecessary. The adductor is freed up off the flexor brevis tendon, and a longitudinal capsulotomy made dorsal to the fibular sesamoid, between it and the metatarsal head and neck. This lateral release of the sesamoid is important, since it should glide under the metatarsal head once correction of the metatarsal is performed. The fibular sesamoid rotates almost 90° with severe hallux valgus, and unless it is completely freed from its scarred attachments in the web space, accurate repositioning of the sesamoid mechanism is not possible. If the deformity is severe, the lateral portion of the flexor brevis tendon has to be cut in order to relax the contracture. The lateral capsule is then perforated with a #15 knife blade, and the hallux is passively manipulated into varus. The range of motion at the hallux MP joint is again assessed in the valgus and corrected neutral position to evaluate for any incongruity.

A third incision is made proximally, medial to the extensor hallucis longus tendon to expose the metatarsocuneiform joint. In the original descriptions of this procedure, a biplanar wedge resection of the joint was recommended. The wedges were lateral and plantar, thereby adducting and plantar flexing the metatarsal (Fig. 6). Although this concept is important to prevent shortening, it is probably more important to remove as little bone as possible. Due to difficulty with fixation, and

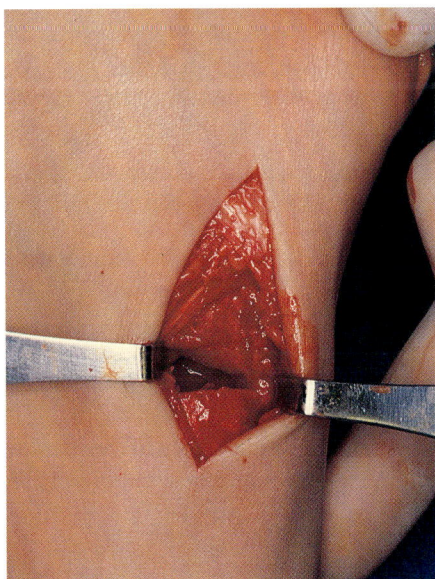

Figure 6. Resection of a biplanar wedge at the metatarsocuneiform joint is demonstrated.

the potential for shortening and malunion of the metatarsal, I became dissatisfied with this wedge resection of the joint. I realized that the position of the metatarsal may be corrected with little if any bone resection. This correction is actually easily accomplished with a more natural movement of adduction, plantar flexion, and slight internal rotation of the first metatarsal (Fig. 7). The correction depends on the slight concavoconvex configuration of this articulation.

The lateral and plantar articular cartilage only is removed; and the medial aspect of the joint is left intact. It is important to plantarflex as well as adduct the first metatarsal. Due to the anatomy of the joint this is not always easy to achieve. The articular surfaces of the metatarsocuneiform joint are not always flat, but occasionally saddle or bean shaped. Numerous configurations of the joint surface are encountered, some of which enhance and some block the repositioning of the metatarsal. Occasionally there are two separate facets on the base of the metatarsal. The plane of this concavity is toward the second cuneiform and the convexity faces medially. The base of the articular surface is extremely deep and sometimes difficult to reach even with a long curette. When resecting any bone from this articulation there is a tendency therefore to remove insufficient bone from the deeper plantar base of the metatarsal and cuneiform. This can only be accomplished by careful repeated inspection and removing the deeper part of the metatarsal with a long rongeur or thin chisel.

The correction should therefore be achieved by sliding the metatarsal, and not by resecting too large a wedge from the joint. Care is taken not to overcorrect the first metatarsal; if a negative intermetatarsal angle is created, a hallux varus deformity may result. I emphasize this point, as it is easy to remove too large a wedge at the tarsometatarsal joint. The metatarsal is held in adduction and plantar flexion and secured with a Kirschner wire for temporary fixation. Intraoperative anteroposterior (AP) and lateral radiographs should be obtained to confirm correction. Particular attention should be paid to overcorrection, undercorrection, and dorsal elevation of the first metatarsal.

Following radiographic evaluation, permanent fixation is performed using 3.5-mm cortical screws. The first screw is introduced dorsal to plantar from the medial cuneiform proximally into the first metatarsal distally using a lag screw technique. When I introduced the screw from distal to proximal, I experienced many problems associated with fixation and I believe that this modification, which was brought to my attention by K. A. Johnson, is far preferable. The second screw is introduced medially from the first metatarsal into the second metatarsal base from slightly plantar to dorsal avoiding the middle cuneiform (Fig. 8). This second screw is not introduced with a lag technique, and is used to control rotation of the joint only. When this second screw is inserted, it is important to ensure that the advancing edge of the screw does not push against the second metatarsal. Not only will this separate the first and second metatarsals, but it affects the stability of the compression at the metatarsocuneiform joint. This can of course be obviated by inserting the second screw in a lag fashion, but this too may create unnecessary compression of the first and second metatarsals, again compromising the arthrodesis.

A burr is used to create two or three small dorsal and medial troughs across the joint, and local bone graft is used to fill these defects.

Once the metatarsal has been stabilized attention is again directed to the distal alignment. The congruity of the MP joint is again evaluated. If there is any potential for medial impingement and incongruity, the range of motion of the MP joint will decrease in the corrected position. It is then preferable to leave the hallux in a slight valgus position and perform a closing wedge osteotomy at the base of the proximal phalanx. The hallux should finally rest in a neutral position and closure made without relying on the capsulorraphy to straighten it. The capsulorraphy is performed as described above by using the L-shaped flap, and attachment with a Kirschner wire hole into the metatarsal neck if necessary. Nonabsorbable 2-0

9 CUNEIFORM–METATARSAL ARTHRODESIS

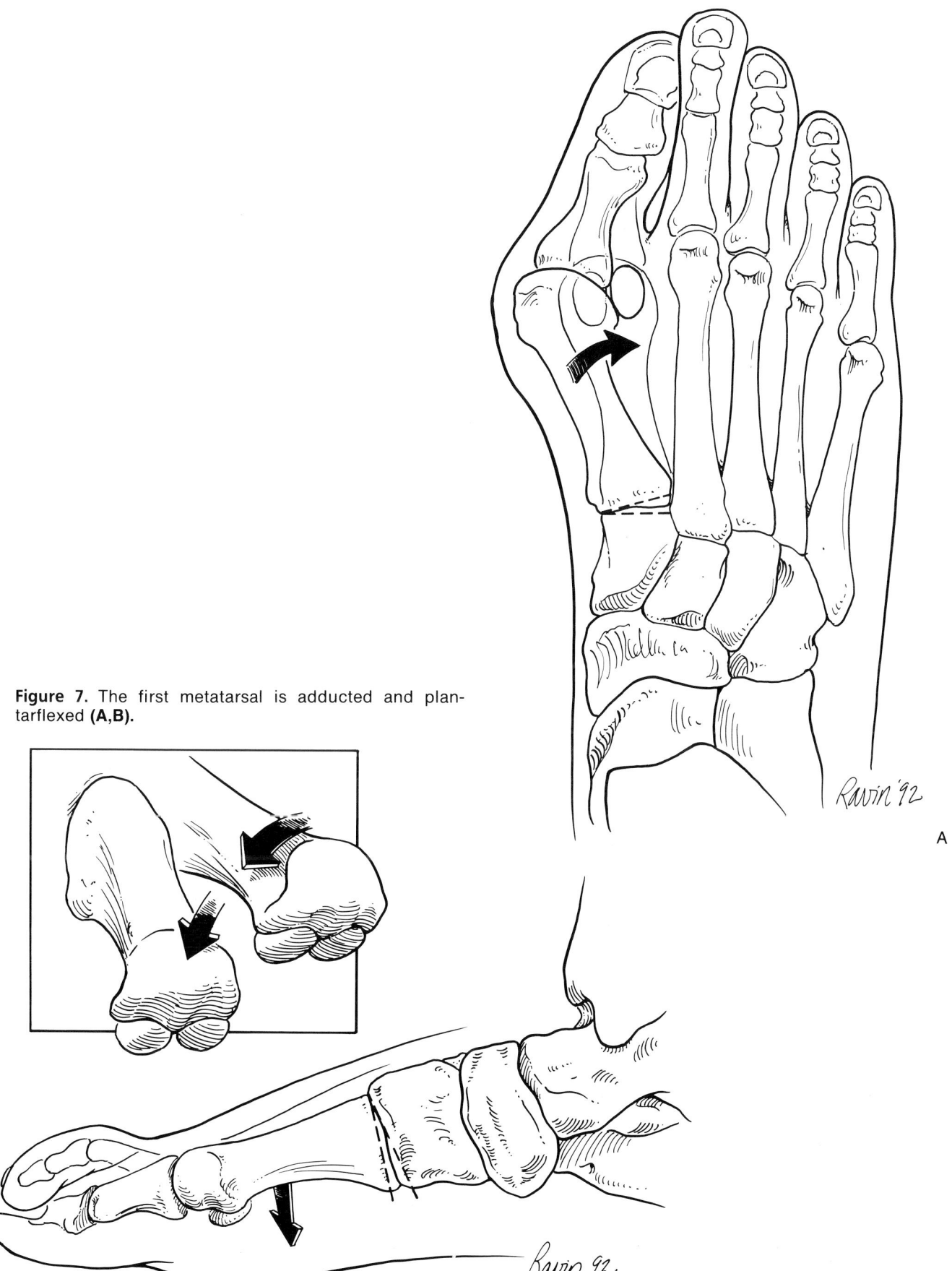

Figure 7. The first metatarsal is adducted and plantarflexed (A,B).

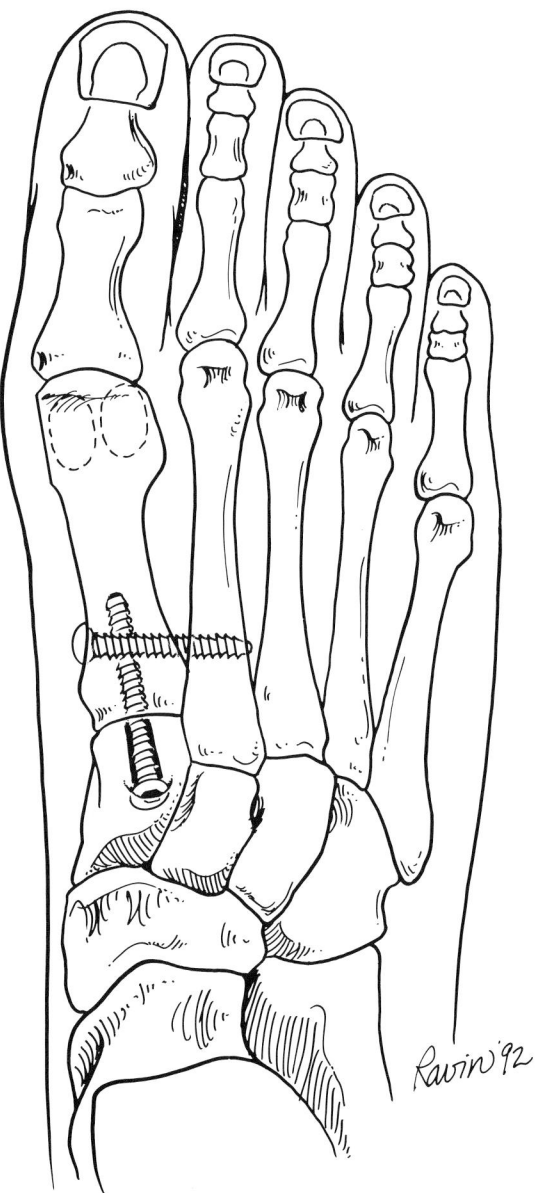

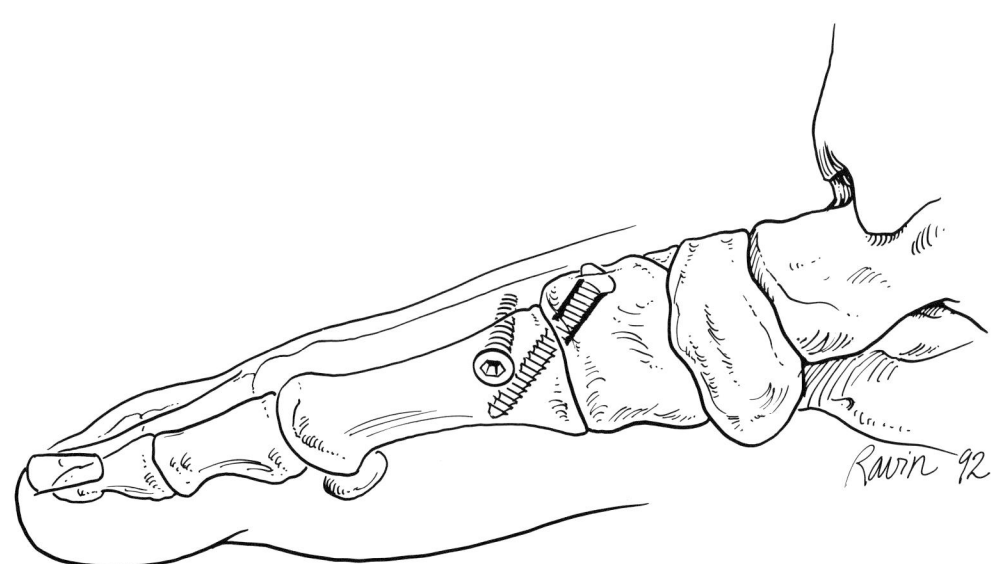

Figure 8. The screw technique is demonstrated (A,B).

suture is used in the capsular structures and nylon mattress or nonabsorbable subcuticular sutures in the skin.

POSTOPERATIVE MANAGEMENT

Patients use crutches until comfortable, followed by weight bearing as tolerated in either a short leg cast or a stiff surgical shoe. If the patient is very active, I would recommend a cast. Generally, the cast may be removed by the sixth week, and progress to a surgical shoe until comfortable, usually a further few weeks. A soft bunion splint to maintain the hallux in neutral alignment for nighttime use is used for an additional 4 weeks. At 8 to 10 weeks patients are allowed to walk in a comfortable sneaker and by 4 months shoe-wear is unrestricted. Most patients find that the foot is still swollen at 3 months and are unable to return to the shoes they had worn preoperatively up until approximately 4 to 6 months. Some swelling, stiffness, and aching persist up until 6 months. During this rehabilitation phase patients are encouraged to ambulate and obtain physical therapy to improve the motion at the MP joint if needed.

An evaluation of patients who have had this procedure indicated that 77% of the patients were totally relieved, 15% partially relieved, and 8% not relieved with respect to pain, comfort, appearance of the foot, and shoe-wear following surgery.

COMPLICATIONS

Pseudarthrosis, stiffness, and dorsal elevation of the first metatarsal are potential problems with this procedure. Although nonunion is a problem, we have reduced the incidence of this problem over the past few years by the different screw techniques, and careful attention to immobilization postoperatively. Nonunion is typically associated with persistent swelling, aching, and intermittent pain, which last approximately 6 to 9 months. A nonunion does not always remain symptomatic, and with further follow-up probably 75% are actually asymptomatic. A dorsal bunion may develop in association with nonunion or malunion of the first metatarsal. Although most are asymptomatic, decreased range of motion of the hallux MP joint may be present, and treated either with cheilectomy or revision of the arthrodesis. Although it may seem that revision of the arthrodesis is a major undertaking, it is easily accomplished by a simple opening wedge osteotomy of the arthrodesis site, and interposition of a tricortical bone graft. This osteotomy-arthrodesis is quite stable, and patients may begin ambulation immediately in a surgical shoe with an elevated heel.

ILLUSTRATIVE CASE FOR TECHNIQUE

This 46-year-old woman presented with marked pain over the medial eminence, and pain and callosity under the second metatarsal head. Shoe fitting was becoming increasingly difficult.

On examination, she had severe hallux valgus, hypermobility of the medial ray, pain under the second metatarsal head, and a painful second hammertoe deformity. Mild pes planus was present. Range of motion of the hallux MP joint was normal in the valgus position, unassociated with any crepitus. With the hallux passively manipulated into the neutral position, motion of the hallux decreased significantly, possibly as a result of a congruent MP joint. The second toe MP joint could not be passively reduced.

The radiographs on the weight-bearing AP view demonstrated an intermetatarsal 1–2 angle of 18°, and a MP angle of 54°. The second toe MP joint was dislocated.

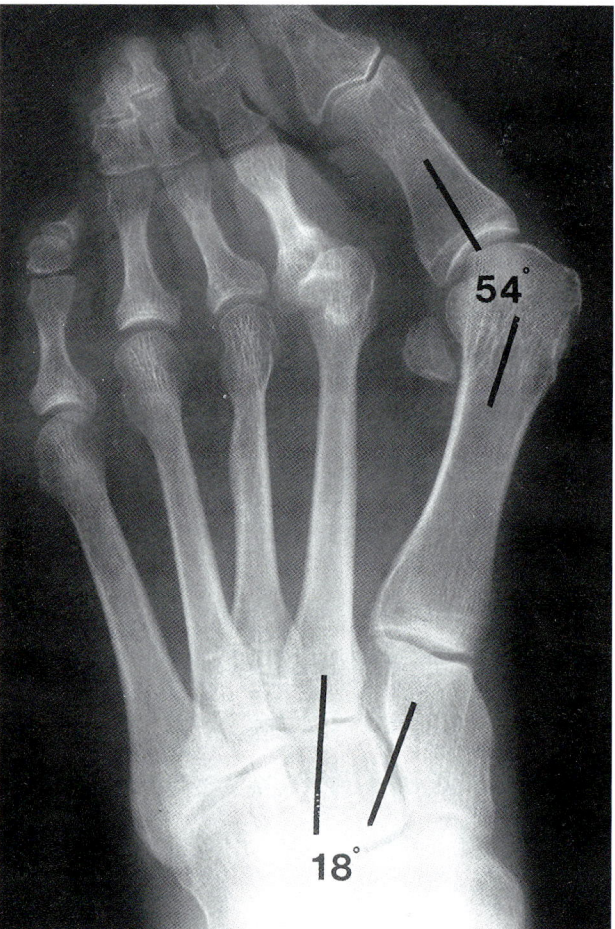
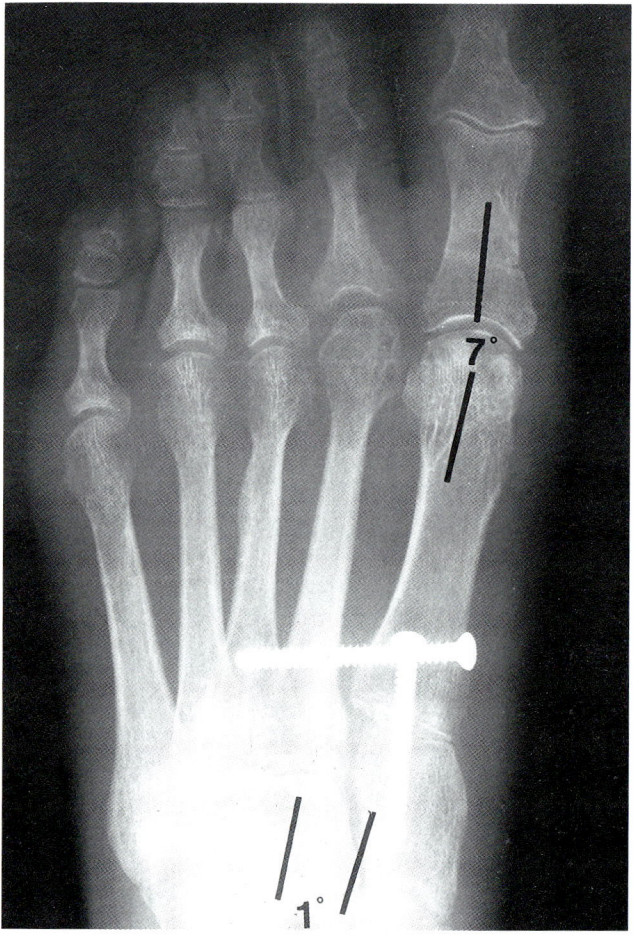

Figure 9. Anteroposterior (AP) radiograph demonstrating severe hallux valgus associated with metatarsus adductus, and hypermobility of the medial ray.

Figure 10. AP radiograph 7 weeks following surgery.

Note generalized metatarsus adductus and slight thickening of the medial border of the second metatarsal shaft (Fig. 9).

A metatarsocuneiform arthrodesis with screw fixation was performed under local anesthesia as an outpatient procedure. This was combined with a lateral soft tissue release, and a medial exostectomy. Following this stabilization procedure, the range of motion of the hallux MP joint was evaluated in its resting (slight valgus) position, and following passive manipulation into neutral. Decreased motion was noted at the joint with the hallux passively manipulated into neutral, and a closing wedge osteotomy of the base of the hallux phalanx was performed.

She remained non–weight bearing for the first 2 weeks following surgery. Following suture removal, a walking cast was applied, and partial weight bearing commenced. Full weight bearing was allowed by 4 weeks in a cast, which was changed to a surgical shoe worn for the following 3 weeks until arthrodesis.

Radiographs obtained at 7 weeks demonstrate an arthrodesis with correction of the intermetatarsal 1–2 angle to 1°, and the MP angle to 7°. The second MP joint is reduced (Fig. 10).

RECOMMENDED READING

1. Clarke, H. R., Veith, R. G., and Hansen, S. T.: Adolescent bunions treated by the modified Lapidus procedure. *Bull. Hosp. Joint Dis.*, 47: 109–122, 1987.

2. Lapidus, P. W.: The operative correction of the metatarsus varus primus in hallux valgus. *Surg. Gyneol. Obstet.*, 58: 183–191, 1934.
3. Lapidus, P. W.: A quarter of a century of experience with the operative correction of the metatarsus varus in hallux valgus. *Bull. Hosp. Joint Dis.*, 17: 404–421, 1956.
4. Lapidus, P. W.: THe author's bunion operation from 1931 to 1959. *Clin. Orthop.*, 16: 119–135, 1960.
5. Myerson, M. S.: Metatarsocuneiform arthrodesis for treatment of hallux valgus and metatarsus primus varus. *Orthopedics*, 13: 1025–1031, 1990.
6. Myerson, M. S., Allon, S., and McGarvey, W.: Metatarsocuneiform arthrodesis for management of hallux valgus and metatarsus primus varus. *Foot Ankle*, 13: 107–115, 1992.

10

Cheilectomy

Glenn B. Pfeffer

INDICATIONS/CONTRAINDICATIONS

Hallux rigidus is a degenerative condition of the great toe metatarsophalangeal characterized by decreased dorsiflexion, osteophyte proliferation, and painful motion. First described by Davies-Colley in 1887, J. M. Cotterill coined the term "hallux rigidus" 1 year later (1). After hallux valgus, it is the most common painful affliction of the great toe, occurring in approximately 2% of the population between the ages of 30 and 60. As the degenerative process progresses, proliferation of bone on the dorsal aspect of the metatarsal head increases the size of the joint and blocks dorsiflexion of the proximal phalanx. These changes are usually unilateral and are possibly initiated by previous occult trauma (5).

Initial conservative treatment attempts to decrease inflammation within the joint and to protect the toe from painful motion. A nonsteroidal antiinflammatory agent, contrast baths, and a stiff-soled, low-heeled shoe are helpful. An intraarticular injection of a steroid preparation may decrease an active synovitis but repeated injections are not recommended. Shoe modification can include a wide toe box or stretching the shoe in the area of the painful dorsal prominence. A rocker bottom, metatarsal bar, or an orthotic device can also be used to decrease stress on the metatarsophalangeal joint. These modifications are often cumbersome, however, and have low patient compliance.

When conservative treatment fails, surgical intervention should be considered. The specific indication for cheilectomy is the painful abutment of the proximal phalanx of the great toe against degenerative osteophytes on the dorsal aspect of the first metatarsal (Fig. 1). The term "cheilectomy" derives from the Greek *cheilos* meaning "lip." The goal of surgery is to excise the proliferative bone on the "lip" of the joint, thereby allowing unrestricted motion. Other surgical options

---

G. B. Pfeffer, M.D.: Department of Orthopaedics, University of California, San Francisco, San Francisco, CA 94143; California Pacific Medical Center, Pacific Campus, San Francisco, CA 94115.

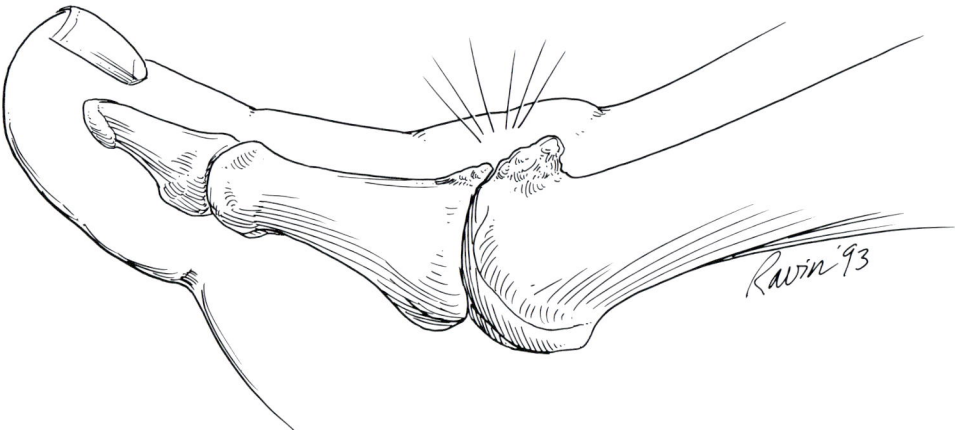

Figure 1. Degenerative osteophytes on the first metatarsal head block extension of the proximal phalanx.

include resection arthroplasty or implant arthroplasty, osteotomy about the joint, and an arthrodesis. Cheilectomy offers the advantage of preserving the length, stability, and power of the great toe that are often sacrificed after these other procedures. An arthroplasty or arthrodesis can always follow a failed cheilectomy, but not vice versa. There are no specific contraindications to a cheilectomy other than very advanced degeneration of the joint.

PREOPERATIVE PLANNING

It is essential to differentiate hallux rigidus from other possible causes of great toe pain. The hallmark of the physical examination of hallux rigidus is restricted active and passive dorsiflexion of the toe with reproduction of the patient's pain (3). The toe is rarely rigid, but a firm end point to dorsiflexion can always be appreciated. Compensatory hyperextension at the interphalangeal joint may occur. Plantar flexion of the toe is usually not restricted, although passive motion may cause dorsal pain by stretching the inflamed capsule or extensor tendon over a prominent osteophyte (4) (Fig. 2). A large osteophyte along the dorsal aspect of the metatarsal head may irritate the sensory nerve to the first web space and cause dysesthesias with palpation.

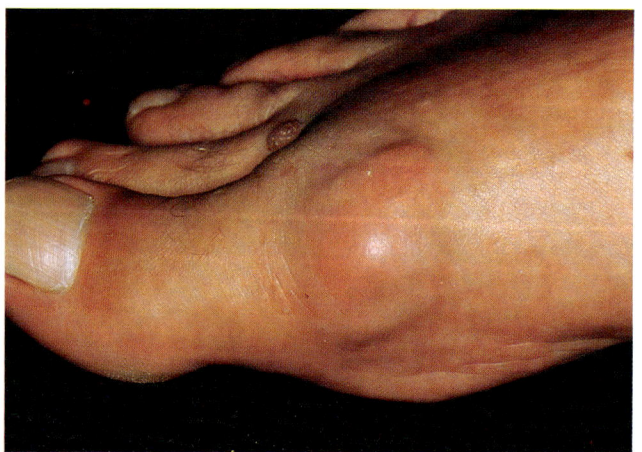
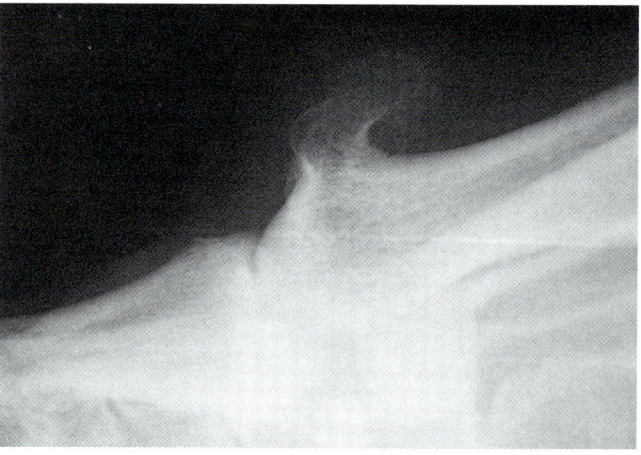

Figure 2. A: Inflamed dorsal skin and bursa overlying degenerative dorsal osteophyte of metatarsal head. **B:** Large prominent dorsal osteophyte.

Radiograph evaluation should include standing anteroposterior (AP) and lateral views. The standing lateral view is most helpful as it demonstrates the dorsal osteophyte and reveals the extent of joint space narrowing. The upper portion of the joint may be destroyed while the lower one-half is preserved. If the inferior portion of the joint space is not preserved, a cheilectomy will not be successful. The AP radiograph demonstrates the typical formation of medial and lateral osteophytes, as well as subchondral sclerosis and in advanced cases cyst formation. Occasionally an oblique view of the great toe will help visualize early joint space narrowing. The sesamoids are rarely involved in the degenerative process of hallux rigidus and an axial view to visualize them is not required.

Based on the radiographic findings the grade of hallux rigidus should be determined. Grade I is mild to moderate osteophyte formation with joint space preservation (Fig. 3). Grade II is moderate osteophyte proliferation with joint space narrowing and subchondral sclerosis (Fig. 4). Grade III changes consist of marked osteophyte formation and loss of a visible joint space, including the inferior portion of the joint as seen on a lateral radiographic view. Marked sclerosis and cyst formation are also present (Fig. 5). Patients with grades I to II changes are excellent candidates for cheilectomy (2). Patients with grade III change should be considered for an alternative procedure such as an arthrodesis or a Keller resection arthroplasty. On occasion, the decision can only be made at the time of surgery. The patient should be counseled preoperatively that the appropriate procedure will be chosen after the joint cartilage is examined.

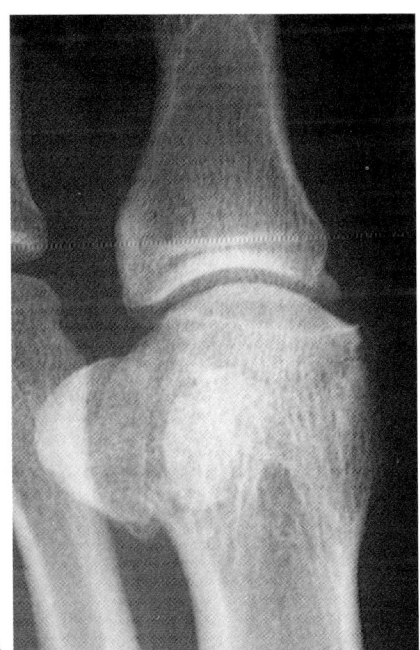
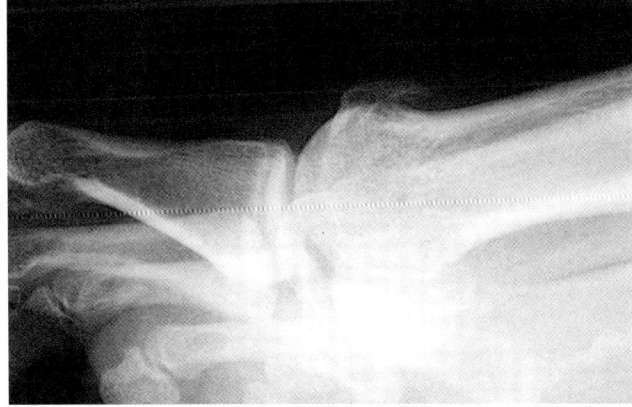
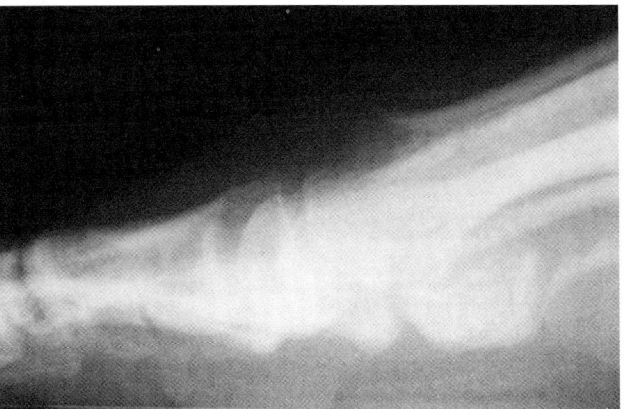

Figure 3. A and **B:** Mild hallux rigidus with minimal spurring and no joint space narrowing. **C:** Lateral view following cheilectomy.

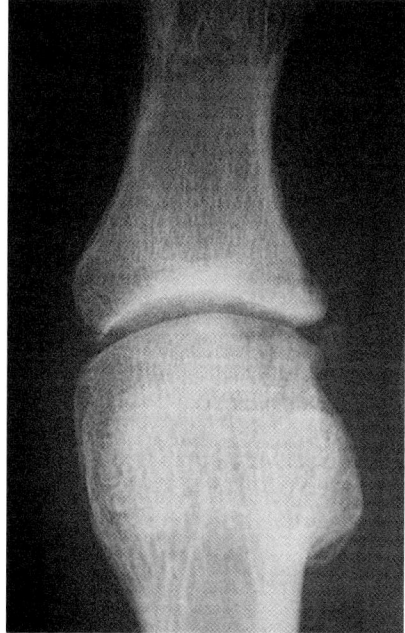
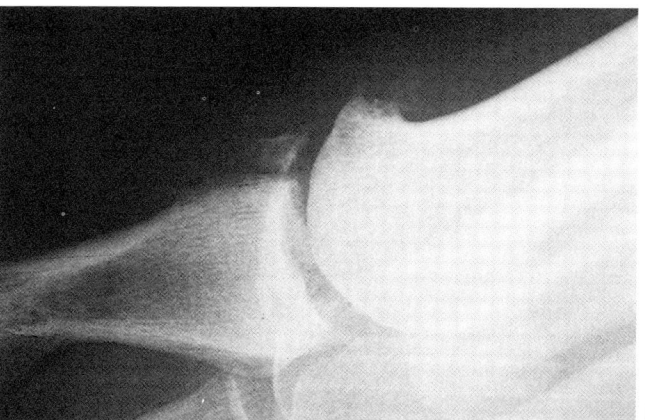
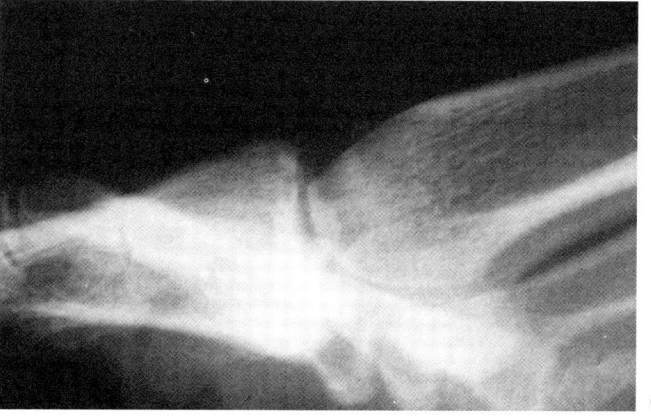

Figure 4. A and **B:** Moderate hallux rigidus with spurring and joint space narrowing. **C:** Lateral view following cheilectomy.

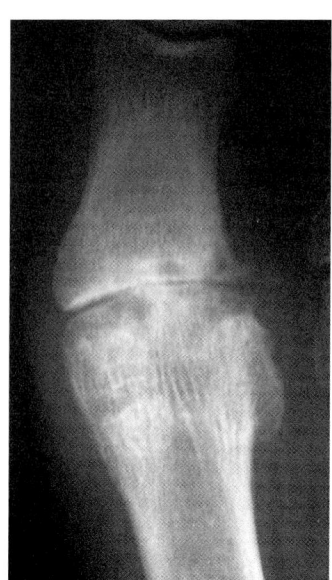
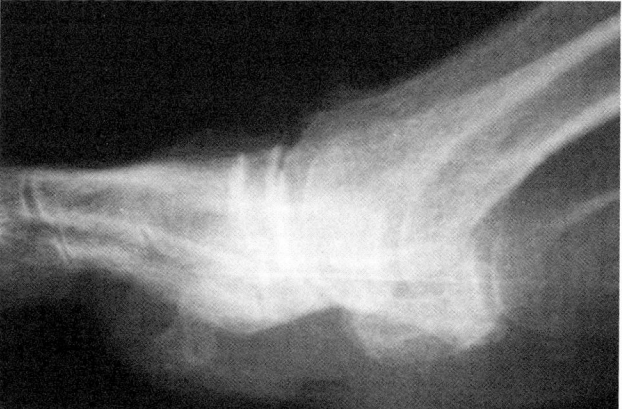
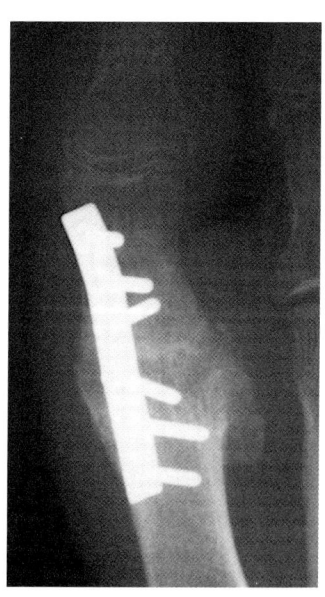

Figure 5. A and **B:** Advanced hallux rigidus with significant degeneration and loss of joint space. **C:** This patient required a fusion of the metatarsophalangeal joint.

SURGERY

A cheilectomy is usually performed under regional anesthesia with intravenous sedation. An ankle block using a 20-cc solution of 0.25% bupivacaine hydrochloride (Marcaine) and 1% lidocaine, both without epinephrine, is appropriate. The patient is placed supine on the operating table. A pneumatic ankle tourniquet is applied over two or three layers of cast padding. After the foot in exsanguinated with a 3-inch Esmarch bandage, the tourniquet is inflated to 250 mm Hg.

Technique. Using a #15 blade, a 5- to 6-cm incision centered over the first metatarsophalangeal joint is made along the medial border of the extensor hallucis longus tendon (Fig. 6). Care is taken to protect the dorsocutaneous sensory nerves, although they are not routinely visualized in this approach (Fig. 7). The extensor hood is divided 2 mm medial to the border of the extensor hallucis longus, thereby keeping the tendon within its sheath (Fig. 8). This will minimize postoperative adhesions. The tendon is retracted laterally and the joint capsule is divided longitudinally. A proliferative synovitis is often encountered and a plane between the capsule and the synovium is developed. A complete synovectomy is performed. A cartilaginous loose body may be present. A #15 blade or a #64 Beaver blade is then used to carefully dissect the joint capsule and expose the medial, dorsal, and lateral aspects of the metatarsal head and the base of the proximal phalanx (Fig. 9).

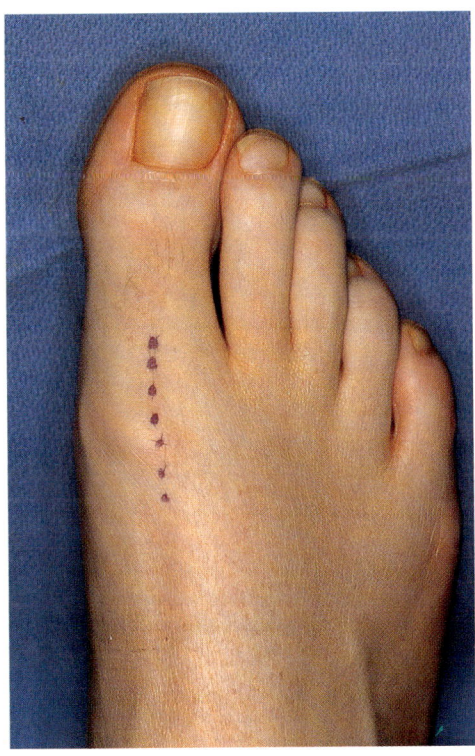

Figure 6. A 5- to 6-cm incision along the medial border of the extensor hallucis longus tendon.

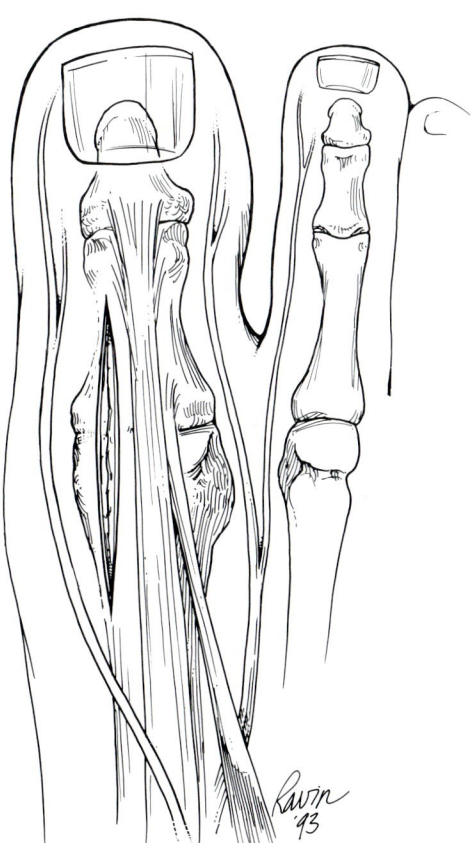

Figure 7. Care should be taken to protect the dorsal sensory nerves although they are not routinely visualized in this approach.

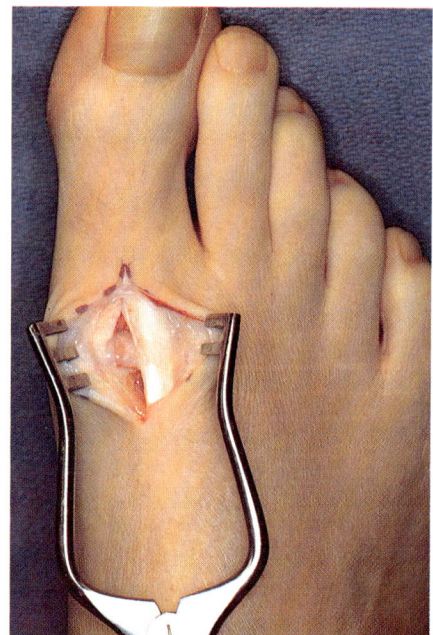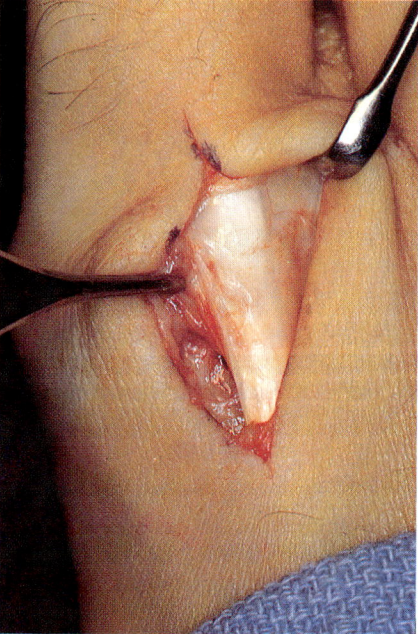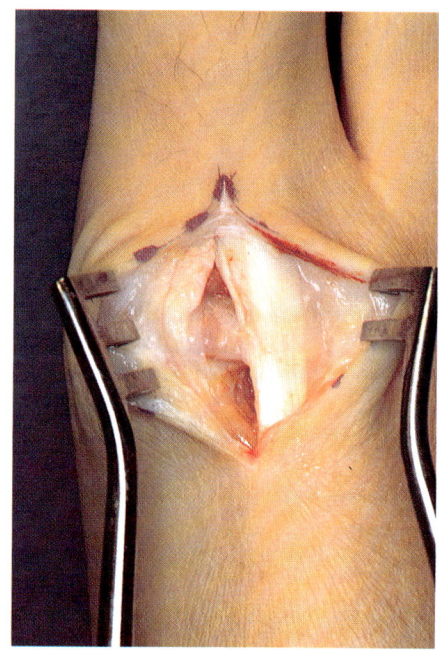

Figure 8. A: The extensor hallucis longus sheath is divided 2 to 3 mm medial to the border of the tendon, thereby keeping the tendon within its sheath. **B:** The medial border of the extensor hallucis longus sheath is held in the forceps. **C:** The capsule is divided longitudinally.

The toe is plantar flexed at the metatarsophalangeal joint approximately 45° to allow complete inspection of the metatarsal head (Fig. 10). Further dissection of the capsule may be required in order to gain adequate exposure. The large dorsal ridge of arthritic bone and the predominant lateral osteophytes are readily apparent (Fig. 11). The pathologic changes of the cartilage on the metatarsal head can now be appreciated fully. The changes are often worse than expected as based upon

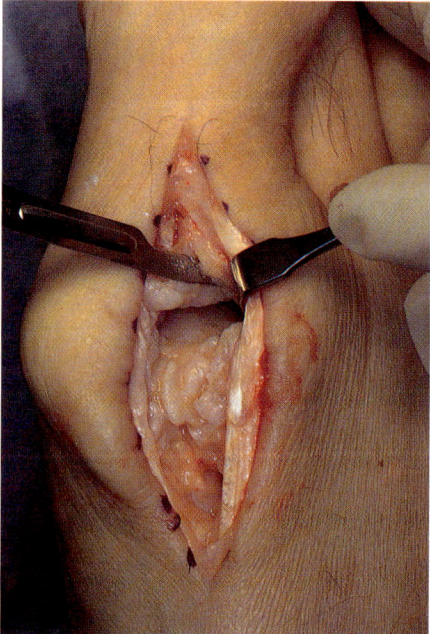

Figure 9. The capsule is dissected off the metatarsal head and the base of the proximal phalanx to expose medial and lateral osteophytes.

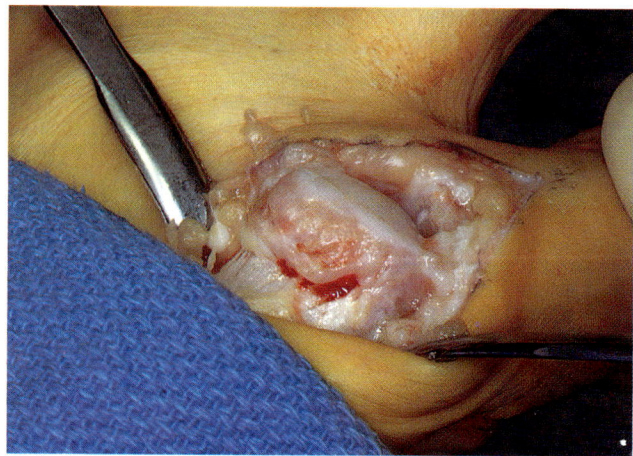

Figure 10. The toe is plantar flexed 45° to expose the metatarsal head.

preoperative radiographs. The cartilage on the proximal phalanx is usually intact although central fibrillation and slight dorsal loss can occur. A prominent dorsal ridge of bone at the base of the proximal phalanx is frequently present. This is removed with a needle-nosed rongeur.

The dorsal bony prominence of the metatarsal is excised along with up to 35% of the metatarsal head (Fig. 12). The amount of metatarsal head that is excised is dependent upon the degree of cartilage destruction and the amount of bone removal that is required to allow passive dorsiflexion of the toe. Even in the mildest of cases, at least 20% of the dorsal metatarsal head should be removed to adequately decompress the joint. From distal to proximal the line of resection slopes upward, extending from just dorsal to the edge of viable cartilage to just proximal to the dorsal prominence (Fig. 13). Any exposed bone that remains on

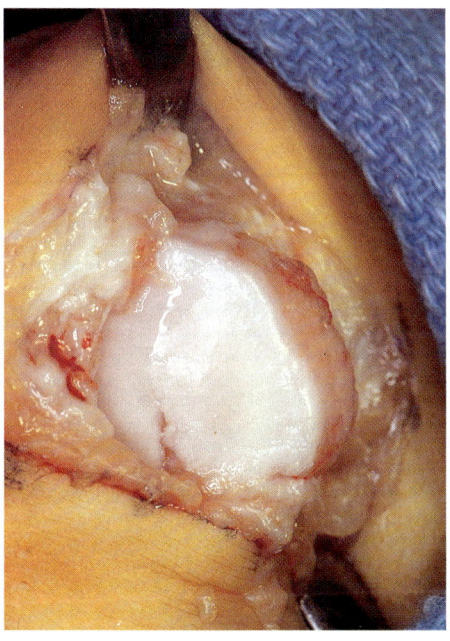

Figure 11. The large dorsal ridge of arthritic bone is visualized. In this case, approximately 35% of the metatarsal head is damaged with fissuring and softening of the dorsal cartilage.

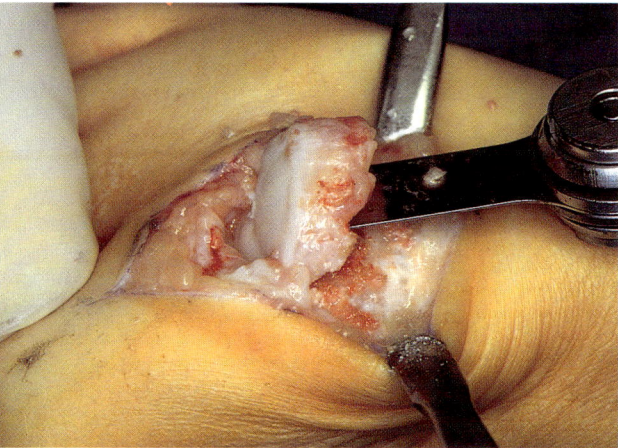

Figure 12. The involved portion of the metatarsal head is excised using a saw cut from distal to proximal.

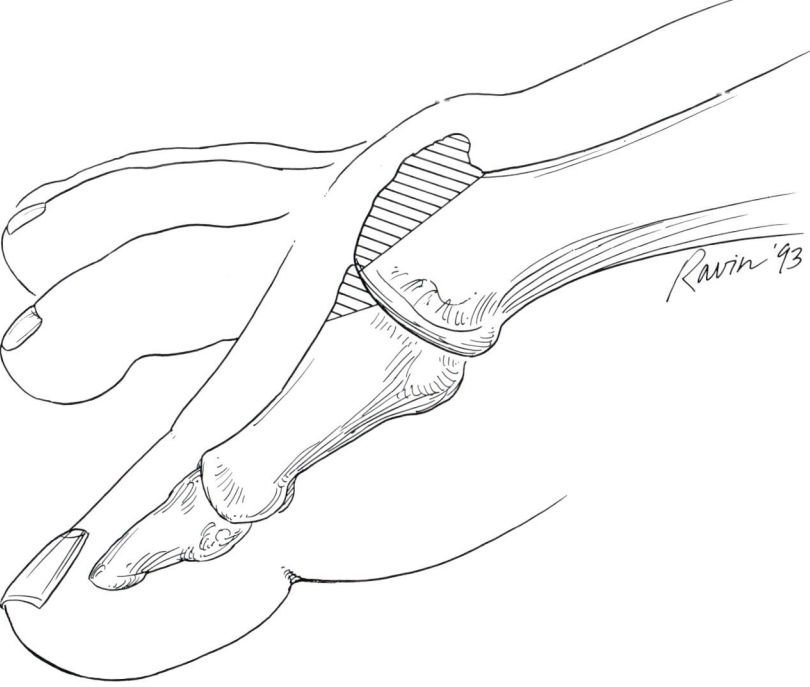

Figure 13. The line of resection extended from just dorsal to the edge of the viable cartilage to just proximal to the dorsal prominence.

the metatarsal head should be drilled multiple times with a small K-wire to induce fibrocartilage growth postoperatively. Any small irregularities along the cartilage edges should be carefully trimmed using a #15 blade or small rongeur.

I prefer to use a Zimmer Microaire saw (Zimmer, Co., Warsaw, IN) with a fine-toothed sagittal blade (#ZS-038), which is approximately 1.25 inches long, 0.37 inches wide, and 0.015 inches thick. A small amount of irrigation may be used so as not to burn the articular cartilage. A 6-mm osteotome can also be effective, although fragmentation of the bone more commonly occurs. The bone cut is most easily done from proximal to distal, especially if 25% or more of the head is to be removed. When less of the head is excised it is difficult to place a power saw sufficiently parallel to the metatarsal shaft. In such a case, the cut is better made from distal to proximal (Fig. 14).

Once the metatarsal prominence is excised, the marginal osteophytes are addressed. Two small Homan retractors provide exposure of the metatarsal head while protecting the tendons and neurovascular structures. Once again, a microsagittal saw is used. The osteophytes should be excised flush with the metatarsal

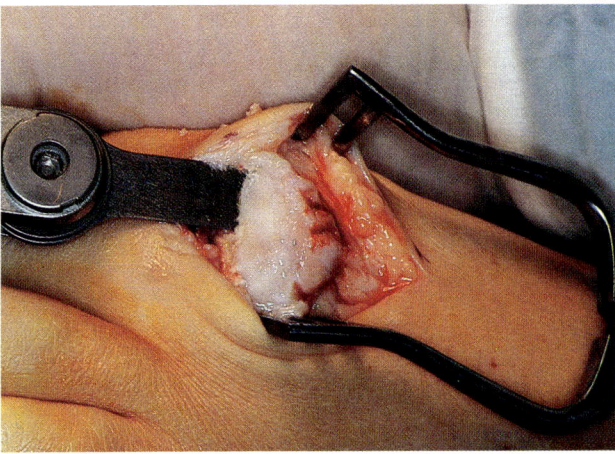

Figure 14. If only a small portion of the metatarsal head is resected the cut can be easily made from a distal to proximal direction.

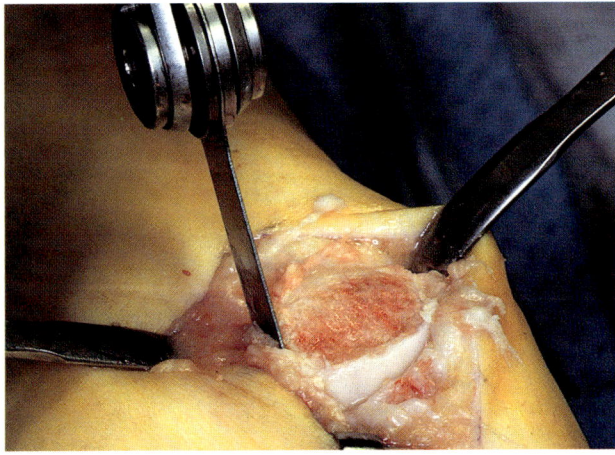

Figure 15. Lateral osteophytes along the metatarsal head should be excised. Homan retractors are used to protect the neurovascular structures and tendons. If there is loss of articular cartilage on the lateral aspect of the joint, that portion of the metatarsal head should be excised as well.

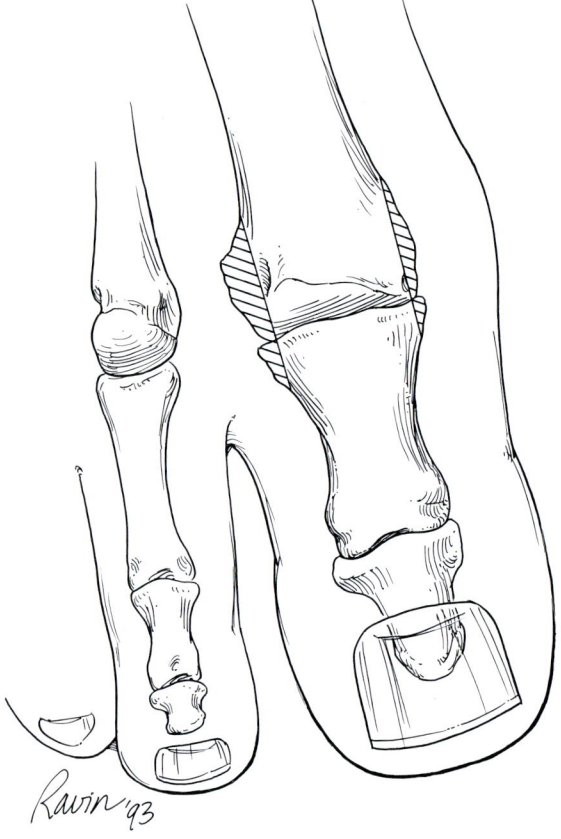

Figure 16. Excision of lateral osteophytes and a portion of metatarsal head with cartilage loss.

shaft unless there is loss of medial or lateral cartilage (Fig. 15). In such a case 2 to 3 mm of the metatarsal head should be removed in the sagittal plane. If such articular cartilage loss occurs it is usually on the lateral aspect of the joint where the most prominent osteophytes occur (Fig. 16). Significant medial osteophytes, in fact, are unusual and can easily be excised with a small needle-nose rongeur. The sharp borders left by the saw cuts should be rounded using a rongeur or preferably a microreciprocating rasp. A prominent dorsal lip on the proximal phalanx should be trimmed down in a similar fashion, using rongeur and microreciprocating rasp.

After the bony cuts have been made, the sesamoid metatarsal complex should be examined. There are rarely any degenerative changes present. A small Freer elevator is used to break up any adhesions of the plantar aspect of the metatarsal head. At this point, one should be able to passively dorsiflex to 70° (Fig. 17). If this degree of dorsiflexion is not obtainable, the joint should be reassessed for probable further bony resection (Fig. 18). The joint is then copiously irrigated with antibiotic solution and the capsule closed using absorbable suture. A nonabsorbable suture would cause less of an inflammatory reaction postoperatively but the suture knots are often uncomfortable in shoe-wear. One or two 4-0 absorbable sutures are used to repair and realign the extensor mechanism, sewing into the medial border of the extensor hallucis longus sheath that remains from the operative approach. The tourniquet is deflated and hemostasis obtained with compression and cautery. No subcutaneous sutures are required. The skin is closed with

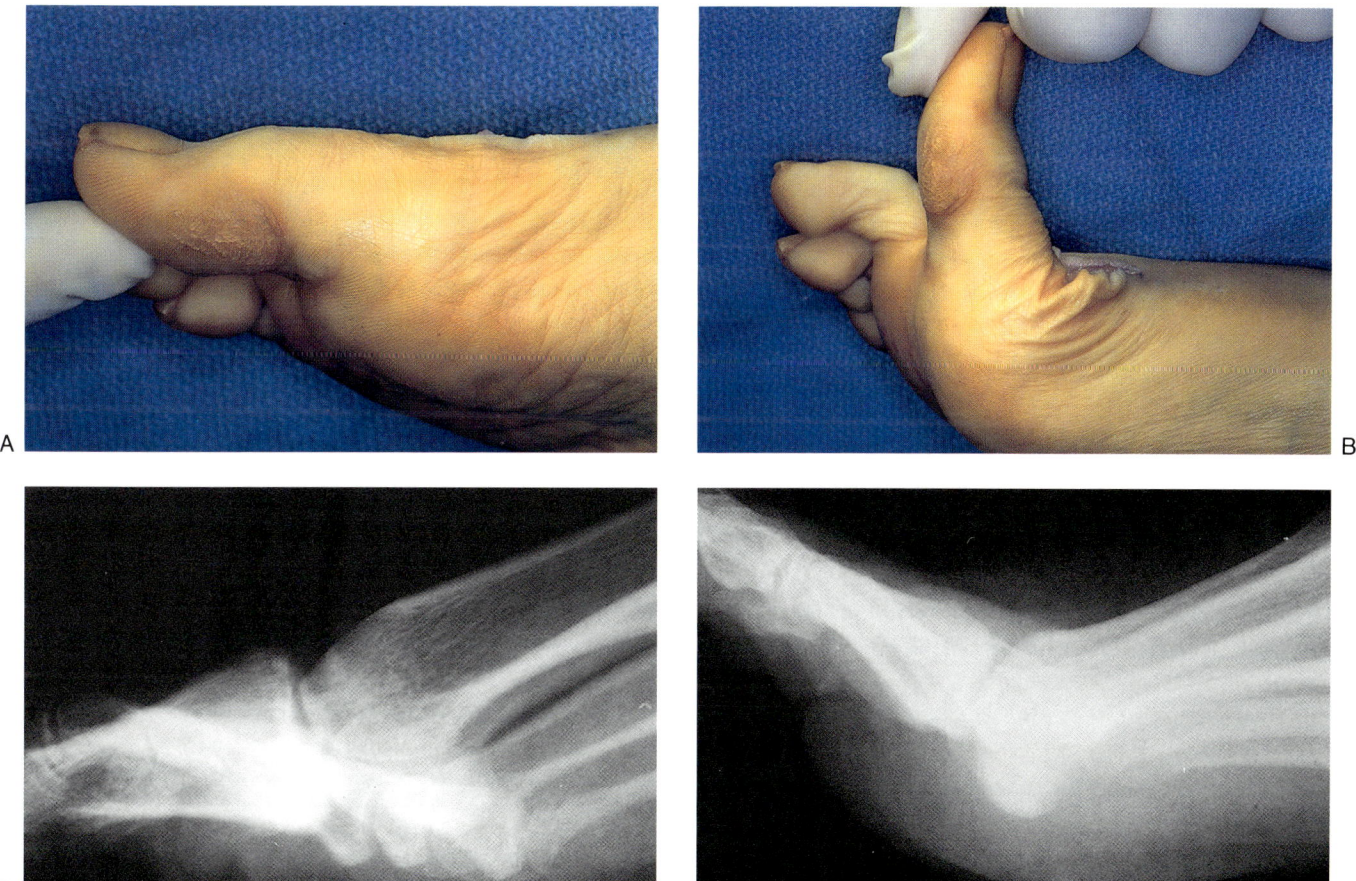

Figure 17. A: There is 20° of passive motion preoperatively. **B:** Almost 90° of passive dorsiflexion postoperatively. **C:** Approximately 30% of the metatarsal head has been excised. **D:** Postoperative film of dorsiflexion. The proximal phalanx can now glide freely on the metatarsal head, no longer blocked by a prominent dorsal osteophyte.

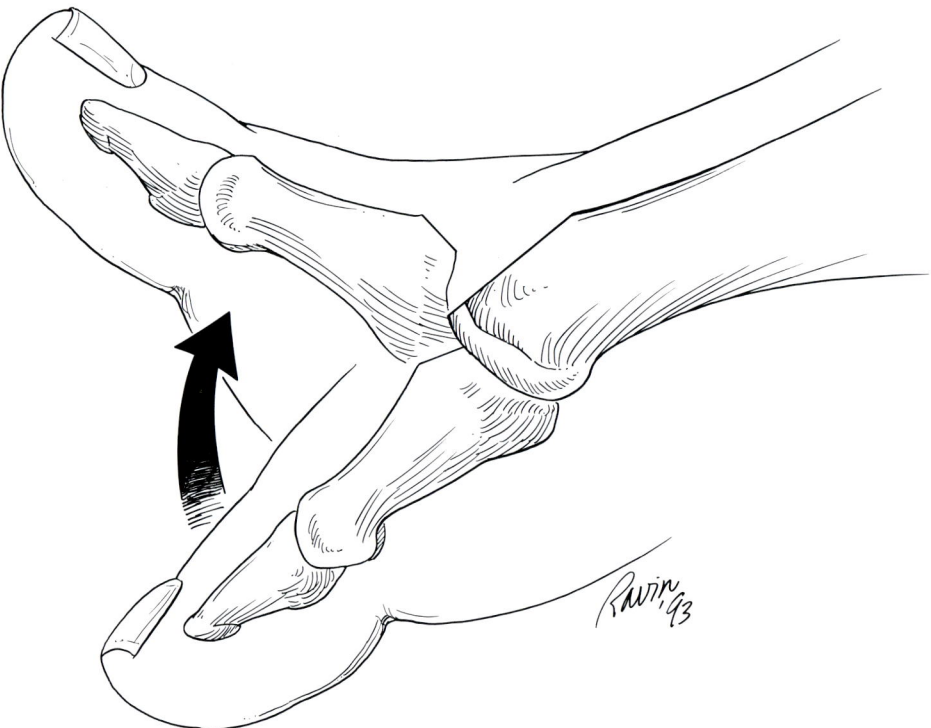

Figure 18. Adequate resection of the metatarsal head is essential in order to gain relief of pain and adequate motion.

interrupted 4-0 horizontal nylon mattress sutures. An antibiotic ointment and nonadherent 4 × 4 are placed over the wound and a sterile bulky compressive dressing is applied.

Technically, the cheilectomy is an easy procedure. Variations of the above surgical approach have been recommended by different authors. I would suggest, however, not varying from the following specifics of the procedure. An approach based on the medial side of the extensor hallucis longus tendon provides excellent visualization of the joint and avoids dissection of the extensor brevis tendon. By leaving the extensor hallucis longus in its sheath, postoperative tendinous adhesions are minimized. Aggressive bony resection of the dorsal osteophyte and diseased portion of the metatarsal head is essential. A large portion of the metatarsal head is not visible through this approach and although it may seem that the cheilectomy removes 50% of the joint surface, in fact more than 30% is rarely excised. Excision of the prominent lateral osteophytes with squaring off of the metatarsal is required to adequately decompress the joint.

POSTOPERATIVE MANAGEMENT

Postoperatively the patient is kept in a wooden-soled bunion shoe for 10 days until the wound has healed and the sutures are removed. Gentle range of motion exercises are started by the patient on the second postoperative day as pain allows. The first postoperative visit is at 3 to 5 days, at which time the dressing is changed and a new compressive dressing is applied. Three or four sterile 4 × 4s and a 3-inch Kling are used, beginning the circumferential compressive dressing just distal to the tibialis anterior insertion. By the 14th postoperative day the patient should be back into a flexible soled sneaker.

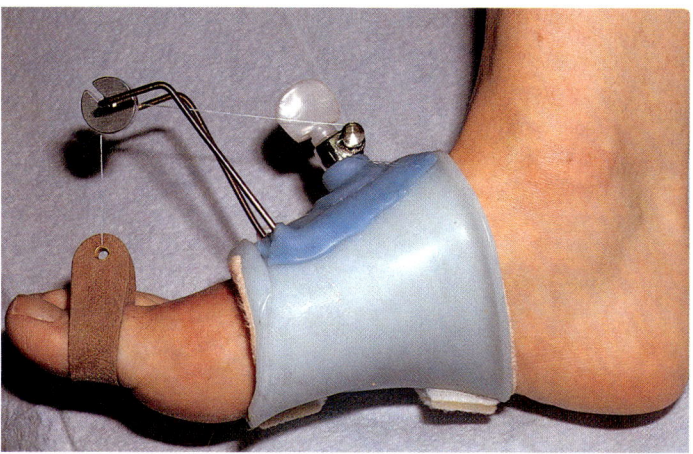

Figure 19. A dynamic extension splint for the great toe metatarsophalangeal joint.

REHABILITATION

Active and passive range of motion is encouraged. A home therapy program of passive motion should include 10 minutes of dorsiflexion exercises every 1 to 2 hours while awake. A nonsteroidal, ice, massage, and contrast baths are helpful to decrease inflammation. The patient may use a mild narcotic rather than forego motion exercises.

If no significant progress is obtained with the home program, formal occupational or physical therapy is ordered at 3 weeks postoperatively. The patient should attend three times a week as needed. I have found that a dynamic extension splint, similar to that used in certain hand surgery, can be very helpful in regaining motion (Fig. 19). The dynamic splint is worn at night and is used for approximately 1 month, as tolerated. Manipulation of the joint in the office under regional block should be considered 8 to 10 weeks after surgery if significant disparity exists between intraoperative and postoperative motion.

Without aggressive therapy, the patient can be expected to gain only approximately 50% of the motion obtained during surgery. While the degree of intraoperative motion is not a prerequisite for a successful outcome, there is certainly no reason to lose what has been gained by a careful surgical dissection. The majority of patients will plateau at their therapy program approximately 4 months postoperatively, with little increase in range of motion seen at that time. The symptoms often continue to abate, however, for up to 6 months after surgery, and in some cases, up to 1 year or more. Most patients have pain relief postoperatively, even if range of motion is not increased significantly (6). There is no clear correlation in fact between the amount of pain relief and the percentage of motion obtained.

COMPLICATIONS

A few patients may continue to be symptomatic and require additional surgery. I would defer a second procedure until 1 year after the first. Rather than have a second operation, the patient may be willing to accept the type of shoe modification discussed under conservative treatment. If not, a Keller resection arthroplasty or an arthrodesis of the joint can be performed. Prior to the original cheilectomy all patients should have been cautioned about the need for a possible second procedure. The cheilectomy relieves the dorsal impingement of the joint but does

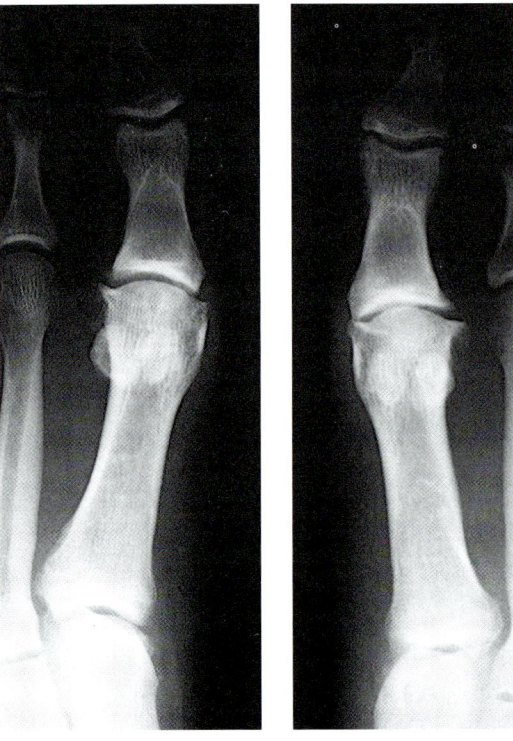

Figure 20. A standing preoperative view of bilateral moderate hallux rigidus.

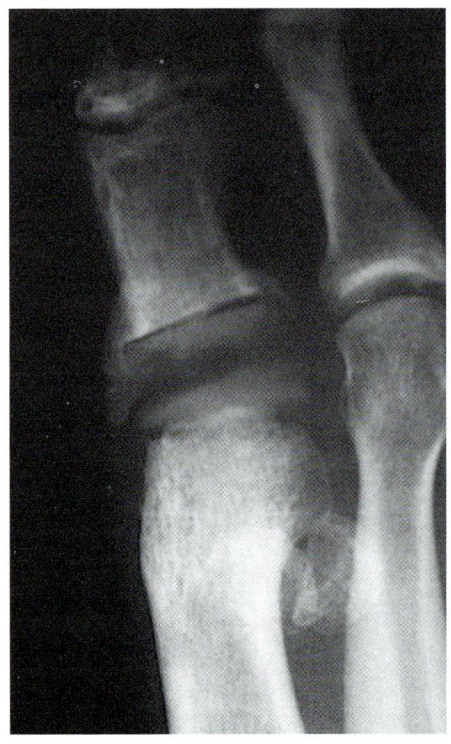

Figure 21. Implant of metatarsophalangeal joint performed elsewhere.

not alter the underlying degenerative process that may require further operative intervention.

There are a few complications reported that are specific to this procedure. Excessive metatarsal head resection can produce an unstable metatarsophalangeal joint that requires an arthrodesis or resection arthroplasty to salvage. Damage to the extensor hallucis longus tendon during the operative procedure is another difficult complication to manage. If the tendon is inadvertently cut it should be repaired with a 4-0 nonabsorbable suture. A rigorous range of motion program postoperatively is comprised as plantar flexion of the ankle and great toe must be avoided while the tendon heals.

ILLUSTRATIVE CASE FOR TECHNIQUE

This 42-year-old heavy laborer with bilateral grade II hallux rigidus (Fig. 20) had an implant arthroplasty of the right metatarsophalangeal joint performed elsewhere (Fig. 21). Preoperatively his range of motion was 20° of dorsiflexion. Six months postoperatively he had 30° of dorsiflexion on the operative side with complete relief of pain. He had continued pain on the left and chose to have a cheilectomy performed. Large dorsal and lateral osteophytes were excised along with approximately 30% of the dorsal metatarsal head (Fig. 22). A small osteophyte on the dorsal aspect of the proximal phalanx was also excised. He obtained 65° of passive dorsiflexion on the operating table. Five months postoperatively he has 40° of active dorsiflexion on the left and is pain free (Fig. 23). He does not prefer one side to the other but in retrospect would rather have had a cheilectomy on the right side than an implant.

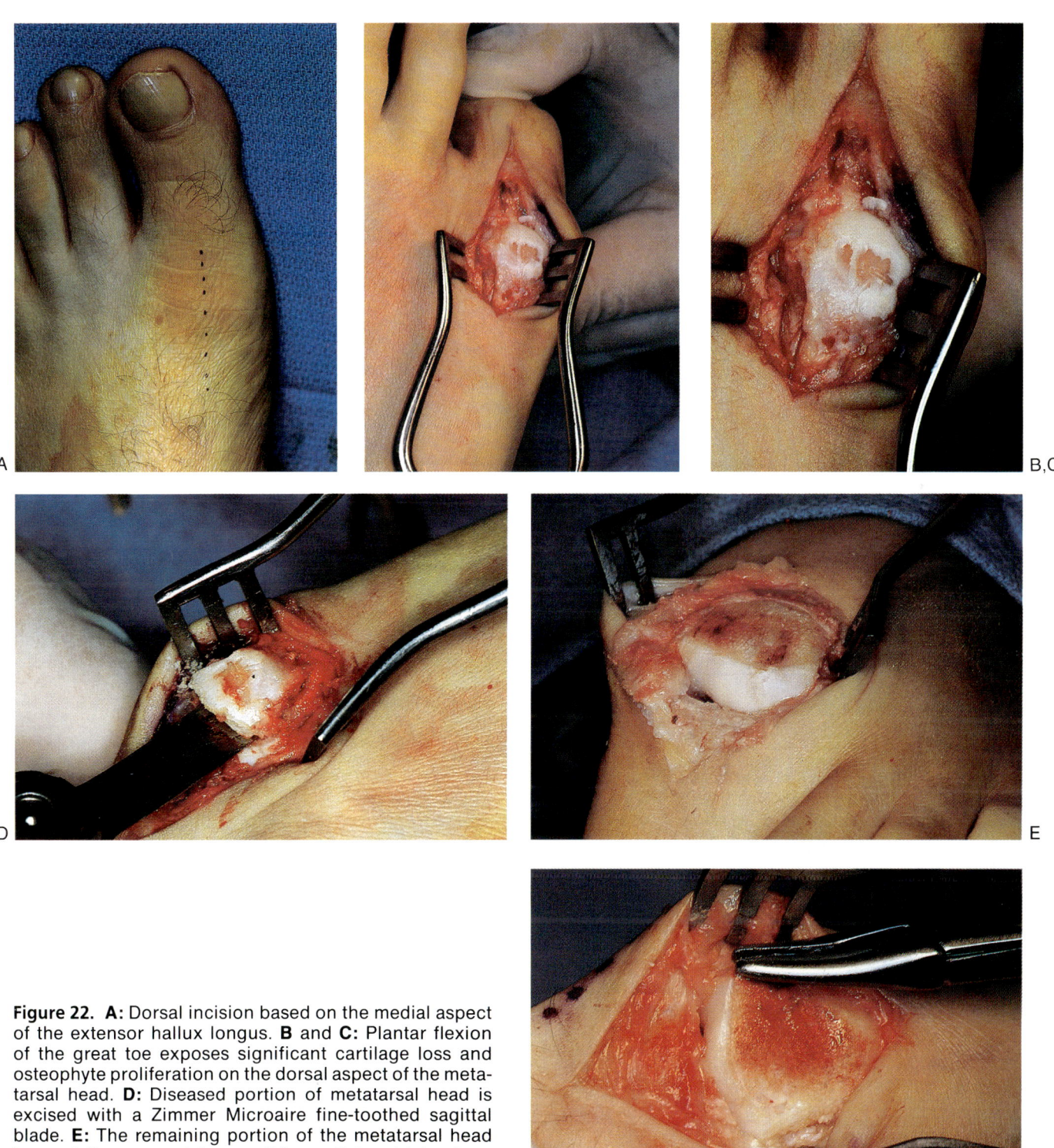

Figure 22. A: Dorsal incision based on the medial aspect of the extensor hallux longus. B and C: Plantar flexion of the great toe exposes significant cartilage loss and osteophyte proliferation on the dorsal aspect of the metatarsal head. D: Diseased portion of metatarsal head is excised with a Zimmer Microaire fine-toothed sagittal blade. E: The remaining portion of the metatarsal head is carefully assessed for possible medial and lateral osteophyte excision or drilling of small cartilage defects. F: Small medial osteophytes are excised with a rongeur.

Figure continues on next page.

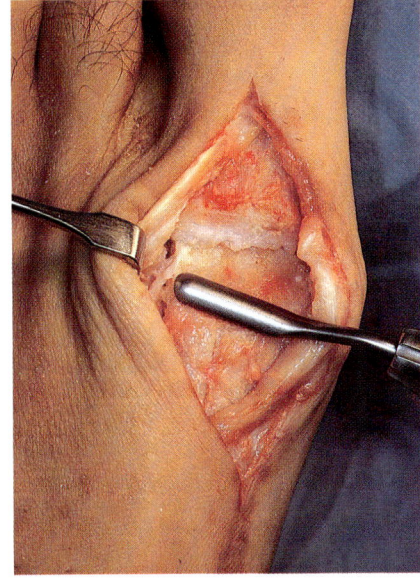
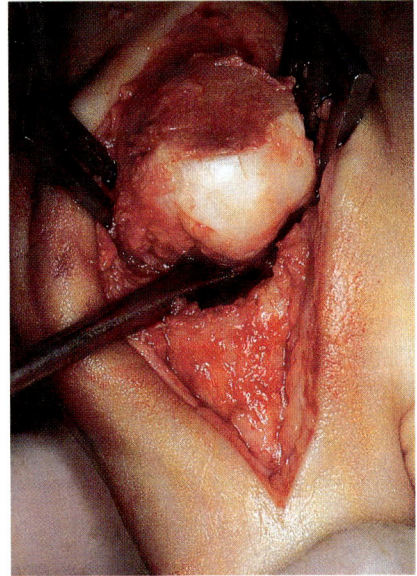
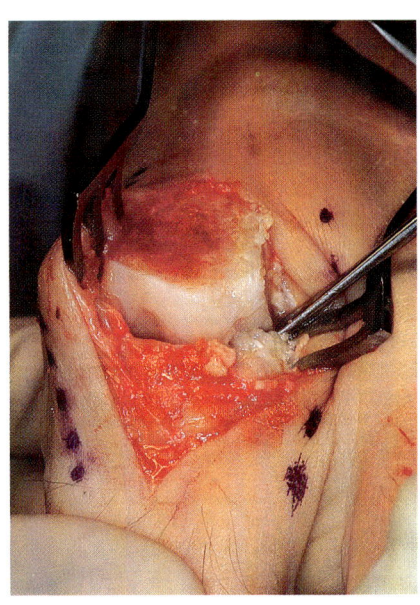

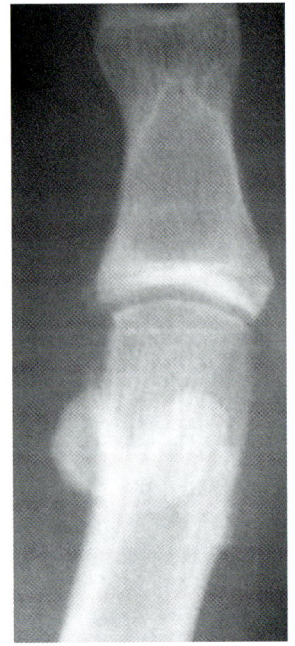

Figure 22. *(Continued.)* **G:** A microreciprocating rasp is used to smooth out prominent edges created by the metatarsal head and osteophyte resection. **H:** A Freer is used on the plantar aspect of the metatarsal head to free up any adhesions that may restrict dorsiflexion of the great toe. **I:** Prominent osteophytes on the lateral aspect of metatarsal head have been removed. **J:** Approximately 70° of passive dorsiflexion has been obtained on the operative table.

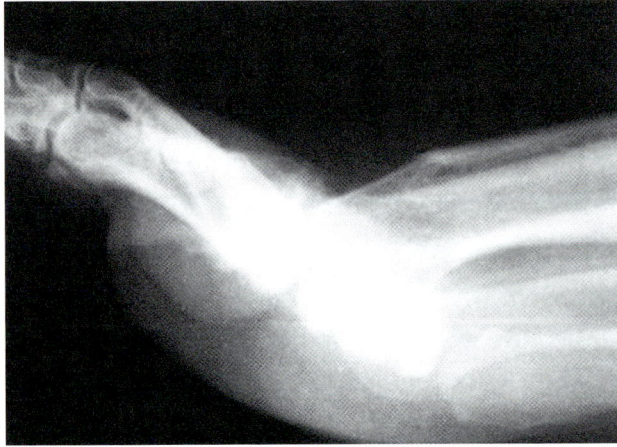

Figure 23. Postoperative AP **(A)** and lateral radiographs **(B)** of the left metatarsophalangeal joint.

RECOMMENDED READING

1. Davies-Colley, N.: Contraction of the metatarsophalangeal joint of the great toe (hallux flexus). *Br. Med. J.*, 1: 728, 1887.
2. Hattrup, S. J., and Johnson. K. A.: Subjective results of hallux rigidus following treatment with cheilectomy. *Clin. Orthop. Rel. Res.*, 226: 182–191, 1988.
3. Hawkins, B. J., and Haddad, R. J.: Hallux rigidus. *Clin. Sports Med.*, 7(1): 37–49, 1988.
4. Karasick, D., and Wapner, K. N.: Hallux rigidus deformity: radiologic assessment. *Am. J. Radiol.*, 157: 1029–1033, 1991.
5. Mann, R. A.: Hallux rigidus. In: *Instructional Course Lectures*, edited by W. B. Green, pp. 15–21, 1990.
6. Mann, R. A., and Clanton, T. O.: Hallux rigidus: Treatment by cheilectomy. *J. Bone Joint Surg.*, 70A: 400–405, 1988.

11

Realignment of the Overlapping Second Toe

E. Greer Richardson

INDICATIONS/CONTRAINDICATIONS

Recognition of the second toe as a primary entity rather than a deformity secondary to hallux valgus is relatively recent and is due, in large part, to the work of Coughlin (1,4), who emphasized and defined this problem (Fig. 1). The indications for surgery vary with the severity of the deformity. There are two common complaints that may require surgery. The first is pain in the second metatarsophalangeal (MP) joint, which may be secondary to chronic synovitis (5). This usually occurs with mild or moderate deformities. The second complaint is mechanical impingement of the toe on the adjacent hallux and the toe box of the shoe. This usually occurs in severe deformities with second MP joint symptoms decreasing while symptoms over the dorsum of the proximal interphalangeal (PIP) joint increase (Fig. 2).

In mild deformities serial taping or splinting of the second toe in a reduced position and selective use of antiinflammatory medications and intraarticular injections of a corticosteroid may avoid the need for surgery.

The pathophysiology of this deformity is more readily explained than the exact etiology. The essential lesion in the overlapping toe is attenuation of the fibular collateral ligament (1) (Fig. 3) that allows subluxation of the base of the proximal phalanx medially, carrying with it the plantar plate. The inciting event is felt to be a synovitis of the second MP joint (Fig. 4). If this synovitis is unchecked, the fibular collateral ligament, lateral capsule, and even the second dorsal interosseous tendons are weakened through incremental attrition. The deformity progresses in direct proportion to the laxity of the lateral supporting capsular structures and finally results in plantar plate insufficiency.

E. G. Richardson, M.D.: Department of Orthopaedics, University of Tennessee, College of Medicine, Memphis, TN 38105; and The Campbell Clinic, Memphis, TN 38103.

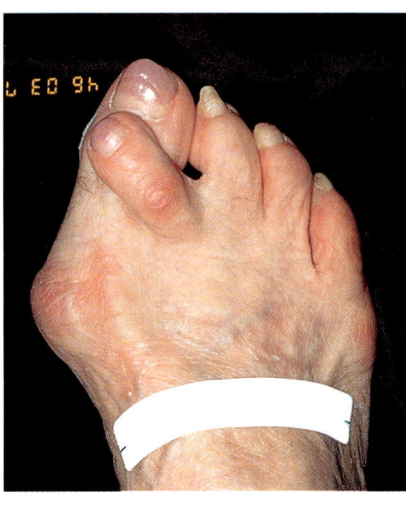

Figure 1. Severe overlapping second toe deformity with associated hallux valgus.

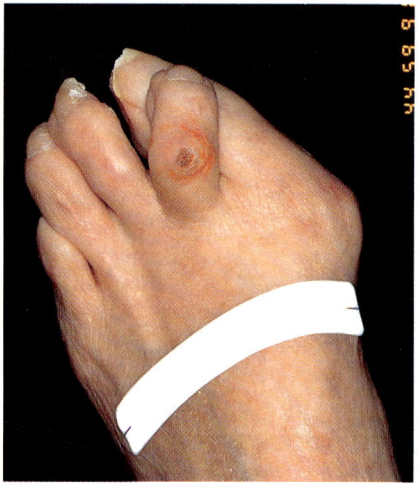

Figure 2. Ulcer over proximal interphalangeal (PIP) joint from toe box impingement in patient with severe overlapping toe deformity.

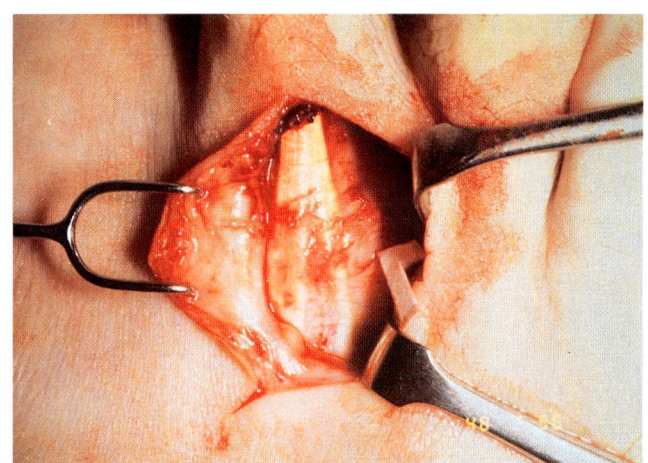

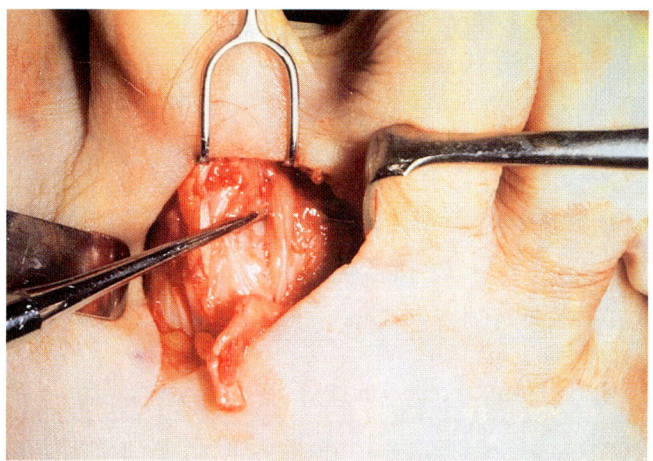

Figure 3. A: Rupture of dorsofibular capsule of second metatarsophalangeal (MP) joint *(arrow).* **B:** Fibular collateral ligament (FCL) is attenuated; tissue under the probe was more synovial than fibrous.

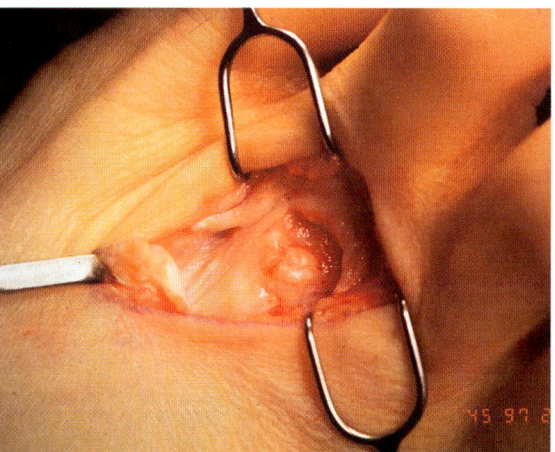

Figure 4. Synovitis of second MP joint with erosion of the dorsal capsule and FCL.

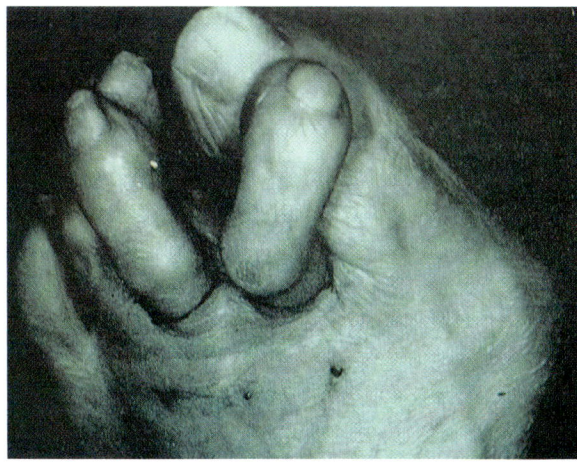 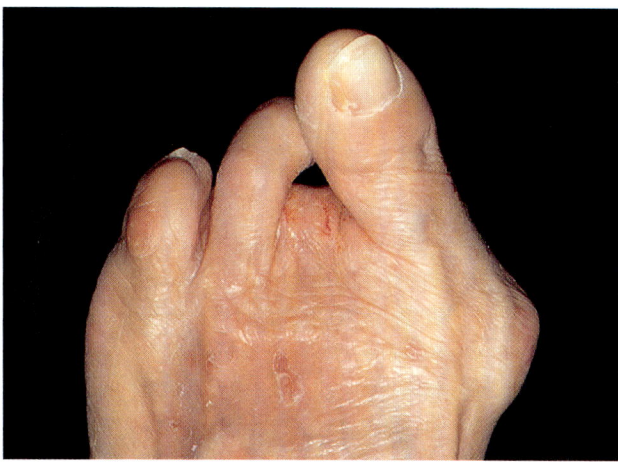

Figure 5. A: Dislocation of second and third MP joints with divergent overlapping. **B:** Several months after amputation of second and third toes; hallux valgus is about the same.

The contraindications for surgical repair of this deformity are insufficient vascular supply to the toe and such severe, long-standing deformity in elderly patients that there is no place to put the toe once it is released. An example would be a severe varus deformity of the rest of the lesser toes for which amputation is probably the best solution (Fig. 5).

PREOPERATIVE PLANNING

The extent of operative repair required for correction depends on the severity of the deformity. The purpose of the classification scheme in Table 1 is to aid in preoperative planning, realizing that there are exceptions that do not fall into this classification scheme; for example, occasionally the MP joint is completely dislocated, causing a marked overlapping deformity, whereas the PIP joint remains supple (Fig. 6).

The physical examination should not only focus on the obvious deformity, but in addition, the hindfoot and midfoot position during weight bearing and the remainder of the forefoot should be examined. A fixed varus deformity of the third toe at the MP or PIP joint may require correction to allow space for placement of the corrected second toe (Fig. 7). If the hallux is in so much valgus that the normal position in the forefoot alignment is unavailable to the second toe, this hallux valgus deformity must be corrected even if it is not a primary complaint

TABLE 1. *Cross-over toe deformity*

Mild	Subluxation proximal phalanx less than one-third of articular surface metatarsal
	No fixed deformities; attenuation FCL
Moderate	Subluxation proximal phalanx one-third to two-thirds articular surface of metatarsal head
	Fixed flexion contracture PIP joint
	Incomplete tear FCL
Severe	Complete dislocation MP joint
	FFC PIP joint
	Complete tear FCL + extensor apparatus

FCL, fibular collateral ligament; FFC, fixed flexion contracture; MP, metatarsophalangeal; PIP, proximal interphalangeal.

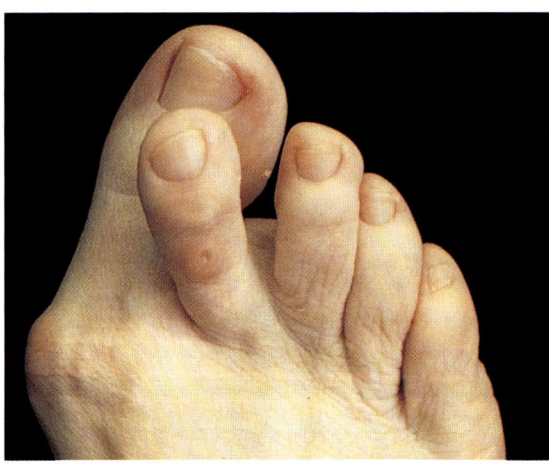

Figure 6. In this patient, the PIP joint was supple even with the severe overlapping of the second toe; this is the exception rather than the rule.

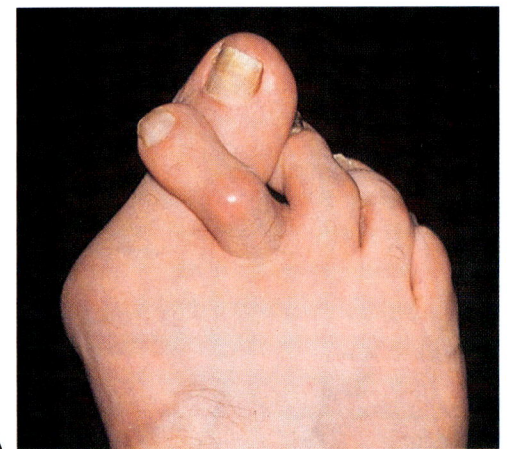 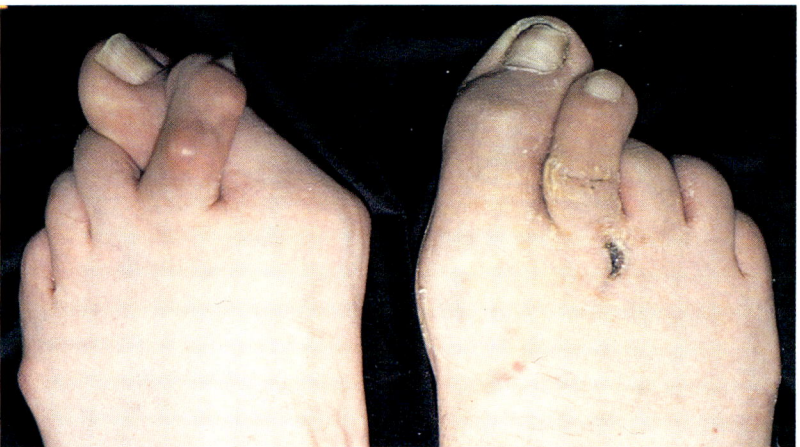

Figure 7. A: Severe overlapping second toe deformity with varus of remaining lesser toes at PIP joints. **B:** Underlapping third toe holds second toe in slight extension.

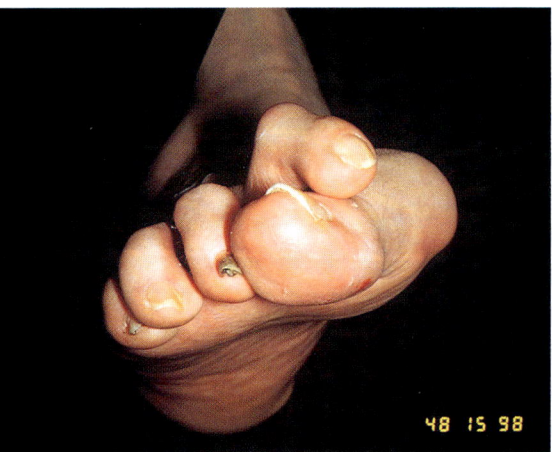

Figure 8. Hallux valgus must be corrected in severe deformity, even if the patient is not complaining of that component of forefoot deformity.

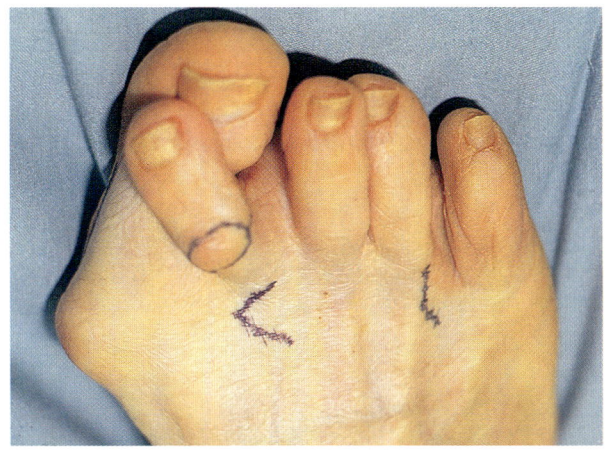 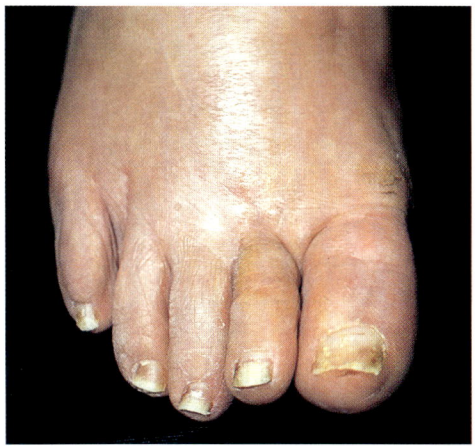

Figure 9. A: Severe overlapping second toe deformity with hallux valgus. **B:** After arthrodesis of the first MP joint, resection of the base of the second toe proximal phalanx (no longer recommended), and arthrodesis of the PIP joint.

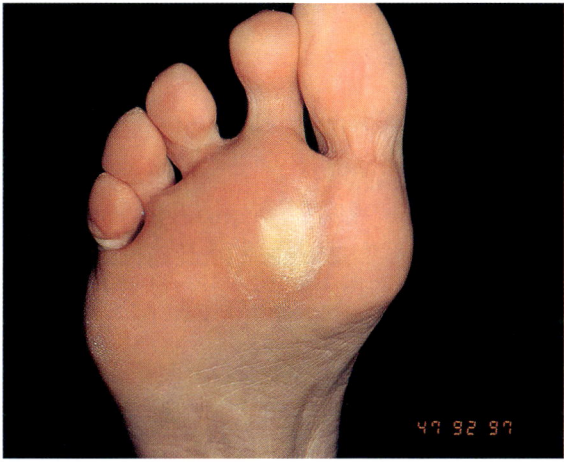

Figure 10. Mild overlapping toe deformity; this patient's primary complaint was of a painful callosity beneath the second metatarsal head.

(Fig. 8). If the hindfoot is in marked valgus because of posterior tibial tendon rupture and the second toe is overlapping a severe hallux valgus deformity, arthrodesis of the first MP joint may produce a better long-term result than would another type of hallux valgus repair (Fig. 9). Any fixed contracture such as MP joint extension or PIP joint flexion should be noted because it will affect the result of the procedure if not corrected.

Weight-bearing anteroposterior (AP) and lateral radiographs and non–weight-bearing oblique views will aid in evaluation of the remainder of the foot.

The test popularized by Thompson and Hamilton (7) for evaluation of the competence of the plantar plate is helpful. This consists of an "anterior drawer" sign elicited by straightening the second ray with one hand and with the other hand grasping the second toe at its base and lifting it dorsally. Occasionally, this joint is lax in the AP plane, so the test should be performed on the uninvolved toe for comparison. The second MP joint should be inspected for subtle changes, such as loss of the extension creases suggestive of joint effusion or slight subluxation/rotation of the second toe, which is best viewed from an end-on, axial perspective.

The examiner should "get a feel" for the ease with which the MP joint can be reduced and how quickly it returns to its subluxed position. Likewise, the remaining MP joints should be tested in the AP (frontal) and mediolateral (transverse) planes to determine the presence of any fixed deformities.

The plantar surface of the foot should be inspected for painful callosities beneath the second metatarsal head. A callosity is one sign of an altered weight-bearing load caused by an extension posture, with or without a fixed contracture, of the second MP joint (Fig. 10).

Occasionally flexion contractures will be present at both the PIP and distal interphalangeal (DIP) joints in the overlapping toe. If a painful end corn is present or the patient complains of pain over the DIP joint, both the PIP and DIP joint abnormalities must be corrected.

SURGERY

The surgery is performed after the use of a local anesthetic consisting of 1% lidocaine and 0.5% Marcaine without epinephrine. A first and second intermetatarsal block is sufficient for correction of the second toe deformity. The patient is supine on the operating table. An elastic Esmarch wrap is used for exsanguination as well as ankle tourniquet. It is removed before skin closure. The steps of the procedure vary with the severity of the deformity.

If there is no fixed flexion contracture at the PIP joint and the tibial subluxation of the proximal phalanx is mild, a transfer of the flexor digitorum longus (FDL) to the extensor hood over the proximal phalanx, combined with advancement of the lateral slip of the longitudinally sectioned tendon to hold the phalanx reduced (as recommended by Coughlin), is a reasonable choice. This procedure is best for the mild deformity. Theoretically, it moves the deforming force (3) to a position that helps maintain correction (1,4,7). It rarely will afford active flexion at the MP joint, but it may be helpful when it is combined with synovectomy and dorsal capsulotomy at the MP joint. I use it infrequently. If the patient has a painful callus beneath the second metatarsal head, with or without a fixed flexion contracture at the PIP joint, this procedure alone is contraindicated; it must be used in conjunction with other surgical steps.

Technique. *Mild Deformity.* For a flexor to extensor transfer a transverse plantar incision is made at the proximal flexion crease of the toe, being careful to preserve the digital arteries and nerves. The skin and subcutaneous tissue are retracted with small hooked retractors to expose the underlying flexor tendons and their fibrous sheaths. The proximal 3 or 4 mm of the pulley is opened to expose the FDL immediately under it. This is best done by opening the pulley to one side and dissecting over the underlying tendons, removing a small segment of pulley. This dissection is made easier by the use of magnification loupes and a small round-end knife. Topographically, this dissection is located at about the middle third of the proximal phalanx. The central tendon should be the FDL, but gentle, passive flexion and extension of the DIP joint while the proximal interphalangeal joint is held straight will confirm this. While lifting the FDL tendon, the vinculum longum, if present, will appear under tension and should be severed after electrocautery. A second transverse plantar incision is made at the DIP joint and a tenotomy of the FDL is performed, being careful to not violate the plantar plate of this joint (Fig. 11A, B).

Returning to the proximal incision, the FDL is hooked (but not clamped) with a small hemostat and the distal segment is delivered into the wound. If the vinculae between the two incisions are tenacious, this step might require force. Once the FDL is delivered from the proximal incision, the wound is inspected again to be certain that the two lateral slips of the flexor digitorum brevis are intact (Fig. 11C).

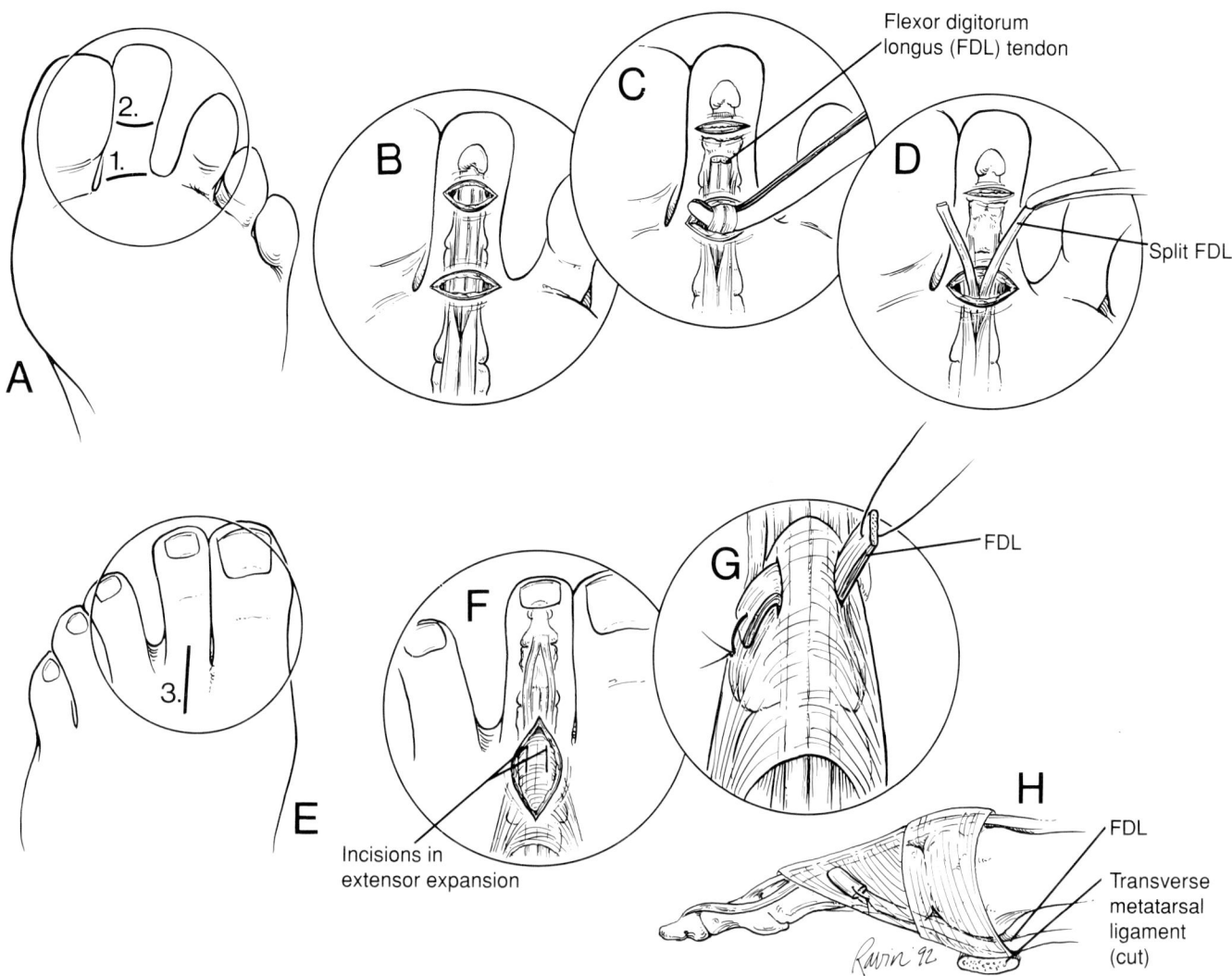

Figure 11. Flexor digitorum longus (FDL) transfer for mild deformity. (From ref. 6.) **A:** Transverse incisions at distal interphalangeal (DIP) and PIP creases. **B:** Flexor tendon is released at DIP joint. **C:** FDL is brought into proximal wound with hemostat. **D:** FDL is split about 2 cm along natural cleavage line in its center. **E** and **F:** A 2-cm longitudinal incision is made over dorsum of proximal half of proximal phalanx. Separate, smaller incisions are placed through the extensor expansion in the distal part of wound for windows through which FDL slips will pass. **G:** FDL slips pass plantar to transverse metatarsal ligament, which is essential for any flexion moment at MP joint. **H:** Tendon slips may be crossed and sutured together, but this may leave a small knot beneath skin.

Careful inspection of the FDL shows a shallow, linear furrow running longitudinally along its plantar surface. Using small forceps, an assistant holds one side of the delivered tendon at its free end and the surgeon holds the other, while splitting the tendon longitudinally along this natural cleavage plane for 1.5 to 2.5 cm (Fig. 11D). The tendon must be pulled distally with the ankle plantar flexed to clearly see both sides of the tendon during this step. This will avoid inadvertent sectioning of half of the tendon. Other helpful points are to hold the two segments apart only enough to fit a small pair of straight scissors in the axilla of dissection and to use the tips of the scissors.

The tendon is moistened with saline and a second skin incision is made longitudinally in the midline on the dorsum of the proximal phalanx, 1.5 to 2 cm in length.

The dorsal digital veins usually are to each side of this incision, but if they are in line with the incision, they should be cauterized. By sharp dissection, the trailing edge of each lateral band of the extensor mechanism is identified while the skin is retracted, including the superficial veins and nerves to either side, using two-pronged skin hooks. A 2- to 4-mm longitudinal incision is made in the extensor mechanism halfway between the midline dorsally and the trailing edge of the lateral band plantarward on each side. These incisions should be at the level of the middiaphysis of the proximal phalanx (Fig. 11E,F). A small hemostat is passed through one incision in the extensor mechanism to emerge in the plantar incision, staying close to bone. This technique will avoid the digital neurovascular bundle. One slip of the split FDL is grasped at its tip with a hemostat and is brought into the dorsal wound through the extensor mechanism. The same procedure is repeated on the other side of the phalanx. With an assistant holding the ankle joint at 90° (neutral dorsiflexion–plantar flexion), the tendon slips are overlapped sufficiently to hold the MP joint in 5° to 10° of plantar flexion. Occasionally, the FDL will need further splitting linearly. If so, the tendon slips *must* be returned to the plantar incision to avoid severing one half. With the tendon slips held at the desired tension, 3–0 or 4–0 nonabsorbable sutures are used to fasten each slip of the FDL under tension to the extensor mechanism, while the assistant continues to hold the ankle in neutral position. Then the tip of each slip is looped back on itself and secured to the trailing edge of each side of the lateral band and to itself (Fig. 11G). Any excess tendon is sectioned. Alternatively, the two tendon slips may be sutured to one another over the dorsum of the phalanx (Fig. 11H). With the ankle extended to neutral, the MP joint should rest in the neutral or slightly flexed position and the PIP joint in neutral or less than 10° of flexion.

Before closing the skin, the tourniquet is removed and hemostasis is obtained by cautery or compression. The wounds are closed with 4–0 monofilament nylon or suture of the surgeon's choice.

Mild–Moderate Deformity. The second MP joint is approached through a chevron incision with its apex at the MP joint. The distal limb of the incision crosses obliquely over the proximal half of the proximal phalanx and the proximal limb crosses the second metatarsal obliquely at the neck–distal metaphysis level (Fig. 12A). The venous and superficial fascial network is cleared from the extensor apparatus 2 cm proximal and 1 cm distal to the second MP joint. The interval between the extensor digitorum longus (EDL) and the extensor digitorum brevis (EBL) is identified in the proximal portion of the wound. The EDB approaches the MP joint from lateral to medial and becomes confluent with the EDL at the level of the metatarsal neck (Fig. 12B); however, it can be severed from the EDL distally over the base of the proximal phalanx. This extra length will be needed later. The EDB is released from the EDL, transected about 1 cm distal to the MP joint, and placed in the depths of the wound. The EDL is freed from its soft tissue bed, and with a #67 Beaver blade a Z-plasty lengthening is performed. The EDL can be lengthened up to 2 cm, but this degree of lengthening is reserved for severe deformities (Fig. 12C). The lengthened tendon is placed to the side of the metatarsal to protect it during the next part of the procedure.

The dorsal capsule is inspected carefully, especially dorsolaterally. Magnification loupes are helpful. With an angled probe, any weakness in the capsule is evaluated by gentle probing. Invariably some difference is found between the integrity of the dorsolateral and medial aspects of the capsule. A weakened dorsal, or more commonly dorsolateral and lateral, aspect of the capsule may have a fibrinous covering or the lateral base of the proximal phalanx and adjacent lateral surface of the metatarsal head may be completely exposed; any degree of disruption between these two extremes may also be found. If the entire lateral capsule is disrupted, the second dorsal interosseous tendon usually is disrupted too because of its intimate attachment on its course to the base of the proximal phalanx.

With small right-angle (Ragnell) retractors placed laterally, the proximal phalanx

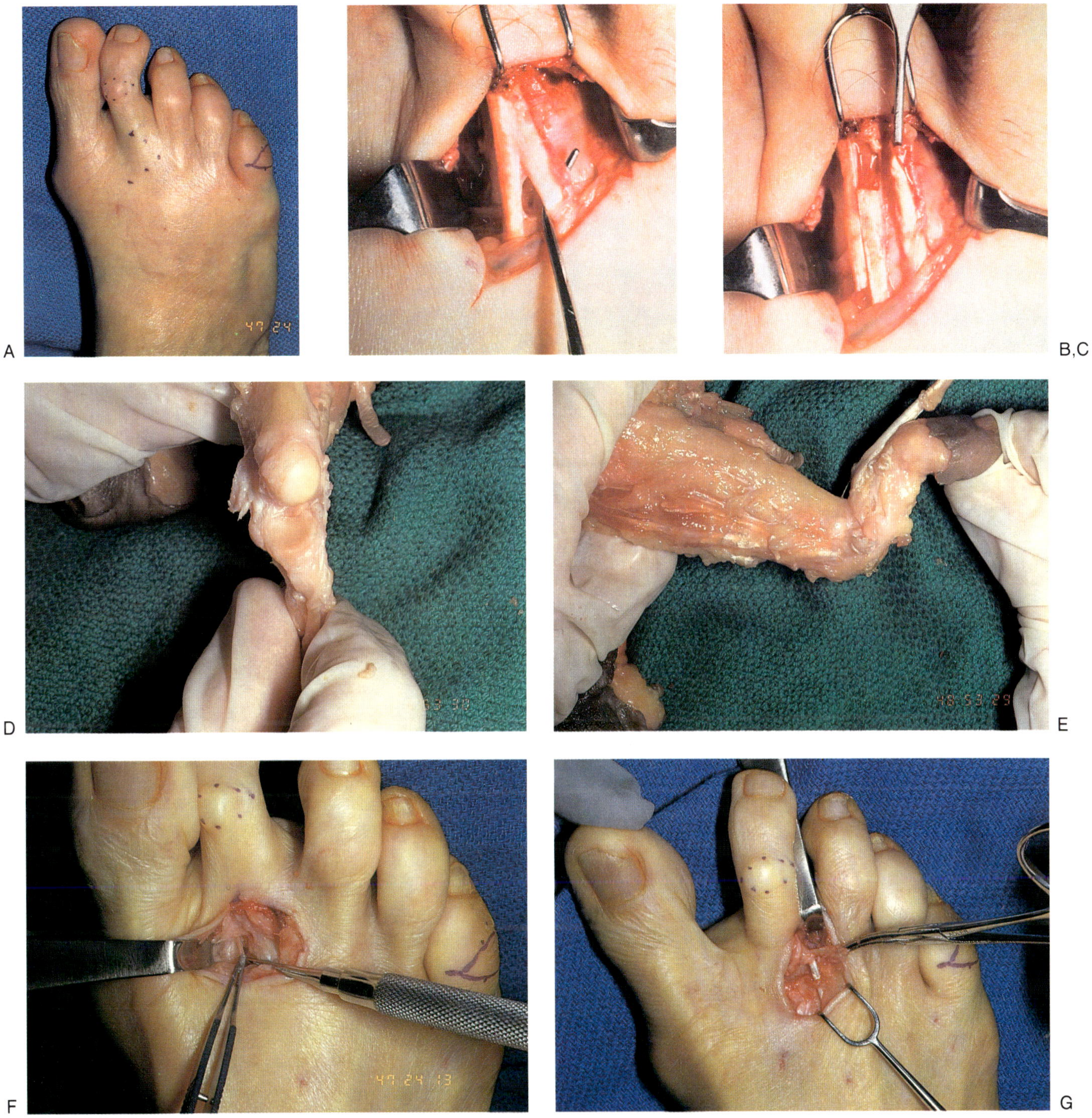

Figure 12. A: Synovitis of second MP joint with mild deformity. The mild hallux valgus and overlapping toe deformities in this forefoot are precursors to the severe deformity shown in Fig. 1. The angled incision has its apex at the fibular border of the MP joint. **B:** Probe beneath the extensor digitorum brevis (EDB) tendon; note the junction with the extensor digitorum longus (EDL) at the MP joint. **C:** The EDL has been lengthened in a Z fashion and the EDB has been dissected and released about 1 cm distal to the MP joint. **D:** Dorsal view of anatomic specimen with all soft tissue except the plantar plate removed from MP joint. **E:** Sagittal view of same specimen demonstrating extreme dorsiflexion allowed without dislocation of the joint. **F:** Probe beneath thickened tibial collateral ligament and intrinsic muscle tendon. **G:** EDB tendon is passed through tunnel in extensor expansion and sutured to itself after remaining fibular capsular structures have been sutured. In severe, long-standing deformities, tissue may not be adequate to hold sutures when tightening fibular side of capsule.

is displaced medially and dorsally, and the joint is inspected and palpated with the probe to evaluate the integrity of the plantar plate. In my experience, if the plantar plate is disrupted from the neck of the metatarsal (its weakest mooring and the usual site of disruption), no soft tissue realignment procedure will maintain long-term reduction. Soft tissues seem to work because an intact plantar plate will allow extreme dorsiflexion without disruption (Fig. 12D,E).

The phalanx is reduced congruously on the metatarsal head and its stability is evaluated. If it springs back into a dorsomedial deformity, the medial capsule is examined. In severe, long-standing overlapping this part of the capsule may be very thick (Fig. 12F). The medial capsule should be released if necessary. Because this also releases the first dorsal interosseous, the joint is held congruously reduced in 0° of flexion and the tibial collateral ligament is stressed before releasing the medial capsule. If the tibial collateral ligament is tight, it also must be released. The dorsal capsule is incised transversely if the second MP joint cannot be easily brought into 20° of flexion.

Even with the capsule released from "plantar plate to plantar plate" (medially and dorsally by scalpel and laterally by the pathologic process), the toe frequently assumes a dorsotibial deformity. This is perplexing and most difficult to treat without limiting MP joint motion by a fibrous arthroplasty.

Any fixed contractures of the PIP joint must be released. The PIP joint is approached through a dorsal elliptical incision that measures 5 to 6 mm wide and has a 2 or 3 mm lateral extension on either side. Initially only the skin is removed and the vessels are cauterized. A slightly smaller segment of extensor tendon and dorsal capsule of the PIP joint is removed, leaving a 2 mm remnant of extensor tendon attached to the base of the middle phalanx. The proximal end of the extensor tendon usually retracts beneath the proximal skin flap, but can be easily pulled distally at the appropriate time. The PIP joint is flexed about 20° while traction is placed on the distal and middle phalanges. Then with a small-blade knife, the collateral ligaments are sectioned from outside in on both sides of the joint by placing the blade between the skin and the ligament and then turning the cutting edge toward the joint. Now the PIP joint can be flexed to 90° and the head and neck of the proximal phalanx is clearly exposed. A tongue of the EDL is raised for later suture stabilization of the PIP joint. With a rongeur or small-blade power saw, the head and neck of the proximal phalanx are removed, and any sharp points of bone are smoothed with a rasp or rongeur. The toe is extended to neutral position at the PIP joint and tightness with abutment of the articular surface of the middle phalanx on the distal end of proximal phalangeal remnant is sought. If it feels tight, 2 or 3 mm more of bone are removed. The proximal skin edge is entered with 4–0 nonabsorbable suture, which is then passed through the proximal end of the extensor tendon. Next, the distal remnant of the extensor tendon is entered on its joint surface and the suture exits through the skin. By canting the stitch, a few degrees of lateral deformity also will be corrected. The corners of the wound are sutured with a simple stitch. An initial mattress stitch may be used if deemed appropriate.

After all contracted tissues have been released, the EDB tendon is transferred through a tunnel in the lateral extensor hood as far plantarward as possible. Having an assistant translate the toe dorsally while the tunnel is made and the tendon is transferred makes this step easier (Fig. 12G). Once the tendon is through the tunnel of tissue on the lateral base of the proximal phalanx, the MP joint is overreduced about 10° laterally, the tendon is brought proximally, and sutured back to itself with 4–0 Vicryl on a #P-3 plastic needle. Placing more curve in this small needle makes the next step (capsular imbrication) easier. A stout two-tooth retractor is used to pull the third metatarsal head laterally and a suture is placed as far plantar as possible toward the plantar plate, beginning proximally and passing the needle distally to tissue near the lateral side of the base of the proximal phalanx. If possible another suture is placed in the same tissue but dorsal to the EDB transfer, which is in the midline.

After the EDB transfer and repair of the lateral capsule, the reduction is examined. If the toe rests congruously reduced on the metatarsal head, the toe is held in 10° to 20° of flexion and the EDL is sutured in this lengthened position. Side-to-side suturing will supply additional strength. The dorsotibial capsule is left unsutured. The skin is closed with interrupted absorbable sutures with the knots buried.

This is my preferred technique for the mild to moderate deformity. Removing the head and neck of the proximal phalanx relatively lengthens the FDL and aids correction of the flexion at the PIP joint. The tendon-capsule procedure at the MP joint corrects the AP and mediolateral deformities.

The previously described procedures are for mild and moderate deformities. If the second MP joint is completely dislocated, with the second toe resting on the dorsum of the metatarsal, reduction should be attempted. If it reduces easily and redislocates easily (as is usually the case), soft tissue stabilization alone should not be used to maintain reduction.

The DuVries arthroplasty consisting of a partial metatarsal head resection is useful after complete capsulotomy and collateral ligament release. The plantar plate has been disrupted to allow the complete dislocation and a soft tissue procedure alone usually will not maintain reduction.

For the MP resection arthroplasty (DuVries), the metatarsal head and base of the proximal phalanx are exposed through an angled incision over the second MP joint. Usually the metatarsal head is covered by the proximal phalanx. The EDL tendon is released with a step-cut incision and a transverse tenotomy of the EDB, and both collateral ligaments and the dorsal capsule are severed. Transfer of the EDB is not necessary. Longitudinal, manual traction is placed on the second toe to relocate it if possible. By relocating the toe and reducing the joint congruously, a better "mind's eye" view is obtained as to the shape of the metatarsal head and the final desired resting position of the phalanx after removing part of the head.

The toe is redislocated to its former position. That spot is marked and again traction is placed on the toe while rounding of the metatarsal head with a 6 to 7 mm wide osteotome or a small rongeur. I prefer the latter. The second toe must rest in the reduced position without abutting against the metatarsal head remnant. This usually requires removal of 5 to 6 mm of the head. If the dislocation is severe and long-standing, and the joint cannot be reduced despite extensive soft tissue release, the metatarsal must be resected at the level where the phalanx rests.

I do not use a pin to maintain reduction, but do stress fastidious application of the dressing, which is maintained for 3 weeks and is followed by use of a hammer-toe pad for another 3 weeks (Fig. 13). If a pin is used to maintain reduction, it is removed at 3 to 4 weeks. Vascular compromise of the digit is more common

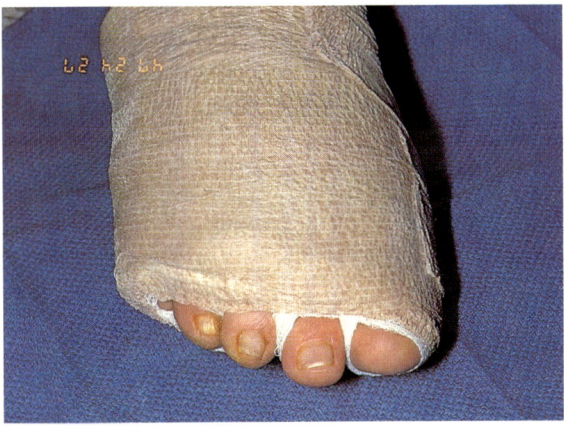

Figure 13. Form-fit dressing for maintaining position. Use of longitudinal pin is optional.

when a pin is used and prompt removal of the pin is required if this complication develops.

POSTOPERATIVE MANAGEMENT

A wooden-sole shoe is worn for 3 weeks, then a soft-soled shoe with a deep, wide toe box is worn for 4 to 6 weeks. Tape or a commercial pad to hold the toe

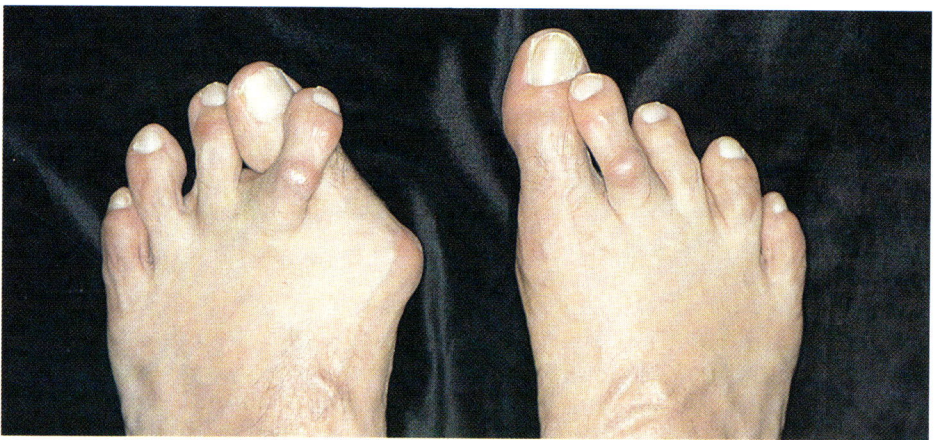

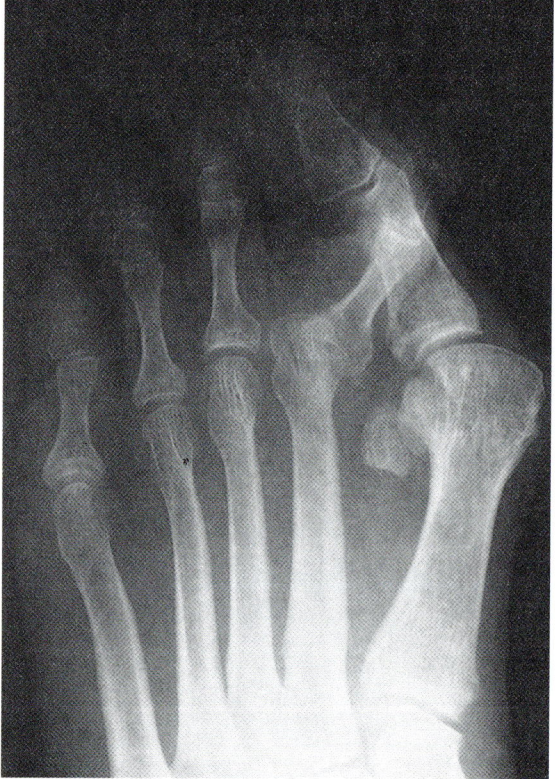

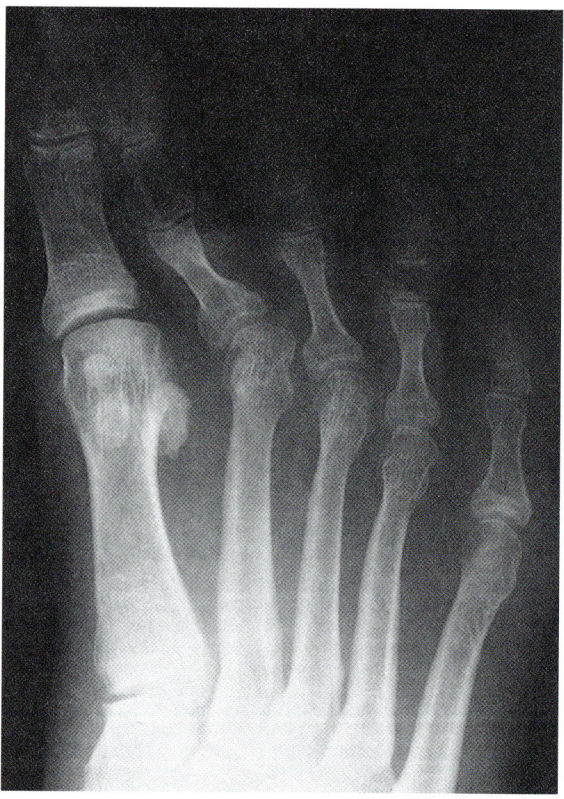

Figure 14. Severe overlapping toe deformity on left foot and moderate deformity on right foot. **A:** In clinical photograph, note hallux valgus on left foot and straight or slightly varus position of right hallux. This patient had no history of previous surgery or trauma. **B:** Note dislocation of second MP joint of left foot (severe deformity). **C:** Note second toe pulling third toe into varus on right foot (moderate deformity). This may become a fixed deformity and should be evaluated before surgery. If it is fixed in any degree of varus, this joint also must be released by release of tibial collateral ligament.

reduced is used during this time. The toe remains swollen for 3 to 6 months, and active control of the digit always is less than normal, but may approach what it was preoperatively if the deformity was severe and control was limited anyway.

COMPLICATIONS

Recurrence of the deformity and reduced voluntary control of the digit are common. Delayed wound healing and vascular compromise of the digit are less common but more troublesome complications.

Recurrence of the deformity probably is caused by failure of the procedure to hold the plantar plate under the metatarsal head. The extrinsic flexors (longus and brevis) may pull the second toe tibialward, especially in patients with pes planus, a valgus hindfoot, and abducted forefoot. This may occur after transfer of the FDL dorsally or even after tenotomy of the FDL. If this develops, a fibrous arthroplasty using the DuVries is the treatment of choice. The toe is held in the corrected position for 6 weeks.

Reduced voluntary control of the digit is almost inevitable and should probably not be thought of as an operative complication. Nonetheless, the patient will notice this and must be advised before surgery that loss of control is the compromise required for correction of the deformity. However, if the patient is shown how much voluntary control actually is present at each joint of the toe *before surgery* compared to the other toes, this "complication" usually is more acceptable.

Delayed wound healing at the MP incision is most common in moderate and severe deformities if the joint is not decompressed by an arthroplasty. Once the toe is reduced, a good deal of tension remains at the skin edges. Intermittent debridement of the skin edges in the office and the use of a removable short leg cast-brace to reduce tension from movement of the ankle and toes usually allows healing in 6 to 12 weeks. A split-thickness skin graft rarely may be required.

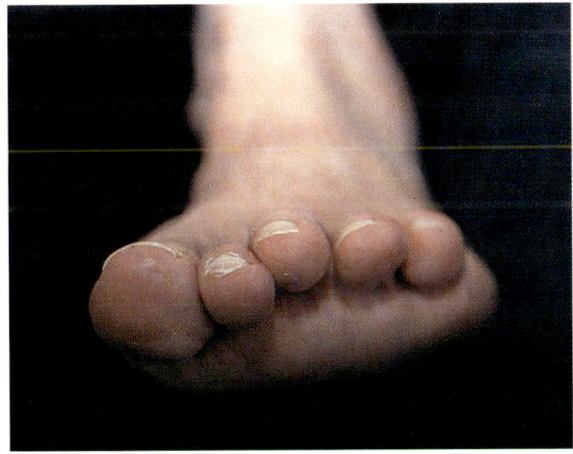
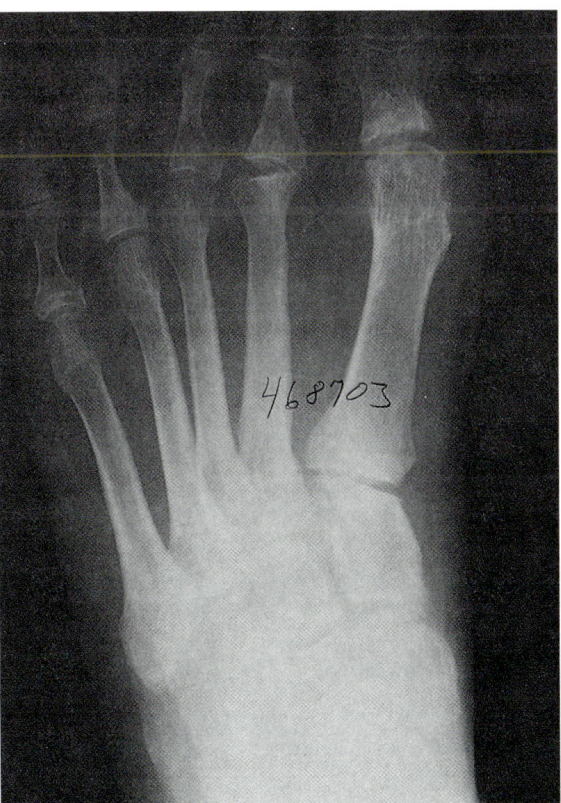

D and E: Clinical (D) and radiographic (E) appearance of left foot (severe deformity) several months after Keller procedure for hallux valgus, resection arthroplasty at second MP joint, and resection of head and neck of proximal phalanx.

Vascular compromise of the digit almost always is seen after the use of an intramedullary pin. Should the toe not "perk-up" 5 to 10 minutes after the tourniquet is released, the pin should be removed and a dressing should be used to maintain position.

ILLUSTRATIVE CASE FOR TECHNIQUE

This 58-year-old man has a severe deformity of his left foot that had developed over many years. The second toe was completely on top of the great toe, and a similar deformity to a lesser degree was present in his right foot (Fig. 14A–C).

Several months after his surgical correction the foot was satisfactory to the patient (Fig. 14D,E). An arthrodesis of the first MP joint may have even been a better procedure because there was still some "crowding" of his toes from the residual great toe deformity.

RECOMMENDED READING

1. Coughlin, M. J.: Crossover second toe deformity. *Foot Ankle*, 8: 29–39, 1987.
2. Jahss, M. H.: *Disorders of the Foot and Ankle*, 2nd ed, vol 2. W. B. Saunders, Philadelphia, 1991, pp. 1217–1221.
3. Johnson, J. B., and Price, T. W.: Crossover second toe deformity: etiology and treatment. *J. Foot Surg.*, 28: 417–420, 1989.
4. Mann, R. A., and Coughlin, M. J.: Lesser toe deformities. *AAOS Instr. Course Lect.*, 36: 137–159, 1987.
5. Mann, R. A., Mizel, M. S.: Monarticular nontraumatic synovitis of the metatarsophalangeal joint: a new diagnosis? *Foot Ankle*, 6: 18–21, 1985.
6. Richardson, E. G.: Lesser toe abnormalities. In: *Campbell's Operative Orthopadics*, 8th ed, edited by A. H. Crenshaw. Mosby Year Book, St. Louis, 1992.
7. Thompson, F. M., and Hamilton, W. G.: Problems of the second metatarsophalangeal joint. *Orthopedics*, 10: 83–89, 1987.

12

Resection Arthroplasty of the Second and Third Toes

Robert D. Teasdall

INDICATIONS/CONTRAINDICATIONS

Resection arthroplasty of the second and third metatarsophalangeal joints is used to treat deformities of these articulations. These deformities can usually be categorized into one of three types.

The most common deformity to be treated by resection arthroplasty is a subluxation or dislocation that occurs at the second and/or third metatarsophalangeal joints. Usually the second metatarsophalangeal joint is the most severely affected, but the third metatarsophalangeal joint will follow the deformity of the second after a period of some months to years in most instances. This condition seems to have become more common in the past several years. It may be that the dorsiflexed position at the metatarsophalangeal joint with high-heeled shoe-wear may be a contributing factor, since the deformity is most often seen in women. Men who develop this problem are usually quite physically active and participate in repetitive dorsiflexion motions at the metatarsophalangeal joint to the longer second and third rays by activities such as long-distance running.

Acquired extension contractures at the metatarsophalangeal joint 2 and 3 area are another indication for resection arthroplasty. Most often these deformities are termed severe hammer or claw toes. With such deformity, the metatarsophalangeal joint does not dislocate, but the extension contracture does occur. This idiopathic deformity is associated with aging as it occurs in the older population. Such extension contractures can also occur following severe foot trauma and increased closed compartment pressures in the foot.

Another indication for this procedure is the spreading deformity between the second and third toes. The patient notes the spreading between the toes with the

---

R. D. Teasdall, M.D.: Department of Orthopaedics, The Bowman Gray School of Medicine, Winston-Salem, NC 27157-1070.

second toe usually overlapping the great toe. Such deformity probably occurs as a result of a rupture of the collateral ligament of the metatarsophalangeal joint allowing the toe to go into a deviated position. Usually this deviation is mainly at the second metatarsophalangeal joint with the fibularward collateral ligament being the site of capsular disruption of the joint.

A mild deformity does not warrant this procedure. Treatment can be by other less ablative measures, such as a flexor to extensor transfer and release of the dorsal joint capsule. This would not be the appropriate procedure for a patient overly interested in cosmetic appearance. The toes are shortened and show the webbing between the toes when the procedure is completed. The webbing between the toes is not as much of a cosmetic concern as the shortening of the toes. Finally, a contraindication to resection arthroplasty is when there are significant functional needs for flexion at the metatarsophalangeal area. A highly competitive sports-oriented patient or a physically active person who has a significant functional need for the second and third toes should not be considered a candidate for this procedure.

PREOPERATIVE PLANNING

The typical patient with a subluxation or even dislocation at the second and third metatarsophalangeal joint is an older woman. The pain is located at the plantar aspect of the second metatarsophalangeal joint and is made worse with activity and relieved by rest. The toe may appear in a dorsiflexed position, but this is usually of a milder degree. By clasping the proximal phalanx between the thumb and index finger, while stabilizing the forefoot with the other hand, a repetitive dorsiflexion stress at that joint will usually elicit a grimace from the patient (Fig. 1). Putting direct pressure on the dorsal and plantar aspects of the second metatarsophalangeal joint is also painful. A standing radiograph shows changes ranging from a very mild double shadow on the dorsal aspect of the metatarsal head as the proximal phalanx rides dorsalward to a frank dislocation with overriding of the proximal phalanx completely above the metatarsal head and neck region.

If an extension contracture is the deformity present, this will be apparent on the physical examination. Usually the pain with a contracted toe is due to rubbing of the footwear on the dorsal aspect of the proximal interphalangeal joint. It is not possible to manipulate the metatarsophalangeal joint into a straight position. A callus over the dorsal aspect of the proximal interphalangeal joint is evident. The standing radiograph will show the second and third toe deformity, but a dislocation at the metatarsophalangeal joint does not occur.

Spreading between the second and third toes is usually accompanied by a mild pain at the metatarsophalangeal joint area. The subluxation stress test is also painful but not as much as a pure subluxation dislocation. The patient can usually describe approximately when the change in appearance of the second and third toes began and trauma is usually not a factor. Again the radiograph will show this deformity, which can probably be attributed to a rupture of the fibularward collateral ligament at the metatarsophalangeal joint.

The amount of phalanx to be resected should be determined prior to the surgical procedure. In mildly subluxed or spreading toes, the proximal one-third of the proximal phalanx needs to be resected. When the deformity is greater, such as with a frankly dislocated base of the proximal phalanx on the metatarsal head or with a severe claw toe, then up to two-thirds of the proximal phalanx bases of toes two and three need to be resected to allow relaxation of the deformity. The patient should be informed of the expected outcome. Relief of pain is usually quite good, but the toes do lose their plantarward flexion ability and become somewhat "floppy" as well as shortened. The principle of the procedure is to allow the toe to relocate into an improved position (Fig. 2).

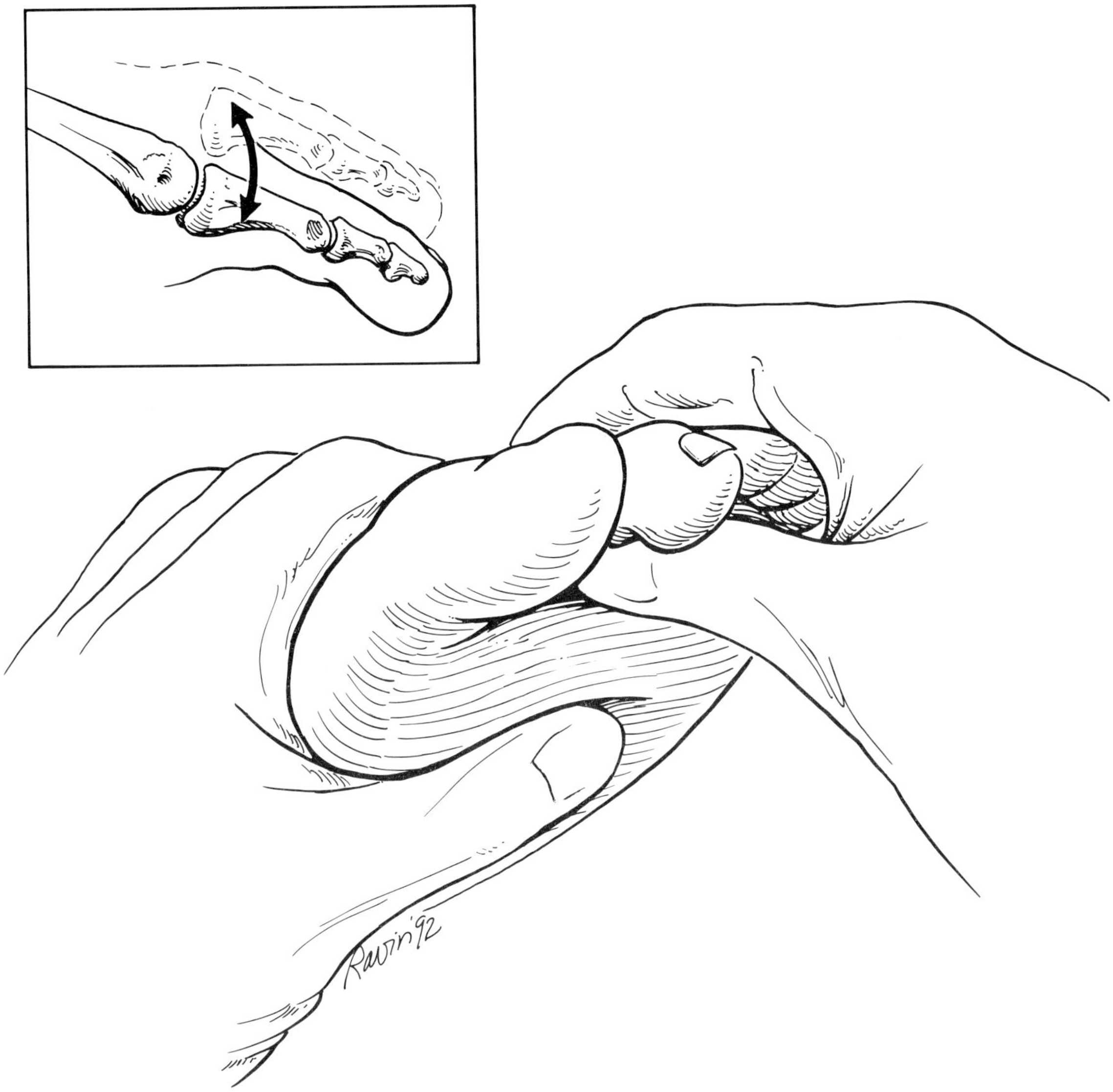

12 RESECTION ARTHROPLASTY

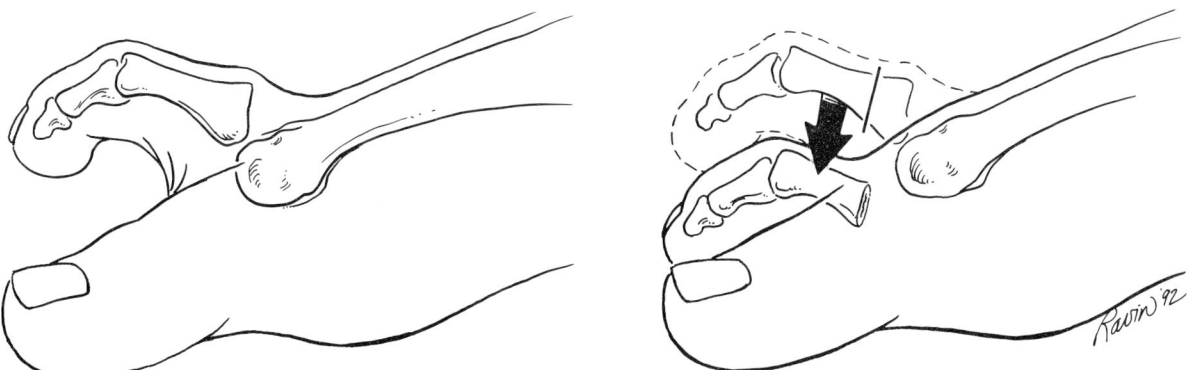

Figure 1. Position of the examiner's hands for instability testing at the metatarsophalangeal joint. Motion of the phalanges with the metatarsal *(inset)*.

Figure 2. The principle of resection arthroplasty is to allow the displaced or deformed toe to relax back into a more normal position.

SURGERY

The patient is positioned supine on the operating room table draping out just the foot and ankle region. The surgeon sits at the end of the table with an assistant when available at the side of the table closest to the foot.

Regional block anesthesia of the second and third toes at the mid-metatarsal shaft area is utilized. A combination of a long- and short-acting anesthetic such as Marcaine 0.25% and lidocaine 1% in 50/50 solution is used. The dorsal cutaneous nerves are blocked across the midshaft of the second and third metatarsals and the deep common digital nerves are reached by inserting the needle down between the metatarsal heads at the first, second, and third web spaces and injecting the anesthetic solution below the level of the intermetatarsal ligament. Local anesthetic in the operative area is not desired since this makes surgical dissection difficult. An Esmarch bandage is used to exsanguinate the foot and then wrapped around the ankle. Beneath the Esmarch bandage at the ankle, a folded towel is wrapped around the ankle to increase the patient's comfort. With a 3-inch Esmarch bandage, about three turns with moderate pressure around the leg are sufficient to control bleeding. Intravenous sedation is helpful to the patient in tolerating the ankle tourniquet as well as the insertion of the local metatarsal block anesthesia.

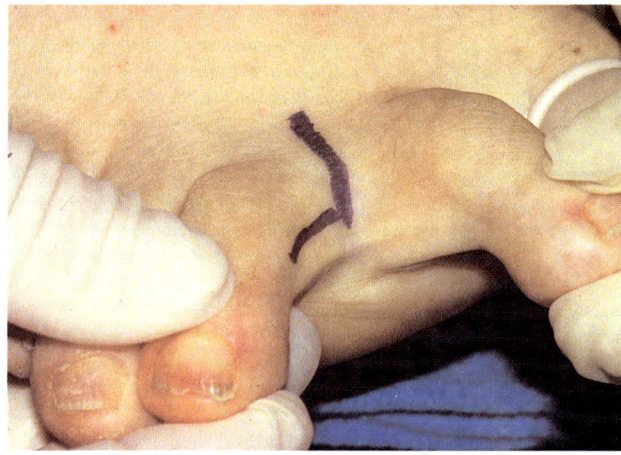

Figure 3. The skin marker is drawn extending the arm of the marked incision out on the shorter third toe.

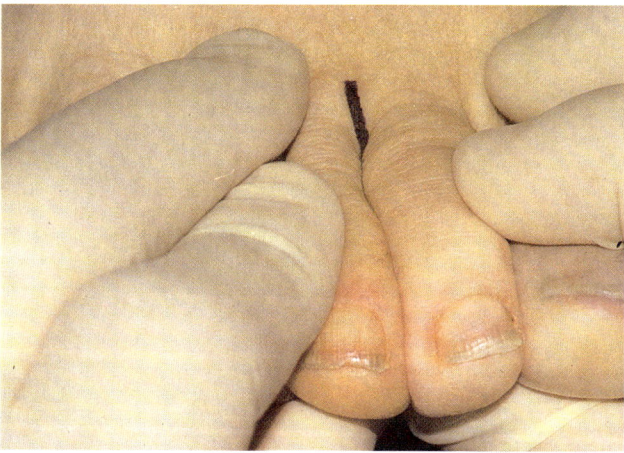

Figure 4. The toes are pressed together, trying to hold them in an anatomically correct position.

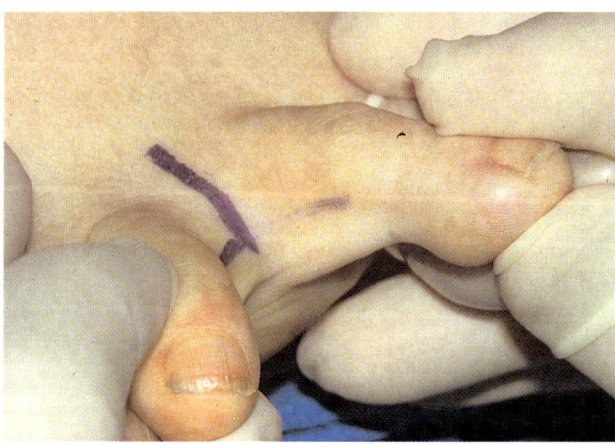

Figure 5. The faint marking of the ink on the longer second toe is seen.

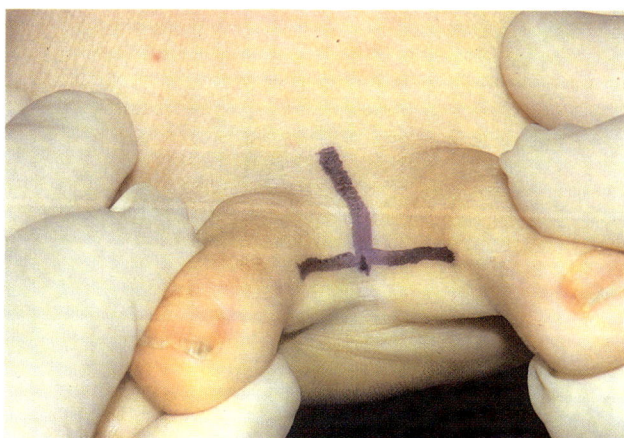

Figure 6. This faint line is then marked clearly with the marking pen.

Initially the shorter third toe is marked with a marking pencil in the midline between the dorsal and plantar aspect of the toe (Fig. 3). The length of webbing is determined by the amount of proximal phalanx to be resected. When only the proximal one-third of the proximal phalanx is to be resected, then the toe is webbed approximately one-half the length of the toe to about the level of the midportion of the middle phalanx. When two-thirds of the proximal phalanx is to be resected, the toe will be marked to the midportion of the distal phalanx to provide the added stability for the more extensive phalanx resection. While the marking pencil ink is still moist on the shorter third toe, the toes are manipulated into an anatomically and cosmetically satisfactory position and the second and third toes are pressed against each other (Fig. 4). This leaves a fainter ink imprint on the second toe indicating the appropriate length and location of the second toe skin incision (Fig. 5). This ink shadow is then drawn in, along with an extension proximally in the web space, to outline a Y-shaped incision (Fig. 6). Particular care should be given to marking out the ink lines on the toes. If the ink is made too far dorsal in the web space the toes will tend to rotate inward toward each other. If the line is made too far plantarward the toes will tend to rotate outward from each other (Fig. 7). Also, if the relative lengths of the two arms of the incision are not in the proper relative positions, one toe will tend to protrude out further than the other.

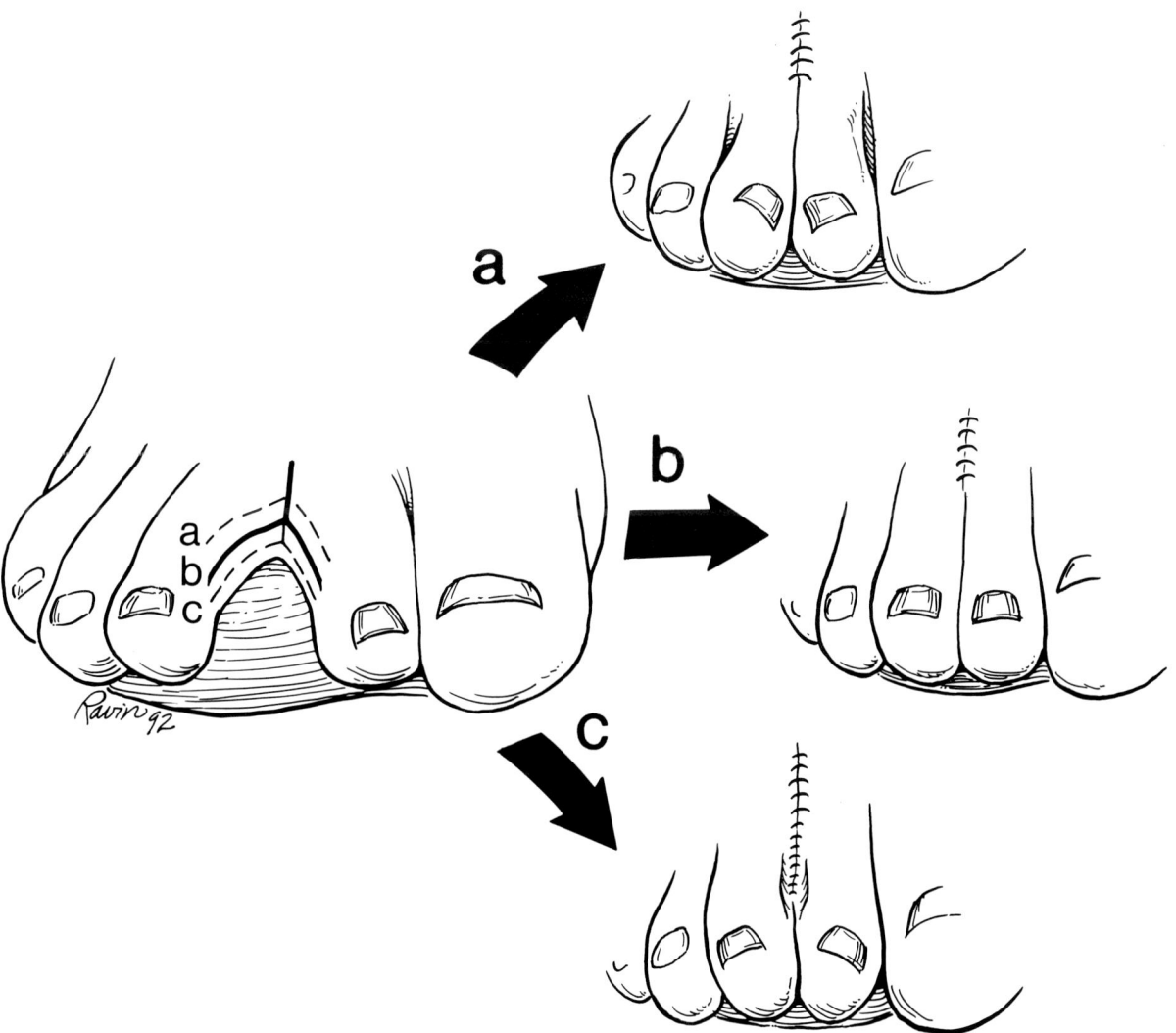

Figure 7. The effects of improper marking between the toes and the final appearance of the toes is shown. **a:** Incision too dorsal; **b:** incision correct; **c:** incision too plantar.

Technique. Using a #15 blade, the incision is made along the lines drawn. Because the incision is in the midline, the proper digital nerves to the second and third toes are essentially split and taken off the phalanx with the dorsal and plantar flaps. The proximal phalanx is identified and its articulation with the metatarsal head is seen (Fig. 8). If the proximal phalanx is dislocated completely off the metatarsal head region, the base of the proximal phalanx will be quite dorsalward and located above the metatarsal neck region. The periosteal elevator elevates the periosteum from the medial, dorsal, and plantar aspects of the proximal phalanx. Care at this point is taken to preserve the flexor tendons to the toe. These flexor tendons come through a depression at the base of the proximal phalanx and aggressive sharp dissection in that area can easily sever the tendons. By elevating the flexor tendons from the midportion of the proximal phalanx and then working proximally to the base such a severing of the flexor tendons can be avoided. An inadvertent severing of the flexor tendons will decrease the plantarward pressure on the toe after the surgical procedure. This may lead to an undesirable dorsiflexion deformity. A Hall microsaw 100 sagittal with a 5053-232 blade is used to cut the phalanx perpendicular to the shaft (Fig. 9). The amount of bone resected from the base of the proximal phalanx should be approximately equivalent on the two toes so that equal relaxation occurs. There should be enough of the proximal phalanx removed to provide a feeling of excessive floppiness at the time of surgery. These toes tend to firm up during the healing period more than would at first experience be expected. A small towel clip is then placed in the fragment with one tong in the articular surface and the other tong in the freshly cut surface of the proximal phalanx base. With this small towel clip, the proximal phalanx base can be maneuvered so as to allow clean transection of the capsular and collateral ligament tissues on the side of the proximal phalanx away from the incision (Fig. 10).

When both the second and third phalanx bases have been excised (Fig. 11), a tenotomy of the respective extensor tendons to these toes is performed. By going into the subcutaneous tissues on the dorsal skin flap, the extensor tendon is easily identified and an approximately 5-mm section removed from the extensor tendon of both the second and third toes. Removing a section of the extensor tendon is suggested because these tendons have a strong propensity to reconstitute themselves and cause later deformity.

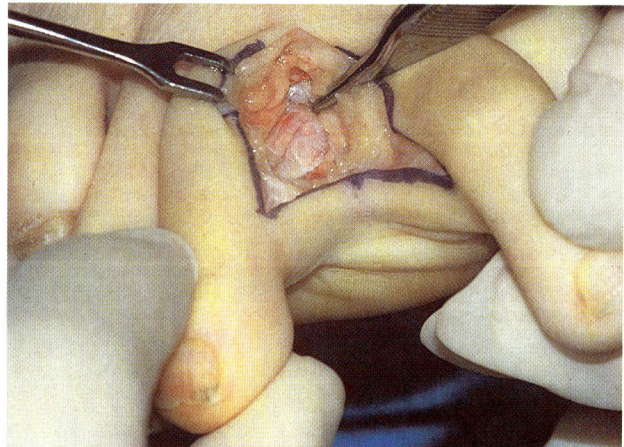

Figure 8. A straight midline incision allows exposure of the base of the proximal phalanx. The point of the thumb forceps is at the articular surface of the proximal phalanx base.

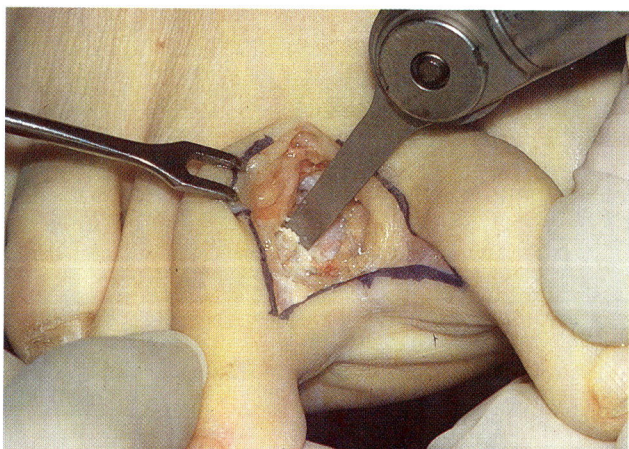

Figure 9. The sagittal saw is used to transect the proximal phalanx above the flare of the proximal phalanx. Usually about one-third to one-half of the proximal phalanx is removed.

Closure of the wound starts on the plantar aspect of the wound attaching the plantar skin of the second toe to the plantar skin of the third toe with a simple 4-0 absorbable suture (Fig. 12). The suture line is then brought to the apex of the incision and this suture is made particularly strong, taking more of the skin tissue since it is the suture that receives the most stress. Continuing a bury-the-knot technique, the suture line is extended to the dorsal skin flaps of the toes attaching that of the second toe to that of the third toe to complete the webbing (Fig. 13). Each suture is made with three knots. The first knot just approximates the skin edges. The second knot is squared and locks the first knot, but does not press the skin edges. A third square knot is pulled tight to cinch the suture and the suture is cut close to the knot. By only using three knots on the sutures the strength of the knot is sufficient and yet there is not so much suture material left in the wound as to cause prolonged suture reaction. This skin closure is very important and is the most time-consuming aspect of the surgical procedure. When this suture line is completed, the toes should be cosmetically acceptable lying side by side in a normal position with the majority of the suturing not visually apparent except in the proximal arm of the Y (Figs. 14 and 15).

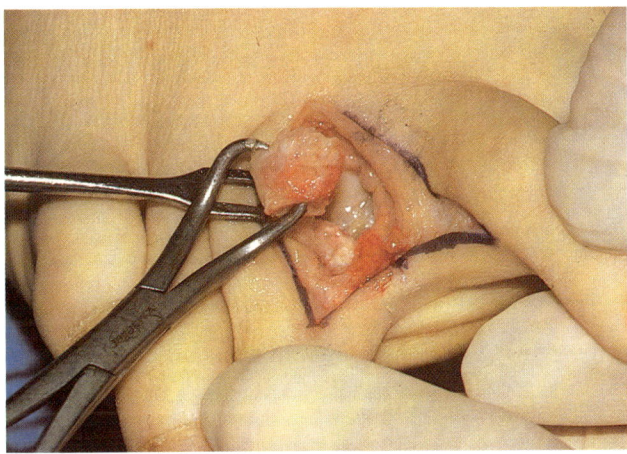

Figure 10. This transected proximal phalanx is grasped with a towel clip and removed.

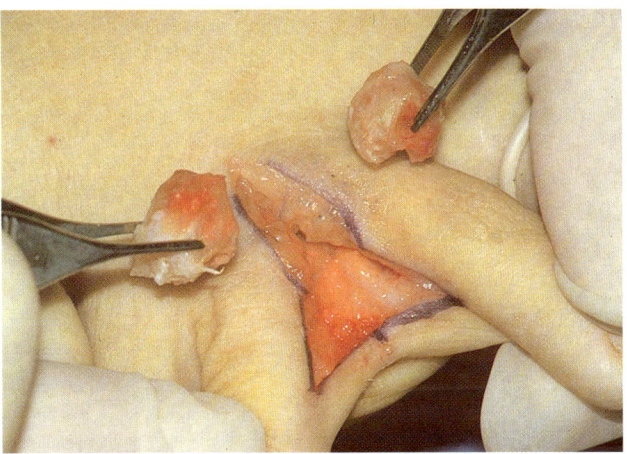

Figure 11. The portions of proximal phalanx removed from the second and third toes are shown.

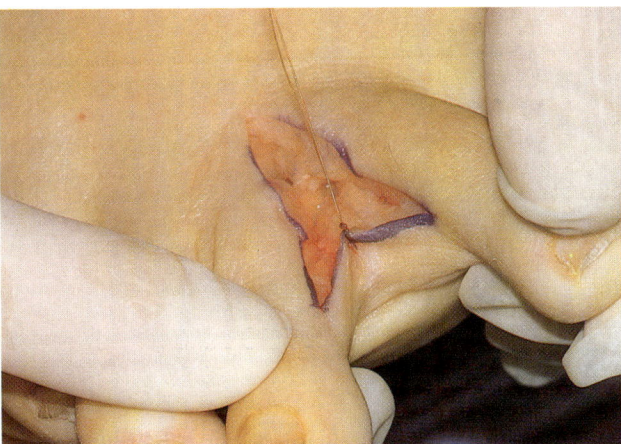

Figure 12. The suture line is begun, taking the inferior portions of each toe and apposing them with absorbable suture.

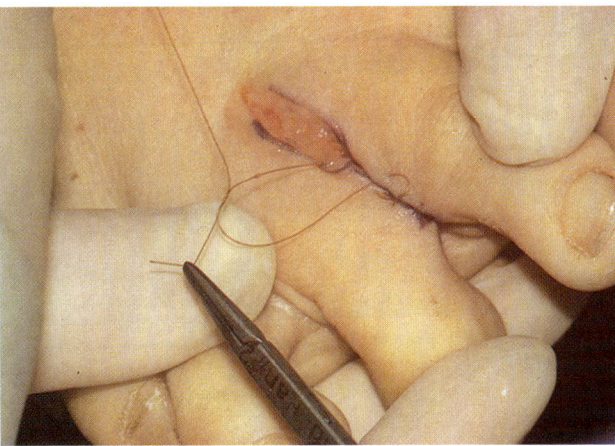

Figure 13. Suture line is continued along the plantar flap to the apex of the wound and then dorsally as shown.

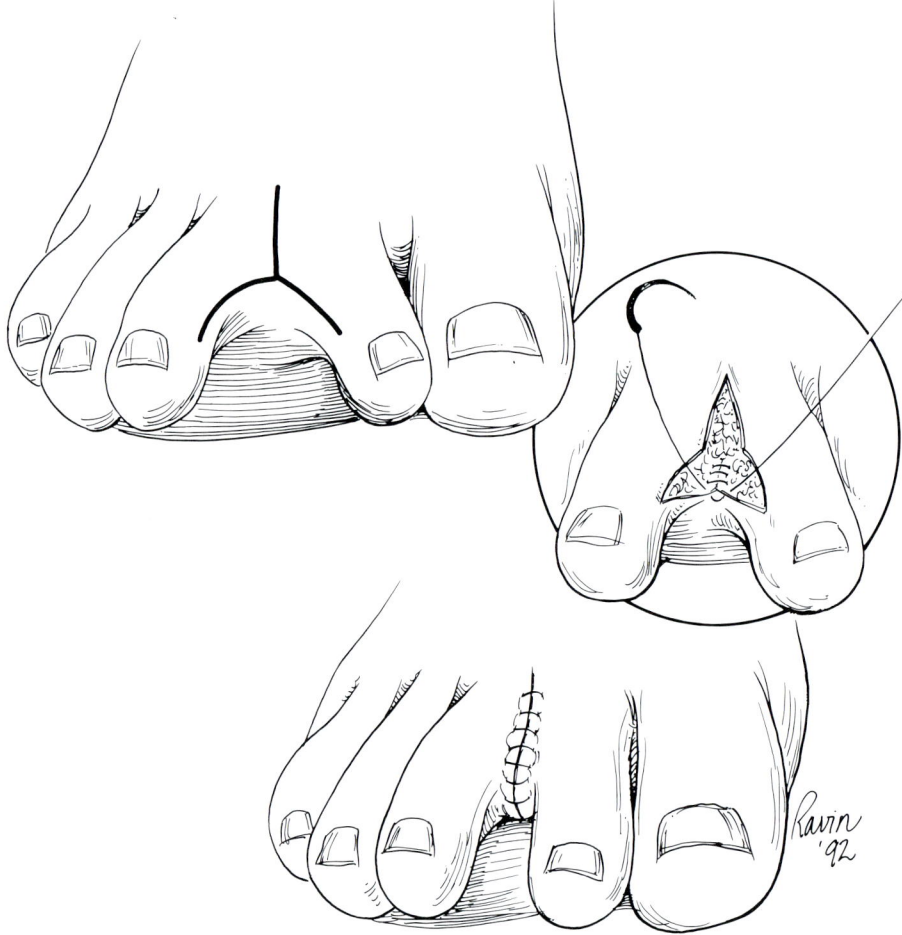

Figure 14. The progression of the suture line to final webbing is shown.

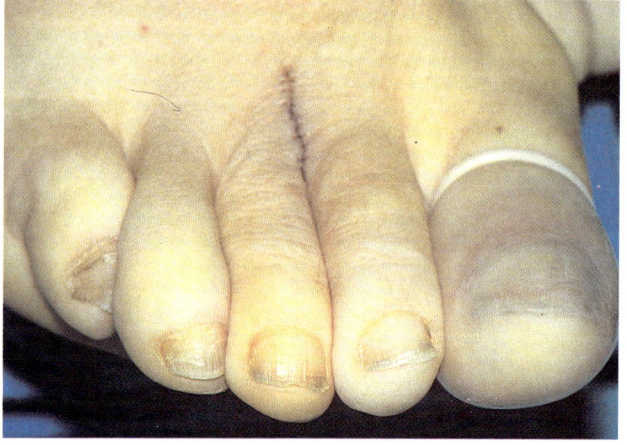

Figure 15. With completion of the sutures, the toes should lie in a cosmetically satisfactory position with only a small portion of the wound visible.

POSTOPERATIVE MANAGEMENT

The 4″ × 4″ gauze is doubled on itself and placed on top of the two toes. Then using a 2-inch Kling bandage, a spica-type dressing is applied to the second and third toes with just one width of Kling bandage between the second and third toes

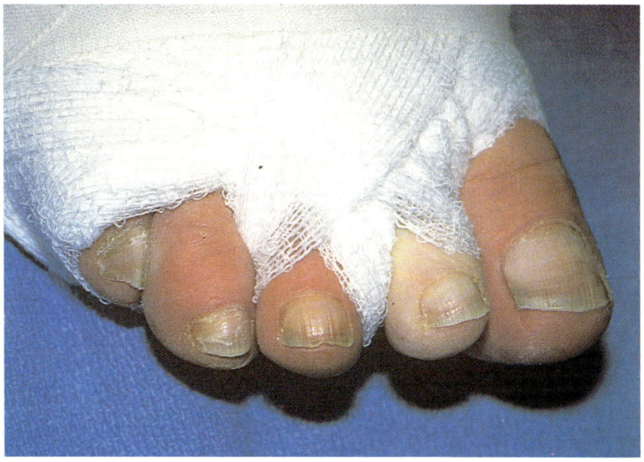

Figure 16. A soft dressing is applied stenting the toes in a proper position with slight displacement plantarward.

up to the apex of the webbing (Fig. 16). This soft tissue dressing should support but not compress the toes into a slightly downward position at the site of the resection arthroplasty. In this dressing, the toes should lie in the position that is ultimately desired. Analgesics are given to the patient and a postoperative recuperation-type shoe is used. The first evening after surgery the patient makes a special effort to keep the foot elevated and the following day returns to the clinic for a dressing change. Hemorrhage into the dressing is not uncommon and the dressing is changed the following day, again holding the toes into the proper position. The dressing is then kept in place for 10 days for a total of about 11 days postoperative. At that time the dressing can be removed. Occasionally at several weeks following the procedure, the sutures, although absorbable, will not have been spontaneously released and need to be coaxed out with a suture removal kit. Once the dressing has been removed, the patient is encouraged to work back toward normal footwear. A wide pair of tennis shoes can usually be worn at about 2 to 3 weeks postoperative, but the swelling may remain for a period of a few months before the exquisite high-heeled shoe might be used.

The expectations for this procedure based on the report by Daly and Johnson (1) are that approximately 80% of the patients will be satisfied with the procedure. Of course those patients who had the most severe deformity preoperatively will have the greatest satisfaction rate. The remainder of the patients (20%) will have concerns about loss of toe function, decrease in toe length, or a dorsiflexion of the toes. Even these patients will usually derive some benefit from the operative procedure.

COMPLICATIONS

Complications following this procedure may include dorsiflexion of the metatarsophalangeal joints, shortening of the toes, loss of toe stability, and cosmetic concerns.

Dorsiflexion deformity can occur at the metatarsophalangeal joints. With the modified procedure, the extensor tendons are tenotomized and particular care is given to preserve the flexor tendons. Also keeping the toes in a slightly plantar-flexed position during the period postoperatively helps to obviate the dorsiflexion toe deformity.

Excessive shortening can occur. This has not been a major problem, but may occur if overly aggressive resection of the base of the proximal phalanx is done.

Because both the proximal phalanges of the second and third toes are done, these toes retract proximally in an even fashion and still are cosmetically satisfactory.

Some floppiness of the second and third toes is to be expected with resection of the proximal phalanx base. By preserving the flexor tendons, however, and not resecting an excessive amount of proximal phalanx, this floppiness and ability to flex the toes into a plantarward direction is maintained as much as possible.

By placing the webbing between the second and third toes, the webbing is not readily apparent. Also if the webbing is made an appropriate length, this is of help cosmetically. It has been pointed out that the more the proximal phalanx is excised, the further the webbing goes out in the toes. Very rarely does the webbing extend out so far that it reaches as far as the tip of the toe.

Uneven resection occurs at the base of the proximal phalanx. If the base of the proximal phalanx is not resected in an even manner, one toe may have a tendency to protrude longer than its partner. This is an unusual situation, however, and if both proximal phalanges are resected equally, it is not a problem.

ILLUSTRATIVE CASE FOR TECHNIQUE

A 45-year-old woman complained of pain at the distal second metatarsal of the right foot for 6 months. The pain was associated with activity. Physical examination of her foot was essentially normal except she had a spreading of the second and third toes and there was some erythema over the proximal interphalangeal joint of the second toe (Fig. 17). She had a positive subluxation test. Anteroposterior radiographs showed mild subluxation at the second metatarsophalangeal joint (Fig. 18).

A partial resection of the proximal one-third or the proximal phalanges of toes two and three was performed as well as an extensor tenotomy and subtotal web-

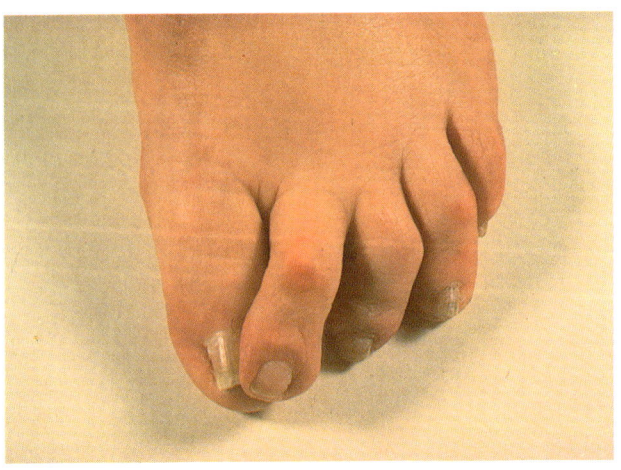

Figure 17. Preoperative status of the patient's foot with spreading of the second and third toes most evident on weight bearing.

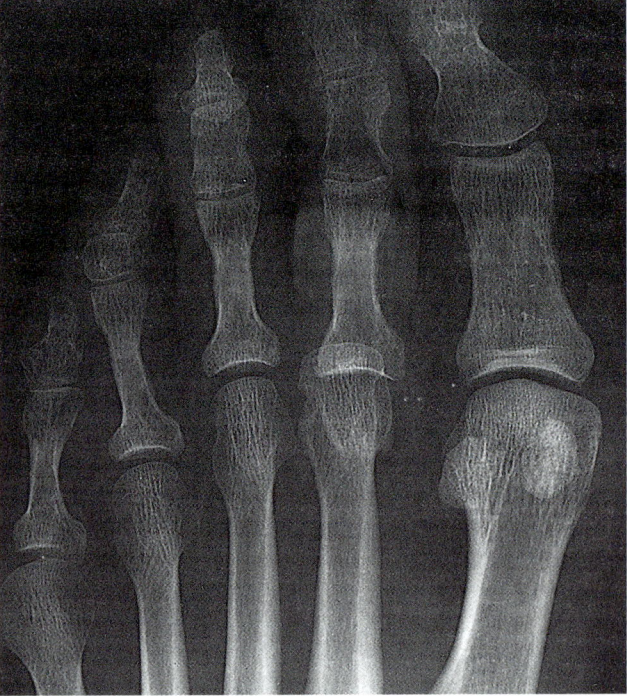

Figure 18. This radiograph shows subluxation at the second metatarsal phalangeal joint.

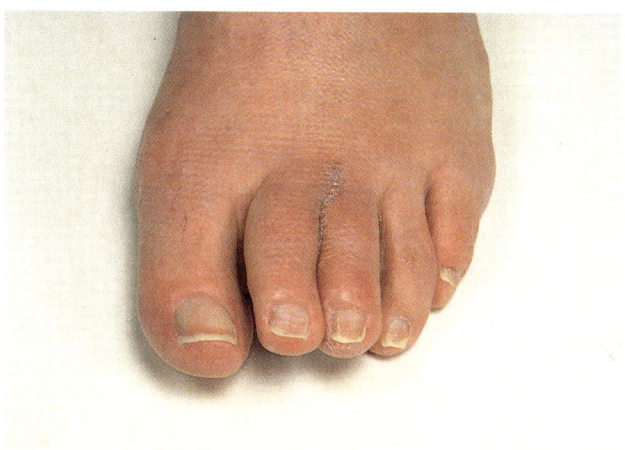

Figure 19. Postoperative appearance of the toes is seen. Notice the shortening, but overall satisfactory position.

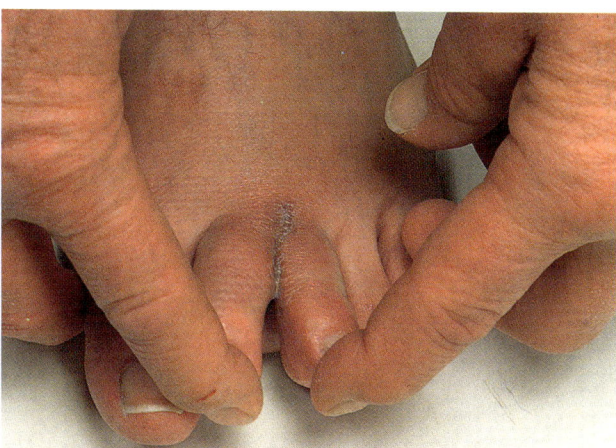

Figure 20. The webbing between the toes is minimal and seems to decrease with time because of the overall toe retraction.

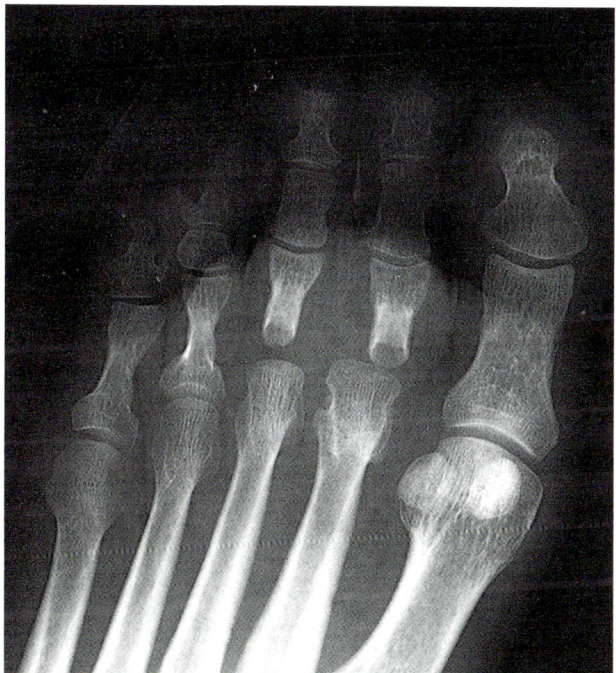

Figure 21. Radiographic appearance showing the extent of proximal phalanx resection.

bing of toes two and three. The surgery was done in the outpatient surgery center under local anesthesia. She went home the same day with the foot in a soft tissue dressing and a postoperative shoe. She returned to the clinic the following day and the foot was redressed holding the second and third toes approximated and in a down position for 2 weeks. Weight bearing was allowed as tolerated in a postoperative shoe. The foot at 3 months postoperative (Figs. 19 and 20) shows the wound well healed with the toes in an acceptable position. The postoperative radiograph (Fig. 21) shows the excision of the base of the second and third proximal phalanges.

At follow-up 12 months later, she described no pain and was satisfied with the cosmetic appearance.

RECOMMENDED READING

1. Daly, P. J., and Johnson, K. A.: Treatment of painful subluxation or dislocation at the second and third metatarsophalangeal joints by partial proximal phalanx excision and subtotal webbing. *Clin. Orthop.*, 278: 164, 1992.
2. Johnson, K. A.: *Surgery of the Foot and Ankle.* New York: Raven Press, 1989.
3. Kelikian, H., Clayton, L., and Loseff, H.: Surgical syndactylia of the toes. *Clin. Orthop.*, 19: 208, 1961.
4. Scheck, M.: Etiology of acquired hammertoe deformity. *Clin. Orthop.*, 123: 63, 1977.

PART III

Metatarsals

13

Primary Interdigital Neuroma Resection

James A. Amis

INDICATIONS/CONTRAINDICATIONS

In general, the indications that would result in the resection of an interdigital neuroma are quite simple. Web space pain in the forefoot that is diagnosed as an interdigital neuroma (a.k.a. Morton's neuroma) that is recalcitrant to conservative measures would require surgical excision. Therefore, the prerequisites leading up to resection would include failure of conservative treatment and a proper diagnosis.

The third web space is by far the most common web space involved, representing 80% to 85% of interdigital neuromas (Fig. 1). The second web space accounts for the other 15% to 20%. It is never present in the first or fourth web space. When considering this diagnosis involving the second and especially the first or fourth web space, other etiologies masquerading as an interdigital neuroma must be considered.

Conservative measures for a Morton's neuroma commonly include shoe-wear modification, adhesive fixed metatarsal pads (Hapad) for existing shoe-wear, formal orthotics or inlays, and cortisone injection in the web space. Despite these conservative measures, it has been estimated that 50% to 80% of patients ultimately require excision of the interdigital neuroma as a definitive solution to their pain.

While there are no absolute contraindications to removal of an interdigital neuroma, there are relative contraindications. The largest relative contraindication includes other processes that may be masquerading as an interdigital neuroma. Any process that is inflammatory or compressive about a normal interdigital nerve

---

J. A. Amis, M.D.: Department of Orthopaedics, University of Cincinnati Medical College, Cincinnati, OH 45220.

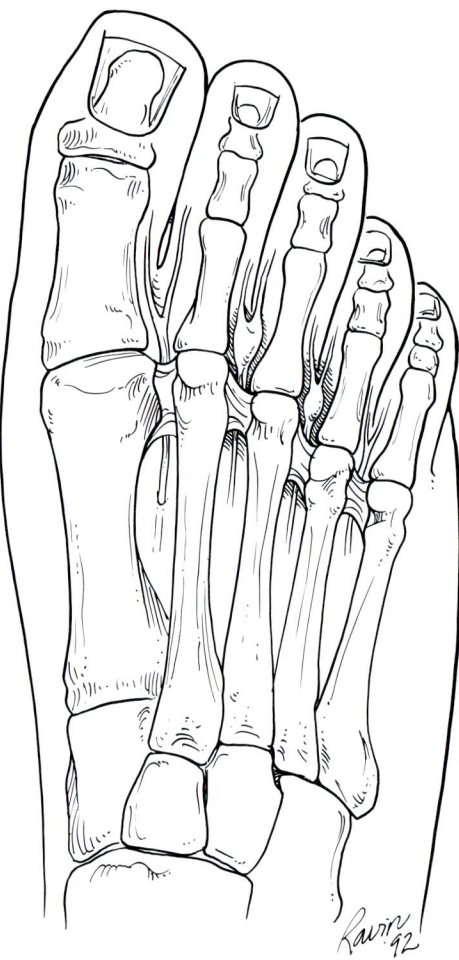

Figure 1. Anteroposterior (AP) view of foot showing a neuroma in the second and third web space and its relative location to the intermetatarsal ligaments.

may irritate the nerve, giving symptoms similar to an interdigital neuroma. Examples include an adjacent inflammatory synovitis such as rheumatoid arthritis, synovial cyst formation from the adjacent metatarsophalangeal joint, or a local infection.

Whenever symptoms of an interdigital neuroma are considered, thought should be given to the possibility of a more proximal neurologic cause to the patient's symptoms. For example, a lumbar radiculopathy, tarsal tunnel syndrome, or any other variety of neurologic causes resulting in forefoot pain may be manifest as symptoms consistent with interdigital neuroma.

PREOPERATIVE PLANNING

It is essential that the proper diagnosis is confidently confirmed prior to a resection of an interdigital neuroma. The spectrum of history of neuroma pain can be broad and vague.

The classic presenting symptoms of a patient with an interdigital neuroma include pain that is worse when wearing shoes, especially confining shoes when walking or standing. It is usually described as a burning pain that is slowly relieved by resting the foot. An almost pathognomonic sign of interdigital neuroma is the

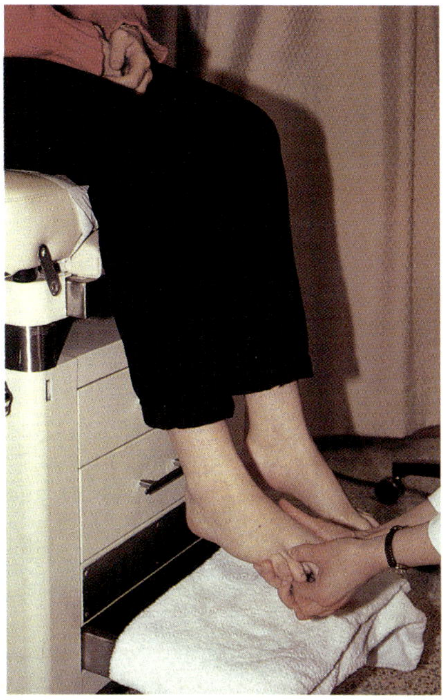

Figure 2. Preferred general method of foot examination.

patient's description of removing the shoe and getting relief from rubbing the foot. However, absence of this historical description certainly does not exclude interdigital neuroma as the diagnosis.

These patients will describe a vague, slowly progressive forefoot pain anywhere from a few months to many years duration prior to their presentation. They quite often have great difficulty in localizing the pain and may describe it by pointing to the entire forefoot or, less commonly, the pain may be pinpointed to the exact web space. The lateral or medial toe of the involved web space may be the only areas where the patient perceives pain. Other complaints may be the sensation of a mass under the forefoot or that the stocking or sock is folded, only to find out upon removal of the shoe that there is no fold present.

One presenting complaint that can be particularly misleading is that of lateral ankle pain. This can be the result of avoiding the interdigital neuroma pain on a prolonged basis by weight bearing on the lateral border of their foot, straining the lateral ankle, while having since forgotten about the interdigital neuroma pain that promoted the abnormal gait many months past. A primary problem should be sought by careful history taking and physical examination.

The physical examination should begin by observing the feet in a standing position. With larger neuromas, the corresponding toes to the involved web space may physically spread from the bulging neuroma. The patients may also show evidence of prolonged lateral weight-bearing habitus when observing the gait. Any lateral shoe-wear, especially when not present in the contralateral shoe, as well as lateral plantar callousing pattern on the foot may be indicators.

I prefer to examine the patient while he or she is in a sitting position with the foot relaxed, dangling from the examination table. I ask the patient to move back until the posterior aspect of the calf actually contacts the examining table so that the entire thigh is supported by the table and the patient is fully relaxed (Fig. 2).

It is extremely important to perform an anatomy-based examination on the forefoot rather than random palpation or, more importantly, going straight to the web space in determining that the patient has pain in that area. Multiple structures in the forefoot can cause pain, and therefore, to the best of the examiner's ability, the anatomy should be considered when palpating. Furthermore, what must be sought is recreating the patient's presenting pain in contrast to producing other unrelated painful stimuli when examining the patient.

I prefer to go from metatarsal head to metatarsal head comparing them anatomically to the web space. One particular trick that I use is a method of palpation that is based just distal to the metatarsal heads, almost underneath the toes, directing force from that portion of the forefoot straight to the heel instead of a straight plantar palpation with the force directed dorsally (Fig. 3). This method of palpation localizes the metatarsal nerve and any neuroma that may be present and recreates the patient's symptoms more consistently.

A Mulder's click should be tested but is not always found. A Mulder's click is elicited by palpating from the distal portion of the forefoot toward the heel as previously described, thereby trapping the nerve between the metatarsal heads. At the same time, the metatarsal heads are compressed with the other hand from medial to lateral "spitting" the nerve out as one would a watermelon seed when extruded from between the fingers. This can give a palpable "click." It is important to note that Mulder's click can be present in perfectly normal feet and can even be present in adjacent web spaces such as the second web space when the third web space is the area of concern. It is the presence of the click in association with recreation of the patient's symptoms that makes this a finding of clinical significance. Therefore, a Mulder's click is of help when it is present, but when it is not present a diagnosis of an interdigital neuroma is not excluded. Repeat examination or several occasions can help assure accurate localization of the web space pain.

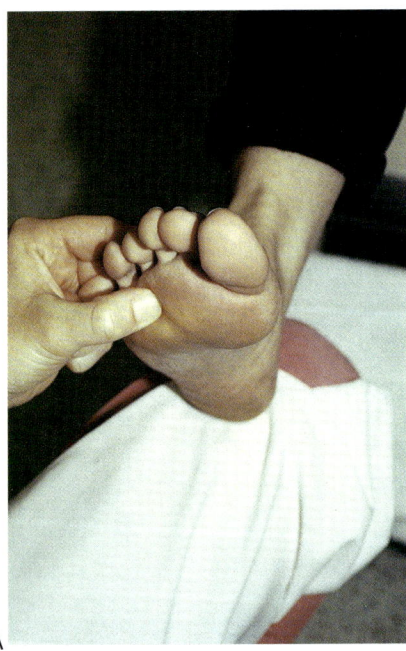
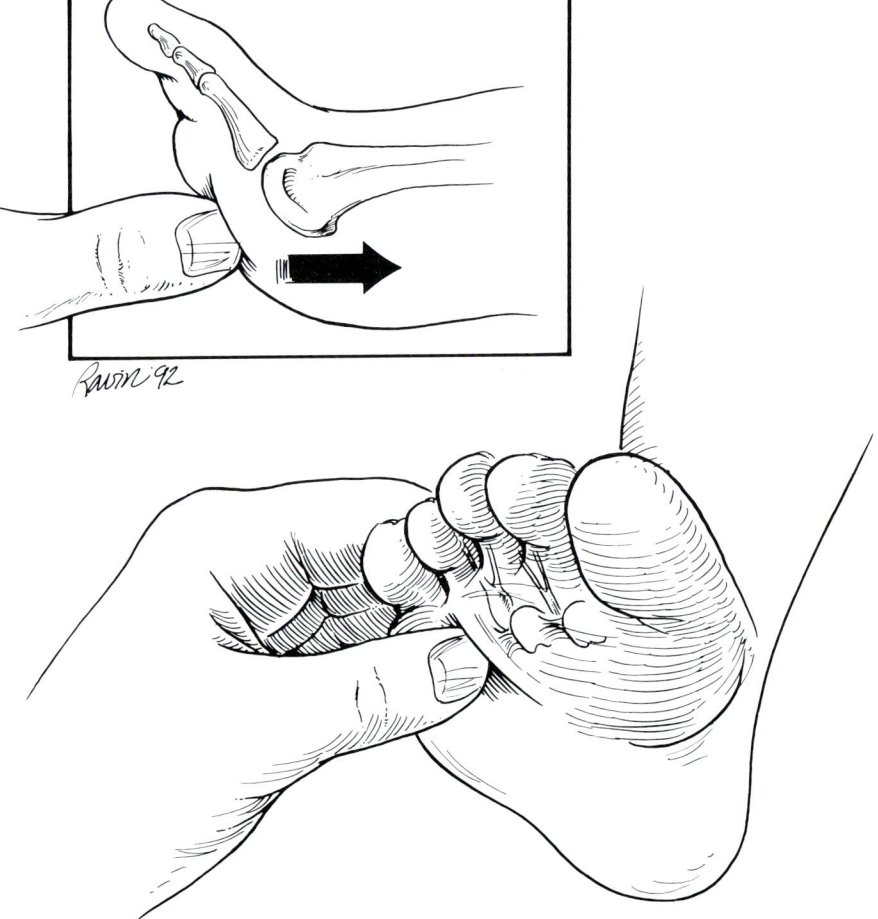

Figure 3. A: Notice that the palpation is done distally almost in the web space and is directed toward the ankle. **B:** Pressing the thumb proximal in the web space will elicit pain of an interdigital neuroma.

Sensation testing is extremely variable and usually of uncertain value; however, I always test it with light touch and at times with Semmes-Weinstein monofilaments. Percussion testing is usually unfruitful in the web space area but may be of value when considering a tarsal tunnel syndrome as an alternate diagnosis.

Standing radiographs of the foot, anteroposterior (AP), lateral, and oblique, are essential to rule out any bony pathology that may be present. On more difficult cases a bone scan may be helpful to rule out occult bony processes that may be suspected, such as an early Freiberg's infraction. Magnetic resonance imaging is dubious and costly in the routine diagnosis of interdigital neuroma. It has not been shown to be highly effective in the diagnosis of a Morton's neuroma. Electromyogram (EMG)–nerve conduction studies may be helpful in ruling out other neurologic causes of the presenting pain, but are rarely indicated.

Diagnostic injections are essential in my practice for the diagnosis of interdigital neuromas. I consider these injections to be a final diagnostic confirmation of the patient's problem. The injection is done from dorsal to plantar in the web space between the adjacent metatarsal heads. I generally use a longer-acting anesthetic such as mepivacaine or bupivacaine. Cortisone may be used at the same time if a longer-term conservative result is being sought in addition to the diagnostic information from the injection. The total amount of the injection should be approximately 1 cc and no more. The needle is palpated subcutaneously as it is brought through the foot to the plantar aspect. If cortisone is injected, make sure that the needle is palpated plantarly and that a collateral ligament is not injected, as crossover toe deformities have been reported from injection of cortisone directly into the collateral ligaments and subsequent ligament rupture.

When using a diagnostic injection, it is very important that the patient be clearly instructed as to the purpose and goals of this test. The injection, in my practice, is critical due to the fact that if you cannot alleviate the patient's symptoms, at least temporarily, by means of an accurately performed injection, then the hopes of alleviating the problem permanently by properly excising the affected nerve may be fruitless. Diagnostic injections may also help differentiate pathology if two web spaces within the same foot are painful. It is imperative, therefore, that the patient have consistent pain, present at the time of injection, or at least be able to consistently recreate it, so as to verify that the injection at least temporarily relieved the symptoms. Otherwise, the patient will not be able to offer any valuable information regarding the diagnostic nature of the injection. If the injection does not alleviate the pain or other symptoms it is possible that either the injection was not accurately placed or an interdigital neuroma in that web space may not be the proper diagnosis.

SURGERY

This type of surgery can be done either in an ambulatory surgery center or in a formal operative suite. The patient is placed in the supine position facilitating the dorsal approach. If a tourniquet is used, as is my preference, either an ankle (supramalleolar) or a thigh tourniquet may be utilized. It is recommended that the prep extend to the tourniquet so that an elastic Martin bandage may be used to exsanguinate the extremity to the level of the tourniquet.

Anesthetic chosen must be discussed with the patient, taking into consideration the patient's age, medical status, preference for anesthetic methods, or any other important issues. I prefer an ankle block that is performed by the anesthesiologist after giving the patient a short-acting intravenous anesthetic that lasts briefly while the ankle block anesthesia is performed. This protocol avoids most of the complications of a true general anesthetic while making the patient comfortable, thereby reducing their anxiety regarding having an ankle block anesthesia.

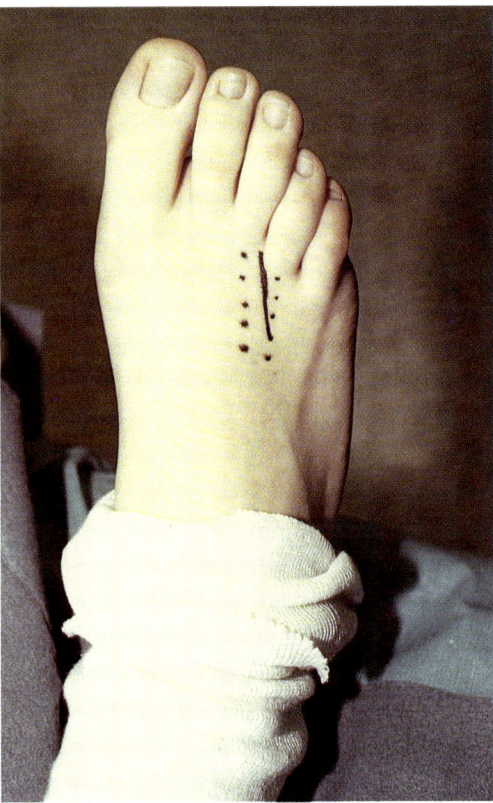

Figure 4. Proper position of incision just proximal to the affected web space.

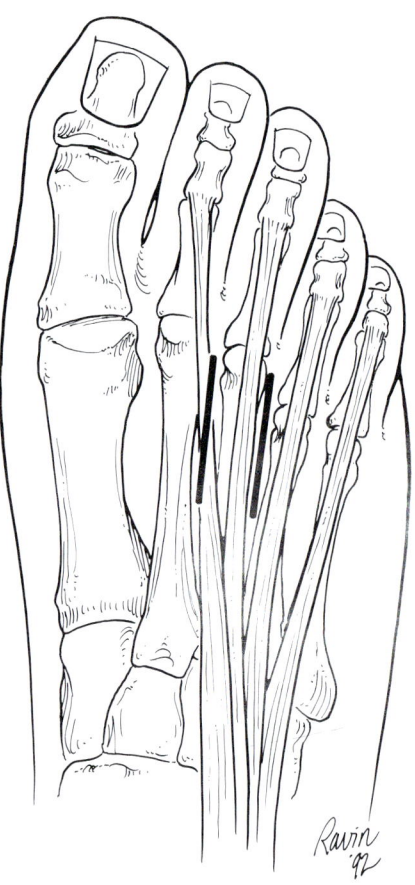

Figure 5. Diagram showing that the skin incision is intermetatarsal and does not generally follow the course of the superficial extensor tendons.

The position of the surgeon should be one of comfort. I find it best to place my back toward the patient's head thus facing toward the dorsum of the foot.

Technique. This surgery is done under loupe magnification, preferably 2.5×. A dorsal longitudinal incision is used starting at the proximal portion but not into the web space and coursing approximately 3 to 4 cm (Fig. 4). It is important not to follow the extensor tendons, as they take a direction more laterally (Fig. 5). Therefore the incision will be slightly oblique and medially directed in relationship to the course of the extensor tendons when made properly in reference to the metatarsal shafts.

As the dissection is deepened, the dorsal sensory nerves should be identified and retracted to the side of least resistance. Avoidance of these nerves may prevent a painful neuroma within the scar. The dissection should first be deepened more proximally until the dorsal interosseous fascia is identified. The dorsal interosseous fascia and muscle should be followed distally leading you directly to the bursa overlying the intermetatarsal ligament (Fig. 6). When the bursa is opened the intermetatarsal ligament is easily identified.

After identifying the intermetatarsal ligament, the surgeon should sweep back proximally and subperiosteally on the medial border of the lateral metatarsal so that the corresponding dorsal interosseous muscle may be retracted medially, thereby opening the web space for better visualization proximally (Fig. 7). A baby Inge 6½-inch lamina spreader is placed between the metatarsal necks, spreading them apart, further facilitating visualization. The deep blade of a Senn retractor

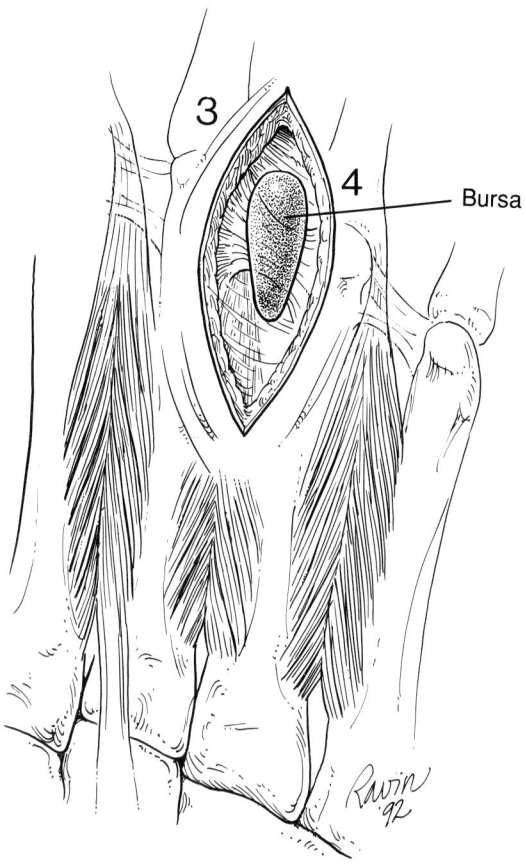

Figure 6. The more proximal dorsal interosseous compartment is key to finding the intermetatarsal ligament (IML) dorsally. A bursa commonly will lie over the intermetatarsal ligament.

is used to retract the web space fat pad distally. At times, a larger interdigital neuroma can be identified at this point. It is common, but not recommended, that during this surgery the surgeon or an assistant press up beneath the foot to extrude the neuroma distal to the intermetatarsal ligament. It is my opinion that pressing the plantar aspect of the foot dorsally to present the nerve allows for a false sense of exposure and is probably one major reason why incomplete resection or recurrence occurs.

The intermetatarsal ligament must be dissected free at its distal portion and divided along its entire length longitudinally. The intermetatarsal ligament is released by using either the scissors in hand or a #15 blade while protecting the structures beneath. Pay careful attention not to damage the underlying lumbrical tendon beneath. Once the distal portion of the intermetatarsal ligament is identified, I prefer to use the scissors to spread beneath the intermetatarsal ligament from distal to proximal to free up the neurovascular bundle. At this point, I am unconcerned about the status of the neuroma and make no attempt to try to identify it until I have released the intermetatarsal ligament. After the intermetatarsal ligament is released, a finger is used to rake back proximally, in order to identify any remaining intermetatarsal ligament that may not have been released. A complete release of the intermetatarsal ligament is essential to the success of this surgery.

It is extremely important at this point that the surgeon understands that the size of the intermetatarsal nerve may not be enlarged to any great degree. Unfortunately, textbooks traditionally show the largest nerve possible and so we feel that if a "whopper" is not found we may not be dealing with a Morton's neuroma.

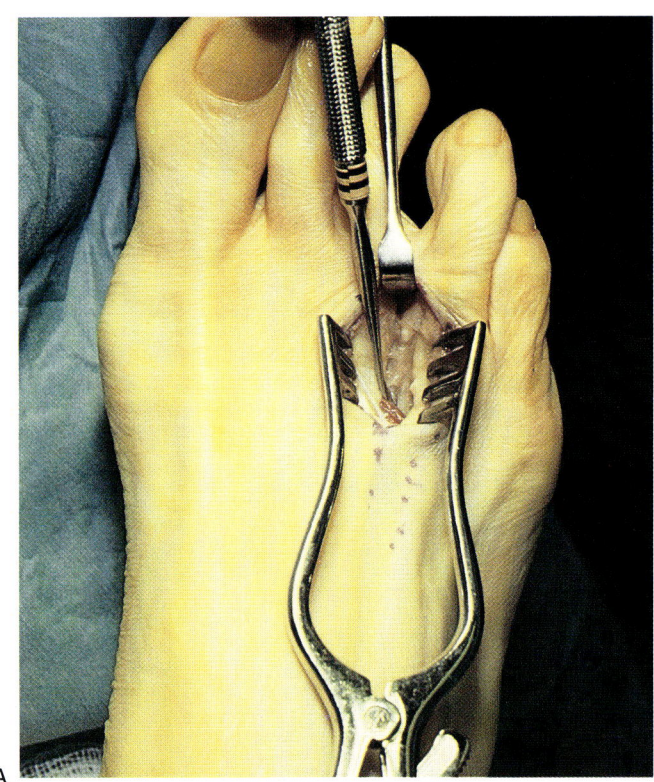
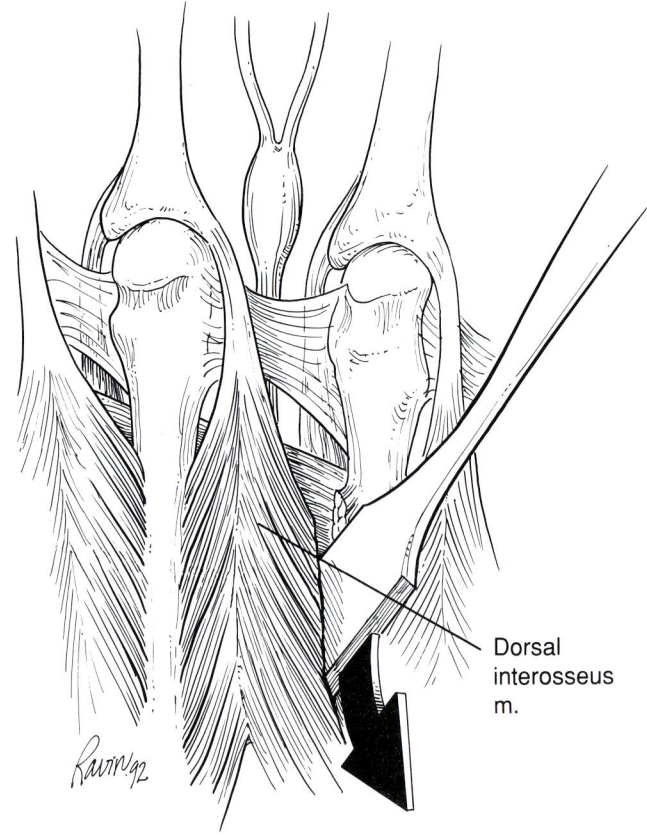
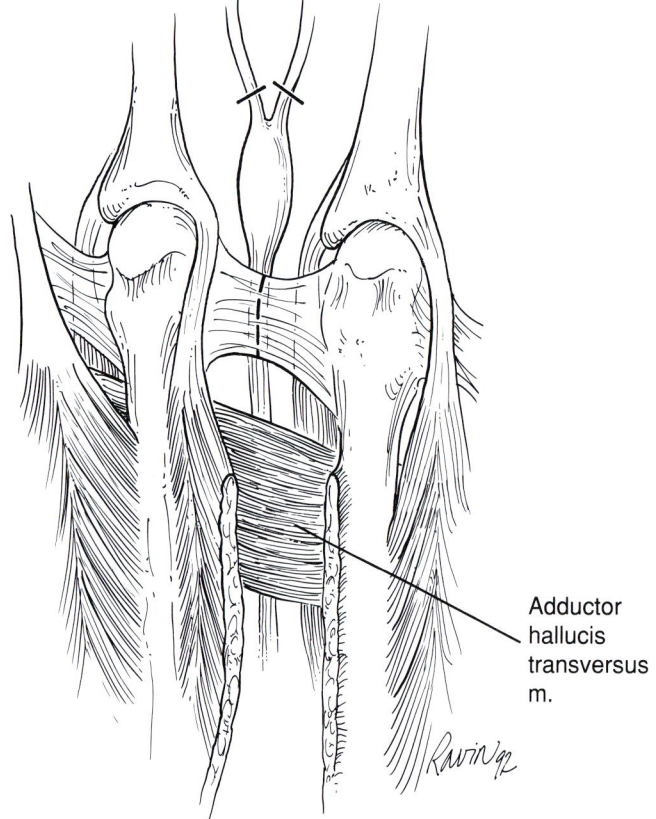

Figure 7. A: The dorsal interosseous muscle is lifted medially away from the lateral metatarsal. This facilitates placement of the baby Inge lamina spreader prior to dividing the IML. **B:** Stripping of the interosseous origin from the metatarsal. **C:** The transverse head of the adductor hallucis is then exposed.

Second-guessing at this point should not be entertained. If the diagnosis is correct, and it should be, the surgeon should dissect out the nerve and resect it as planned, regardless of its size.

Structures that should be looked for and that could be mistaken for the nerve in the web space include the lumbrical tendon that passes to the medial portion of the adjacent proximal phalanx, and the artery, which usually crosses proximal medial to distal lateral lying dorsally over the nerve (Fig. 8). Quite often the artery comes out from under the medial metatarsal neck. If the artery is identified, it must be dissected away from the nerve and preserved.

The nerve at this point, having been identified, should be dissected more distally, but not necessarily out to the two proper digital branches. The neuroma is usually present at or just distal to the intermetatarsal ligament distal border. The dissection can be extended to the distal aspect of the neuroma, dividing the neuroma at that point.

The nerve is then dissected in a circumferential manner to approximately 3 to 3.5 cm proximal to the neuroma. Quite often, this deeper proximal dissection takes the surgeon through a transverse muscle belly, identified as the adductor hallucis muscle (Fig. 9). This muscle can either be partially divided or retracted dorsally using the ragnel retractor. The plantar-directed branches of the intermetatarsal nerve should be divided cleanly so that the nerve is easily traced proximally (Fig. 10). Make sure that the area of transection will correspond to a region of the non–weight-bearing portion of the foot 1 to 2 cm proximal to the weight-bearing pad of the forefoot (Fig. 11). This is accomplished by placing a blunt

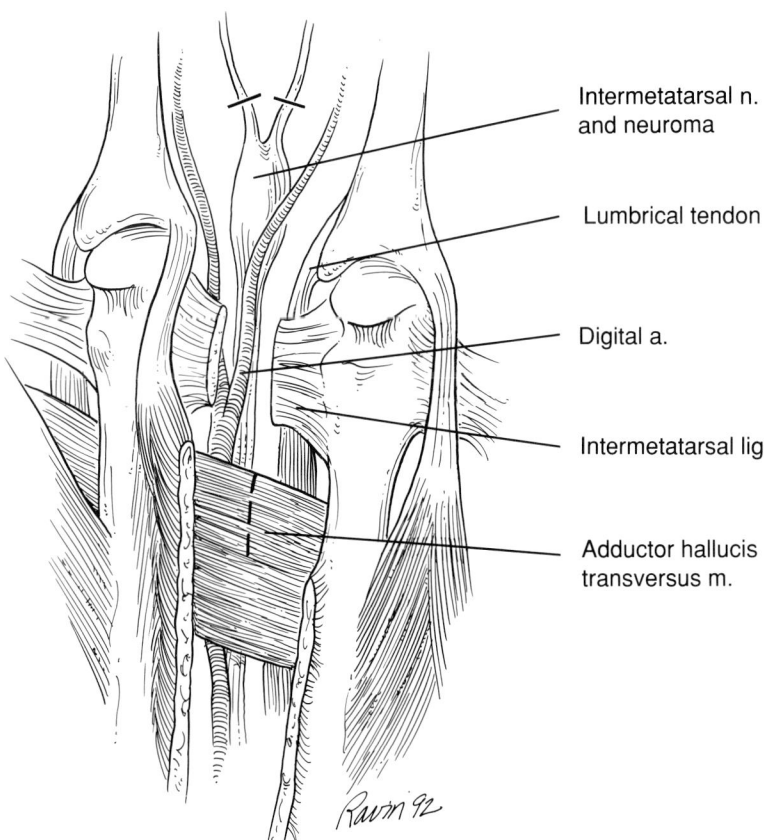

Figure 8. Full view of the base of the incision following IML sectioning. Note the lumbrical tendon and common digital artery and the proximal adductor hallucis transversus and its transversely directed muscle fibers.

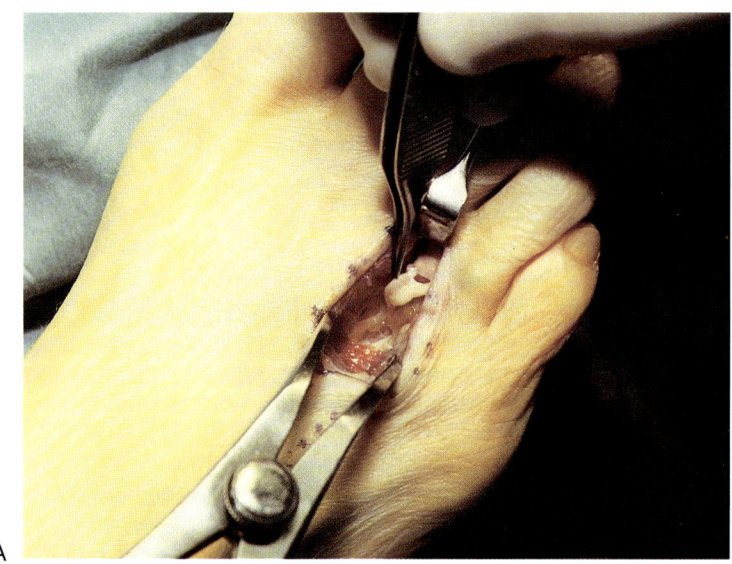

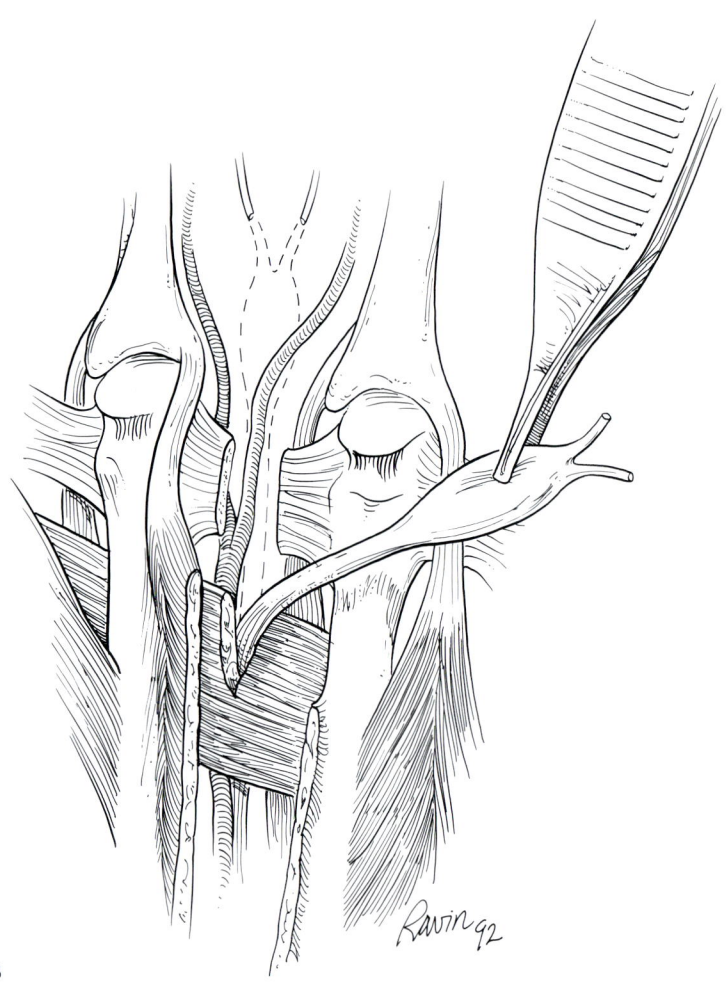

Figure 9. A: Placement of the lamina spreader is essential for deeper exposure. **B:** The distal portion of the adductor hallucis transversus is divided to facilitate dissection to free up the common digital nerve more proximally.

13 PRIMARY INTERDIGITAL NEUROMA RESECTION

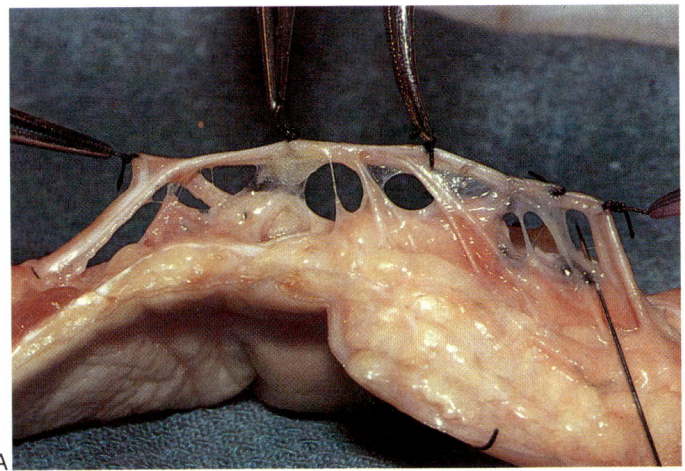
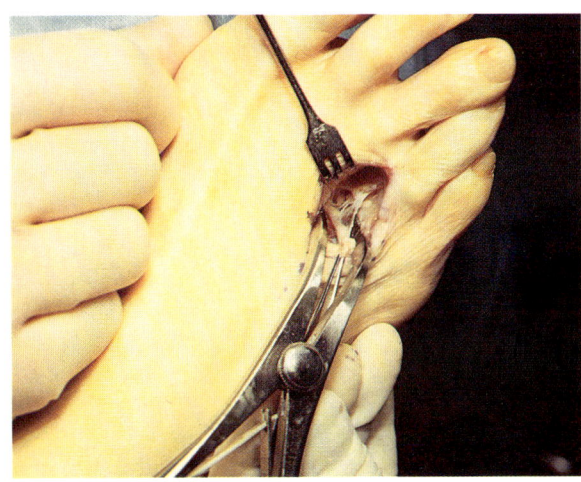

Figure 10. A: Cadaveric dissection of the third common digital nerve showing plantar-directed sensory branches. Note how proximal (left) these nerve branches take off of the common digital nerve. **B:** Intraoperative photograph showing the plantar-directed sensory branches.

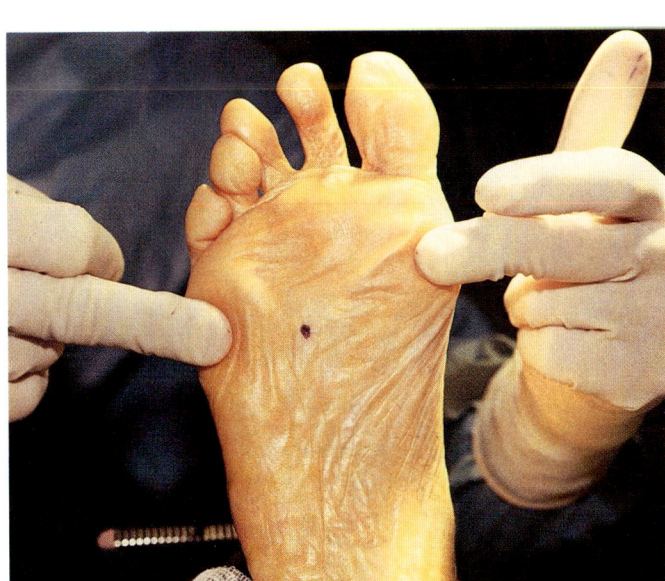
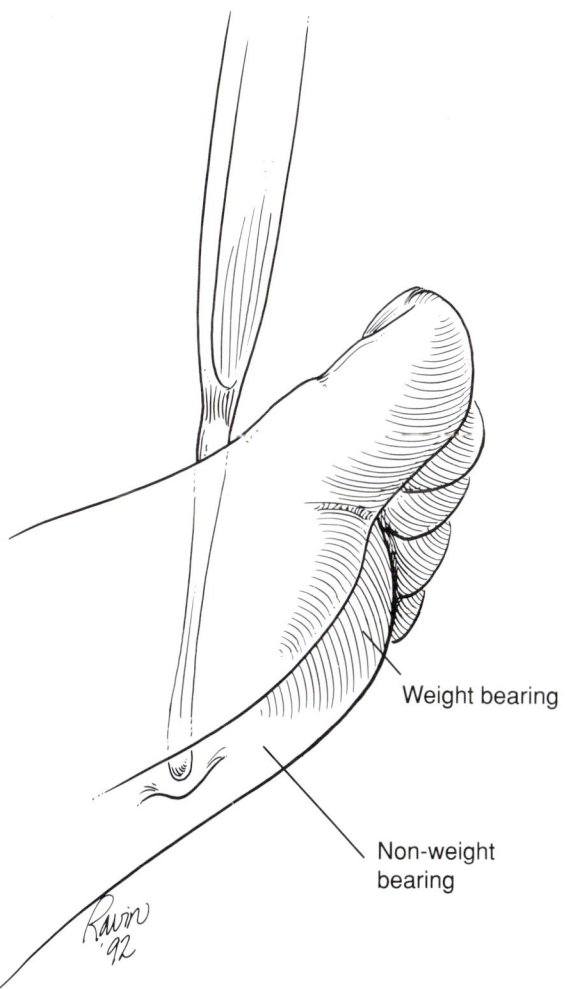

Figure 11. A: Area where distal end of remaining stump of divided common digital nerve will lay just proximal to the weight-bearing area of the forefoot. **B:** The resulting stump neuroma will not be in a weight-bearing part of the foot.

instrument, such as a Joker elevator, in the same location in which the nerve will be transected and by palpating it in the plantar aspect of the foot. If this non–weight-bearing area is not obtained, a more proximal dissection must be continued. The nerve is then divided at its proximal resting place and the neuroma and the more proximal nerve that has been circumferentially dissected out is removed. This is sent to the pathology department for a biopsy.

I prefer to let the tourniquet down at this point with the lamina spreader still in place. If any arteries or larger vessels have been transected inadvertently during this procedure, they can be easily identified when the tourniquet is released, thus facilitating cauterization as blood flow is restored to the foot.

Next, the lamina spreader is removed and light compression is placed on the forefoot for 5 to 10 minutes while the reactive hyperemia time passes. Closing the wound under tourniquet and then allowing the tourniquet to be released following placement of sterile dressings is a reasonable option, and depends on the surgeon's preference. After the reactive hyperemia time has passed, the skin alone is loosely closed using 4-0 nylon in a horizontal mattress fashion suture. Precautions must be taken not to gather the dorsal sensory nerves within the closure, especially if any subcutaneous closure is performed. For this reason I perform only a skin closure. A slightly bulky "sandwich" dressing over a Vaseline-impregnated gauze is placed on the foot followed by an Ace bandage with only mild compression (Fig. 12).

If general anesthesia is used, I prefer to use on all foot procedures a subcutaneous injection of 0.5% bupivacaine along the wound margins. This allows the patient to wake up with less incisional pain and in my opinion provides much improved results.

Several features of my surgical technique have been revised with experience. These changes deal primarily with circumferential dissection of the nerve and visibly transecting the nerve proximally. During past surgeries I have noted that there were plantarly directed nerve branches passing into the sole of the foot that I felt would tether the nerve and keep the common digital branch from retracting proximally. This method of proximal perineuroma division and dependence on a subsequent "retraction" of the nerve proximally is widely practiced. My approach to revision Morton's neuromas is directed dorsally. I have found all of the nerves to be either not resected at all or resected too distally. Thus, I believe that the recurrence, indeed, was just an amputation neuroma retained in the weight-bearing area. For this reason I have since included in the routine of my procedure placement of the nerve in the non–weight-bearing area as described above.

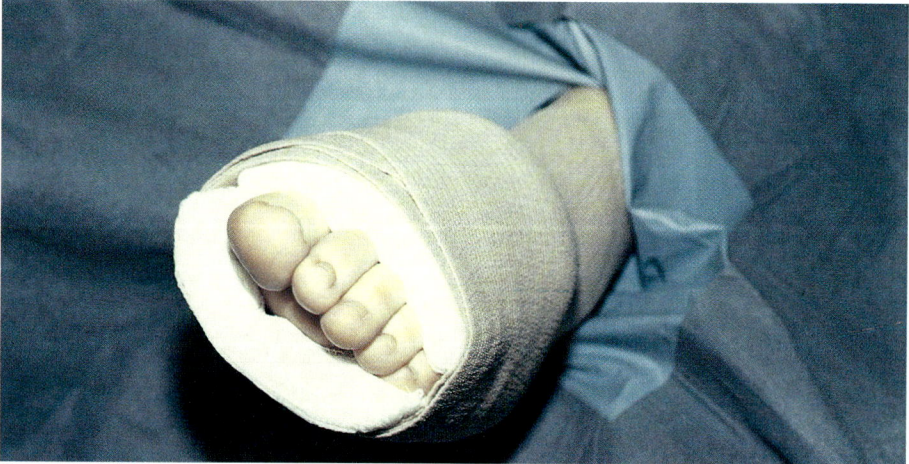

Figure 12. This simple dressing of dorsal and plantar 4" × 4" sterile gauze sponges provides optimal compression.

POSTOPERATIVE MANAGEMENT

Patient management following an interdigital neuroma excision is quite simple. Patients are instructed to undergo strict elevation of the affected extremity for approximately 2 to 3 days to avoid swelling as well as to assist in pain management. Patients are allowed to weight bear as tolerated, preferably on the heel or lateral border of the foot in a postoperative wooden-soled shoe. My patients are allowed to remove their dressing after 48 hours, being instructed that there may still be slight oozing at that time. They may bathe after 48 hours and even swim in a chlorinated pool.

The patient should be followed up at 10 to 14 days postoperatively and the sutures removed at that time. I prefer to apply Steri-strips over benzoin to be maintained for approximately 7 to 10 days following suture removal. The patient is instructed and encouraged to do cross-frictional massage of the area where the nerve was left plantarly as well as over the dorsal incision for approximately 2 to 3 months following surgery. We prefer to do cross-frictional massage for all incisions on the foot and ankle area to maintain mobility of the skin as well as to help reduce any incisional pain afterward.

Between 2 and 4 weeks postoperatively the patient is allowed to discard the postop shoe and return to shoe wear as tolerated. It is extremely important that the patients be forewarned that it may take months for them to be able to get their foot into a more fashionable shoe due to the postoperative swelling. Unrestricted use of the foot and athletics may be allowed approximately 6–8 weeks following the surgery.

Once the diagnosis of an interdigital neuroma has been made confidently and surgery has been planned, it is essential that the patient understand the process of the surgery and the length of time to recover. It is my finding that most patients today are expecting more than they can get and that it will come faster than is realistic. Patients' expectations about how they may benefit as a result of this surgery must be tempered by complete discussion of potential complications as well as the sometimes lengthy recovery following foot and ankle surgery.

My expectations following an interdigital neuroma resection are that better than 95% of the patients will get relief from their pain but will certainly be left with a permanent numbness between the adjacent toes. Reported rates of recurrence are as high as 30%. I feel it is a direct result of the described method of resection outlined in each particular report. The patients' results will match the expectations only if the expectations are realistic. These expectations must be honed by discussing the process of this surgery with the patient preoperatively, as well as to continue counseling and answering questions following the surgery in a reassuring manner.

COMPLICATIONS

Potential complications of interdigital neuroma surgery must be discussed preoperatively. Even a problem that is of minor consequence following surgery can be perceived as very irritating and concerning to the patient, especially if he or she was unaware of the possibility before surgery. On the other hand, even large postoperative complications, if discussed and understood preoperatively, may be perceived as expected occurrences and thus are better tolerated by the patient.

The most important and common complication following an interdigital neuroma excision is its recurrence. After reviewing several reports in the past few years, it is now felt that recurrence more likely represents failure to resect the nerve or inadequate proximal resection leaving an amputation neuroma in the weight-bearing area (see Chapter 27 by Jeffrey Johnson).

Some patients, following interdigital neuroma resection, may complain of an "annoying" sensation in the toes or the plantar aspect of the forefoot where the neuroma was resected. Usually this result is admittedly much more tolerable than the neuromatous pain, and if discussed preoperatively is well accepted by the patient. If the annoying numbness is a major complaint, a recurrence or a failure to completely excise the nerve may be partly responsible.

Another complication following an interdigital neuroma resection involves misdiagnosis prior to surgery. If there has been a misdiagnosis the patient will continue to have their preoperative symptoms following an adequate excision of the nerve. An accurate and confident diagnosis of an interdigital neuroma is essential.

Tenderness of the dorsal incision is a relatively common but usually temporary result following not only interdigital neuroma excision but other foot and ankle procedures as well. This expected phenomenon should be discussed prior to surgery and can be minimized by early and aggressive cross-frictional massage to the incision as described above.

Loss of a toe following an interdigital neuroma surgery can occur even in younger patients; however, older patients with vascular disease are more at risk. Another cause of loss of toe is simultaneous dorsal exposure of adjacent web spaces such as the second and third with resultant damage or spasm to the arteries thereby leaving an inadequate vascular supply to the third toe. Most commonly, if the artery is disrupted in a single web space, the other contributing artery to the adjacent toe will be sufficient to meet the demands of both toes for vascular supply.

The above complications of recurrence versus incomplete excision, "annoying" sensations, and painful dorsal scar following an interdigital neuroma resection must be followed for a prolonged period of time prior to acting upon them. It is important to note that these annoying symptoms or the perception of recurrence quite often resolve up to a year after this type of surgery. Therefore, intervening earlier than 1 year in most cases will be unnecessary. Truly a "tincture of time" is an important treatment modality following interdigital neuroma resection and its complications. The complication of a nonviable toe must be addressed promptly and appropriately.

ILLUSTRATIVE CASE FOR TECHNIQUE

A 43-year-old woman presents to the office with a history of left forefoot pain that has been present for approximately 3 to 4 years. She is a housewife who occasionally wears fashionable shoes but for the past year has begun wearing wider toe boxed, tennis type of shoe. Despite the change to wider shoes, her symptoms have continued to worsen. In the past few months, prior to presentation, she had started to develop left anterolateral ankle pain especially with increased activities. The patient's quality of life was deteriorating due to the inability of the foot to perform to her expectations.

Physical examination revealed separation between the third and fourth toes on the left foot when compared to the opposite foot. Her gait pattern showed her to bear weight on the lateral border of her left foot. On sitting examination her ankle was noted to be stable to anterior drawer testing and she was nontender in the area of her perceived pain. The patient at this point admitted that the ankle pain always followed the forefoot pain and never occurred on its own. Deep palpation in the forefoot revealed nontender metatarsal heads but showed a positive Mulder's click, recreating the patient's symptoms in the third web space of the left foot. A provisional diagnosis of Morton's neuroma was made. The patient was given felt metatarsal pads as a conservative trial of management.

The patient, upon returning in 2 months, noted that the metatarsal pads were of little benefit. She continued to have symptoms. At that point, the patient inquired about surgery and an injection of 1 cc of 0.5% bupivacaine hydrochloride was given in a sterile fashion in the third web space. At the time of the injection, the patient was having symptoms in the web space. The patient left the office and reported back the next day by telephone that for approximately 2½ hours her symptoms were completely relieved and that this temporary result if given permanently would be satisfactory. A preoperative repeat examination reconfirmed a third web space Morton's neuroma provisional diagnosis.

Subsequently the patient underwent excision of her interdigital nerve and neuroma. This was done under ankle block anesthesia as an outpatient. The patient had an uneventful postoperative recovery but did have approximately 2 to 3 months of incisional tenderness that was resolved with cross-frictional massage. At the 1-year follow-up the patient was completely free of symptoms.

RECOMMENDED READING

1. Alexander, I., Johnson, K. A., and Parr, J. W.: Morton's neuroma: a review of recent concepts. *Orthopedics*, 10(1): 103–106, 1987.
2. Amis, J. A., Siverhus, S. W., and Liwnicz, B. H.: An anatomic basis for recurrence after Morton's neuroma excision. *Foot Ankle*, 13(3): 153–156, 1992.
3. Bradley, N., Miller, W. A., and Evans, J. P.: Plantar neuroma: analysis of results following surgical excision in 145 patients. *South. Med. J.*, 69: 853–854, 1976.
4. Johnson, J. E., Johnson, K. A., and Unni, K. K.: Persistent pain after excision of an interdigital neuroma. *J. Bone Joint Surg.*, 70A: 651–657, 1988.
5. Mann, R. A., and Reynolds, J. C.: Interdigital neuroma—a critical clinical analysis. *Foot Ankle*, 3(4): 238–243, 1983.

14

Secondary Interdigital Neuroma Resection

Jeffrey E. Johnson

INDICATIONS/CONTRAINDICATIONS

Pain is the primary indication for reoperation of an interdigital neuroma following failed primary resection. Recent reports have noted continuing complaints of pain in the affected interspace by 10% to 20% of patients after the first attempt at excision of a primary interdigital neuroma (3–5,8). The location and quality of the pain are important determinants in deciding whether the presenting pain symptoms are due to a surgically treatable cause such as an incompletely resected primary interdigital neuroma or a painful amputation stump neuroma versus pain from an unrelated cause. Reoperation for persistent web-space pain should only be undertaken when the surgeon is convinced that the persistent pain symptoms are secondary to a surgically treatable nerve lesion. This determination can only be made after a thorough history and physical examination accompanied by the appropriate supporting tests or imaging studies, as indicated by each individual case, to rule out the other potential causes of web-space pain.

The contraindications to reoperation for persistent pain following a primary interdigital neuroma excision include significant peripheral vascular disease, peripheral neuropathy, pain not characteristic of a recurrent neuroma of the interdigital nerve (i.e., pain at multiple areas, inconsistent physical findings), reflex sympathetic dystrophy syndrome, long history of chronic pain, and unrealistic patient expectations.

Friscia et al. reported in a large series of primary interdigital neuroma excisions that if the preoperative symptoms could be localized to either the second or the third web space that 80% of the patients were either completely satisfied or satis-

---

J. E. Johnson, M.D.: Department of Orthopaedic Surgery, Medical College of Wisconsin, Milwaukee, WI 53217.

fied with minor reservations following neuroma resection (5). However, when there were symptoms in both feet, or when more than one web space in the same foot was symptomatic, the satisfaction rate dropped significantly (5). Therefore, a relative contraindication to reoperation of a neuroma would be pain at more than a single web space, or pain at other than the second or third web space.

Reexploration for a neuroma would also be contraindicated if the pain was not due to a surgically treatable nerve lesion, i.e., diffuse peripheral neuritis, musculoskeletal pain, or neoplasm. Reflex sympathetic dystrophy syndrome is a relative contraindication to reoperation and is controversial. If it can be determined that there is a reflex sympathetic dystrophy syndrome superimposed on well-localized, characteristic symptoms of a recurrent interdigital neuroma at a previously operated web space, then it may be indicated to reexplore and excise the neuroma in the carefully selected patient in an attempt to remove this focus of irritation. However, this should not be undertaken without aggressive multidisciplinary treatment of the reflex sympathetic dystrophy during the preoperative, intraoperative, and postoperative periods.

Dorsal web-space pain and hypersensitivity due to an incisional neuroma of the dorsal sensory branches of the superficial peroneal nerve would obviously also not respond to reexploration of the interdigital nerve for a neuroma. An incisional neuroma may respond to nerve exploration with neurolysis or neurectomy if initial nonsurgical treatment fails.

A relative contraindication to reoperation is the patient who has a chronic pain syndrome with the abnormal personality traits or the patient who, despite appropriate counseling, has unrealistic expectations regarding the results of surgery. Both of these types of patients have a high rate of dissatisfaction despite a technically appropriate surgical procedure.

The patient with a multiply operated neuroma may have little to gain by a third or fourth nerve exploration unless they have all previously been done through the dorsal incision and there is a likelihood that an incompletely resected neuroma is the cause of the continued pain. In the absence of a discrete neuroma in the multiply operated foot, nonsurgical treatments are indicated. In recalcitrant cases, an implantable tibial nerve stimulator or spinal cord stimulator may provide significant relief from pain (6).

PREOPERATIVE PLANNING

The most common etiology of persistent pain following excision of an interdigital neuroma is incomplete initial excision (7). Other causes of persistent pain that should be considered are a painful amputation stump neuroma, a second neuroma in the same foot (12), surgery on the wrong web space (12), and surgery for pain due to some cause other than an interdigital neuroma (i.e., metatarsalgia, metatarsophalangeal synovitis, flexor digitorum longus tenosynovitis, Freiberg's infraction, metatarsal neck stress fracture, neoplasm, or a diffuse peripheral neuropathy).

The history of the pain and the physical examination are the most helpful tools in distinguishing between the various sources of persistent pain following primary interdigital neuroma excision. Pain from an incomplete neuroma excision and an amputation stump neuroma can often be distinguished by the history. If the pain in the affected interspace was still present soon after the initial surgery (within a few days to weeks) then it is more likely that the neuroma was incompletely removed. If there was a pain-free interval after the initial surgery for at least several weeks to months, it is more likely that the neuroma was removed but that a painful amputation stump neuroma developed at the (proximal) cut end of the interdigital nerve. Approximately two-thirds of patients with persistent pain after an interdigital neuroma excision will have had an inadequate initial excision (7).

The quality of the pain due to a recurrent neuroma is often different than the initial presenting pain of a primary neuroma. In addition to the web space pain and burning that radiates into the adjacent toes, there is often a significant hypersensitivity to the plantar skin in the metatarsal head region. Even light touch or stroking of the plantar skin in this area causes significant discomfort. This hypersensitivity is localized to the distribution of the operated nerve and should be distinguished from the more diffuse hypersensitivity that may accompany a peripheral neuropathy or reflex sympathetic dystrophy syndrome. There may be exquisite tenderness that is greater than the web space tenderness present preoperatively. The pain may be centered beneath the fourth metatarsal head after a 3–4 web space neuroma excision, especially if the communicating branch from the lateral plantar nerve (Fig. 1) courses close to the fourth metatarsal head rather than joining the medial plantar nerve branch more proximally. In this situation, transection of the 3–4 interdigital nerve will allow the cut end of the communicating branch to retract into the area beneath the fourth metatarsal head and develop a painful amputation stump neuroma in a weight-bearing area.

If the persistent pain is localized to another interspace in the same foot and the symptoms are still characteristic of a primary neuroma, the wrong web space may have been operated on or a second neuroma in the same foot may be present. Thompson and Deland reported that a second neuroma in the same foot was a

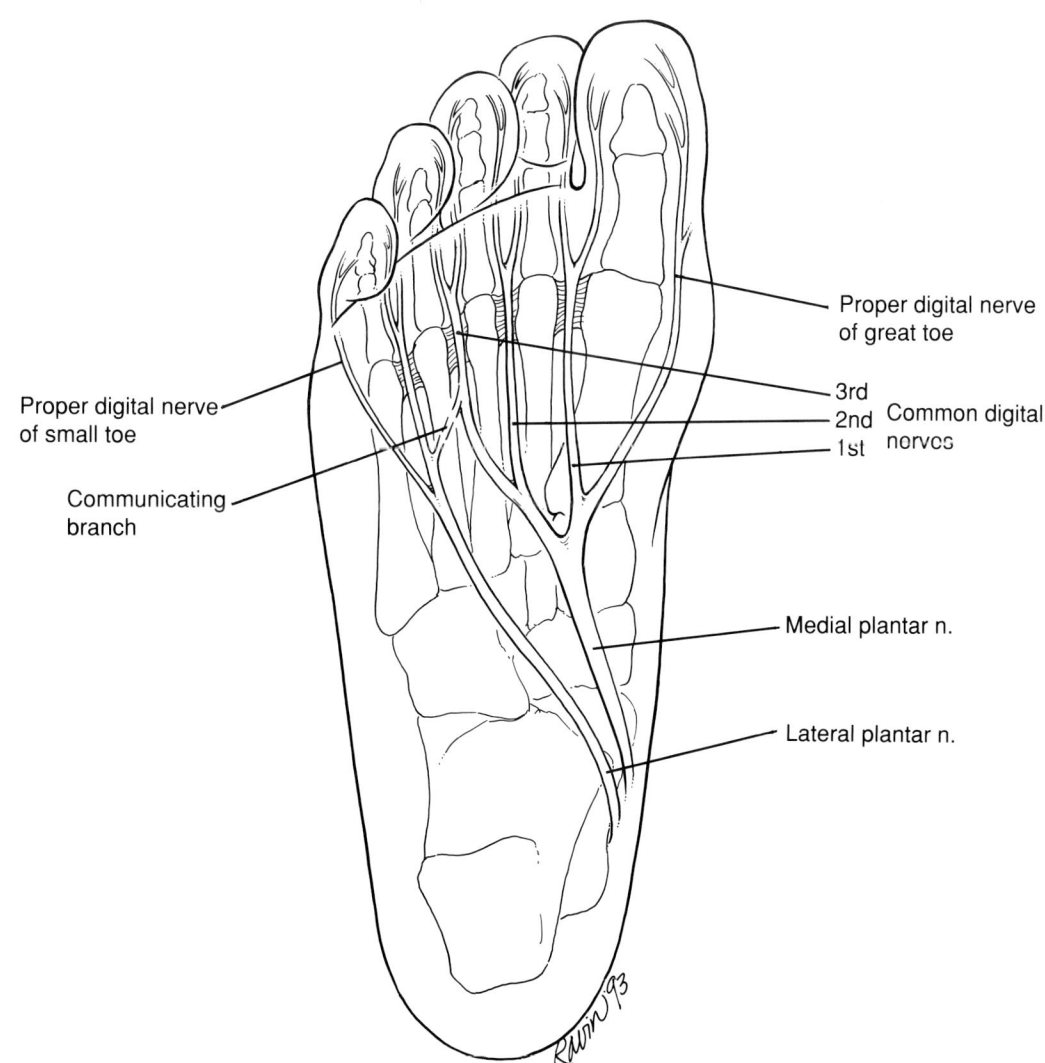

Figure 1. Anatomy of the plantar (tibial) nerve branches of the foot.

rare entity occurring in only 3 (3.8%) of 80 patients studied (11). However, they also reported that two of the five (40%) failed neuroma resections were due to the initial surgery having been done on the wrong interspace (12).

Hypersensitivity of the dorsal scar is usually due to an incisional neuroma of the cutaneous branch of the superficial peroneal nerve supplying the dorsal web space and may have no relation to a recurrence of the interdigital neuroma. If dorsal hypersensitivity and pain is the major symptom causing dissatisfaction after primary neuroma excision, web-space reexploration would not provide relief and treatment of the incisional neuroma would be indicated.

Given normal radiographs of the foot, lack of a history of trauma and absence of a palpable interspace mass, it may be necessary to obtain other diagnostic tests to rule out other causes of persistent pain if the history and physical examination findings are not characteristic for a recurrent neuroma. A bone scan is helpful to rule out an occult bone or joint abnormality in the foot. An electromyogram and

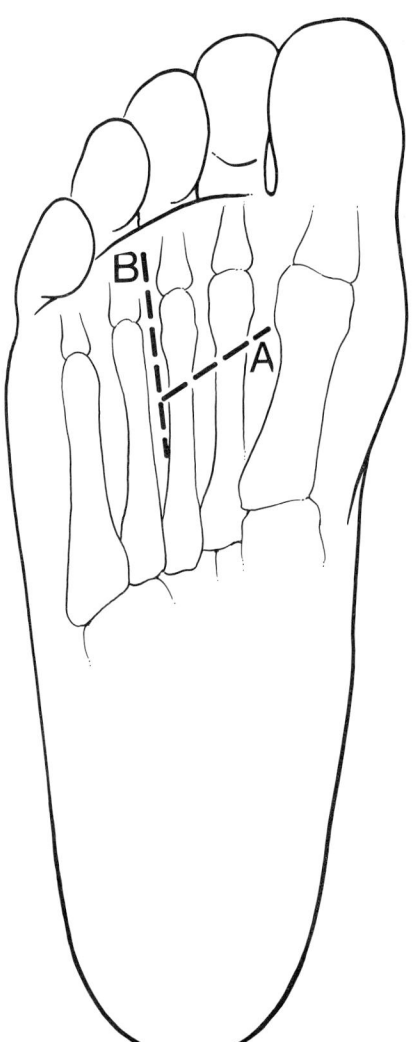

Figure 2. Examples of plantar incisions used for excision of a recurrent interdigital neuroma following primary excision. *A,* Oblique/transverse incision to 2–3 common interdigital nerve. *B,* Longitudinal (extensile) incision to 3–4 common interdigital nerve.

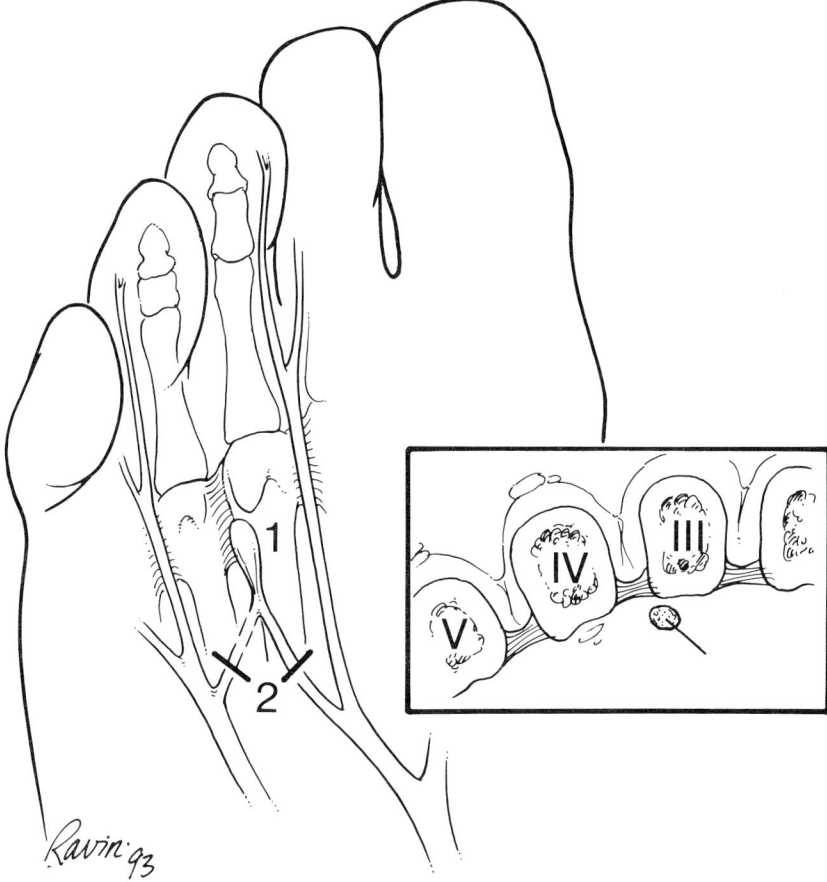

Figure 3. "Amputation stump" interdigital neuroma. *1,* Site of nerve transection following primary neuroma resection. Note location of end bulb "stump" neuroma. *2,* Site of nerve transection for removal of a recurrent neuroma.

nerve conduction study (EMG/NCS) or Semmes-Weinstein monofilament sensory examination may be needed to determine if a peripheral neuropathy is present. A magnetic resonance imaging (MRI) scan may be necessary to rule out a neoplasm or other space-occupying lesion. However, an MRI scan is not very helpful in determining if a recurrent neuroma is present in the area of the previous surgery due to the difficulty in distinguishing neuroma from scar tissue. An MRI scan using a small forefoot surface coil might detect a neuroma at an adjacent web space but correlation with clinical symptoms would be needed to recommend reoperation.

Once the decision has been made to reoperate on a recurrent interdigital neuroma, the surgeon must decide whether to utilize the dorsal or plantar approach to the nerve. Reexploration of the nerve through the original dorsal approach may be useful when the initial incision was made very distal in the web space, the history is consistent with an inadequate primary excision of the neuroma, and the tenderness is at or distal to the metatarsal head level. In this case, the recurrent neuroma may be visible through a dorsal exposure. Proponents of the dorsal approach have reported good results using this technique, and it precludes the need for an incision on the weight-bearing surface of the foot (8). However, good results have also been reported by using the plantar approach without significant problems with the plantar incision (1,7). If there is doubt about being able to locate the neuroma from the dorsal approach, a plantar approach should be used.

The other role for a dorsal approach is the rare case when the "recurrent neuroma" is at an adjacent interspace. In this case the procedure would be performed similarly to a primary neuroma excision. If a completely normal-appearing nerve was found in the adjacent interspace, the transverse intermetatarsal ligament is divided and a section removed to decompress the nerve. The "normal" interdigital nerve may not be excised in this case because it would needlessly denervate the third toe.

Plantar incisions (Fig. 2) are either oblique/transverse (1) or longitudinal (7). The advantage of the oblique/transverse is that the incision is placed proximal to the weight-bearing area of the metatarsal heads and gives easy access to more than one interdigital nerve if necessary. The advantage of the longitudinal incision is the ability to extend it as far as necessary to locate the nerve lesion. Another major advantage of the longitudinal incision is the ability to find a "normal" plantar nerve trunk proximal to the site of the neuroma and trace its path to the abnormal region (Fig. 3). If significant scarring is present around the cut end of the nerve, it may be difficult to identify a neuroma unless the dissection is begun proximal to the scarred portion of the nerve. In most cases the (extensile) longitudinal plantar incision is the approach of choice and is the single incision with the most utility.

SURGERY

The patient is positioned prone on the operating table. It is preferable to do the surgery under some type of regional blockade (spinal, epidural, femoral/sciatic block, knee block, or ankle block). The advantage of a regional block is that the dorsal horn of the spinal cord is protected from the noxious stimuli of manipulating the already excitable nerve lesion (preemptive analgesia).

If general anesthesia is chosen, there is good evidence to support the use of *preoperative* ankle block or other regional anesthetic (in addition to the general anesthetic) for use as analgesia (Fig. 4). The ankle block has an advantage over the spinal or epidural for preemptive analgesia in that long-lasting postoperative anesthesia can be obtained by using bupivacaine as the anesthetic agent. The ankle block may last for 12 hours, allowing patients significant comfort until they are back at home. Other types of regional blocks must "wear off" and motor power return to the lower extremities before the patient is allowed to return home after this outpatient procedure.

A tourniquet is used at the thigh or ankle and a bipolar cautery is used to limit potential injury to the nerve caused by conduction of current through the nerve that occurs when a nearby blood vessel is cauterized using conventional electrocautery. Loupe magnification is helpful in identifying nerve structures.

Technique. A 3- to 4-cm longitudinal incision is made in the plantar surface of the forefoot between the metatarsal heads in the affected interspace (Fig. 5). Dissection is carried through the skin and plantar fat and the digital nerve is identified (Fig. 6). The nerve is found just deep to, and often between, the distal extensions of the plantar fascia that are fanning out to attach to the plantar aspects of the metatarsophalangeal joints (Fig. 7). The digital nerve is identified proximally

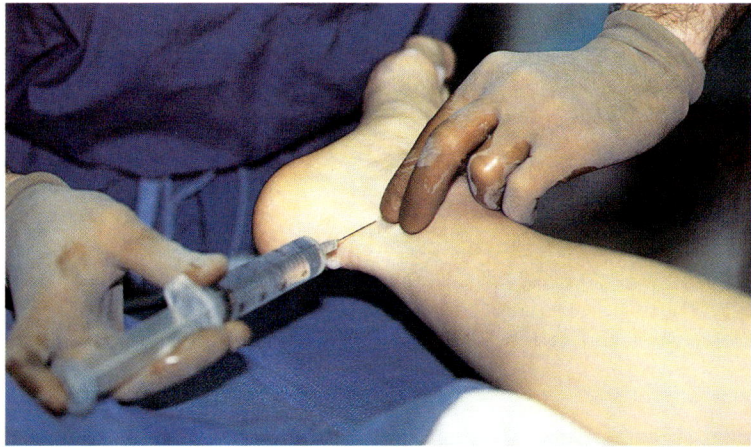

Figure 4. Ankle block being administered as pre-emptive analgesia prior to placing patient in the prone position for plantar exposure of the recurrent neuroma.

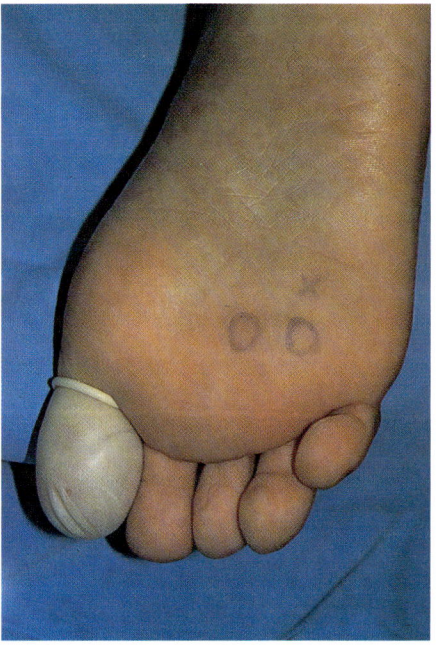

Figure 5. Third and fourth metatarsal head landmarks outlined.

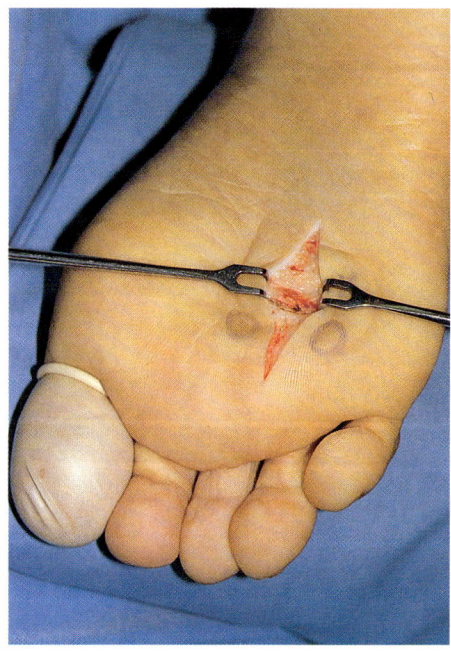

Figure 6. Plantar dissection through skin and subcutaneous tissue.

and traced distally to the site of the neuroma (Fig. 8). The intermetatarsal ligament is not routinely divided since the interdigital nerve lies superficial to the ligament when viewing it from the plantar approach. The digital nerve is divided, under gentle traction, as far proximally as possible, so that it retracts from the weight-bearing area of the fore part of the foot (Fig. 9). The skin only is then closed with interrupted vertical mattress sutures of 3-0 nylon (Fig. 10). No subcutaneous sutures are used. Great care is taken to approximate the edges of the skin evenly without inverting, everting, or overlapping the incision. A short leg compressive dressing is applied (Fig. 11).

POSTOPERATIVE MANAGEMENT

The postoperative short leg compression dressing is used with crutches, non–weight bearing on the operated leg for 2 to 3 days. The dressing is then changed and a short leg cast with a rubber walking heel is applied. Weight bearing as tolerated is allowed. The cast and sutures are removed at 3 weeks postoperatively, and walking is continued using a cushioned-soled shoe.

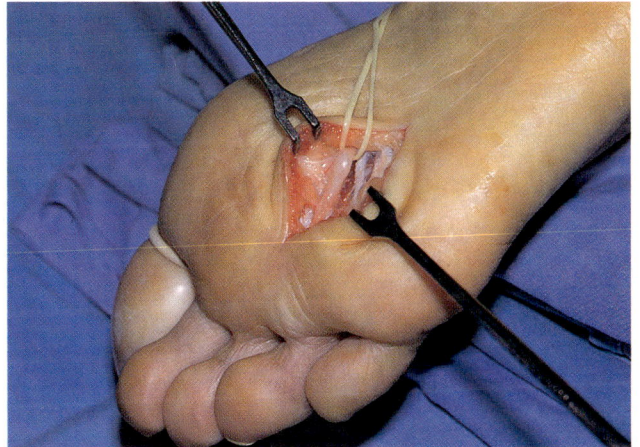

Figure 7. Third web-space interdigital nerve isolated proximally. (From ref. 7.)

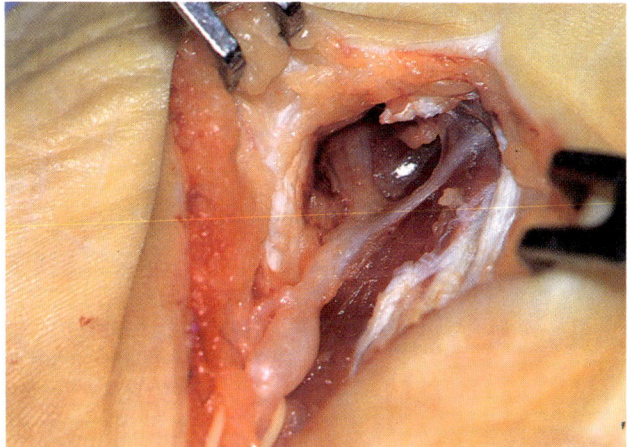

Figure 8. Nerve traced distally to neuroma. Note apparent incomplete initial excision. (From ref. 7.)

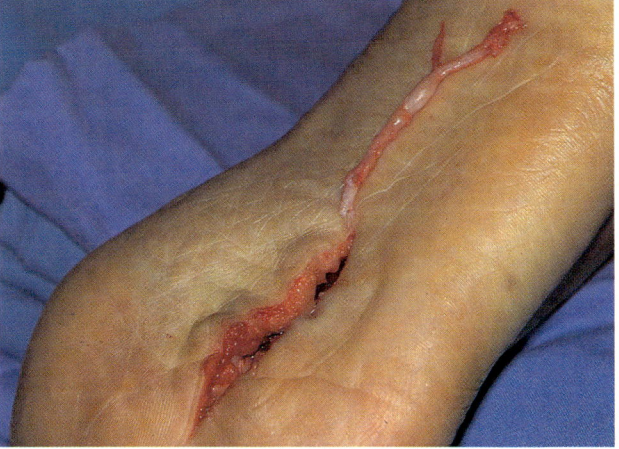

Figure 9. Nerve divided distally and ready for proximal transection.

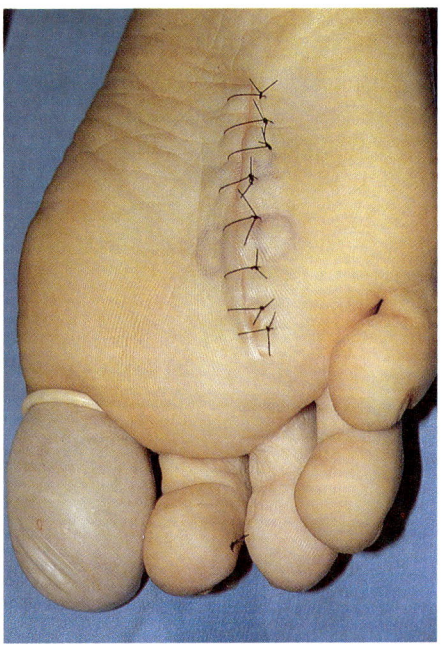
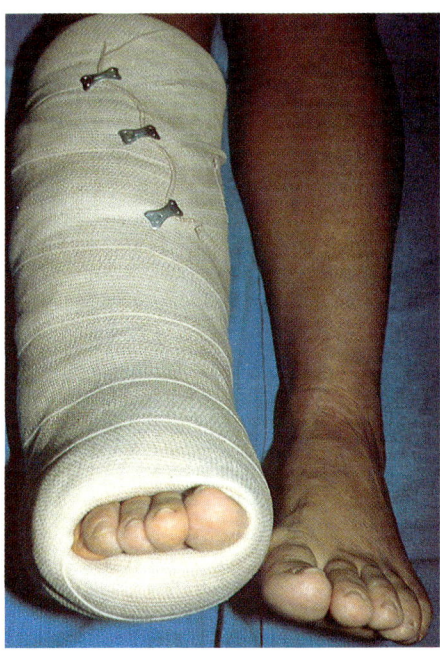

Figure 10. Skin edges closely approximated with 3-0 nylon sutures. (From ref. 7.)

Figure 11. Short leg compression splint applied immediately postoperative.

If there is significant incisional pain or metatarsalgia, a custom-molded total contact insert is fabricated for an in-depth shoe. A rocker bottom sole may be added if additional relief of metatarsal head loading is needed.

If there is a significant component of hypersensitivity to the incisional area at the time of cast removal, a manual desensitization program is begun, supervised by a physical therapist skilled in this technique. If pain and hypersensitivity do not respond within several weeks, oral medication and other nonsurgical treatments of neurogenic pain may be instituted. It is important for the surgeon to be watchful for the development of a pain syndrome and begin treatment early and aggressively if one develops.

Clearly, reoperation for recurrent or persistent pain following a primary interdigital neuroma excision is a worthwhile procedure in the carefully selected patient. However, the patient and the surgeon should understand that although a significant percentage of patients are "satisfied," many patients continue to have some type of symptoms at the involved interspace. A small group of patients are either not improved or worse.

Johnson et al. reported 66% "complete satisfaction or satisfaction with minor reservations" following reoperation of 37 feet in 34 patients using the technique described here (7).

Beskin and Baxter used a dorsal incision or an oblique/transverse plantar incision proximal to the metatarsal heads and reported approximately 80% of 30 patients with 39 recurrent neuromas were "satisfied" (1). Fifty-eight percent of patients still had difficulty with certain types of footwear. Of note, they reported fewer failures using the plantar approach than the previous dorsal incision (8% vs. 21%) (1).

Mann and Reynolds, using the previous dorsal incision, reported 9 of 11 patients with recurrent neuromas were "significantly improved" (8). However, 7 of 11 still had some plantar tenderness.

COMPLICATIONS

The most common complication following reoperation for a recurrent interdigital neuroma is failure to obtain relief in the preoperative pain symptoms. The reasons for this area similar to the reasons why the initial procedure failed (wrong diagnosis, wrong web space operated, unrealistic patient expectations, inadequate surgical excision). A more difficult complication is the development of a chronic localized pain syndrome or a reflex sympathetic dystrophy. Both of these problems can cause more pain and functional limitation than the isolated recurrent neuroma for which the surgery was performed. In general, the treatment for persistent pain following the second attempt at neuroma excision is nonsurgical and includes the modalities discussed previously including medication, physical therapy, local injections, and sympathetic blocks. In recalcitrant cases unresponsive to these modalities, an implantable tibial nerve stimulator or spinal cord stimulator may provide significant relief in pain as a salvage procedure (6).

A potential complication is development of a painful plantar scar due to hypertrophic changes and callus formation in the plantar incision. The series in the literature that used the plantar longitudinal incision, including primary and secondary neuroma excisions, have not reported problems other than a rare instance of mild tenderness at the site of the scar (2,3,7,9,10). In fact, most patients in one series stated they had difficulty finding the site of the previous plantar incision at the time of follow-up examination (7).

ILLUSTRATIVE CASE FOR TECHNIQUE

This 22-year-old woman underwent a primary interdigital neuroma excision 1 year prior utilizing a dorsal web-space incision between the third and fourth metatarsal heads (Fig. 12). She never obtained a significant amount of pain relief from the initial procedure. In addition, she complained of a "burning and tingling" pain on the plantar aspect of the foot in the area just proximal to the fourth metatarsal head. The plantar skin was very hypersensitive to even light touch and any weight

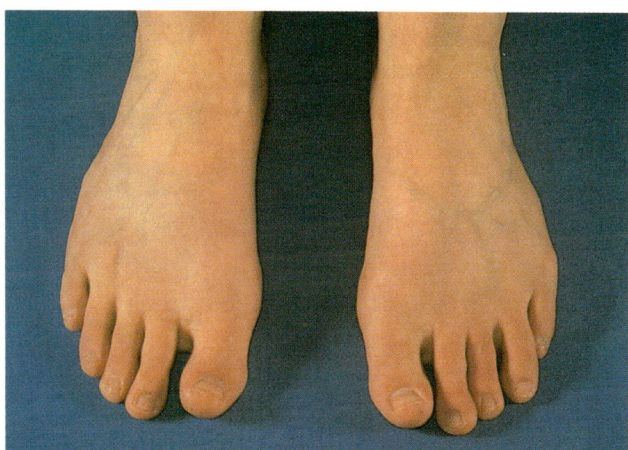

Figure 12. Previous dorsal incision from failed 3–4 interdigital neuroma excision, right foot.

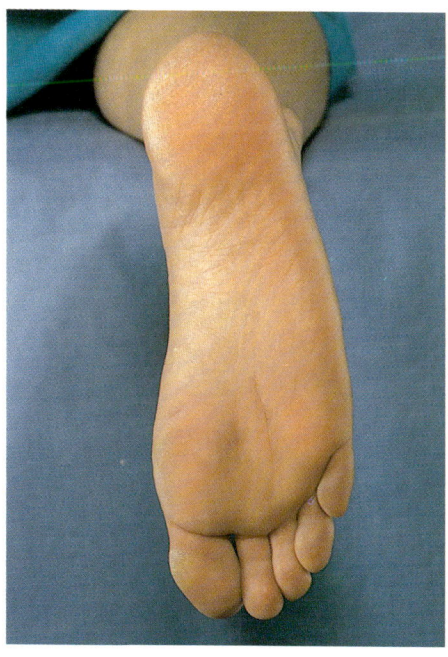

Figure 13. Appearance of pain-free plantar scar at 2 years postoperative. (From ref. 7.)

bearing on the metatarsal head region was painful. Molded polyethylene foam shoe inserts provided some relief but the pain was disabling in any type of shoe.

There was exquisite tenderness proximal to the area between the third and fourth metatarsal heads. There was some loss of sensation in the third web space. Radiographs were normal. A local injection into the painful area gave 90% temporary relief in pain during the action of the local anesthetic.

The patient chose a general anesthetic. After this was induced, an ankle block was placed in the tibial nerve prior to rolling her into the prone position. A plantar longitudinal incision was used to expose the plantar interdigital nerve proximally. The nerve was traced distally and a bulbous thickening of the nerve was found. The nerve was transected distally and then proximally under moderate tension to allow retraction into the forefoot. Skin sutures were placed to carefully approximate the skin edges. A short leg compression splint was applied, which was changed to a walking cast and worn for 3 weeks. At 2-year follow-up she was completely satisfied with no restrictions in her activity level. Her only complaint was occasional plantar "soreness" after strenuous activity and she preferred soft-soled shoes with an accommodative total contact insert. She had no complaints regarding the plantar scar (Fig. 13).

RECOMMENDED READING

1. Beskin, J. L., and Baxter, D. E.: Recurrent pain following interdigital neurectomy—a plantar approach. *Foot Ankle*, 9(1): 34–39, 1988.
2. Betts, L. O.: Morton's metatarsalgia: neuritis of the fourth digital nerve. *Med. J. Aust.*, 1: 514–515, 1940.
3. Bickel, W. H., and Dockerty, M. B.: Plantar neuromas, Morton's toe. *Surg. Gynecol. Obstet.*, 84: 111–116, 1947.
4. Bradley, N., Miller, W. A., and Evans, J. P.: Plantar neuroma: analysis of results following surgical excision in 145 patients. *South. Med. J.*, 69: 853–854, 1976.
5. Friscia, D. A., Strom, D. E., Parr, J. W., Saltzman, C. L., and Johnson, K. A.: Surgical treatment for primary interdigital neuroma. *Orthopedics*, 14(6): 669–672, 1991.
6. Gould, J. S.: Treatment of the painful nerve in-continuity. In: Gelberman, R. H., ed. *Inoperative Nerve Repair and Reconstruction*. Philadelphia: J. B. Lippincott, pp. 1541–1550, 1991.
7. Johnson, J. E., Johnson, K. A., and Unni, K. K.: Persistent pain after excision of an interdigital neuroma—results of reoperation. *J. Bone Joint Surg.*, 70A(5): 651–657, 1988.
8. Mann, R. A., and Reynolds, J. C.: Interdigital neuroma—a critical clinical analysis. *Foot Ankle*, 3: 238–243, 1983.
9. Morris, M. A.: Morton's metatarsalgia. *Clin. Orthop.*, 127: 203–207, 1977.
10. Mulder, J. D.: The causative mechanism in Morton's metatarsalgia. *J. Bone Joint Surg.*, 33B(1): 94–95, 1951.
11. Thompson, F. M., and Deland, J. T.: Second neuroma same foot. Presented at American Orthopaedic Foot and Ankle Society, sixth annual summer meeting, Banff, Alberta, Canada, June 22, 1990.

15

Osteotomy of the Fifth Metatarsal

Harold B. Kitaoka

INDICATIONS/CONTRAINDICATIONS

Pain over the lateral condylar process of the fifth metatarsal is the main indication for fifth metatarsal osteotomy in patients with bunionette (tailor's bunion). There may be associated bursitis, intractable plantar keratosis of the fifth metatarsal head, and difficulty tolerating most footwear (6). While there is usually varus malalignment of the fifth toe associated with the bunionette, the malalignment alone is not a consistent source of symptoms. Patients with bunionettes often have significantly increased metatarsophalangeal 5 and intermetatarsal 4–5 angles (7).

The distal chevron fifth metatarsal osteotomy has been success for the treatment of hallux valgus (2) and a similar technique has been applied to the bunionette. It may be applied to patients with a painful bunionette including those with marked splaying (increased intermetatarsal 4–5 angle), lateral bowing of the metatarsal, and increased head to neck ratio. Unlike the chevron first metatarsal osteotomy for hallux valgus, the operation may be successfully used in patients that have more severe deformities, as there is no correlation between the degree of fifth metatarsal splaying and the clinical results (5). This operation may be successful in adults of all age groups. It is appropriate if there is satisfactory fifth metatarsophalangeal joint function. In some instances this operation may be performed as a salvage procedure following failed lateral condylar process resection if most of the fifth metatarsal head remains.

Contraindications of distal fifth chevron metatarsal osteotomy are the absence of pain, and presence of stiffness and/or arthrosis of the fifth metatarsophalangeal (MP) joint. Another contraindication is skin ulceration or infection, which may occur in patients with bunionette and sensory neuropathy. Peripheral vascular

---

H. B. Kitaoka, M.D.: Department of Orthopaedics, Mayo Clinic and Mayo Foundation, and Mayo Medical School, Rochester, MN 55905.

disease is also a contraindication. In cases where there are severe juxtaarticular erosions associated with an inflammatory disease, osteotomy at the distal level may not be possible.

PREOPERATIVE PLANNING

It is appropriate to carefully assess the patient's symptoms and signs in order to determine whether operative treatment is indicated. It should be considered in patients who have failed nonoperative treatment such as use of footwear with a wider toe box, softer leather upper, and shoes in which the leather is stretched over the lateral forefoot prominence. Based upon the patient's symptoms (pain, restricted footwear, restricted activities), medical evaluation, radiologic studies, and appropriate patient expectations, the decision regarding surgery can be made.

On physical examination the alignment of the fifth toe should be assessed. Fifth MP joint range of motion in the dorsiflexion–plantar flexion plane should be determined, as well as whether this motion is painful. The presence of intractable plantar keratosis beneath the fifth metatarsal head should be documented. One should also observe evidence of abnormal forefoot loading in other regions such as under the fourth metatarsal head. The presence of other lesser toe or great toe deformities should be noted. Other associated fifth toe problems such as dorsal subluxation at the MP level or hard corn formation at the interphalangeal level should be noted. A general medical examination is necessary to identify regional or general conditions that may be the source of problems such as peripheral vascular disease, diabetes mellitus, and systemic inflammatory diseases. Standing anteroposterior and lateral weight-bearing radiographs and an oblique view of the foot should be obtained to assess the level of arthrosis at the MP joint, juxtaarticular erosions, and alignment with respect to intermetatarsal 4–5, and metatarsophalangeal-5 angles. Fifth MP subluxation also should be assessed on the radiographs.

While this chevron-type metatarsal osteotomy has application for most bunionette problems including those with severe deformities, it is appropriate for the surgeon to be aware of alternative procedures that may be useful in specific situations. Removing the prominent lateral condyle is simple and has the advantages of preserving joint function and metatarsal length. Fixation and immobilization are not required. This operation has application in patients in which the simpler operation is preferred but one must accept the possibility of residual pain in a higher percentage of patients than the distal chevron osteotomy (4). The midshaft osteotomy proposed by Coughlin (1,2) has application particularly in patients who have failed previous bunionette surgery. While it has the potential of achieving a larger degree of correction of the intermetatarsal 4–5 angle, it requires more extensive exposure, fixation, and postoperative cast immobilization.

Finally, fifth metatarsal head resection (3) is a useful procedure in patients who have significant juxtaarticular erosions in which the joint is not salvageable and an osteotomy operation is not possible at the distal level. It is useful in patients with stiffness and/or arthrosis of the fifth MP joint, selected patients who have failed bunionette operations, and patients who have a neurotrophic ulcer with extension of the infection to the distal fifth metatarsal and MP joint.

SURGERY

This preferred chevron type fifth metatarsal osteotomy can be done utilizing ankle block, spinal, or general anesthesia. It is usually performed as an outpatient procedure and it is also possible to perform the operation on both feet at the same time.

15 FIFTH METATARSAL OSTEOTOMY

With the patient placed in the supine position the foot is exsanguinated with a rubber bandage. In most cases when ankle block anesthesia is administered a rubber bandage is wrapped at the ankle level for hemostasis. A sterile tourniquet may also be used at the ankle level. In patients who have general or spinal anesthesia a thigh tourniquet may be utilized.

Technique. The skin incision is made in a dorsal lateral longitudinal fashion centered at the distal fifth metatarsal level and is 3 cm in length (Fig. 1). The subcutaneous tissues are retracted.

An incisional neuroma may be avoided by identification of the small dorsal lateral sensory nerve following the skin incision and prior to the capsulotomy. While hypesthesia in a small area of the dorsal lateral aspect of the fifth toe may not be particularly bothersome, local irritation with footwear due to an incisional neuroma can be symptomatic.

A longitudinal incision of the MP joint capsule is made. Care is taken to identify the dorsal lateral sensory nerve, which should be protected. Care should also be taken to avoid excessive removal of soft tissues about the distal fifth metatarsal as this may have an effect on osteotomy union, the occurrence of osteonecrosis of the fifth metatarsal head, and stability of the osteotomy.

Performing an osteotomy with an angle approaching 90° rather than 50° to 60° creates an osteotomy that is less stable and may require fixation. Similarly an osteotomy that is performed too proximally at the neck level may be less stable as the thicker cortical bone at the neck level may not impact to the same degree as the largely cancellous bone at the head level. If the lateral condylar process resection is excessive it may affect the stability of the osteotomy as well.

The lateral condylar process should be removed approximately parallel to the lateral border of the foot utilizing a microsagittal saw with a small saw blade (Figs. 2 and 3). A chevron-shaped osteotomy is made at the metatarsal head level at an angle of 50° with the apex facing distally (Figs. 4 and 5). The distal fragment is displaced medially 3 to 4 mm (Fig. 6). Care is taken to orient the plane of the osteotomy parallel to the plantar foot in order to avoid displacement of the osteotomy in the dorsal-plantar plane. The residual lateral prominence of the metatarsal head and neck is resected (Fig. 7) and the osteotomy is impacted by axial compression of the phalanx on the metatarsal head (Figs. 8 and 9). Stability is tested by metatarsophalangeal joint motion. If it is determined that the osteotomy is not

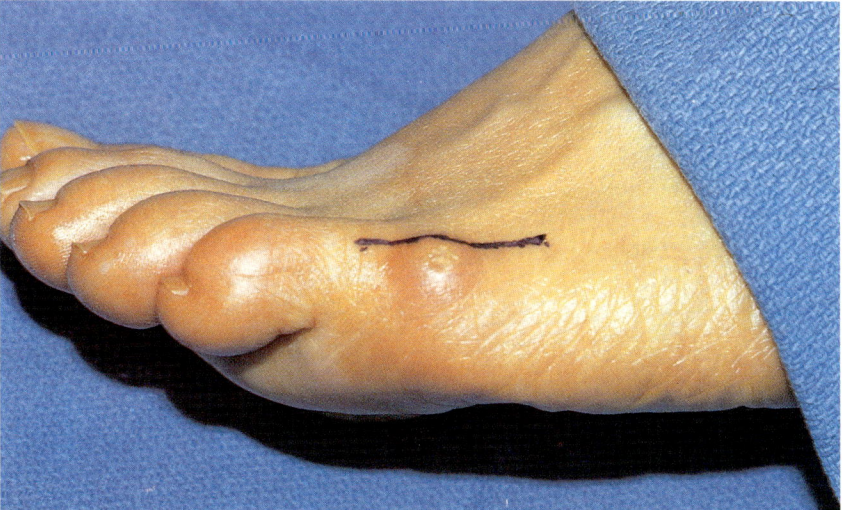

Figure 1. Clinical photo of a 47-year-old female with a painful bunionette. Note the callus overlying the prominent lateral condylar process of the fifth metatarsal. The figure shows the dorsolateral skin incision.

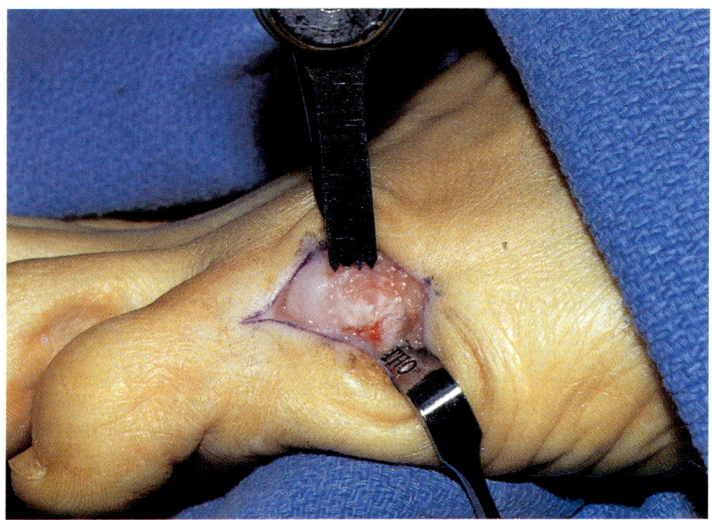

Figure 2. Following longitudinal capsulotomy, the prominent lateral condylar process was resected with a microsagittal saw in a plane paralleling the lateral border of the foot.

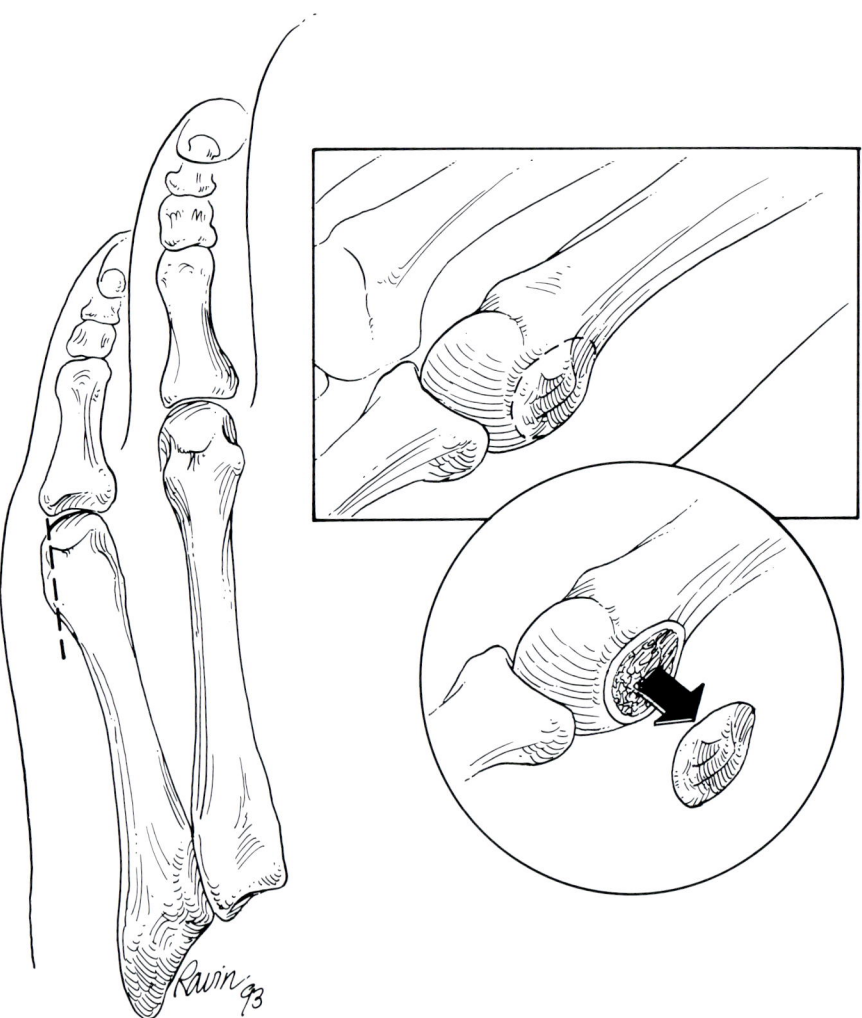

Figure 3. Through a dorsal lateral approach centered at the distal fifth metatarsal level the lateral condylar process is resected at a level parallel to the lateral border of the foot.

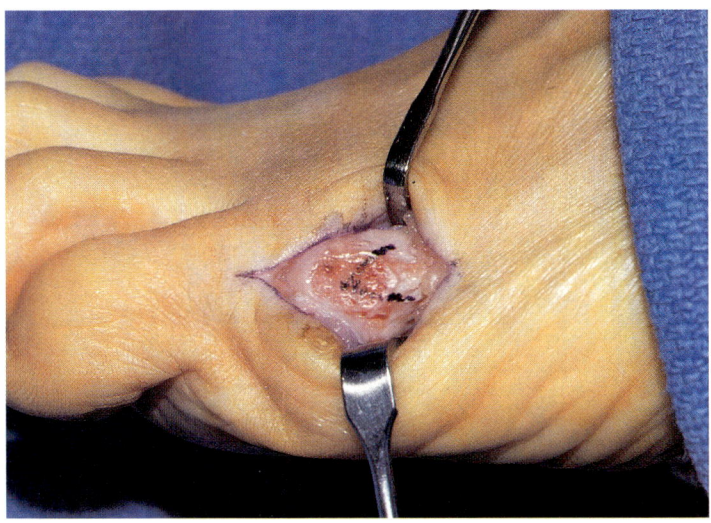

Figure 4. Following resection of the lateral condylar process, the osteotomy is marked with the apex facing distally and centered 1 to 2 mm distal to the center of the metatarsal head with the osteotomy angle of 50°.

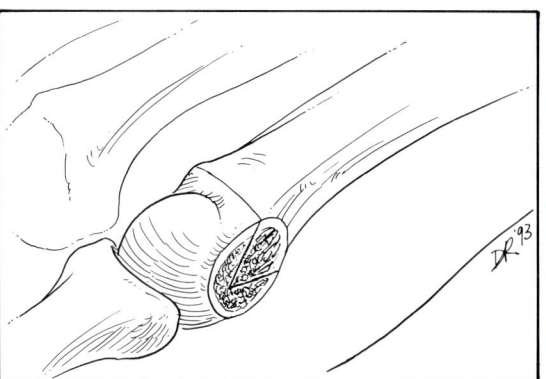

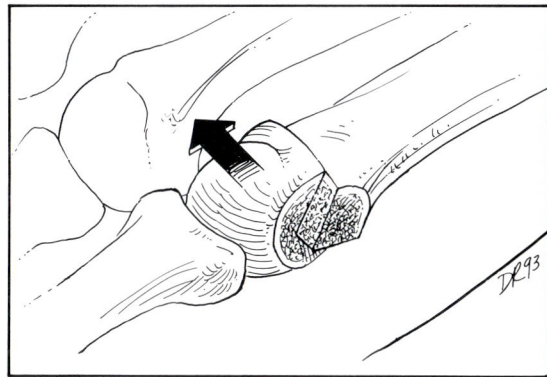

Figure 5. A chevron-shaped osteotomy is made with a microsagittal saw at an angle of 50°. Note the apex of the osteotomy is 1 to 2 mm distal to the center of the metatarsal head. Displacement of the distal fragment is 3 to 4 mm. *Arrow* indicates displacement in the medial direction. Care is taken to avoid any dorsal displacement.

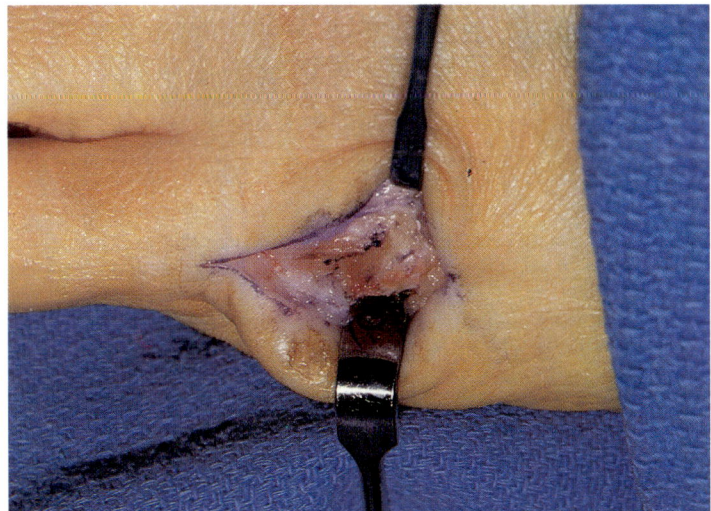

Figure 6. Following the chevron osteotomy utilizing a microsagittal saw, the distal fragment is displaced medially as seen in this dorsolateral view. The remaining head and neck prominence is then removed with the microsagittal saw.

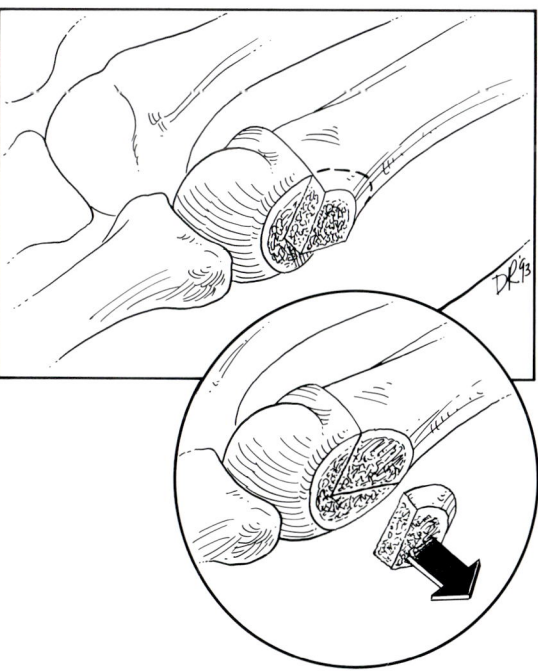

Figure 7. The removal of the remaining head and neck fragment with microsagittal saw.

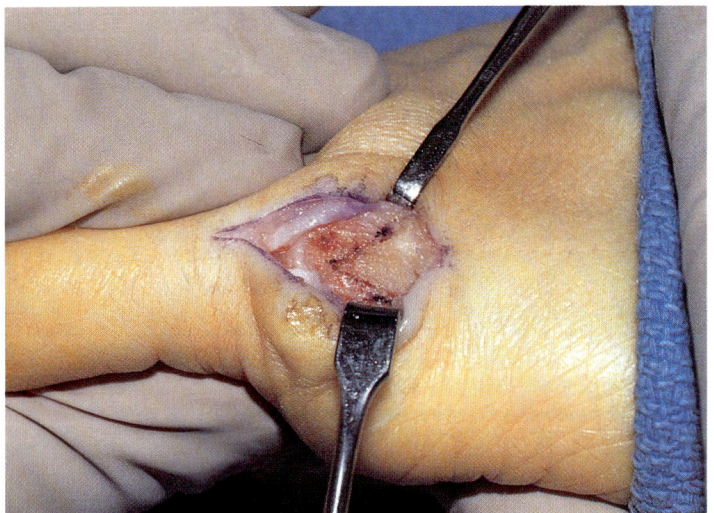

Figure 8. Following removal of the remaining head and neck fragment, the osteotomy is impacted with longitudinal compression. Osteotomy stability is then tested by passive motion of the metatarsophalangeal joint. If this is found to be stable, then no fixation is required. A portion of the redundant capsule is excised followed by skin closure.

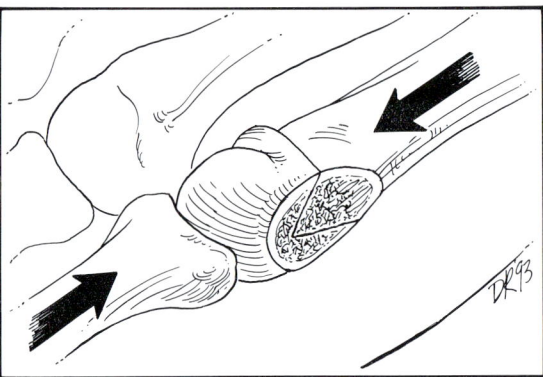

Figure 9. Impaction of the osteotomy by longitudinal compression *(arrows).* The stability is then tested by metatarsophalangeal joint motion.

stable, then a percutaneous Kirschner wire could be added, directed obliquely from the proximal dorsal to the distal plantar aspect across the osteotomy. In general, however, the osteotomy is stable particularly if performed at an angle of 50° and therefore does not require supplemental fixation. Additionally, the apex of the bone cut could be made 1 to 2 mm distal to the center of the metatarsal head rather than the neck level, as the more distal osteotomy tends to be more stable. Care should be taken to avoid performing the osteotomy too far distally or impacting it too vigorously, which has the potential of splitting the distal fragment. It is not necessary to perform a medial capsulotomy in order to adequately correct the toe alignment. The distal chevron osteotomy has been modified since the clinical series reported earlier (5). The main modification is performing an osteotomy at a 50° angle rather than 60°.

The capsule is then closed tightly and a portion of the redundant capsule is excised. The skin is closed in the usual fashion in layers. During capsular and skin closure it is helpful to place a sponge between the fourth and fifth toes to assist in obtaining a tight capsular closure. One will notice that after the wound is closed, the lateral prominence will be reduced and fifth toe alignment improved. The wound is dressed with 4" × 4" sponges and 2-inch Kling bandage that may be applied in a toe spica pattern. A stiff postoperative shoe is applied and anteroposterior and lateral radiographs are obtained in the recovery room.

POSTOPERATIVE MANAGEMENT

A toe spica type of soft tissue dressing is applied followed by application of a postsurgical shoe. On occasion it is beneficial to immobilize the foot in a short leg walking cast particularly when the operation is combined with other foot procedures. The patient is allowed to bear weight in the postsurgical shoe or cast; however, crutches are useful initially as an ambulatory aid. The dressing is changed in several days and the sutures removed at 2 to 3 weeks postoperatvely. If a percutaneous Kirschner wire is utilized it is removed at that time as well. The stiff postoperative shoe is then worn for an additional 2 to 3 weeks at which time anteroposterior and lateral radiographs are obtained to judge alignment and osteotomy union. If radiographs appear to be satisfactory the patient can resume the use of a closed toe shoe with a wide toe box. There is often some degree of swelling for an additional month. As the patient mobilizes the forefoot, gentle range of motion exercises can be started at 3 weeks postoperatively and more vigorous exercises at 6 weeks, particularly at the fifth MP joint.

The results are generally satisfactory for this operation. In a series of 19 procedures performed with a 7-year average follow-up, the overall results were considered good in 17 feet, fair in 2, and there were no failures. Complications such as transfer metatarsalgia occurred in one foot and there was a wound infection in one foot (5). There was a high satisfaction rate and pain over the lateral condylar process was usually relieved. A wider range of footwear was tolerated. The fifth toe varus malalignment was significantly improved.

COMPLICATIONS

Various complications may occur after a fifth metatarsal chevron osteotomy for a bunionette deformity. Displacement of the osteotomy is a possibility that can be prevented by appropriate surgical technique. Avoiding excessive soft tissue stripping of the osteotomy site, making the angle of the osteotomy about 50°, providing supplemental fixation if the osteotomy feels unstable at the completion of the procedure, as well as tight capsular closure all decrease the possibility of osteotomy displacement.

Transfer metatarsalgia to the fourth metatarsal head region is a possibility if the metatarsal head was displaced in a dorsal position. Again, the stability of the osteotomy against dorsiflexion is an inherent advantage of this particular procedure. Being aware of this possibility and providing adequate fixation where necessary is important.

The possibility of avascular necrosis of the fifth metatarsal head is present. The vascular supply, however, is probably similar to that of the first metatarsal and excessive medial stripping of the soft tissues from the metatarsal head should be avoided.

ILLUSTRATIVE CASE FOR TECHNIQUE

This 22-year-old woman presented with pain over the lateral condylar region of her fifth metatarsal in the left foot. She did not have satisfactory relief with symptoms with appropriate footwear. The appearance of the fifth toe was not particularly bothersome to her. Radiographs show some degree of splaying of the fifth metatarsal relative to the fourth (increased in intermetatarsal 4–5 angle) on the standing anteroposterior view (Fig. 10). A distal chevron osteotomy without fixation was performed. She was immobilized in a short leg walking cast. Her cast and sutures were removed at 3 weeks postoperatively and she was placed in a postsurgical shoe for an additional several weeks. Radiographs show the degree of correction of the prominent distal fifth metatarsal with medial displacement of the distal fragment (Fig. 11). The lateral border of the foot was no longer prominent distally. Additionally the fifth toe alignment was improved. At follow-up 6 years later the patient had a good result with no pain, no restriction of activities, and no support requirement; some stylish shoes were tolerated and there was no tenderness or painful callus, stiffness, or objectionable alignment.

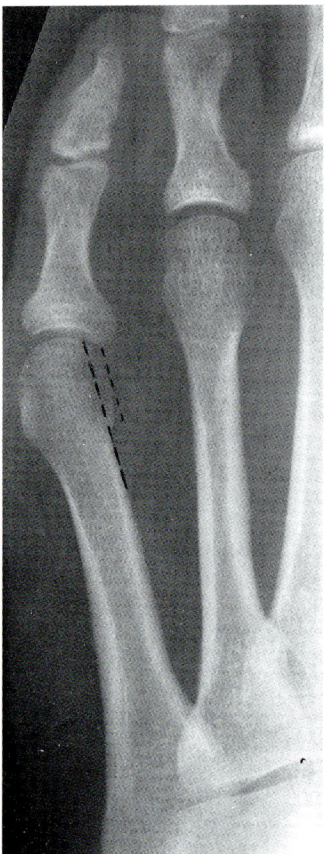 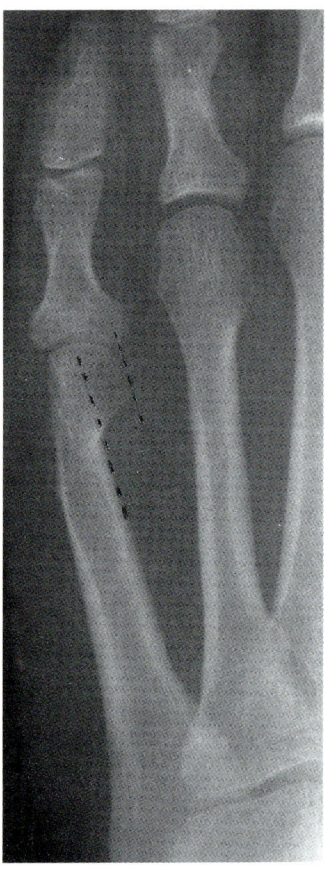

Figure 10. Preoperative radiograph of a 22-year-old woman with painful bunionette.

Figure 11. Six years following successful distal chevron osteotomy. Note the displacement of the metatarsal head medially *(dotted lines)*.

RECOMMENDED READING

1. Coughlin, M. J.: Correction of the bunionette with midshaft oblique osteotomy. *Orthop. Trans.*, 12: 30, 1988 (abstract).
2. Johnson, K. A., Cofield, R. H., and Morrey, B. F.: Chevron osteotomy for hallux valgus. *Clin. Orthop.*, 142: 44–47, 1979.
3. Kitaoka, H. B., and Holiday, A. D., Jr.: Metatarsal head resection for bunionette: long-term follow-up. *Foot Ankle*, 11(6): 345–349, 1991.
4. Kitaoka, H. B., and Holiday, A.D., Jr.: Lateral condylar resection for bunionette. *Clin. Orthop.*, 278: 183–192, 1992.
5. Kitaoka, H. B., Holiday, A. D., Jr., and Campbell, D. C., II: Distal chevron metatarsal osteotomy for bunionette. *Foot Ankle*, 12(2): 80–85, 1991.
6. Kitaoka, H. B., and Leventen, E. O.: Medial displacement metatarsal osteotomy for treatment of painful bunionette. *Clin. Orthop.*, 243: 172–179, 1989.
7. Nestor, B. J., Kitaoka, H .B., Ilstrup, D. M., Berquist, T. H., and Bergmann, A. D.: Radiologic anatomy of the painful bunionette. *Foot Ankle*, 11(1): 6–11, 1990.
8. Sponsel, K. H.: Bunionette correction by metatarsal osteotomy: preliminary report. *Orthop. Clin. North Am.*, 7: 809–819, 1976.

16

Rheumatoid Forefoot Reconstruction

Charles L. Saltzman

INDICATIONS/CONTRAINDICATIONS

The indications for surgical reconstruction of the rheumatoid forefoot are (a) pain unrelieved by nonoperative means and (b) impending ulceration. The goals of surgery need to be considered in light of the natural history of rheumatoid arthritis (RA). Although there may be temporary lulls in the progression of this devastating disease, it never truly "burns out." Consequently, the results of surgery naturally deteriorate over time. Factors that influence outcome include patient selection, surgical timing, and operative technique.

Virtually all patients with long-standing disease have metatarsophalangeal (MP) joint involvement. Initially these joints are swollen and painful. The swelling permanently stretches surrounding ligaments. When this acute phase of synovitis resolves, the residual joint laxity leads to subluxation and dislocation. Although any possible deformity can occur, the most common problems are hallux valgus and lesser toe clawing. Patients complain of pain under the central metatarsal heads, around the medial eminence, and on the dorsum of the toes.

Initial care includes the use of extradepth shoes constructed from a soft pliable or temperature moldable material. Custom inserts with metatarsal pads and a surface interface of medium-density Plastizote are frequently beneficial. If the patient develops severe metatarsalgia, a rocker bottom or metatarsal bar can be added to the sole of the shoe to unload the forefoot.

The primary indication for surgery is pain unrelieved by nonoperative means. Contraindications include severe soft tissue fragility, vascular insufficiency, and ongoing deep infection. Relative contraindications are cervical spine instability, gait unsteadiness, and long-standing steroid dependence.

C. L. Saltzman, M.D.: Department of Orthopaedic Surgery, University of Iowa, Iowa City, IA 55242.

PREOPERATIVE PLANNING

A complete history and physical examination should be done on every RA patient prior to surgery. A history of increasing unsteadiness or the physical finding of lower extremity hyperreflexia can indicate a cervical myelopathy and deserves prompt attention. Lateral flexion-extension radiographs of the cervical spine are routinely obtained. Patients with documented cervical instability should have a regional or spinal anesthetic. If general anesthesia is required, an awake fiberoptic intubation is recommended. Patients with significant instability or myelopathy may be advised to consider cervical spine stabilization prior to foot surgery. Patients on methotrexate are asked to discontinue its use 1 week before surgery until 2 weeks after surgery. Prednisone-dependent patients are given a steroid burst in the perioperative period. Patients with upper extremity arthritic involvement benefit from preoperative instruction in the use of Canadian crutches or a walker with wheels. The ease of postoperative recovery can be enormously facilitated by arranging home care or physical therapy in advance of surgery.

The optimal timing of surgery for patients with bilateral problems is a matter of debate. My preference is to stage procedures with a minimum of 6 months between operations. With this approach, the patient has the nonoperated foot on which to bear weight after surgery and, as result, less postoperative morbidity. Moreover, the patient is able to judge the true benefits of surgery before having both feet reconstructed. In rare circumstances (e.g., patients with bilateral plantar ulcerations or with severe anesthetic risks) it may be wiser to treat both feet simultaneously.

In addition to the general history and physical examination, a focused evaluation of the foot is necessary. The physical examination documents the condition of the peripheral vasculature, the severity and location of skin calluses, as well as the patient's location of pain. The radiographs include a weight-bearing anteroposterior (AP), lateral, and a non–weight-bearing oblique view. From these radiographs, the degree of osteoporosis, joint deformities including subluxation or dislocation, as well as the amount of rheumatoid joint destruction is visualized. No single operative approach suffices for all patients. For example, consider derangements of the hallux in RA. The great toe can drift into valgus or varus at the MP joint, have interphalangeal (IP) arthritis or dislocation, develop clawing from intrinsic imbalance or tendon attrition, and be endowed with either soft or hard bone stock. Although arthrodesis of the first MP joint is generally preferred (5), a resection arthroplasty may be a better procedure for a patient with insufficient bone stock, extrinsic tendon rupture, or significant IP symptoms.

Similarly, treatment of the lesser toes should be individualized. Variable degrees of deformity can develop—ranging from mild MP subluxation to fixed MP dislocation with rigid clawing. The prevailing surgical approach to these problems is MP resection arthroplasty (1). The extent of resection, however, may be modified to accommodate each patient's particular problems. Mild deformities are treated with minimal resections, whereas severe deformities require more bone removal. In borderline clinical decisions, I tend to remove more rather than less bone since attaining soft tissue relaxation through an adequate bony excision is fundamental to the procedure's success (1).

SURGERY

The patient is positioned supine with the operative table inclined in mild, reverse Trendelenburg. The foot is positioned with the heel within inches of the end of the table. This enables the surgeon to have full access to the forefoot from a seat at the end of the table.

A 12-inch inflatable tourniquet is wrapped above the ankle. After the foot is sterilely prepped, a toe cot is placed on the hallux. For patients with marginal skin, the foot is exsanguinated by gravity; for all others, a 3-inch Esmarch is used. The tourniquet pressure is set at 100 mm Hg greater than the systolic pressure. Complete reconstruction of the rheumatoid forefoot can be time-consuming. After 2 hours, the tourniquet pressure is released to reduce the potential of neurovascular complications.

Meticulous, atraumatic technique is essential when performing rheumatoid forefoot surgery. This can be accomplished with single- and double-pronged skin hooks, Boyes-Goodfellow retractors, and Adson forceps. Self-retaining retractors are to be used only sparingly as they can crush the fragile capillary networks of the rheumatoid forefoot.

Technique. Many different incisions have been advocated. These vary from transverse to longitudinal approaches across plantar or dorsal surfaces, with or without soft tissue excision. I prefer to use simple, extensile and longitudinal incisions that avoid neurovascular bundles. A direct medial incision works well for the hallux and two Y-shaped longitudinal incisions are sufficient for the lesser toes (Fig. 1). When doing a first MP fusion the lesser toe procedures are completed first to protect the arthrodesis construct.

The placement of incisions is partially determined by the desired final toe position. At the completion of the bony procedures there should be adequate soft tissue relaxation. Residual lesser toe floppiness is controlled with partial syndactylization. Subtotal webbing also reduces the risk of postoperative infection as compared to use of temporary longitudinal percutaneous pins.

Ordinarily, the second and fourth web spaces are partially syndactylized. The initial incision is placed in the second web space. With toes spread apart, a line is drawn with a surgical skin marker on the second toe. This is started at the natural webbing, slightly plantar to the midline and then J'd dorsally as it is continued distally. For toes with mild deformities, the line ends proximal to the proximal interphalangeal (PIP) joint; for those with greater deformity requiring greater bony resection, it extends more distally. After the first line is drawn, the second and third toes are squeezed together with the nails aligned. This leaves a mirror image shadow line on the medial side of the third toe due to residual ink from the skin marker. The toes are separated and the V line between the toes is extended proximally in a Y fashion between the second and third metatarsal heads. A similar

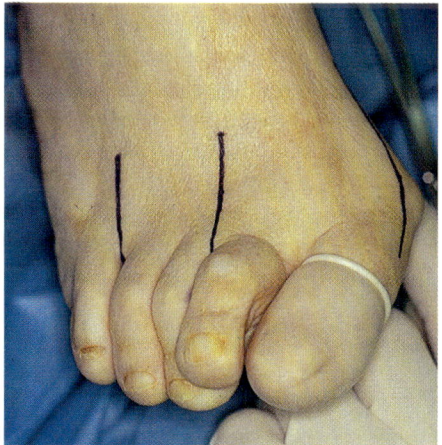

Figure 1. Dorsal view of the incisions used for rheumatoid forefoot reconstruction.

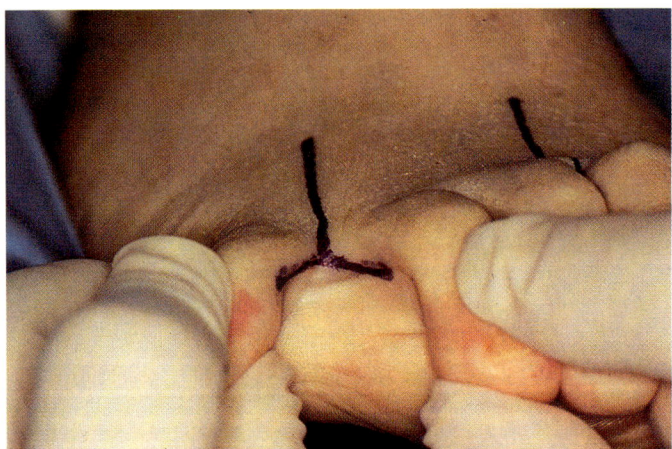

Figure 2. Clinical appearance of the Y-fashioned web-space incision.

procedure is performed in the fourth web space, with the fifth toe serving as the template for drawing the incision (Fig. 2).

The most deformed toe is approached first. Thick flaps are developed by sharp dissection directly down to bone with the neurovascular bundle remaining in the plantar flap. The periosteum is stripped from the MP to the level of planned proximal phalanx transection (Fig. 3). For mild deformities, this level is at the mid-diaphysis; for moderate deformities the level is more distal; and for severe deformities, the entire proximal phalanx is removed. Furthermore, the amount of bony excision can be varied between toes of the same foot depending on the degree of deformity. For example, I commonly remove more than half of the second and third proximal phalanges, slightly less than half of the fourth, and none of the fifth. This usually relaxes the soft tissues and leaves a stable lateral border to the foot.

Osteoporotic forefoot bones in rheumatoid disease require delicate handling. Bony excision is facilitated by removing as much investing soft tissue as possible. The MP plantar plate should be sharply released prior to bony transection. After the neurovascular structures are protected, a small hand-held oscillating saw is used to cut across the diaphysis of the proximal phalanx. With a towel clip the proximal fragment is stabilized by placing one pincer through the proximal articular surface and the other through the cut end of the proximal fragment. The remainder of the soft tissue attachments to the proximal fragment are sharply released and the fragment delivered out of the wound. The extensor tendons are then identified, isolated, and released. This can be done either in a Z fashion or, more typically, by removal of a 1-cm tendon segment just proximal to the extensor hood. The exact same procedure is repeated on the adjacent toe through the other limb of the web-space incision.

At this point I customarily make the Y incision in the fourth web space, remove the base of the fourth proximal phalanx, and perform extensor releases of the fourth and fifth toes. While usually not necessary, for severe deformities the base of the fifth toe is also removed. Excessive bony relaxation of the fifth ray can lead to lateral deviation of the lesser toes

The metatarsal head resections are done with both Y incisions open simultaneously. The key points are (a) to resect an adequate amount of bone to relax the surrounding soft tissues, (b) to develop a cascade of metatarsal lengths that mimics the natural metatarsal break, and (c) to leave no plantar spikes of bone. The first step is to expose the second metatarsal head by retraction of the capsule and excision of the pannus. A Carroll or McGlamry elevator is positioned proximal

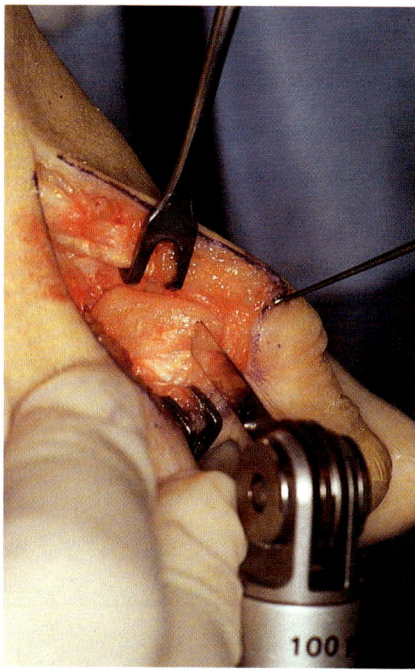

Figure 3. The base of the second proximal phalanx has been cleared of soft tissue and is ready for transection.

to the metatarsal condyle to shield soft tissue and to establish the plantar level of bony transection. Using a small oscillating saw, the cut is started just proximal to the dorsal articular edge and beveled 35° to the metatarsal shaft (Fig. 4). Any residual bony spikes are carefully removed with a small rongeur to avoid propagating a fracture down the shaft. Typically, the third, fourth, and fifth metatarsal heads are sequentially removed. The fifth metatarsal is smoothed laterally to minimize the risk of skin irritation. At the completion of the lesser metatarsal head resections there should be 1 to 2 cm of space between the metatarsals and the phalanges (Fig. 5). If greater bony excision is needed to accomplish tissue relaxation, the proximal phalanges, not the metatarsals, should be shortened further. This is accomplished with a small oscillating saw, rather than a rongeur or bone cutter, to avoid crushing or splintering residual fragments.

Closure of the syndactylization incisions is tedious and time-consuming. There are *no* shortcuts. The flaps must be handled with extreme care. Closure is started at the apex of the V and extended in a side-to-side manner from the plantar aspect around to the dorsum (Fig. 6). For this task, 4-0 PDS-II on a P3 needle works well. Simple, inverted sutures are placed approximately 2 to 3 mm apart. Special concern is given to the most distal stitch, for if it unravels the wound will dehisce.

After the webbing incisions are closed, the first MP joint is arthrodesed using a modification of McKeever's cup and cone technique (7,8). Compared with other approaches, McKeever's method has several advantages. First, it is straightforward and reliable. Second, the IP joint becomes relatively protected as the hallux is shortened functionally. Third, the IP joint is not violated by fixation hardware.

A 4-cm longitudinal incision is placed along the medial border of the first MP joint (Fig. 7). After the dorsal and plantar medial hallucal nerves are retracted, the incision is deepened through the capsule directly to bone. The metatarsal head and most proximal aspect of the phalanx are exposed subperiosteally. The assistant presents the metatarsal head to the surgeon by holding the hallux in

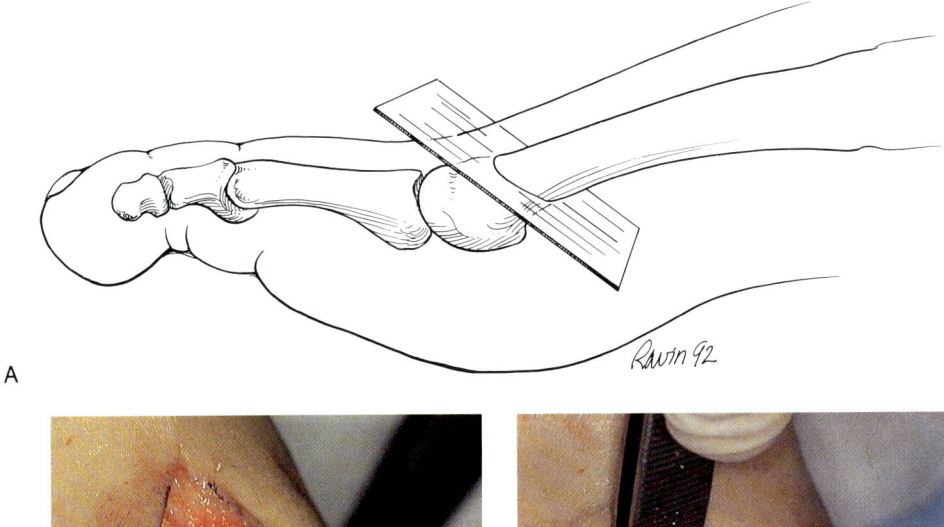

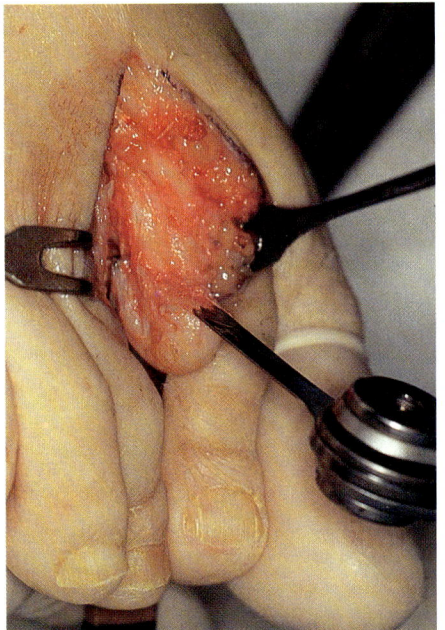
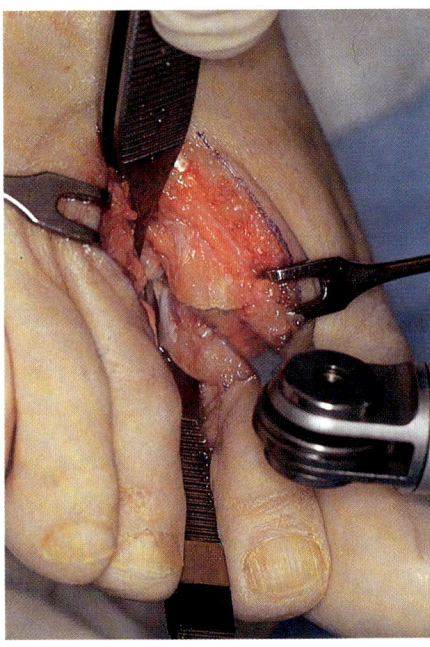

Figure 4. A: The plane of metatarsal neck transection is from distal superior to proximal inferior. **B** and **C:** Clinical photographs showing the metatarsal neck osteotomy orientation.

marked plantar flexion and positioning a Carroll elevator under the lateral lip of articular cartilage. The metatarsal head is now ready to be shaped into a cone.

With the forefoot in neutral position, the surgeon sites down the axis of the first metatarsal and places a mark approximately 3 mm superolateral to its projected intersection with the metatarsal head (Fig. 8). This point will become the tip of the cone. A small oscillating saw is used to roughly define the cone's shape (Fig. 9). More bone is removed medially and inferiorly to protect the superolateral cortex for eventual screw fixation. The metatarsal cone is then hand-finished with a Marin reamer (Sims Surgical Inc., Keene, NH) (Fig. 10).

Next, the proximal phalanx is positioned medial to this newly hewn cone of bone. Impaction of this soft cancellous bone is facilitated by retraction and release of soft tissues from the lateral side of the proximal phalanx. A 4.0-mm oval cutting burr or ¼-inch drill is used to establish access to the intramedullary cavity of the proximal phalanx (Fig. 11). The entrance point is approximately 3 mm inferior to the mid-dorsal articular border. The surrounding cartilage is removed with a Lempert rongeur. The cup is then excavated with the Marin reamer (Fig. 12). The reamer normally can be inserted so that its base is flush with the joint; however, in small

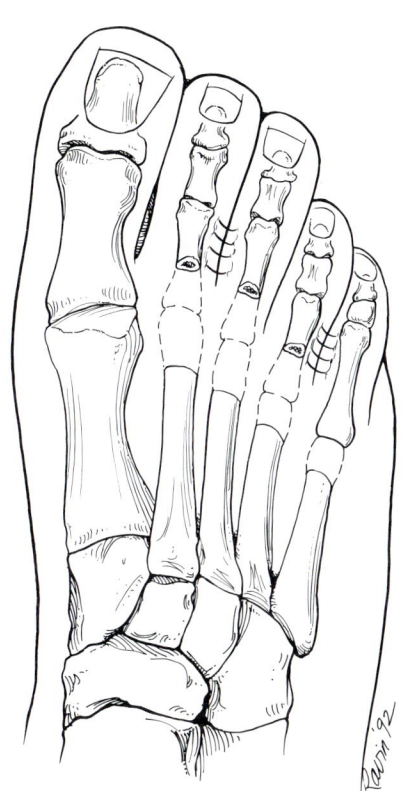

Figure 5. Typical amount of lesser metatarsophalangeal resection arthroplasty needed to correct a moderately deformed rheumatoid forefoot. The base of the fifth proximal phalanx is preserved to stabilize the lateral border of the foot.

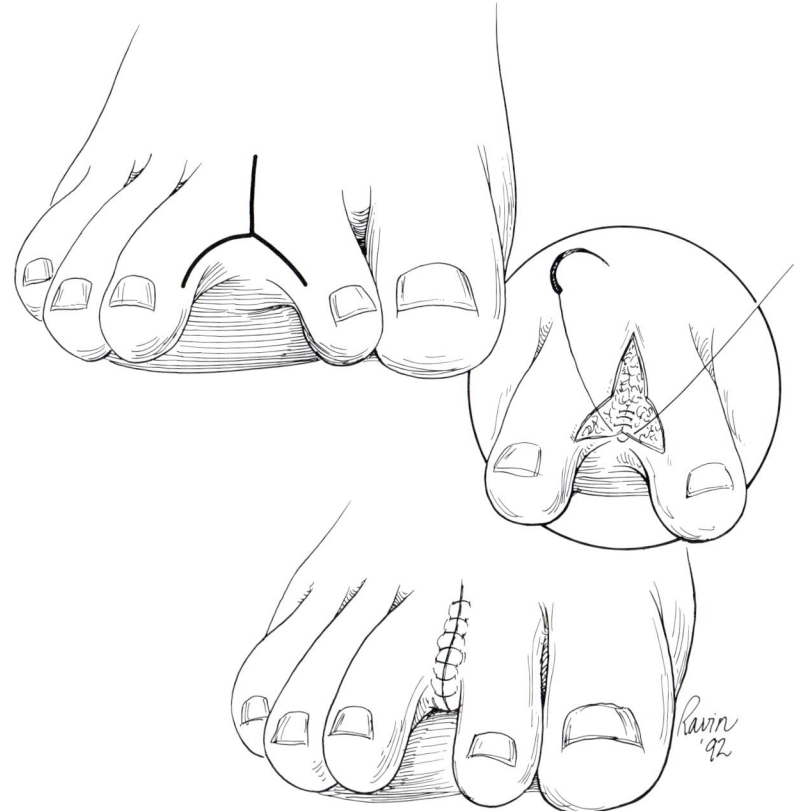

Figure 6. Closure of the subtotal webbings starts at the apex of the V, and is carried around from the plantar side to the dorsum.

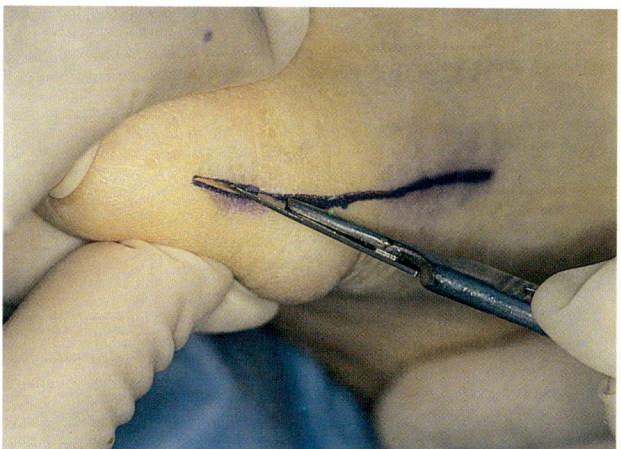

Figure 7. Skin incision for the first metatarsophalangeal arthrodesis.

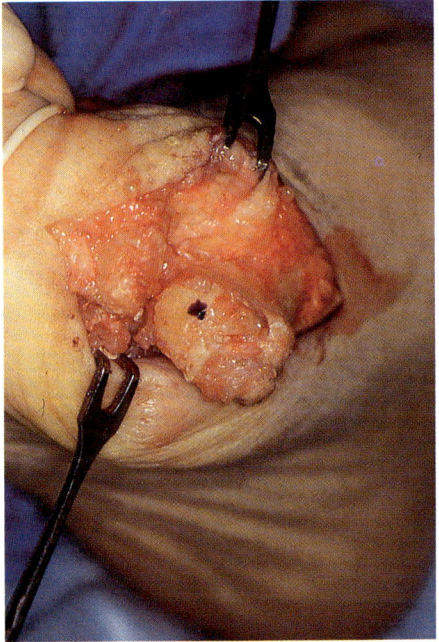

Figure 8. View looking from the head down the shaft of the first metatarsal. A dot has been placed slightly superior and lateral to the projected midline. This will serve as the tip of a cone created from the metatarsal head.

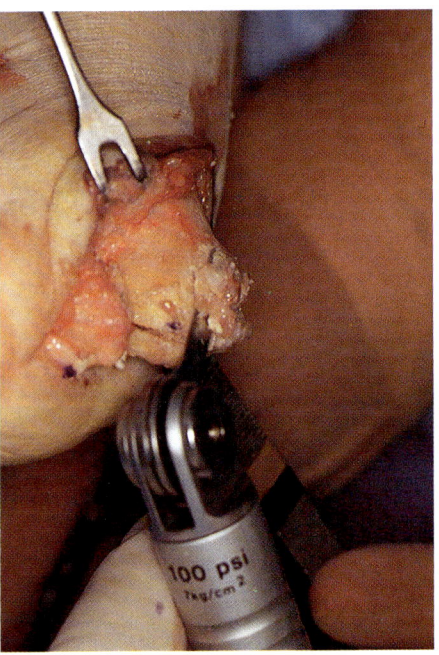

Figure 9. Dorsal view of the initial shaping of the metatarsal cone.

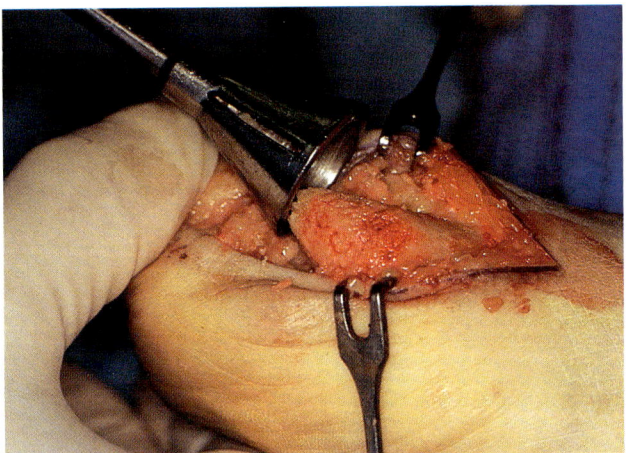

Figure 10. The metatarsal head–shaping Marin reamer is used to complete metatarsal cone sculpting.

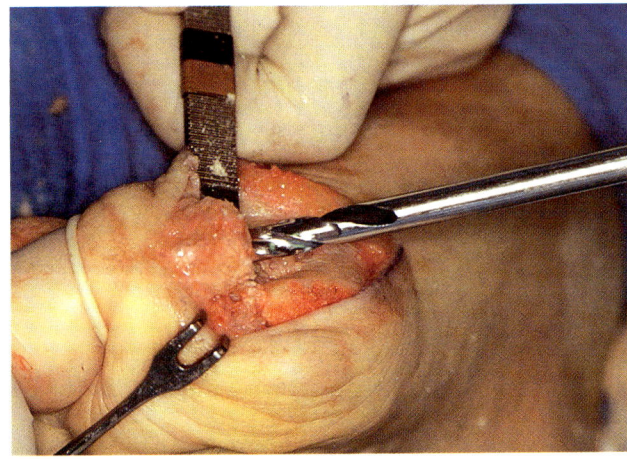

Figure 11. A ¼-inch drill bit helps gain access to the proximal phalangeal medullary canal.

bones this is not feasible. When using the reamer, extreme care must taken to avoid breaking the medial cortex.

The cup of proximal phalanx is then apposed on the cone of the metatarsal (Fig. 13). Typically, at this point some adjustment around the base of the cone is needed to achieve close contact. In order to avoid further shortening of the metatarsal, I prefer to make these modifications with a small rongeur rather than with the Marin reamer. The toe is positioned in approximately 15° of valgus and 25° of dorsiflexion. Temporarily, this alignment is maintained with two parallel 0.035-inch Kirschner (K) wires placed from the superomedial proximal phalanx to the superolateral metatarsal. At this stage hallux position is reassessed. The pulp of the great toe should be parallel or slightly dorsiflexed from the sole of the foot. The hallux should lie within 5 mm of the second toe without touching it.

If the hallux position is satisfactory, permanent fixation is attained using a 4.0 cancellous screw placed from the medial cortex of the proximal phalangeal base to the lateral cortex of the first metatarsal neck (Fig. 14). The entry point is in the center of the concavity just distal to the medial tubercle of the proximal phalanx. A 2.5-mm drill bit is oriented from distal to proximal, medial to lateral, and slightly inferior to superior. With rheumatoid bone, use of the tap and countersink is usually not necessary. A partially threaded 4.0 cancellous screw is inserted with the K-wires removed immediately prior to final screw tensioning.

If the position shifts during screw tightening, it is probably caused by surface incongruity between the cup and cone. In this situation there are two possible solutions. When working with hard cortical bone, the construct can be taken down and the cup and cone reshaped. When working with soft bone, however, fixation can be compromised by repetitive screw insertion. In this situation, it is better to back the screw up a few turns, realign the hallux, reintroduce a K-wire, and retighten the screw. The K-wire can be cut flush with bone and left in permanently.

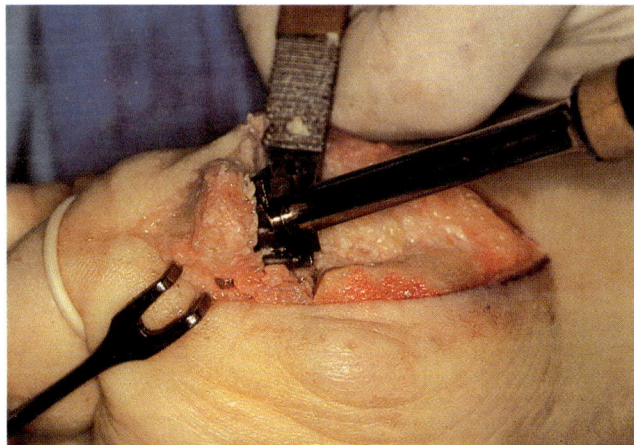

Figure 12. The phalanx base–shaping Marin reamer is rotated down the shaft of the proximal phalanx skirting inadvertent penetration of the medial cortex.

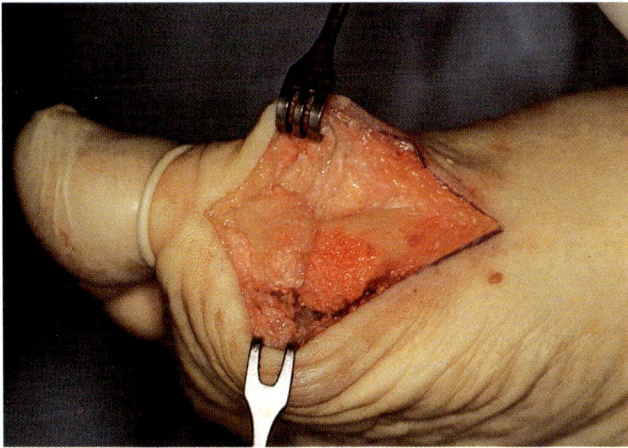

Figure 13. The cup of proximal phalanx is seated on the metatarsal cone.

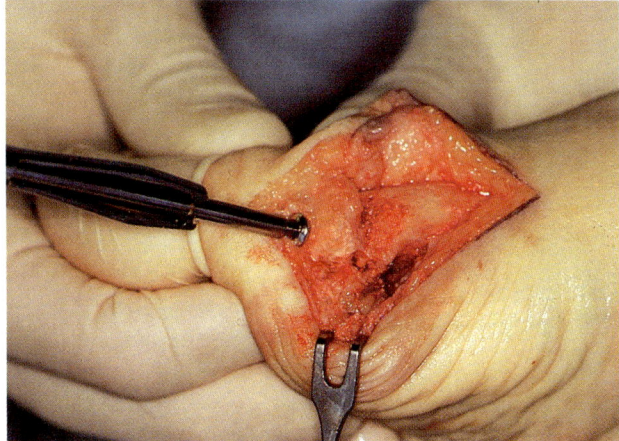

Figure 14. With the proper position maintained by an assistant or temporary K-wires, a 4.0 cancellous screw is tightened for permanent fixation.

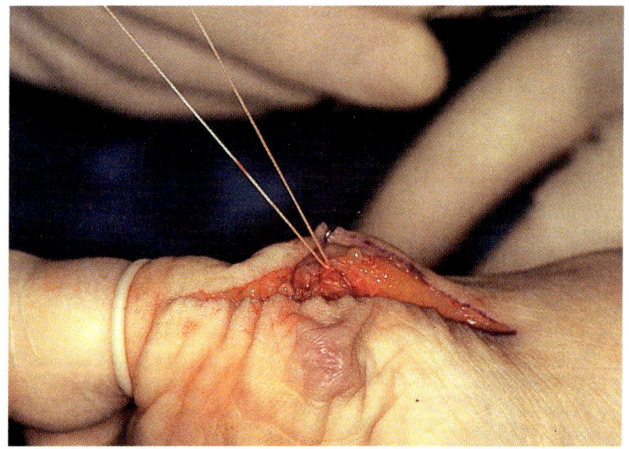

Figure 15. The medial joint capsule is closed tightly with interrupted, inverted 2-0 Ethibond sutures.

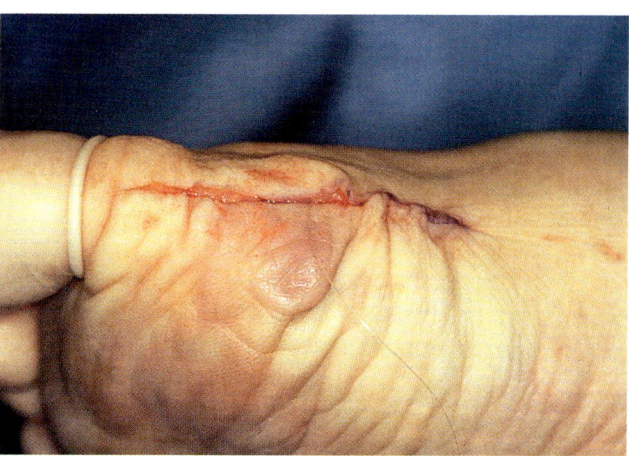

Figure 16. A running absorbable subcuticular suture is used for skin.

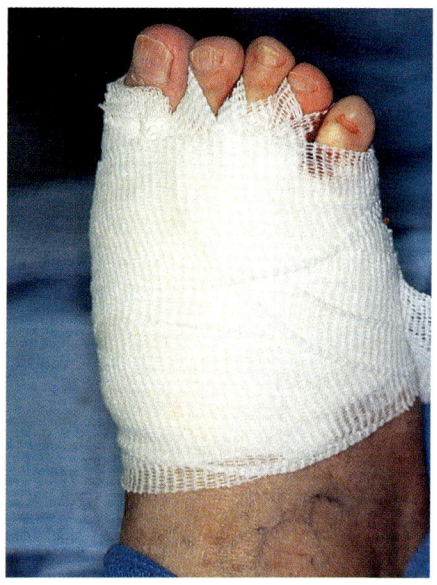

Figure 17. The dressing gently holds the webbed toes together in slight plantar flexion.

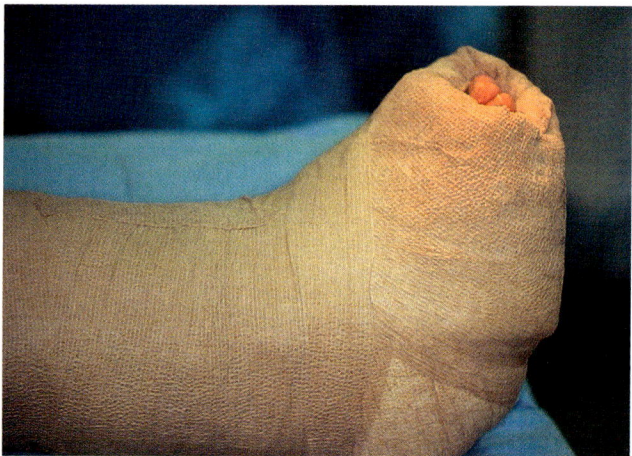

Figure 18. A large Jones compression dressing reduces postoperative swelling and protects the arthrodesis.

The capsule of the first MP joint is closed with 2-0 braided, nonabsorbable inverted sutures (Fig. 15), and skin is closed with a running 4-0 PDS-II suture (Fig. 16). A nonadherent dressing with a single 4″ × 4″ gauze is placed over each wound and the forefoot is carefully wrapped with a 2-inch Kling (Fig. 17). The postoperative dressing determines the final alignment of the lesser toes. After anchoring the Kling with several wraps around the midfoot, it is passed around pairs of syndactylized toes to hold them in slight plantar-flexion. Part of the dressing is placed into the second and fourth web spaces to wick moisture. The entire foot is then protected in a compressive Robert Jones dressing (Fig. 18). At the time of tourniquet release a few toes may show delayed arterial refill. If this persists for several minutes, the bandages should be teased out from between the toes to release any direct compression.

POSTOPERATIVE MANAGEMENT

The patient is placed in a hospital bed with the foot elevated. Intravenous antibiotic coverage is continued for 24 hours. Dressings are removed after 48 hours at which time the wounds are inspected, a new dressing is placed and a short leg cast with a walking heel is applied. Patients are restricted from weight bearing in the cast but are allowed to rest the heel on the ground when seated.

Four weeks later, the cast is removed and radiographs are taken. Usually, there has been sufficient consolidation of the arthrodesis site to permit ambulation in a hard postop shoe. Again, the syndactylized toes are meticulously rewrapped for 4 more weeks. Radiographs are repeated at 8 weeks postoperatively. At this point, the dressings are removed. Most patients have achieved an adequate MP fusion to allow them to begin wearing lose sneakers or extradepth shoes.

Rheumatoid reconstructive surgery changes the forefoot anatomy considerably. It can take several months before the postoperative swelling resolves. Patients often have some initial difficulties with balance. First metatarsophalangeal arthrodesis limits heel height and shoe selection. Patients often require new orthotics or shoes after surgery. Formal rehabilitation is generally not necessary.

In terms of pain relief, the results of surgery average 90% satisfactory at 2 years and 80% satisfactory at 5 years (2,4,10). Wound problems occur in approximately 10% of patients (3,6). Shoe-wear needs rarely change (2,6); thus the desire to wear more fashionable shoes is not a reasonable expectation or an indication for surgery. Gait unsteadiness can be exacerbated by procedures that shorten the functional length of the foot (4,9).

COMPLICATIONS

Reconstructive surgery of the rheumatoid forefoot is palliative, not curative. Although there may be periods of relative inactivity, rheumatoid disease never truly goes away. Continued functional deterioration is expected.

The natural history of the disease needs to be considered when evaluating the results of surgery. Not all bad results are complications of surgery. Those complications directly related to surgery are the following:

1. *Incisional problems.* Both superficial and deep wound infections occur at a much higher rate than for most other forefoot surgeries. The key factors to minimizing the risks of developing wound problems are (a) proper patient selection, (b) meticulous handling of tissues (so-called hand surgery of the feet), (c) the use of longitudinal dorsal incisions, and (d) elevating the foot in a compressive postop dressing. Deep infections are treated with surgical debridement and intravenous antibiotics. Wound dehiscences are treated with b.i.d. soaks in lukewarm tap water, wet-to-dry dressing changes, and oral antibiotics (usually first generation cephalosporins). Healing of syndactylization dehiscences by secondary intention typically takes 6 to 8 weeks.
2. *Neurovascular problems.* Permanent hypoesthesia or vascular compromise can occur from inadvertent transection of a neurovascular bundle. There are two critical moments in the operation when this damage can occur. First, it can occur during the approach to the proximal phalangeal shaft. Neurovascular damage can be averted at this juncture by keeping the incision dorsal to the midline. Second, it can occur during bony transection. This risk can be reduced by shielding all soft tissues from the oscillating saw blade.

   After tourniquet reversal it is not uncommon for the lesser toes to take a few minutes to regain full circulation. Toes with continued impaired vascular status should have all restrictive wrappings released or removed. Venous engorgement is treated with elevation. Persistent and complete loss of arterial inflow is an indication for immediate operative exploration and arterial repair. Marginal arterial inflow causing mild cyanosis and decreased turgor usually responds to strict bed rest with the foot maintained at, or slightly below, the level of the heart. A transcutaneous oxygen monitor can help with early surveillance of vascularly compromised toes.

3. *Callus formation.* It is not uncommon for patients to develop plantar calluses or palpable bursae several years after surgery. The early return of these painful prominences, though, is typically caused by technical mistakes. The most common errors involve irregular bony resection. Sharp plantar spikes left under the metatarsals and an uneven cascade of metatarsal shaft lengths are the two major causes of recurrent callus formation. The offending bony prominences sometimes need to be surgically excised.

4. *Gait instability.* Resection of the metatarsal heads functionally shortens the foot. Some patients report difficulties with gait due to unreliable push-off. When extensive excision of bone is necessary to relax soft tissues it is, therefore, better to remove more of the proximal phalanges than the metatarsals. For patients with established instability, it is helpful to use a shoe with a full-length steel spring insert and slight roller sole.

5. *First metatarsophalangeal nonunion.* Fortunately, first MP nonunion occurs infrequently in rheumatoid patients. Factors responsible for nonunion are (a) insufficient bone stock, (b) incomplete bone apposition, (c) inadequate fixation, and (d) too short a period of protected immobilization. If poor bone stock is encountered intraoperatively, I perform a resection arthroplasty involving removal of the medial eminence and distal metatarsal head (modified Mayo procedure). Bony apposition should be evaluated at the time of surgery. Not uncommonly, a lip of cortical bone from the metatarsal is found to block full contact between the cup and cone. The stability of the arthrodesis construct should always be assessed intraoperatively. The options for improving stability depend on the quality of bone. With hard bone, the screw can be either replaced with a slightly longer one or repositioned after reshaping the cup and cone. With moderately hard bone, the construct can be strengthened by placing an additional screw from the medial metatarsal neck to the lateral phalangeal base. For soft bone, it is often best to use supplementary 0.035 K-wires. These can be left in permanently or removed after bony consolidation. Radiographs should reveal trabecular bridging prior to resumption of unprotected weight bearing.

Established MP nonunions are usually painless and need no treatment. A painful nonunion can sometimes be converted to a painless one by removing the hardware. Continued symptoms may necessitate an attempt at refusion. If, as a result of the initial procedure, first ray length has been shortened considerably, a corticocancellous interpositional graft may be necessary to restore function. Unfortunately, consolidation of these grafts can be slow and unpredictable. Non–weight-bearing immobilization averaging 3 months is required. This is extremely difficult for RA patients with polyarticular involvement. Those patients may be better served by conversion of the first MP nonunion into a resection arthroplasty.

ILLUSTRATIVE CASE FOR TECHNIQUE

A 58-year-old woman with a 17-year history of RA presented with persistent central metatarsalgia. Her initial treatment included fabrication of a heat moldable extradepth shoe with a soft, metatarsal head unloading insert. Eighteen months later she returned with increasing symptoms. The insert was remade, but her pain persisted. A metatarsal bar was then added to the sole of the shoe with temporary, mild improvement. Three months later the severe central metatarsal discomfort returned. She said she felt like she was "standing on marbles." Simple tasks such as walking to the mailbox or shopping at a grocery store were reported as being excruciatingly painful.

Examination revealed normal skin turgor, toe vascularity, and sensation. Static examination showed the hallux IP joint without subluxation or dislocation and the MP joint fixed in severe valgus (Fig. 19A). The lesser toes were all medially deviated and dorsally subluxated at the MP joint. The second and third toes were hammered at the PIP joints. The metatarsal fat pad seemed atrophic with the central metatarsal heads protected from plantar ulceration only by a thin veil of subcutaneous tissue. Dynamic examination revealed that hallux IP motion was full and painless, hallux MP motion was limited to 5° of dorsi-plantar flexion, lesser MP motion was similarly restricted, and the hammering of the second and third PIP joints was passively correctable. The patient's gait was slow with decreased stride length, prolonged double-limb support phase, and loss of normal

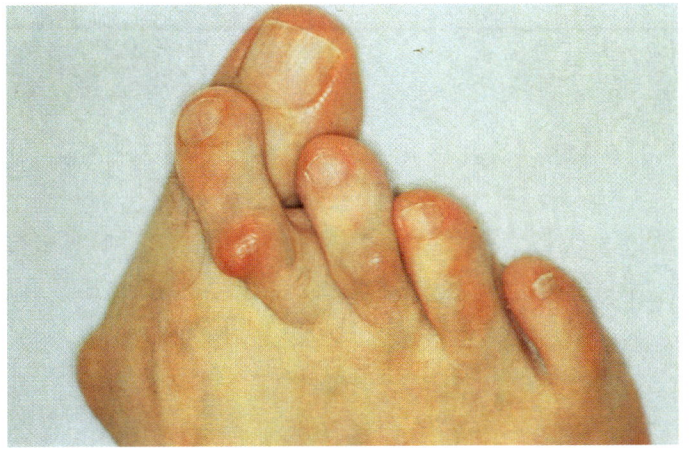

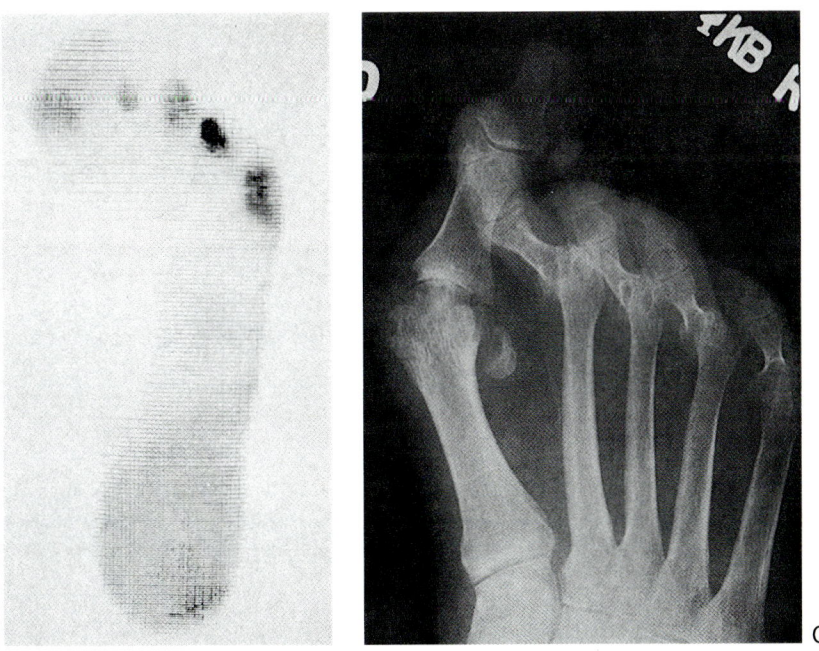

Figure 19. A: Preoperative photograph. **B:** Harris mat imprint. Note the lack of toe loading on the pressure image. **C:** Preoperative standing AP radiograph.

toe-off. The foot was placed flat on the floor and appeared to be used more as a pedestal than a lever (Fig. 19B).

The anteroposterior weight-bearing radiographs demonstrated several key findings (Fig. 19C). The hallux had minimal periarticular osteoporosis around the first MP joint. Juxtaaarticular erosions of the metatarsal head fortunately involved regions that would be excised with arthrodesis surgery. The medial cortex of the proximal phalanx had one small erosion at the insertion of the abductor hallucis tendon, but otherwise appeared intact. The IP joint of the hallux was well located without joint space narrowing but did have medial juxtaarticular erosions. All the lesser MP joints were dislocated and the lesser PIP joints appeared normal. Prominent penciling of the fifth metatarsal head was noted.

A forefoot reconstructive procedure was performed involving hallux metatarsophalangeal arthrodesis, lesser metatarsal head resections, partial proximal phalangectomies, and subtotal webbings. The patient was maintained non–weight bearing in a short leg cast for 4 weeks, followed by 4 more weeks in a hard-sole postoperative shoe.

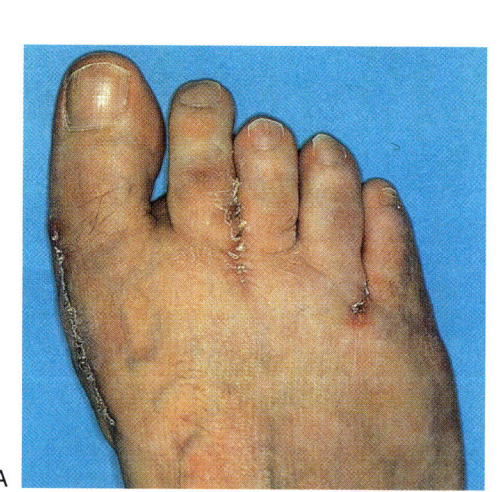
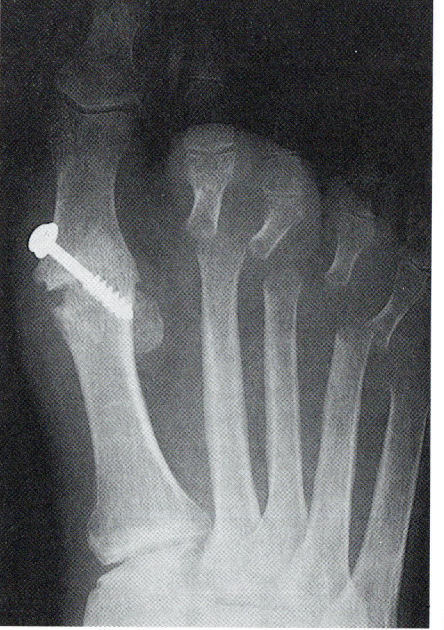
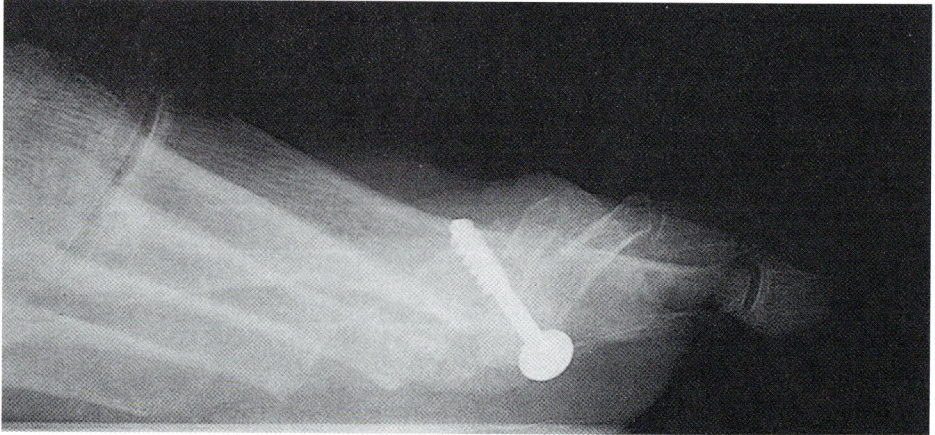

Figure 20. A: Appearance of the foot. **B** and **C:** Standing radiographs taken 8 weeks after surgery.

Standing clinical photograph taken at 8 weeks shows improved forefoot alignment (Fig. 20A). Although there was some crusting around the sutures at the time of final dressing removal, the overall appearance of the partially syndactylized toes was considered acceptable. Moreover, since all the toes had been shortened, their relative lengths seemed normal. The hallux was situated next to, but not contacting, the second toe.

Standing radiographs illustrate several operative points (Fig. 20B,C). On the anteroposterior view you can see that a washer has been used to supplement fixation of tenuous medial cortical bone. The amount of proximal phalangeal resection can be appreciated by comparing the pre- and postoperative radiographs. More bone was removed from the hammered medial toes than the less involved lateral ones. Preservation of the normal cascade of metatarsal lengths can also be seen. The lateral radiograph shows the hallux to be aligned with the sole of the foot. Additionally, the beveled angle of metatarsal head resections can be observed.

RECOMMENDED READING

1. Clayton, M. L.: Surgery of the forefoot in rheumatoid arthritis. *Clin. Orthop.*, 16: 136–140, 1960.
2. Craxford, A. D., Stevens, J., and Park, C.: Management of the deformed rheumatoid forefoot: a comparison of conservative and surgical methods. *Clin. Orthop.*, 166: 121–126, 1982.
3. Faithful, D. K., and Savill, D. L.: Review of the results of excision of metatarsal heads in patients with rheumatoid arthritis. *Ann. Rheum. Dis.*, 30: 201–202, 1971.
4. Hasselo, L. G., Wilkens, R. F., Toomey, H. E., Karges, D. E., and Hansen, S. T.: Forefoot surgery in rheumatoid arthritis: subjective assessment of outcome. *Foot Ankle*, 8: 148–151, 1987.
5. Mann R. A., and Thompson, F. M.: Arthrodesis of the first metatarsophalangeal joint for hallux valgus in rheumatoid arthritis. *J. Bone Joint Surg.*, 66A: 687–692, 1984.
6. McGarvey, S. R., and Johnson, K. A.: Keller arthroplasty in combination with resection arthroplasty of the lesser metatarsophalangeal joints in rheumatoid arthritis. *Foot Ankle*, 9: 75–80, 1988.
7. McKeever, D. C.: Arthrodesis of the first metatarsophalangeal joint for hallux valgus, hallux rigidus, and metatarsus primus varus. *J. Bone Joint Surg.*, 34A: 129–134, 1952.
8. Moynihan, F. J.: Arthrodesis of the metatarso-phalangeal joint of the great toe. *J. Bone Joint Surg.*, 49-B: 544–551, 1967.
9. Newman, R. J., and Fitton, J. M.: Conservation of metatarsal head in surgery of rheumatoid arthritis of the forefoot. *Acta Orthop. Scand.*, 54: 417–421, 1983.
10. Saltzman, C. L., Johnson, K. A., and Donnelly, R. E.: Surgical treatment for mild deformities of the rheumatoid forefoot by partial phalangectomy and syndactylization. *Foot Ankle, 1993 (in press)*.

17

Transmetatarsal Amputation

James W. Brodsky

INDICATIONS/CONTRAINDICATIONS

The primary indication for a transmetatarsal amputation is the presence of nonviable toes with or without loss of viability of the most distal forefoot. In practice, this usually translates into the clinical diagnosis of gangrene. Distal forefoot means involving the tissue no more proximal than the distal one-half of the metatarsals. The causes of the gangrene can be multiple or variable, including, but certainly not limited to, diabetes, arteriosclerotic peripheral vascular disease, nondiabetic peripheral neuropathy, severe trauma, or embolic phenomena caused by sepsis or other causes.

The most common indications for transmetatarsal amputation in decreasing order of frequency are diabetic foot problems, vascular insufficiency in the absence of diabetes, and trauma. Because many of these procedures are done for the reason of tissue death due to poor circulation, a special set of circumstances are presented with regard to the applicability of the operation. Patients who need the amputation because of trauma, such as a boating accident, or because of embolism frequently do not have the problems with healing that the former group demonstrates.

The transmetatarsal amputation is the partial foot amputation that is most easily accommodated in shoe-wear, requiring the least amount of special insoles and special shoe-wear. It has the limitation of being applicable only for cases with the most distal kind of dry or wet gangrene, or trauma. Many patients with infection or local tissue death have involvement far too extensive to be treated with this procedure. Choosing this procedure inappropriately only condemns the patient to additional, possibly unnecessary operations. The choice of a transmetatarsal

---

J. W. Brodsky, M.D.: Department of Orthopaedic Surgery, University of Texas Southwestern Medical School, Dallas, TX; Department of Orthopaedic Surgery, Baylor University Medical Center, Dallas, TX 75246; and *private practice*, Orthopaedic Associates of Dallas, 411 N. Washington #7000, Dallas, TX 75246.

amputation should be made based upon the presence of margins of bleeding and viable tissue at the time of closure.

Transmetatarsal amputation is not indicated for the nonambulatory patient when the level of healing is doubtful. For a patient who will not weight bear because of paralysis, dementia, or severe debility, a more proximal amputation is indicated if the diminished circulation makes the prospect of healing questionable. In other words, one of the principal indications for the transmetatarsal amputation is to preserve the length of the foot so that the patient has maximum function and can wear an easily modified shoe rather than a prosthesis.

Once the amputation is done through the tarsometatarsal joints themselves, rather than being a transmetatarsal amputation, the nature of the amputation and the function of the residual foot are significantly altered. The loss of the attachments, and thus the functions of the peroneus brevis and longus, and the anterior tibialis tendons creates a weaker foot with a notable muscle imbalance. The triceps surae, through the attachment of the Achilles tendon, will produce an equinus deformity of the ankle. If a transmetatarsal amputation is extended proximally, and thus converted to a Lisfranc amputation, or tarsometatarsal disarticulation, the surgeon should try to transfer the insertions of the midfoot tendons proximally to the residual skeletal structure. In addition, or even alternatively, it is usually necessary to do an Achilles tendon lengthening at the same time.

Transmetatarsal amputation is a good procedure to salvage other, more distal procedures that have failed. Examples include failed toe amputations that have not healed because of inadequate circulation or persistent infections, and recurrent soft tissue breakdown, ulceration, or severe metatarsalgia after resection of two or more rays (metatarsal plus corresponding toe).

This operation is also indicated as a salvage procedure in diabetic or other patients with insensitive feet, who have recurrent neuropathic ulcerations, even in the absence of the other factors of infection, gangrene, or vascular insufficiency discussed above. These patients also might be candidates for a modified Hoffmann procedure to remove all of the lesser (and possibly the first, also) metatarsal heads. This might be a patient who had two or three metatarsal heads resected for recalcitrant ulceration or localized infection, now resolved, who is experiencing yet another ulceration due to the concentration of pressure on the remaining metatarsals. While a modified Hoffmann procedure has the advantage of saving the toes, these toes are "floppy" and can be subjected to other recurrent infection and pressure in the shoe, especially if they are elevated by contraction of dorsal scars. A transmetatarsal amputation, especially if it is a proximal one, may have more difficulty in holding on a shoe, but obviates the risk of further recurrent toe lesions.

Age is not an important factor in patient selection for the procedure, provided that the general criteria of adequate perfusion and preexisting ambulatory function are met. Patients with an equinus contracture should not have a transmetatarsal amputation because of the excessive pressure applied to the end of the stump by the plantar flexed ankle, unless a concomitant Achilles lengthening is done. If the equinus is of recent onset, and still relatively flexible (i.e., not a true fixed contracture yet) then the procedure can be followed by stretching in placement of the limb in serial holding casts or by the use of a dorsiflexion ankle foot orthosis. In contrast, the severe equinus contracture may require release of the posterior ankle and subtalar joint capsules as well. At some point, the surgeon should decide if it is worth doing extensive soft tissue releases in order to provide a plantigrade foot with a transmetatarsal amputation, especially if the release requires flexor tendon lengthenings also. At this point, it is usually better to do a more proximal amputation.

Another contraindication for a transmetatarsal amputation is extensive gangrene or infection of the plantar skin, i.e., more proximal plantar than dorsal soft tissue loss, because of the loss of the plantar flap, which is most often used to cover the end of the resected bones. It is relatively contraindicated in patients who have little or no function of the anterior compartment and lateral compartment muscles to oppose the pull of the triceps surae. In these patients, it is necessary to do lengthening of the Achilles tendon, and the permanent use of a polypropylene ankle foot orthosis will probably be required. Even with these caveats, this procedure is still preferable to a proximal amputation, which requires the use of a prosthesis. It is relatively contraindicated in patients who have instability or deformity at Lisfranc's joint, especially diabetics with peripheral neuropathy who have had a Charcot midfoot joint.

PREOPERATIVE PLANNING

In diabetic and in nondiabetic dysvascular patients, it is essential (as in all amputation surgery) to evaluate the preoperative vascular status of the limb. Screening is most easily, and most widely done using the Doppler ultrasound. However, this is only a screening test, and when definitive evaluation is required in cases with marginal vascularity, a vascular surgery consult is usually sought, and other testing is performed, including arteriography. More recent studies have pointed to the efficacy of transcutaneous oxygen (Tco_2) testing for evaluation of viable level of amputation. Tco_2 is widely available technology (it is the form of oxygen monitoring used in newborn nurseries and neonatal ICUs). Experience in its application to dysvascular and diabetic limbs is not nearly so widespread. It is temperature dependent, somewhat cumbersome, and slow. To perform it efficiently requires multiple monitors applied simultaneously.

Radiographs are important in the preoperative routine planning to rule out the extension of osteomyelitis to a level that might preclude the use of this amputation.

It is important to examine the patient for a preoperative equinus contracture. Frequently this is a subtle finding, and the testing needs to be done with the knee in both flexion and extension. Suspect a tight Achilles tendon in patients who have been non–weight bearing for long periods, because the absence of walking and standing easily leads to a tight Achilles tendon. In severe cases of equinus, it may be best not to perform this operation. However, even in moderate degrees of equinus, the transmetatarsal amputation may still be tenable; in these in-between cases, the deciding factor may be the presence of forefoot equinus, which is in addition to and separate from the ankle equinus. Forefoot equinus is caused by plantar flexion contracture at Chopart's joint, i.e., the calcaneocuboid and talonavicular joints. This is frequently overlooked.

SURGERY

Although the transmetatarsal amputation is not commonly performed, it is not technically difficult, either. However, like all operative procedures, proper attention to detail will enhance the quality of the result. Gentle handling of the soft tissues, especially in diabetic and dysvascular patients, is to be kept in mind. Practically, this translates into gentle retraction, and minimal handling of the skin edges with the forceps.

There exists the possibility of transmetatarsal amputations of different length. In general, it is preferable to produce the longest possible stump that is very likely to heal with primary closure of the soft tissue. It is not worthwhile to try to squeeze out a slightly longer stump if the skin and soft tissue will be closed under tension or if the edges are not viable.

Techniques. It is helpful to designate the flaps with a skin marker, measuring out the long plantar flap to correspond to the length of the residual metatarsals. These are basically "fish-mouth" flaps, as illustrated in Fig. 1. While these can be of varied length, the relative proportion is roughly the same. The plantar flap

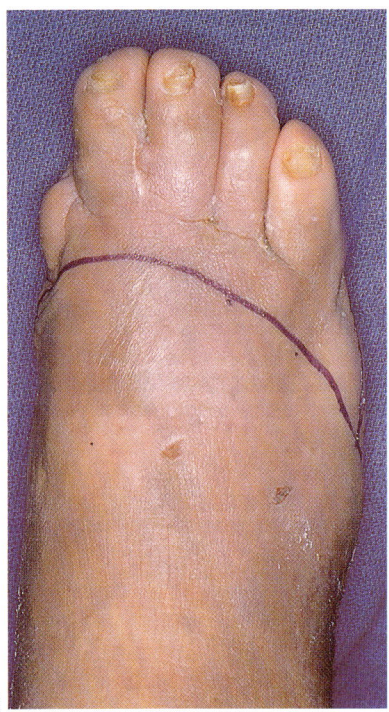
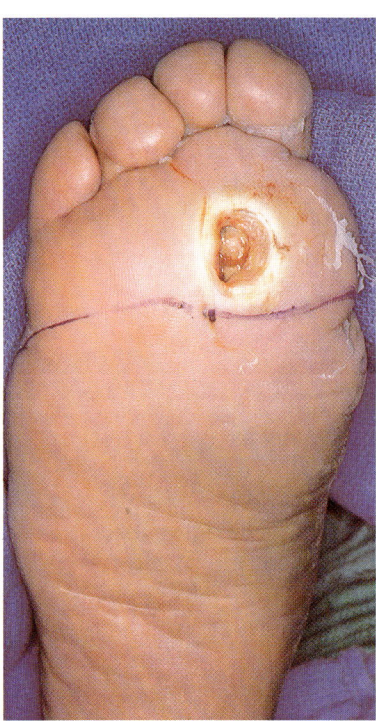
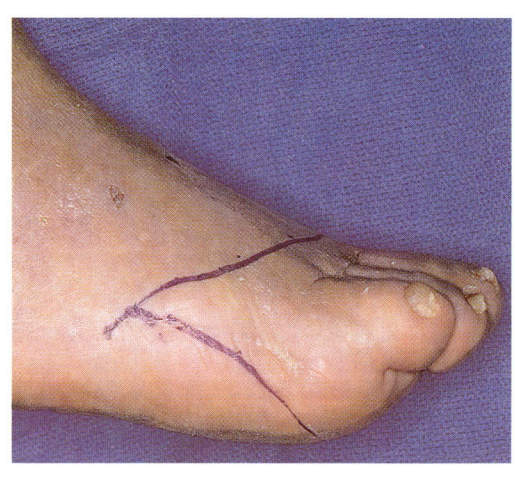

Figure 1. A–C: The skin is marked for the flaps for amputation. Note that the plantar flap is longer whenever possible, and that these have a "fish-mouth" junction on the medial and lateral sides. Note also that the flaps, especially the dorsal flap, are somewhat shorter on the lateral side, corresponding to the pattern of bone resection.

is generally longer, so that it can wrap up around the end of the stump. It is desirable that the posterior flap be long enough to bring the suture line onto the dorsum of the distal stump.

It is also helpful to angle the flaps slightly from medial-distal to lateral-proximal, so that the lateral side of the soft tissue flaps is slightly shorter, corresponding to the pattern of bone resection described below.

Full-thickness flaps are developed cutting from skin down to the bone (Fig. 2). The dorsal flap is fashioned first. Using a large blunt elevator, the soft tissue is elevated in a proximal direction beneath the flap, as shown in Fig. 3. The interosseous muscles are not yet divided because they lay between the metatarsals and below the level of the dorsal cortex. At this point, the dorsalis pedis artery is ligated as needed.

The plantar flap is fashioned next. In a long transmetatarsal amputation, the flap will begin right at the base of the toes on the sole. The incision is carried down to the bone, and soft tissue dissection is done with the elevator right on the plantar cortex of the metatarsal shafts, in order to create a full-thickness flap, as shown in Fig. 4. Hemostasis is usually achieved with electrocautery at this level.

The exposed long flexor and long extensor tendons are now drawn down distally using a sturdy clamp such as a Kocher, and divided so that they retract proximally (Fig. 5). Attention should be paid to the quality of the tendons, to confirm the absence of gross purulence within the tendon sheath. If there is infection that tracks up the extensor or flexor tendon sheath, two changes may need to be made. First, dissection should be extended proximally along the course of the tendon to debride the infected tissue as far up the leg as necessary to aggressively drain the infection. Second, it may be necessary to leave the amputation open and to do local wound care until the wound is clean and granulating, and then return the patient to the operating suite for a delayed primary closure at a later date.

The metatarsals are now divided with a small oscillating saw (Fig. 6). Osteotomes are usually not used because of the splintering that they cause. The dorsal soft tissue flap is held back with rakes or blunt retractors and protected while the bone is cut. The metatarsals are cut from medial to lateral. The angle at which

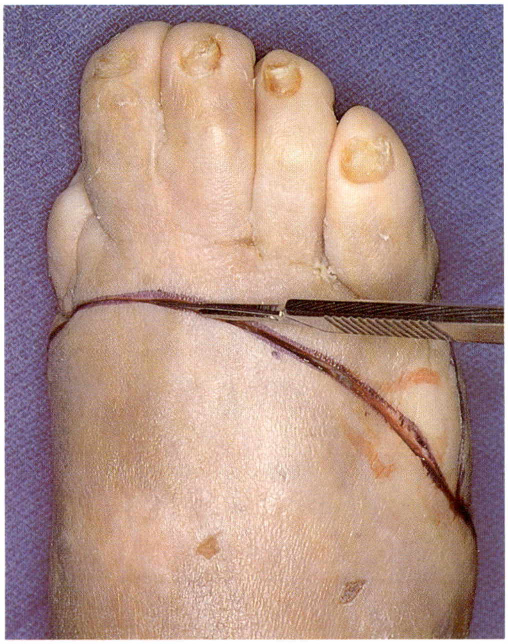

17 TRANSMETATARSAL AMPUTATION

Figure 2. The dorsal flap is developed by cutting down to the bone.

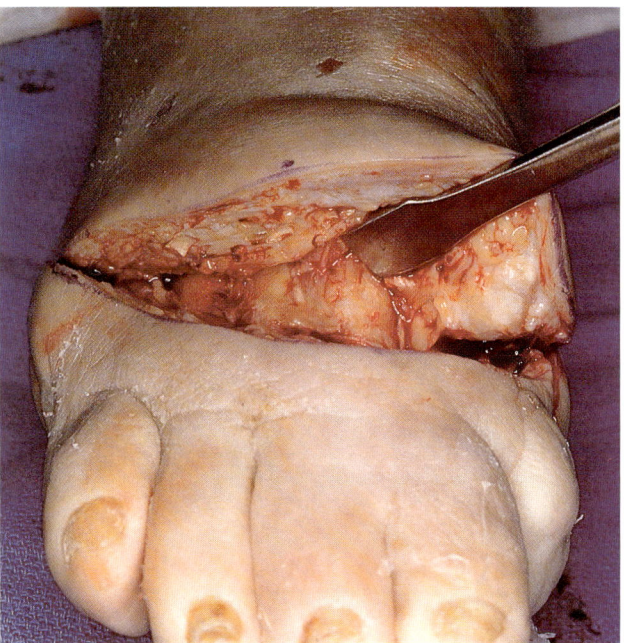

Figure 3. A full-thickness flap is developed with a broad elevator, taking care not to separate the skin and subcutaneous tissue from the deepest layer of the flap.

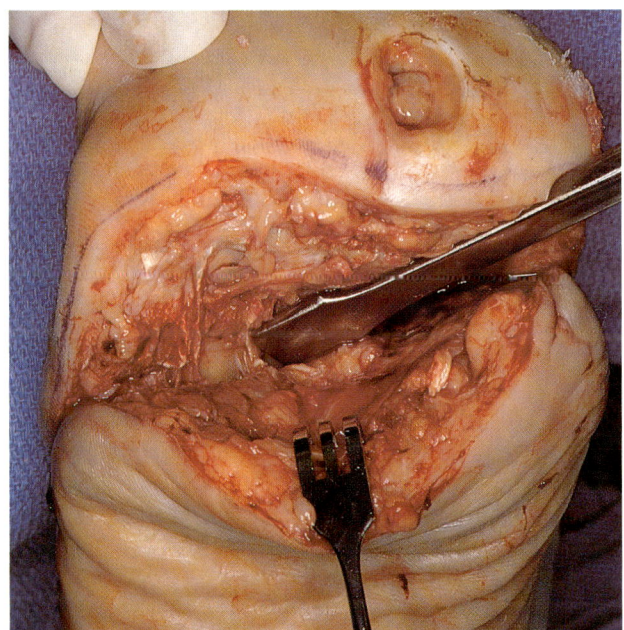

Figure 4. The plantar flap is developed by a similar incision down to the bone, then dissected as a single flap. Note the greater thickness of the plantar flap compared to the dorsal flap, which usually requires thinning of the flap (see Fig. 9).

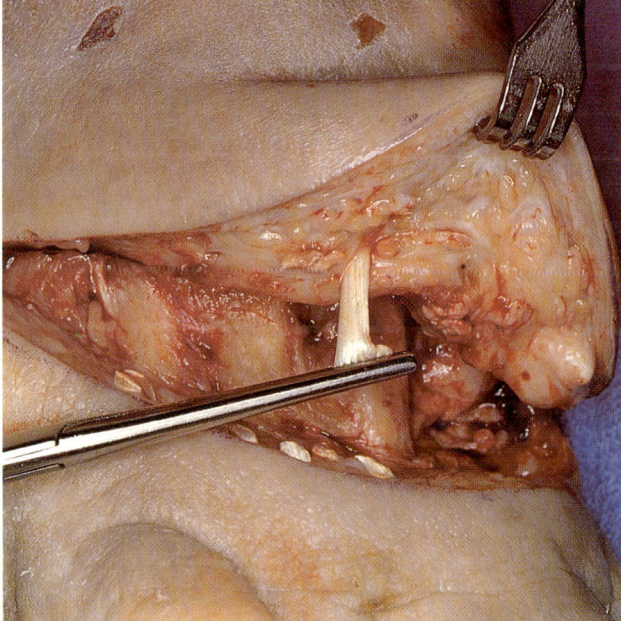

Figure 5. The flexor and extensor tendons are drawn down with a clamp and divided allowing them to retract; the extensor tendons are pictured here.

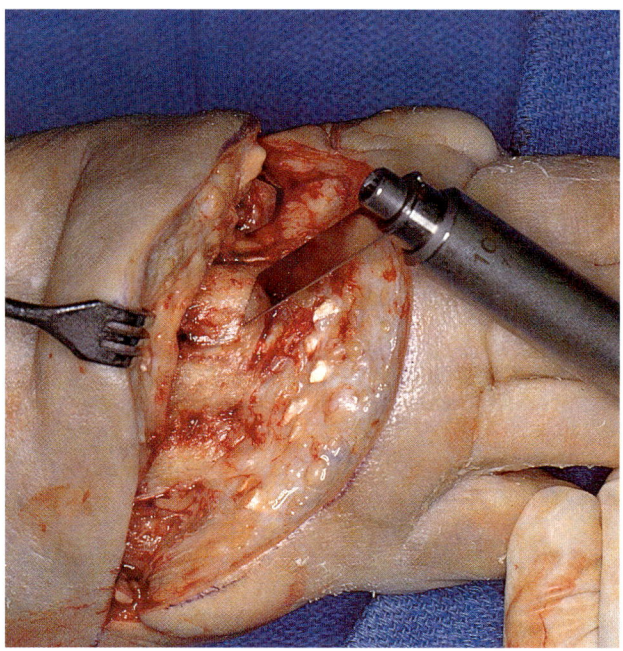

Figure 6. The metatarsals are now divided using a small oscillating saw. Note that the saw blade is angled in two planes.

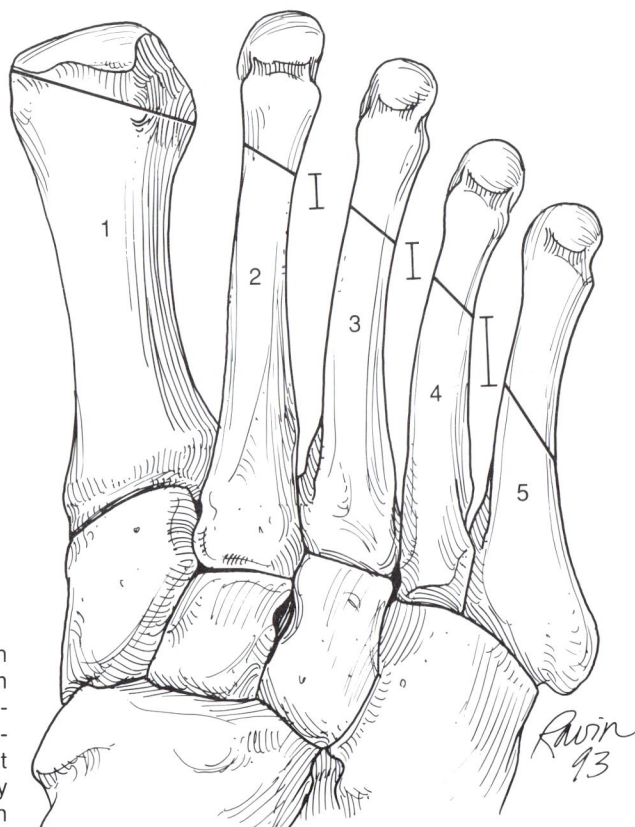

Figure 7. The "cascade" of length as each metatarsal is cut 2 to 3 mm more proximally than the one medial to it. Note that the fifth metatarsal needs a greater increment of shortening, and should usually be at least 4 to 5 mm shorter than the fourth.

the bones are cut and the length of each residual metatarsal are both important. As the surgeon progresses from medial to lateral, each metatarsal is cut in a "cascade" of length, i.e., the metatarsals are progressively shorter as the resections advance laterally. Each metatarsal should be cut 2 to 3 mm shorter than the metatarsal just medial to it, with the exception of the fifth metatarsal, which should be cut at least 4 to 5 mm shorter than the fourth, if not more (Fig. 7). The reason for this is the propensity to develop pressure-related problems under the end of the fifth metatarsal. In a patient with normal sensation, this would be a painful plantar keratosis. In a patient with peripheral neuropathy, such as a diabetic with an insensate foot, a neuropathic ulcer could develop.

In addition to the cascade of length, the angle of the saw blade when the metatarsal is cut is also important (Fig. 8). The blade should be angled from dorsal-distal to plantar-proximal in order to bevel the undersurface of the cut end of the metatarsal. This reduces the pressure under this sensitive spot. The saw blade should simultaneously be angled laterally, i.e., creating a line from distal-medial to proximal-lateral on the metatarsal. This reduces pressure on the end of the metatarsal at the toe-off phase of gait.

A small straight osteotome, which is held against the cut edge of the metatarsal, serves as a simple and practical guide for marking each successive metatarsal to be cut, and improves the accuracy of the cuts. If the edges are rough, do not hesitate to smooth them with a small rasp.

Once the metatarsals have been cut, the dorsal and plantar flaps must be evaluated for the closure. As in all amputations, it is essential to balance the length of residual bone to be covered with the length of viable soft tissue available to close over it. If shorter flaps of viable tissue are available, then the bone must be divided more proximally. It is essential to make every attempt to achieve a primary closure

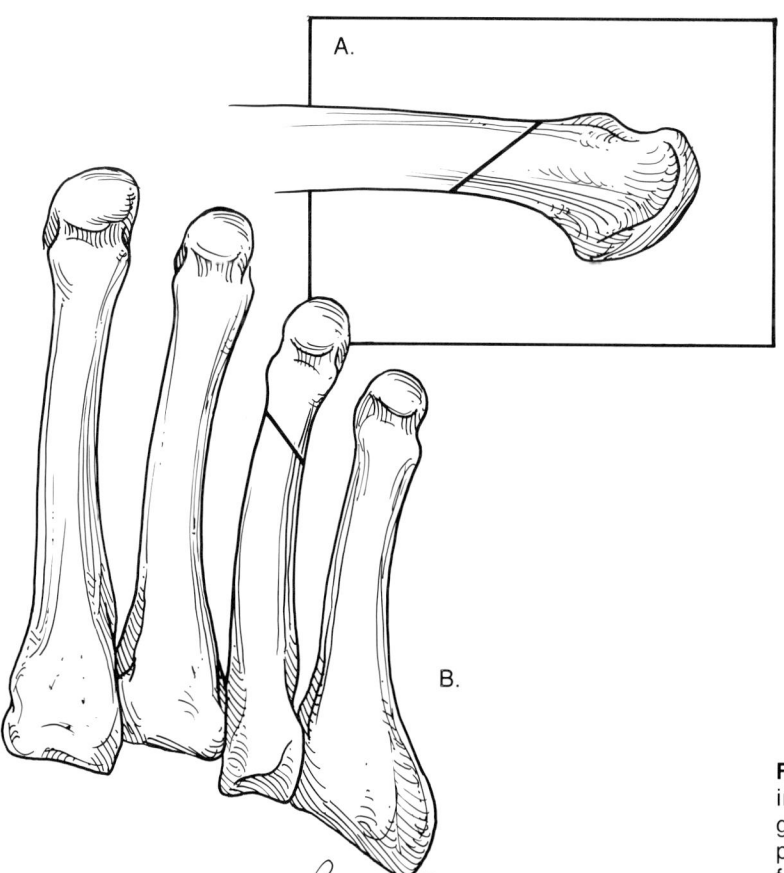

Figure 8. A and **B:** The two planes in which each metatarsal cut is angled: first, from dorsal-distal to plantar-proximal; second, mildly from distal-medial to proximal-lateral.

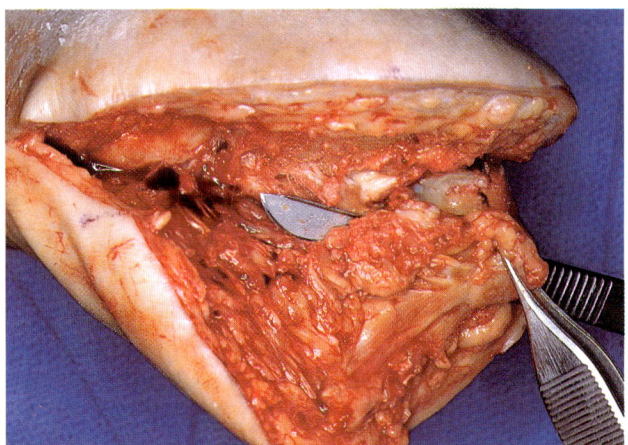

Figure 9. The plantar flap is trimmed to thin the flap. The flap is gently sloped toward the skin edge, taking care not to remove so much tissue distally as to devascularize the skin edge. The flap is smoothed uniformly so that tags and bits of tissue are not left behind.

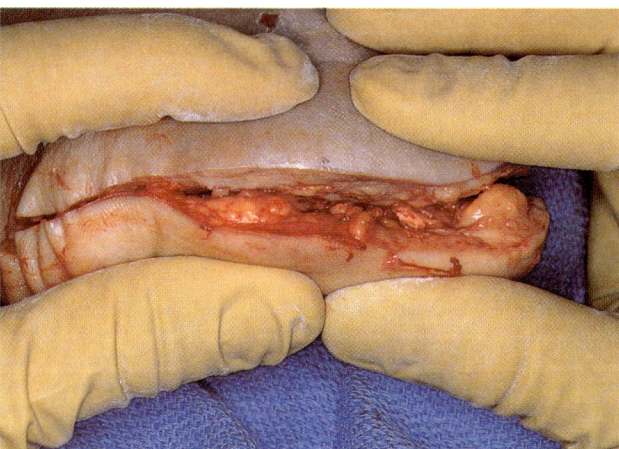

Figure 10. The flaps are gently held together to estimate the ease of closure. The flaps may not readily approximate (see text for three possible reasons). The flaps are too short relative to the length of the residual bones in order to cover, the flaps are improperly shaped, or the plantar flap is too thick and needs to be trimmed further.

without tension on the skin. Not only is it important to balance the amount of soft tissue with the amount of bone, but the shape and thickness of the flaps must be adjusted as well.

The plantar flap almost always needs to be trimmed to facilitate the closure. This should be a gradual, uniform reduction in the thickness of the flap from proximal to distal. Cut the tissue with a #10 blade, making smooth, even strokes in order not to leave tags and projecting bits of tissue. The purpose is to create an even surface and consistent thickness of the flap, while avoiding leaving behind bits of tissue that will necrose (Fig. 9).

Start the closure by holding the dorsal and plantar flaps gently together in order to estimate the necessary trimming for the proper closure (Fig. 10). The flaps may not approximate easily, for three possible reasons: (a) there is inadequate soft tissue to cover the bone, in which case all of the metatarsals need to be trimmed further proximally; (b) the flaps are shaped improperly, e.g., not longer medially than laterally, to match the shape of the underlying bone, in which case further trimming of the bone is required; (c) the plantar flap is too thick and is holding the edges of the skin apart, in which case the plantar flap needs to be trimmed further. This trimming is done by additional "planing" of the intrinsic muscles in the flap, thinning the flap more near the distal edge. Caution must be exercised not to trim the tissue excessively, thereby devascularizing the skin edge inadvertently (Fig. 9).

Once the flaps have been adequately shaped and trimmed and fit easily together while being held with gentle finger pressure, several minor steps are needed before suturing begins. In cases in which the amputation is being performed for infection, a final culture and sensitivity swab or sample should be taken from the wound just prior to closure. This more accurately reflects the risk of infection in the residual limb than a culture of the obviously infected and more distal part.

If a tourniquet has been used, it should be released at about this point in order to check the wound for hemostasis and to evaluate the perfusion of the skin and soft tissue edges. If good bleeding is present, hemostasis is achieved with the electrocautery; sutures can be used for the dorsalis pedis artery and accompanying veins. If there is poor bleeding or no bleeding from the skin edges at this point in the procedure, despite a 5- to 10-minute waiting period, the surgeon has the option to consider proceeding with a more proximal amputation. After release of the tourniquet it takes a minimum of 3 to 5 minutes for the bleeding to reach the edges of the wound.

If a drain is used, it is placed at this point in the operation. In grossly infected wounds, e.g., a distal forefoot abscess in a diabetic, the surgeon may elect to place an irrigation system instead of a suction drain in the wound. The irrigant usually does not require antibiotic. A liter of normal saline or Ringer's lactate solution is used to drip slowly through the wound. This is done by connecting a sterile intravenous extension tubing to a #8 pediatric feeding tube that is placed in the wound through a separate small stab incision proximal to the amputation site (Fig. 11). The solution is run into the wound at a rate of about 40 to 50 cc an hour. The fluid is allowed to exit the wound through the incision and between the loosely placed sutures. When this type of irrigation is used, I customarily do not use deep absorbable sutures, but rather use large mattress sutures of 2-0 monofilament. These mattress sutures are placed full thickness through the flap on the "far" side of the stitch, and then very close to the skin edge on the "near" part of the stitch. These sutures are generally left in place for at least 1 month, and I do not hesitate to leave them in for 6 or 8 weeks if there is a slowly healing area of the incision line. If an irrigation system is used, a very large bulky wrap is applied around the foot for a dressing. All occlusive-type material (petrolatum gauze, etc.) is avoided so as not to impede the efflux of the irrigant through the incision line. The bulky wrap usually consists of 4" × 4" gauze squares, multiple gauze rolls, combine (ABD) pads, and an elastic wrap.

If the wound is not an infected one, then a suction drain is preferable. This is also placed through a small separate stab incision. It is preferable not to use Penrose drains unless they also exit through separate stab incisions. If Penrose drains are brought through the incision itself and in between the sutures, it tends to create a tract that stays open and continues to drain.

Closure is done with a sparing number of 2–0 or 0 absorbable braided sutures placed through the deep fascia. Subcutaneous sutures are usually not used. Skin closure can be either with skin staples or with interrupted vertical mattress sutures of 3–0 or 4–0 monofilament. Regardless of which skin closure is utilized, great care is taken to evert the skin edges. If skin staples are used, the edges are everted with two skin hooks or very gently with a pair of Adson forceps. If sutures are used, the trick is to place the "near" half of the mattress suture very close to the edge of the skin. A dressing is applied beginning with a nonadherent material. I prefer the plastic portion of Telfa, otherwise called "split Telfa dressing," because

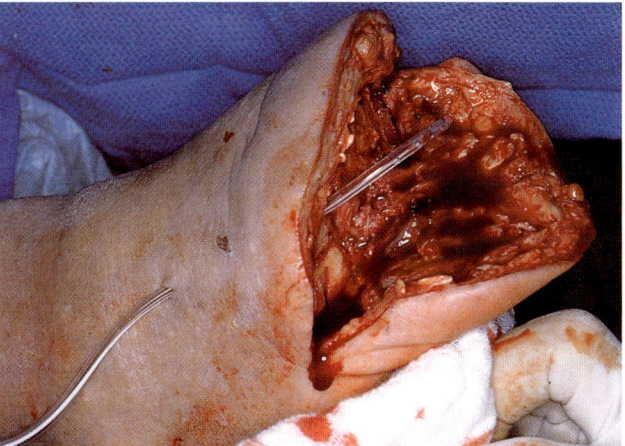

Figure 11. A suction drain is placed in the wound, right on the bone, and brought out through a separate tiny stab incision proximally, avoiding the area of the dorsalis pedis artery.

the material seldom sticks, and if it does, it simply tears and is not painful. It also has perforations to allow bleeding to pass through it. This is followed by gauze squares and gauze rolls, and finally with an elastic wrap, applied as a covering, but with almost no tension at all.

The most common pitfall is to resect too much skin. The surgeon should attempt to maximally conserve skin, cutting right up to the edge of necrotic skin in the case of gangrene. Once the flap has been elevated, the viability can be better discerned, and the flap shortened if necessary. Conservative sparing of the skin can produce the maximal length of the amputation stump.

The next most common pitfall is failing to cut the metatarsals in the cascade of length described above, or failing to cut the metatarsals with the appropriate beveling. This can lead to painful bursae and pressure points in the patients with sensate limbs, and to ulceration and infection in the patient with limb insensitivity.

Failure to maximally utilize the available skin and soft tissue for coverage forces the surgeon to cut the foot to a shorter length in order to produce more "standard" flaps. Very satisfactory results can be produced with irregular flaps provided that the edges approximate well and there is no tension on the suture line.

POSTOPERATIVE MANAGEMENT

After completion of the transmetatarsal amputation, the previously described soft compression dressing is applied. The foot is elevated postoperatively. It is best to elevate the foot in such a way that the heel hangs free in the air, and is elevated off the bed at all times. This is easily accomplished with folded blankets stacked on top of each other, or even taped together. The blankets provide a platform to support the calf and entire lower leg, and the foot hangs off the end. It is inexpensive, universally available, and preferable to pillows, which tend to shift around and require constant rearranging.

If an irrigation system is utilized, it is usually in place overnight and removed the following day. The irrigation tube is removed and a fresh, dry dressing is applied. Although skin appears waterlogged, it quickly dries out.

If a suction drain is utilized, then dressing changes in the early postoperative period are done as needed, depending upon the amount of drainage that appears on the bandage. If a concomitant Achilles tendon lengthening was done at surgery, then the patient is placed in an extremely well-padded cotton wrap, on top of the regular dressing, that extends from toes to knee, over which is then applied plaster splints to hold the foot in dorsiflexion. I prefer the combination of a posterior splint with a "sugar-tong" or stirrup (U-shaped) splint. Posterior splints alone invariably break unless made of synthetic material, and the latter is to be avoided because of the cuts and scratches that its sharp edges can create rubbing against the contralateral limb in the bed. This double plaster splint is applied leaving a space along its entire length anteriorly, and it is wrapped with a moistened gauze roll (Kling bandage); thus the splint could be removed at any time if it is too tight, simply by splitting the gauze anteriorly and spreading the splint apart with the hands.

REHABILITATION

The patient is kept non–weight bearing until the incision is healed and no longer draining. If the patient is debilitated, and unable to do strict non–weight bearing, then touch-down on the heel is allowed, in order to mobilize the patient. Immobilization of the Achilles tendon lengthening is for a minimum of 8 weeks and as long as 12 weeks.

Patients should be warned that some drainage, or a small area of delayed healing is quite common. They should be warned that the exact time until they are fitted in shoes is variable and unpredictable, depending upon the rapidity of their healing. As noted above, the time for removal of sutures is variable, but in amputation surgery 3 to 4 weeks is a minimum time before removal of sutures. In diabetic patients it is often advisable to wait longer; in patients who have had an area of delayed healing, it is even longer, and not uncommon to leave at least some of the sutures in place for 6 to 8 weeks.

Patients must also be counseled regarding the types of shoes that they can wear later, and the limitations in shoe-wear that the amputation imposes. The primary problem for the transmetatarsal amputee in fitting shoes is that the shortened foot is less able to hold on a shoe due to the missing forefoot. This means that a lace-up shoe is almost always necessary, since an open throat, slip-on shoe has inadequate ability to grasp the foot. Moreover, especially in the very short transmetatarsal amputations, a high-top shoe may be required in order to provide the mechanical stability to hold the shoe on. Because of the ever-widening array of available leisure and athletic shoes, this is less of a cosmetic dilemma to patients than in years past.

It is generally advised that diabetic patients be professionally fitted with a shoe with additional depth. This allows fitting a custom, molded insole into the shoe, which serves several purposes. The insole provides a cushioning and weight-distributing function to take pressure off of any residual pressure point on the plantar surface, as would be the case in any diabetic shoe insole. The insole is also modified to attach a toe filler to it, to "block" out the area of the missing forefoot (Fig. 12). This toe filler can even be made to wrap around the forefoot. It serves to reduce or eliminate the side to side and front to back movement of the foot inside of the shoe, which can cause friction leading to further breakdown. This same type of shoe insole is generally used in almost all transmetatarsal amputees. In nondiabetic patients with normal sensation, the option exists that the toe filler can be placed permanently within the shoe, and it does not need to be attached to an insole.

Patients, especially those with insensitive limbs, should be taught to regularly inspect their feet, especially the amputation sites, for evidence of ulceration or skin injury. This is the best way to monitor the durability of the amputated foot, as the patient progressively increases the amount of walking and activity. For the patients with good sensation, the amount of walking they can do is a function of

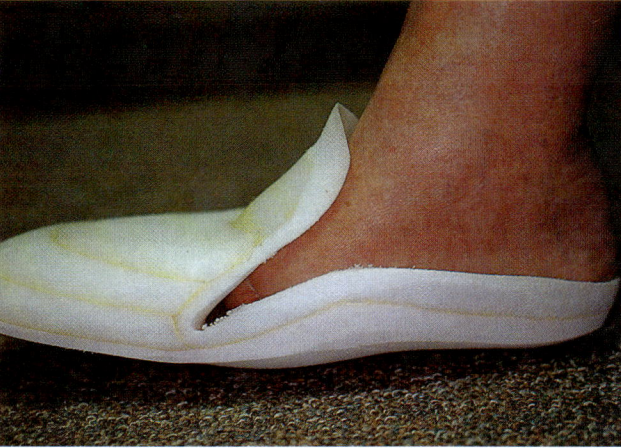

Figure 12. A shoe insole for the patient with a transmetatarsal amputation. The filler or block for the missing part of the forefoot reduces sliding of the foot inside the shoe.

their vascular status and their tolerance. They are advised to build their walking distance gradually and progressively. Consultation with a physical medicine specialist may be helpful in the rehabilitation process.

COMPLICATIONS

Complications of the transmetatarsal amputation are similar to those of other amputations, viz., they concentrate on problems of soft tissue healing or breakdown of the soft tissue, either of which eventually leads to superficial infection, and ultimately osteomyelitis and more proximal amputation. The four main complications—delayed primary healing, failed primary healing, recurrent plantar ulceration or pain, and ulceration or painful blisters on the distal stump—will be discussed separately with consideration of preventive measures and suggestions for appropriate management strategies.

1. *Delayed primary healing:* This is so much a part of the natural history of the procedure as perhaps not even to be a complication. It is often unavoidable. It is usually signified by a small amount of serous, noninfected drainage from a fraction of the suture line. The likelihood *might* be reduced by gentle handling of tissue, and by leaving clean surface without bits and tags of tissue on the flaps of the amputation. It is managed with local wound care in the area of the drainage, including moist-to-dry saline dressings and local debridement. Sometimes one or two sutures need to be removed in order to pack the area gently with the gauze. The surgeon and the patient are counseled to be patient, especially because this is common in the population that most often requires amputation: dysvascular and diabetic patients.
2. *Failed primary healing:* Failure of the wound to heal is usually a function of inadequate vascularity of the tissue, although it can occasionally be attributed to uncontrolled infection. Failure to heal is distinguished from delayed healing by the total absence of wound healing and/or persistent purulent drainage and recurring cellulitis. Management usually requires revision to a more proximal level of amputation. Repeat evaluation of the perfusion of the limb, and repeat cultures for estimation of the adequacy of antibiotic coverage may also be advised.
3. *Ulceration or pain on the plantar surface of the stump:* This is due to inordinate prominence of the end of one of the resected metatarsals. A metatarsal may shift position especially after the destabilizing effect of the amputation on the midfoot tarsometatarsal joints. This can cause a gradually increasing pressure point that leads to pain or ulceration in the sensate or insensitive patients, respectively. More frequently, it is caused by excessive pressure under a metatarsal that has been cut too long. Treatment can begin with conservative measures for nonoperative relief of pressure externally, but if it persists, surgical shortening of the metatarsal is performed. This might be caused by failing to produce the "cascade" of length described above.
4. *Ulceration of the distal stump:* This usually is a manifestation of pressure on the end of the stump that occurs from shoe-wear, is exacerbated by walking, and is caused by an equinus position of the foot. The equinus most often occurs at the ankle, but some of the deformity can also occur at the midfoot (transverse tarsal joint, i.e., talonavicular and calcaneocuboid joints). This is often the sequela of long periods of debility of bed rest. Initial management includes shoe modifications such as a rocker bottom and a stiff sole. If unsuccessful, then Achilles lengthening is done. Rarely, posterior capsulotomies of the ankle and subtalar joints are required as well.

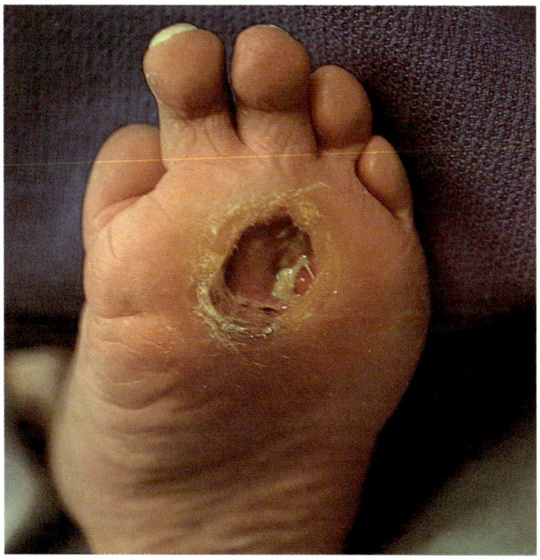

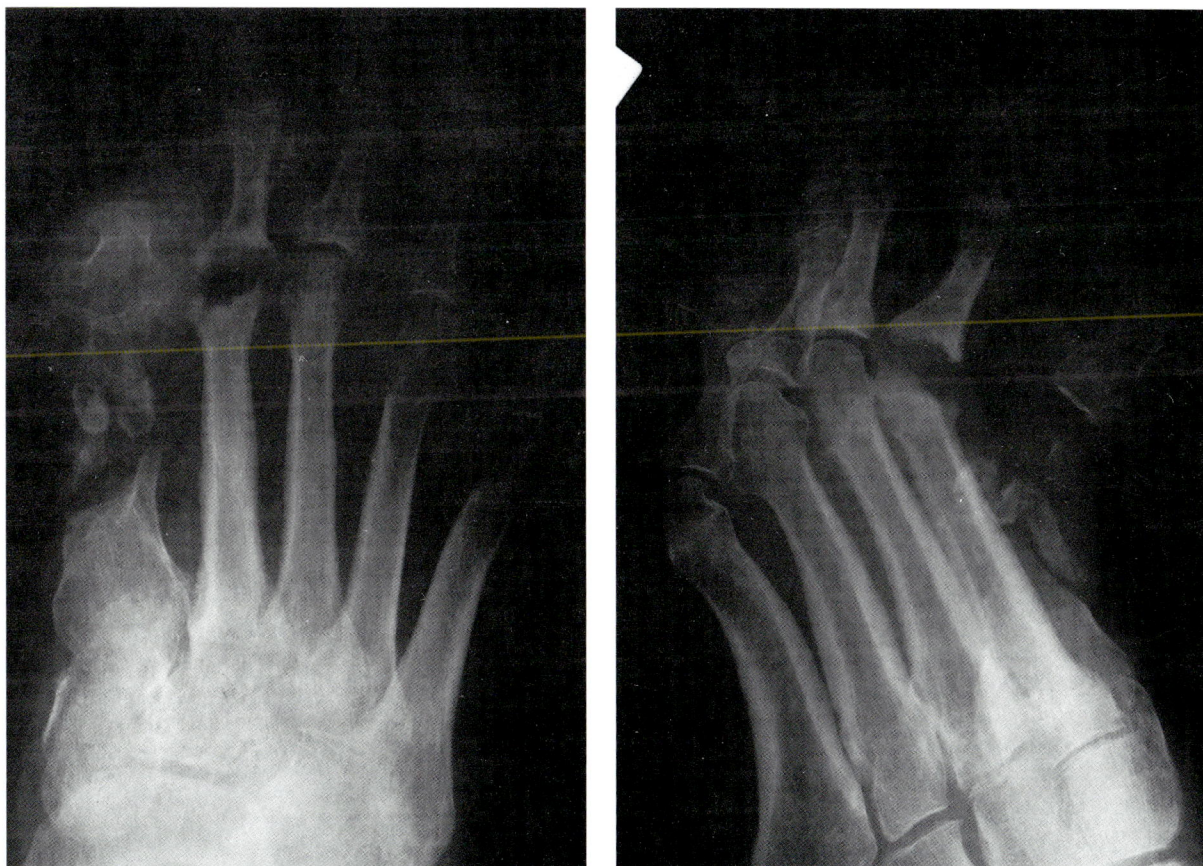

Figure 13. Preoperative appearance with recurrent ulceration prior to transmetatarsal amputation.

Figure 14. Preoperative radiographs demonstrating the previously resected first metatarsal, and most of the second metatarsal head.

ILLUSTRATIVE CASE FOR TECHNIQUE

This is a 68-year-old retired baker with a 20-year history of insulin-dependent diabetes mellitus, who had recurrent ulceration under multiple metatarsals over a period of almost 15 years. Despite conservative treatment with total contact casts and subsequent shoe and insole prescriptions, he developed recurrent ulcerations on both feet. He had been unable to work in his garden or walk in his neighborhood for many years due to the recurrent nature of his problems.

Previous surgical procedures to resect isolated metatarsal heads, debride the ulcers, and amputate an osteomyelitic first ray, provided transient improvement, always followed by recurrent ulceration at an adjacent metatarsal.

Examination of the feet showed recurrent neurotrophic ulceration (Fig. 13). There was no gross purulence or active infection. Severe clawtoes accompanied the increased pressure under the metatarsal heads. Pulses, while somewhat diminished, were present, and preoperative Doppler studies showed satisfactory ankle indices and toe pressures bilaterally. Pulse volume recordings demonstrated pulsatile flow at the toe level on both feet. Radiographs demonstrated the previously resected first metatarsal (Fig. 14), and changes of neuroarthropathy at the second metatarsophalangeal joint, but no evidence of active osteomyelitis.

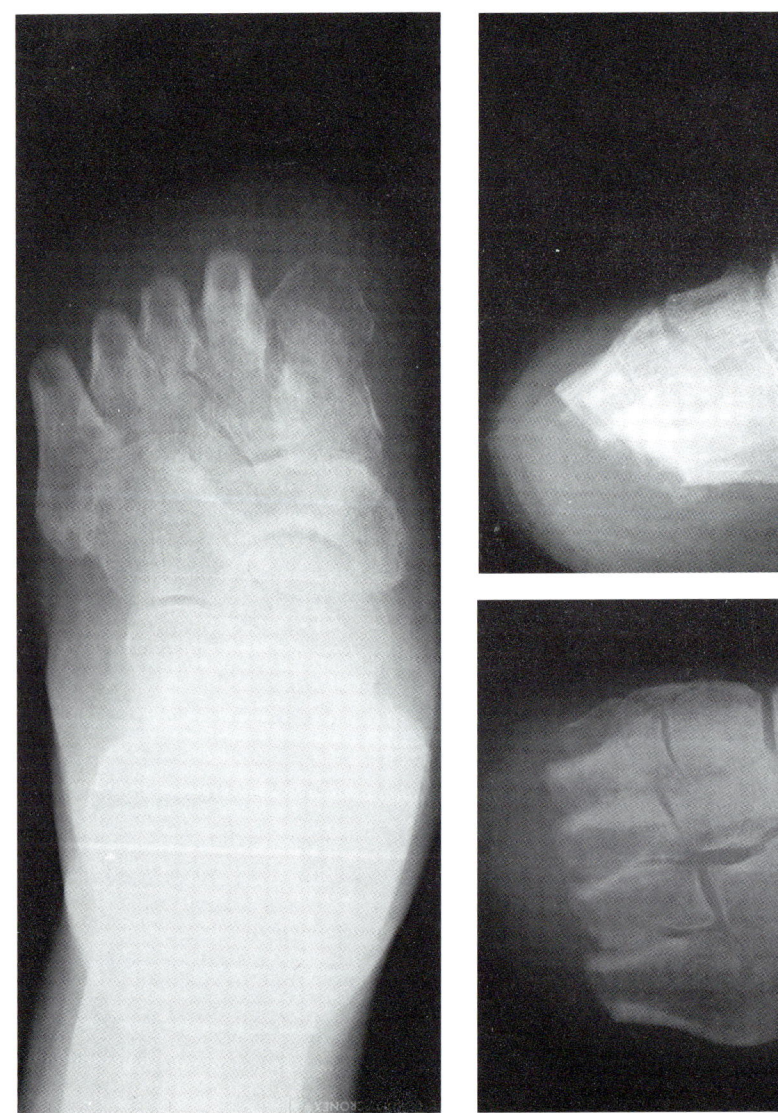
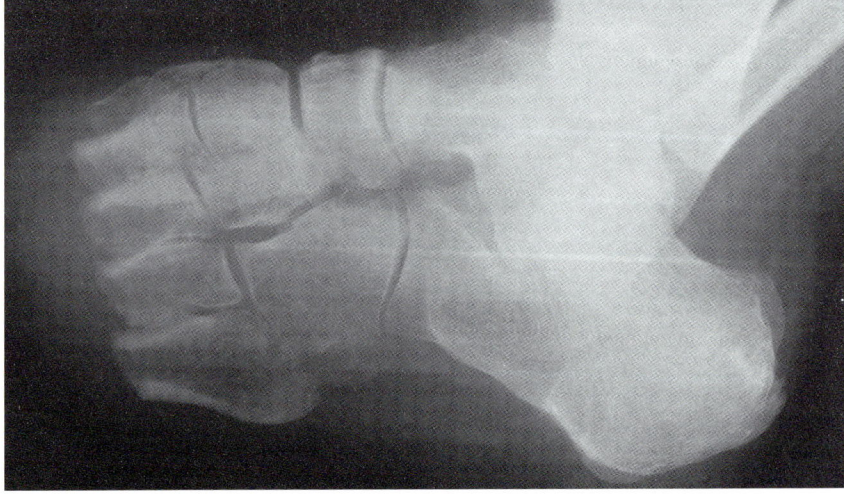

Figure 15. Postoperative radiographs of the transmetatarsal amputation.

A decision to proceed with transmetatarsal amputation was made. The procedure was done bilaterally with the two feet being operated about 2 months apart (Fig. 15). The patient was hospitalized after each one and received a short course of intravenous antibiotics, 72 hours or less, and was discharged home with oral antibiotics for the following 10 days. He was kept non–weight bearing until the stumps healed, averaging 4 weeks. After each foot was healed, the patient was placed in high-top Extra Depth shoes (P. W. Minor Company) with molded insoles that had attached toe fillers. The patient later began taking short walks in his neighborhood, and subjectively was quite pleased with his newfound mobilization. No subsequent skin breakdown was experienced over the ensuing 5 years, up to the present.

This case demonstrates the durability and utility of the transmetatarsal amputation for severe, recalcitrant problems of the forefoot.

RECOMMENDED READING

1. Brodsky, J. W.: Amputations of the foot. In: *Surgery of the Foot and Ankle*, edited by R. A. Mann. M. Coughlin. Mosby, St. Louis, 1992.
2. Brodsky, J. W., and Chambers, R. B.: Effect of tourniquet use on amputation healing in diabetic and dysvascular patients. *Perspect. Orthop. Surg.*, 2: 71–76, 1991.
3. Hodge, M. J., Peters, T. G., and Efird, W. G.: Amputation of the distal portion of the foot. *South. Med. J.*, 82: 1138–1142, 1989.
4. Larrson, U., and Andersson, G. B. J.: Partial amputation of the foot for diabetic or arteriosclerotic gangrene. *J. Bone Joint Surg.* 60B: 126–130, 1978.
5. McKittrick, L. S., McKittrick, J. B., and Risley, T. S.: Transmetatarsal amputation for infection of gangrene in patients with diabetes mellitus. *Ann. Surg.*, 130: 826, 1949.

PART IV

Cuneiform-Metatarsal Joints

18

Cuneiform-Metatarsal Arthrodesis (Lisfranc)

Bruce J. Sangeorzan and Sigvard T. Hansen, Jr.

INDICATIONS/CONTRAINDICATIONS

The midfoot is the region of the foot that extends from the transverse tarsal (Chopart) joint to the tarsometatarsal (Lisfranc) joints. When clinically important instability or arthritis affects the midfoot joints, arthrodesis is the only established salvage procedure. The joints are too small, motion too limited, and the ligaments too complex to respond reliably to reconstructive procedures. Primary osteoarthritis in the intertarsal or tarsometatarsal joints is rare. Most often pathological changes in this area are a result of posttraumatic arthritis or neuropathic midfoot breakdown. When midfoot arthritis or instability cannot be attributed to trauma or neuropathic breakdown, close inspection may demonstrate pes planus with a tight heel cord. Under these circumstances, the inability of the ankle to dorsiflex leads to increasing motion in the midfoot, and, with time, to instability and secondary midfoot arthritis.

Preoperative complaints include pain, fatigue, and instability. Instability may occur during standing but is likely to be most noticeable during the propulsive part of the gait, particularly walking up hills. The patient generally notices that the foot is "turning outward." This tendency to abduct results from a combination of factors. The habitus of a normal limb is slightly externally rotated, and the center of mass of the body is in the midline, medial to the foot. During toe-off, the entire body weight acts medially to the foot to push the forefoot outward. Continued pressure on the forefoot leads to erosion of the dorsal and lateral part of the cuneiforms and progressive abducto-planovalgus deformity (Fig. 1). Although in some cases degenerative changes in these joints may occur in the ab-

---

B. J. Sangeorzan, M.D., and S. T. Hansen, Jr., M.D.: Department of Orthopaedics, University of Washington/Harborview Medical Center, Seattle, WA 98104.

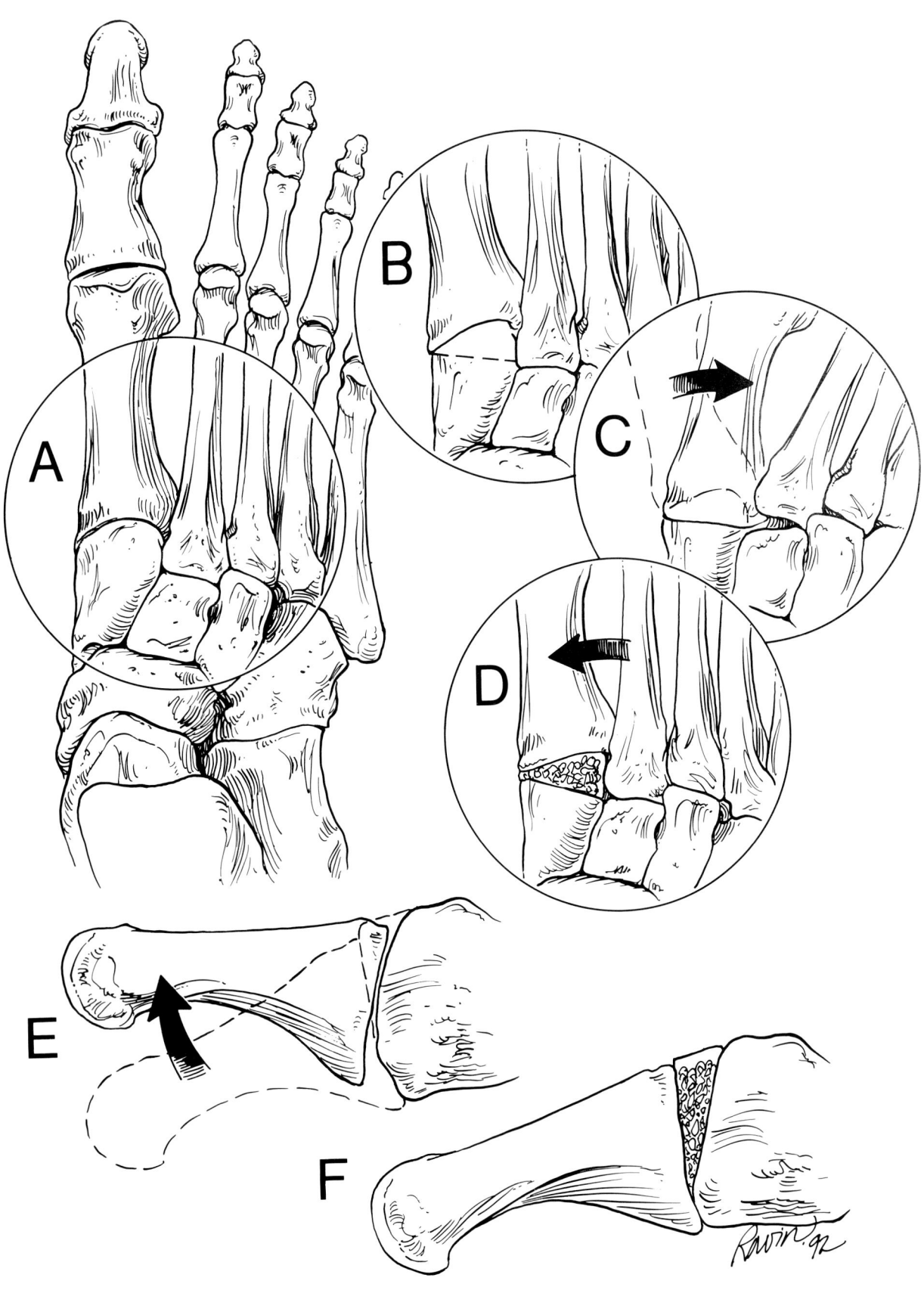

sence of increasing joint instability, more often the degenerative changes are accompanied by increasing mechanical failure.

Nonoperative treatment may be effective in relieving short-term symptoms or an acute exacerbation of low-grade chronic symptoms. External support that diminishes bending forces across the midfoot provides a nonoperative option. A short period of casting is the most effective nonoperative treatment and insures compliance. However, this is not an acceptable long-term treatment and not very well tolerated. An alternative is a rocker bottom sole or a custom molded full-length total contact insole. Though effective, rocker bottom soles are not aesthetic, making compliance unpredictable. In addition, the height added to the treated limb may require a lift on the contralateral side. A less effective but more aesthetic orthotic option is a steel spring between the sole and the shank of the shoe. However, none of these orthotic methods of management seem to function for the long term.

Inadequate soft tissue envelope and inadequate arterial inflow are contraindications to surgery.

PREOPERATIVE PLANNING

The issues to address in preoperative planning include arterial and venous patency, selection of the joints to be fused, placement of surgical incisions, and extent of bony defect. Since this disease predominates in the elderly patient population and in patients with diabetes mellitus, both dorsalis pedis and posterior tibial pulses should be sought. If either is not palpable, preoperative consultation with vascular surgery should be requested to establish the patency of both the vessels and the blood flow into the forefoot. Duplex scanning is an effective noninvasive method of visualizing the vascular anatomy. It is also important to know if an anomaly exists in the vascular anatomy. The dorsalis pedis is at risk during the exposure and reduction of these joints and may be put under tension if substantial reduction has to be performed. This is obviously much greater risk in a patient with no posterior tibial pulse. As a general rule, if both pulses are palpable, no further vascular evaluation is required. Since cigarette smoking has an adverse effect on wound healing, it is banned in the perioperative period and an effort is made to prevent smoking completely during the period of healing.

Roentgenographic examination should include full weight-bearing anteroposterior (AP) and lateral views as well as an oblique view of the foot. Unless the patient is full weight bearing, it is impossible to determine how much breakdown occurs and how much angular correction will be required, particularly in the dorsoplantar direction. An oblique view provides the best perspective of the midfoot joints. The oblique view will help to line up the lesser tarsal articulations with the angle

---

Figure 1. A: The diagrammatic representation of a dorsal view of a right foot. **B:** The *shaded area* of the first cuneiform is the part that becomes eroded. The first metatarsal angles into a valgus position and wears away the lateral aspect of the medial cuneiform *(shaded area)*. Eventually the medial cuneiform assumes a more flattened shape *(dashed line)* that makes the position of reduction uncertain. **C:** The entire forefoot has become abducted. The native position of the medial cuneiform is represented by a *dashed line*. The lesser metatarsals are subluxed laterally. **D:** Restoring the position of the first ray leaves the defect that must be filled with bone graft. The effect is generally wedge shaped and represents the normal contours of the unaffected medial cuneiform *(checkered area)*. **E:** An exaggerated lateral view of the tarsometatarsal articulation of the first ray demonstrating a similar process. The dorsal edge becomes eroded from the repeated dorsiflexion of the first metatarsal. **F:** This up-and-down motion leaves a wedge-shaped defect that must be filled with bone graft. The defect is therefore a two-plane cuneiform shape.

of the beam. Sometimes multiple oblique views have to be done to gather all of the information that is required. Comparison views of the other foot are helpful since alignment in this area varies substantially. If instability is in question, fluoroscopic examination may be required. Computed tomography is generally not required, but may be useful in sorting out problems in the intercuneiform joints.

Preoperative diagrams are used to determine the degree of bony defect, and therefore, the size, shape, and location of corticocancellous bone graft needed. On weight-bearing AP and lateral roentgenograms, tracings are made of the first, second, and third metatarsals and cuneiform bones. The articulations are reduced on the paper tracings by cutting out the metatarsals and placing the bases back in the reduced position. By comparing the resulting diagram to the roentgenograms of the contralateral foot, it is possible to determine whether a block of corticocancellous bone graft will be needed to bring the metatarsals into position and out to length. It will also give the surgeon a good idea of the amount of reduction that will be required.

Though the first, second, and third tarsometatarsal joints are almost always involved, it is often difficult to determine the location of other painful joints in the midfoot. When deciding what joints require arthrodesis, particular attention should be paid to the joint between the medial and intermediate cuneiform. This is a joint with more motion than is generally recognized and also a frequent site of occult injury. Clinical assessment of this joint may reveal whether it is involved. To examine this joint, stabilize the midfoot with one hand, and grasp the first metatarsal head with the other. Plantar flexion and dorsiflexion in the first ray will be painful in the midfoot if the intercuneiform joint is arthritic. If there is any question about pain, selective injection of lidocaine into the joints may be helpful. The use of a miniature fluoroscopy unit such as the Z Scan or HealthMate can help document that the injection is actually in the joint. If it is still unclear after selective injection, we generally will fuse any joint that may be a source of pain. The additional work required to fuse extra joints is small, and the loss of motion negligible. Fusion of an additional intertarsal joint is preferable to continuing pain or having to come back and do a secondary fusion.

SURGERY

The patient is placed supine on the operating table with a roll beneath the hip on the operative side. The roll is placed so as to support the pelvis and greater trochanter. This position helps to internally rotate the limb so that the lateral side of the foot is available for application of a small distractor. The limb is prepped and draped to allow circumferential access. The anterior iliac crest is prepped as well to gain access to autogenous bone graft. The limb is exsanguinated with an Esmarch bandage before the tourniquet is inflated.

Technique. The first skin incision is made over the interval between the first and second tarsometatarsal joints (Fig. 2). A lazy S incision is used that curves laterally and then medially (Fig. 3). This allows exposure of the second tarsometatarsal joint through the lateral curve and the first through the medial curve. Keep in mind that the second tarsometatarsal joint is recessed in relation to the first and both will be expected to be subluxed or dislocated under circumstances of this operative procedure. The medial border of the medial cuneiform can be seen through the medial curve of the S and may be used to align the first ray. The dorsalis pedis artery is in this interval and sends a large branch (the first proximal perforating artery) to the plantar surface of the foot through the first web space. Care should be taken not to injure either artery.

The surgical approach may need to be altered if the soft tissue envelope is abnormal. Scars from initial trauma or ulceration from pressure sores are the most likely to affect the approach. If the deformity has caused a weight-bearing ulcer,

18 CUNEIFORM-METATARSAL ARTHRODESIS (Lisfranc)

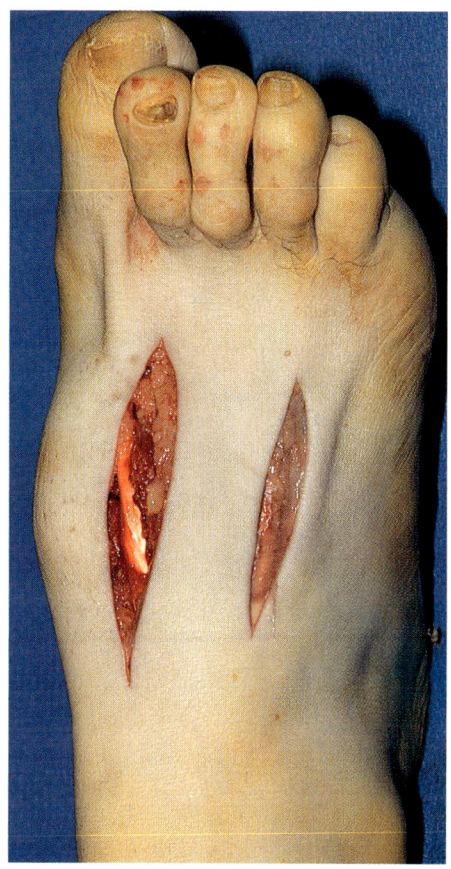

Figure 2. Intraoperative photograph of the surgical approach. The dorsal surface of a right foot is shown. Note the medial dorsal deformity. The incisions allow access to two tarsometatarsal joints each.

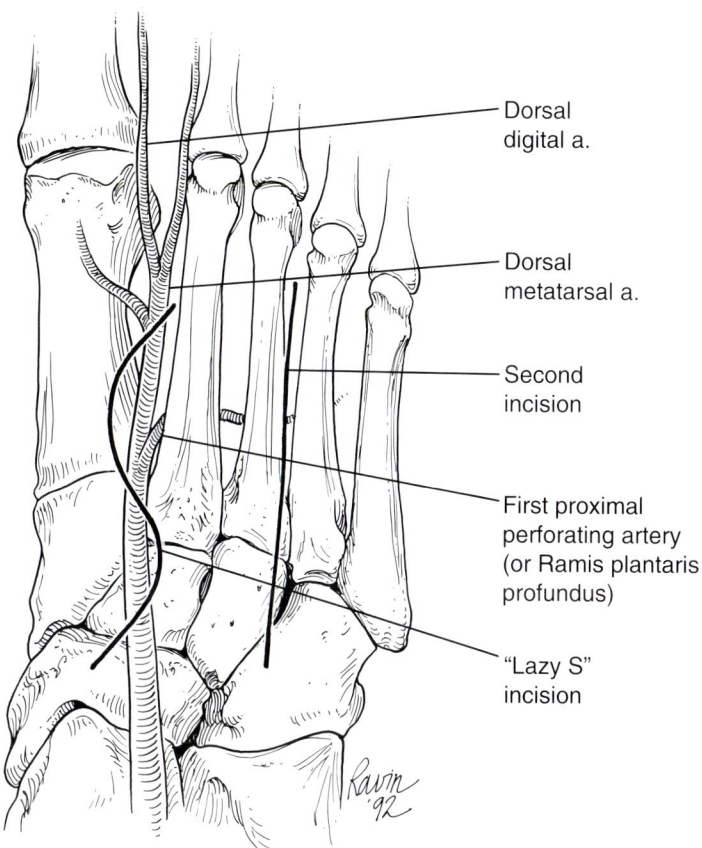

Figure 3. A dorsal view representing the location of the skin incisions and perforating arteries. The lazy S incision is represented by a *line* curving little laterally at the level of the second tarsometatarsal joint and medially at the level of the first tarsometatarsal joint. Note that the incision also exposes the intercuneiform joint. The same net effect can be accomplished by the long straight incision that undermines the skin. The second incision is in the interval between the third and fourth ray. Note the relationship of this incision to the perforating artery and dorsal digital artery. The perforating artery enters the plantar surface of the foot through the first web space.

the most common area is the undersurface of the medial cuneiform. If this ulcer is healed and/or small, the surgical incisions need not be altered. Every effort is made to make sure that the soft tissues are viable and intact before surgical intervention. Before the tourniquet goes up, the dorsalis pedis pulse is palpated and its relationship to the first web space incision is documented.

After the first and second metatarsal joints are debrided, a second incision is made over the medial border of the fourth metatarsal for exposure of the third, fourth, and fifth tarsometatarsal joints. The joints are exposed and scar tissue and debris are removed carefully using a small rongeur curette or osteotome. Each joint is completely debrided so that reduction can be performed. Since the metatarsal bases are connected by ligaments, reduction cannot be performed until all of the joints are mobilized. At times a third dorsal longitudinal incision is needed to completely free the fifth or fourth metatarsal.

If the first tarsometatarsal joint is significantly subluxed and unstable and the disorder has been present for a long period of time, the position of reduction may be in question. The medial cuneiform becomes eroded dorsally and laterally,

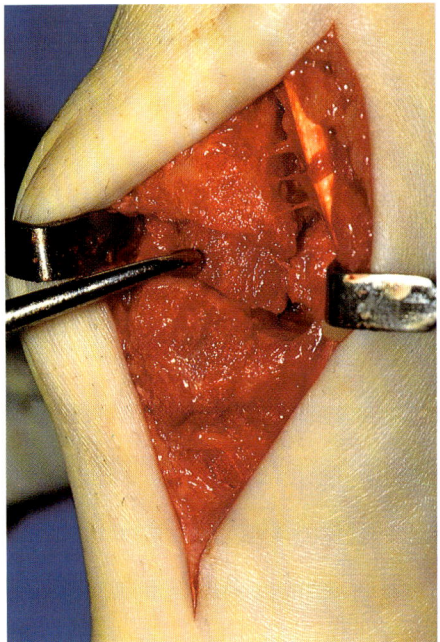

Figure 4. Dorsal surgical exposure of a right foot. Medial is to the left. The bone block is indicated by the Joker. The block of bone is in the dorsolateral tarsometatarsal joint.

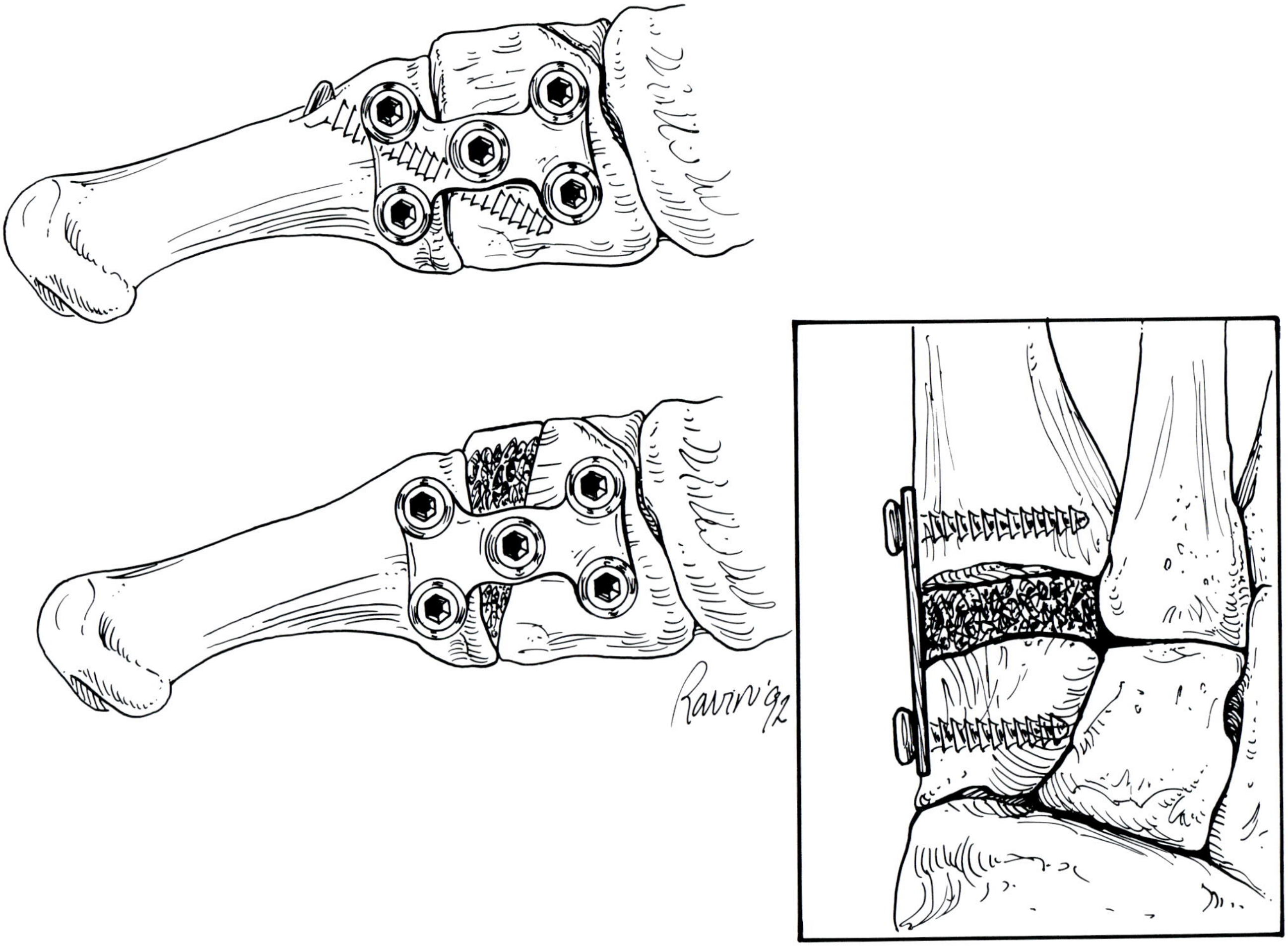

Figure 5. A circumstance in which substantial erosion has occurred in the first tarsometatarsal joint. The relationship of the first metatarsal is restored and held with the combination of a medial tension plate and a 3.5 screw across the tarsometatarsal joint. The defect is then filled with bone graft.

obscuring the native position of the joint (Fig. 4). This joint is reduced before the second through fourth metatarsals for two reasons. Since the forefoot is displaced laterally, the first metatarsal is in the way of the second tarsometatarsal joint. In addition, the first metatarsal is generally not connected to the other metatarsals

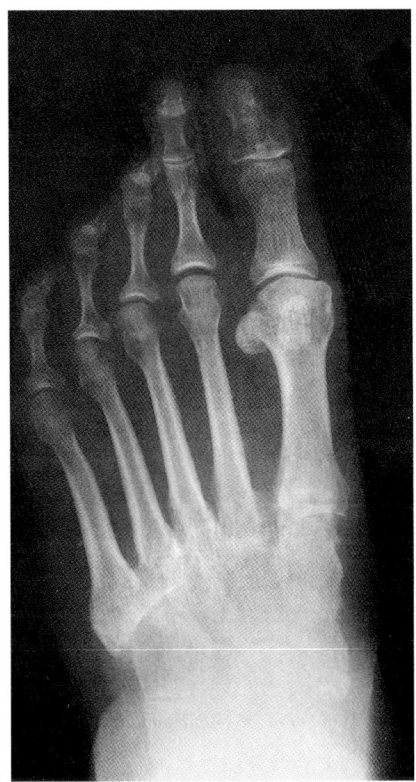

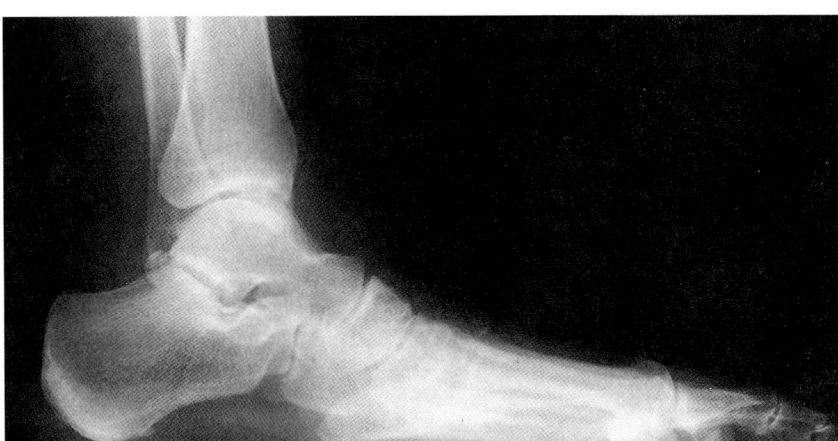

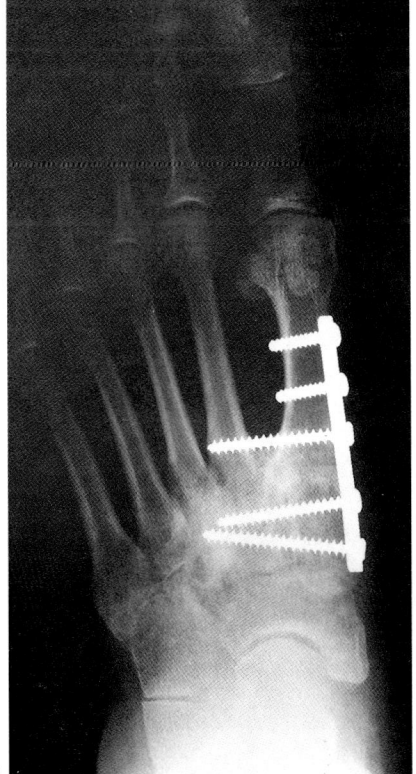

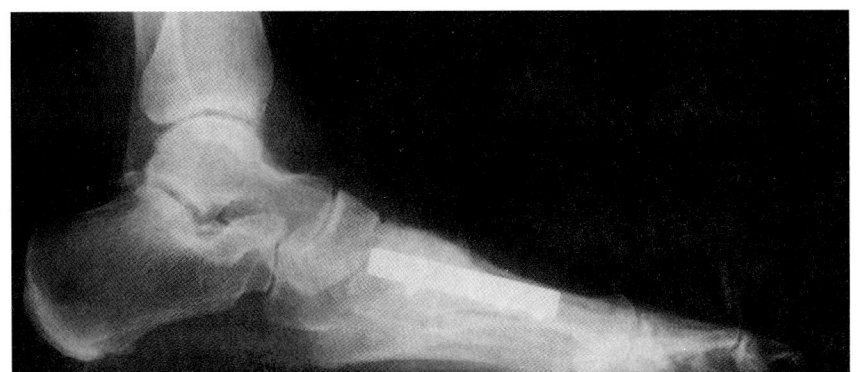

Figure 6. Pre-operative AP **(A)** and lateral **(B)** radiographs of a patient with collapse through the midfoot. Note the abduction of the foot through the Lisfranc joint. **C** and **D**: Postoperatively, the abduction is significantly improved, as is the midfoot sag, by use of a medially applied plate. Note that the intercuneiform articulations have been fused as well. (Case courtesy of Brad Olney, M.D.)

and can be more freely manipulated. A helpful intraoperative method of determining reduction is to reduce and stabilize the joint with provisional fixation, obtain an intraoperative radiograph, and compare it to the radiographs taken of the contralateral foot. More importantly, the clinical appearance of the foot should guide the reduction.

The tendency in the first tarsometatarsal joint is to accept a slightly lateralized or valgus position. It may be counter to instincts honed on hallux valgus surgery to introduce varus to the first metatarsal. But failure to achieve an anatomic varus position may result in residual pronation. A small tension plate may be required along the medial side of the joint to maintain the native position if it has been dislocated for a long period of time (Figs. 5 and 6). A corticocancellous block of bone may also be required to help stabilize this joint. It is important to get both plantar flexion and adduction restored to the joint. The block of bone may be used to fill in a defect that remains when the first metatarsal is positioned appropriately.

After the first tarsometatarsal joint is restored, the entire forefoot needs to be reduced. This is accomplished by use of a laterally placed distractor. The distractor is applied as follows: First, a 2-mm Schanz pin is placed into the calcaneus, perpendicular to the long axis of the foot. A second pin is placed into the proximal fourth and fifth metatarsals. This pin is placed so as to converge toward the first pin

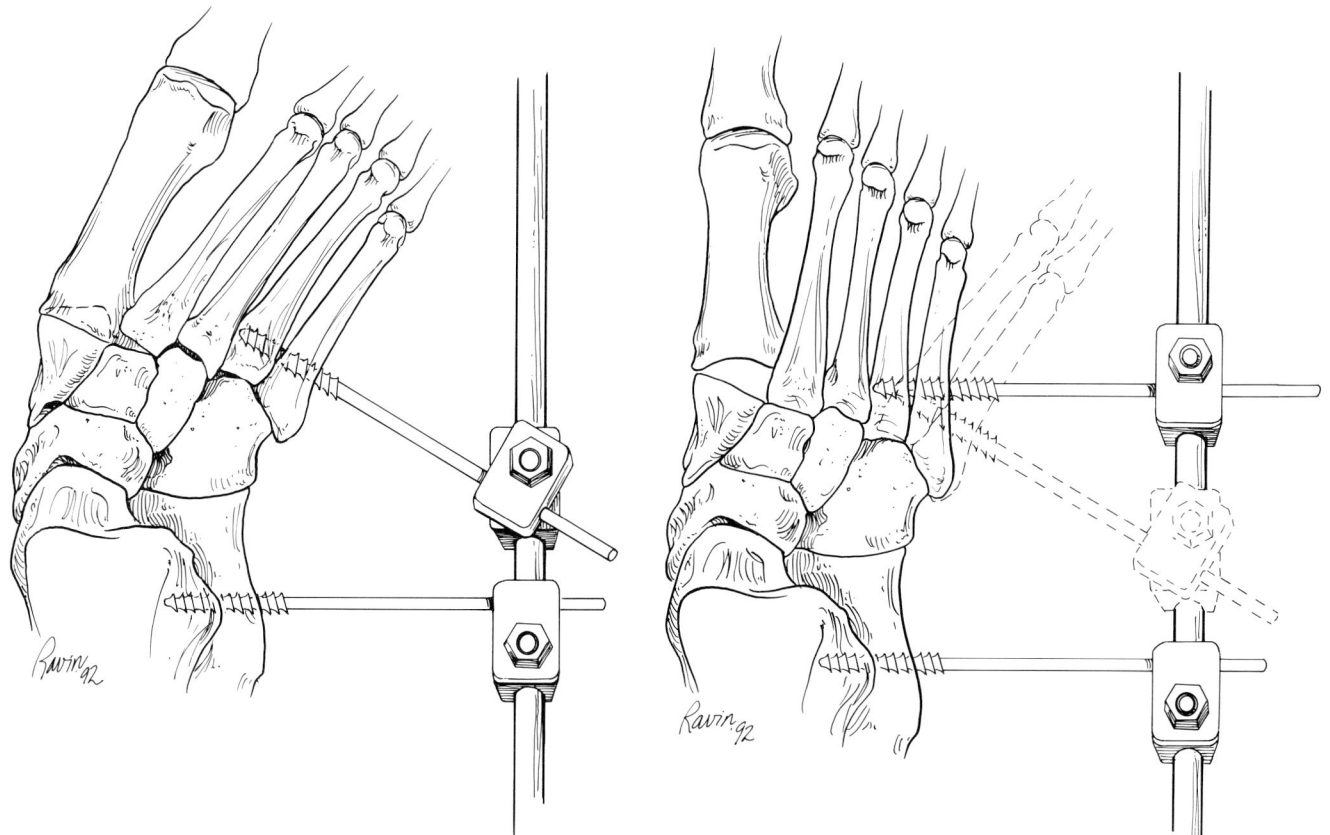

Figure 7. A and **B:** A schematic representation of the use of a small distractor to reduce the forefoot. After all the tarsometatarsal joints have been debrided of scar and the forefoot appears mobile, a laterally placed small distractor is used. A 2-mm Schanz pin is placed into the calcaneus in a position perpendicular to the long axis of the foot. A second pin is placed into the base of metatarsal 5 and 4 and sometimes 3. This pin converges laterally with that placed in the calcaneus. The distractor is then placed across these two pins. As the two pins are distracted, the forefoot is forced out to length, out of abduction and somewhat medially. When enough correction has been restored to get the second metatarsal into its mortise, provisional fixation is performed.

18 CUNEIFORM-METATARSAL ARTHRODESIS (Lisfranc)

laterally. That is, the pin is closer to the proximal pin at its most lateral point than it is at its most medial point (Fig. 7A). The distractor is then placed on the end of these two pins and length is added. As the tissues are stretched by the distractor, the forefoot adducts, and, to some extent, restores the arch (Fig. 7B). It is not uncommon to have to apply this tension in increments over a short period of time with further debridement of each of the tarsometatarsal joints as the position improves. The forefoot is reduced enough to reduce the base of the second metatarsal into its mortise (Fig. 8). Provisional fixation is performed with 0.054-inch Kirschner wires. A lag screw is placed from the base of the second metatarsal into the medial cuneiform, the base of the second metatarsal both proximally and medially. At this point, intraoperative radiographs are taken (Fig. 9).

The third tarsometatarsal joint will frequently be reduced passively as the first and second tarsometatarsal joints are reduced. If not, a large Weber reduction clamp can be placed from the base of the third metatarsal to the medial cuneiform to compress it medially. A 3.5-mm cortical lag screw can then be placed across the base of the third metatarsal into the lateral cuneiform. Under most circumstances, the bases of the fourth and fifth tarsometatarsal joints are not fused because of the mobility needed on that side of the foot for normal walking (Fig. 10).

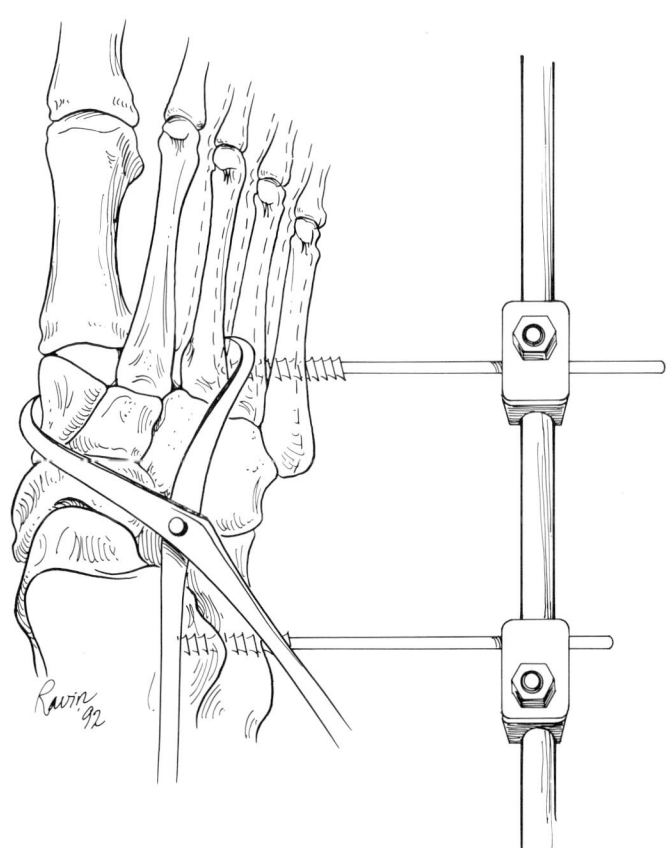

Figure 8. An additional reduction maneuver. At times the disruption is substantial and the third, fourth, and fifth metatarsals do not stay secured when the second metatarsal is secured. Under these circumstances, additional reduction may be needed. Without removing the distractor, a large Weber reduction clamp may be placed from the medial cuneiform to the base of the third metatarsal. Closing the clamp reduces the base of the third metatarsal where it may be secured to the cuneiform.

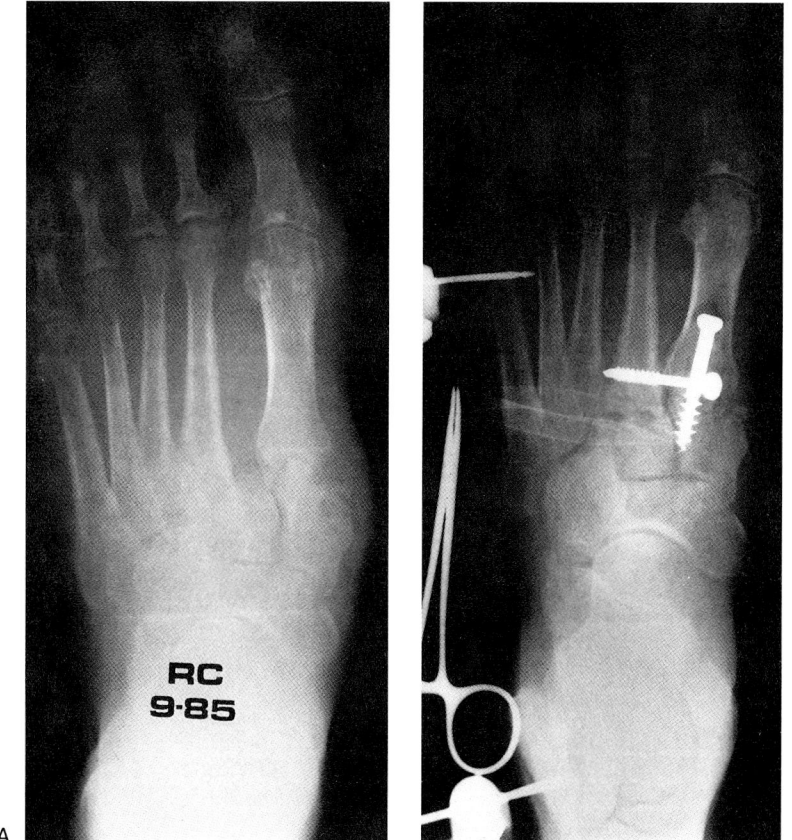

Figure 9. A: The preoperative position with an abducted forefoot and translation through the tarsometatarsal joint. **B:** The laterally placed distractor fixed to the fifth metatarsal and to the calcaneus. The position of the second tarsometatarsal joint has been reduced and held with a malleolar screw crossing from the base of the first metatarsal.

If they have been subluxed or dislocated but the joint surfaces are salvageable, we reduce them and hold the reduction with Kirschner wires that are pulled out at 4 to 6 weeks. If the articular surfaces appear beyond salvage, an "anchovy" procedure is performed and the joint stabilized with Kirschner wires. These joints are fused in the neuropathic foot to prevent late recurrence and to provide improved stability for healing the medial part of the midfoot.

If the intertarsal articulations are to be fused as well, they should be denuded of cartilage and fibrous tissue and fixed. A screw directed laterally from the medial side of the medial cuneiform will compress the lesser tarsal articulations. Cancellous bone graft is used in these joints to facilitate fusion. Routine layer closure of the wound is performed.

A heel-cord lengthening may be performed simultaneously. The indication for the addition of Achilles tendon lengthening is a fixed hindfoot equinus. The hindfoot equinus may be primary, as in the planovalgus foot of long standing, or it may be secondary. When midfoot collapse has been present for more than 6 months, the heel cord may be contracted. Weakening the gastrocnemius also lessens the forces across the midfoot. Radiographic documentation of hindfoot collapse can be achieved by taking a lateral view of the hindfoot in maximum dorsiflexion. This will show that some of the dorsiflexion is occurring through the midfoot. We prefer a closed (percutaneous) three-level slide. It is done before the fusion itself so that dorsiflexion can be applied across the foot without stressing the fixation.

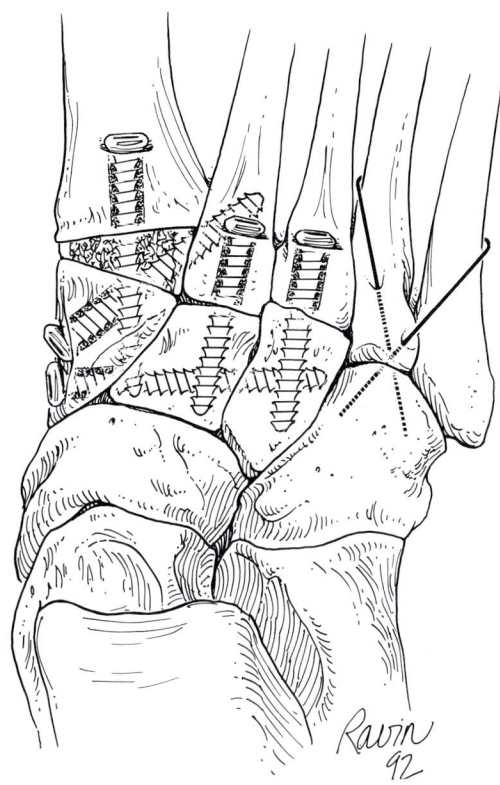

Figure 10. Idealized internal fixation. The building block of this fixation is the cortical lag screw. The near hole is overdrilled, which allows the screw to compress the two bones together. Traditional fixation includes a compression screw across the first, second, and third tarsometatarsal joints supplemented with a screw crossing from the second metatarsal into the medial cuneiform or the medial cuneiform into the second metatarsal. If intertarsal fusion is required, another screw crosses the cuneiform transversely. In feet fused for posttraumatic indications, the fourth and fifth tarsometatarsal joints are temporarily stabilized with Kirschner wires with the expectation of having some continued motion at this level.

POSTOPERATIVE MANAGEMENT

At the end of the surgical procedure, a Marcaine ankle block is done for postoperative pain relief. The patients are placed into a posterior plaster splint or a bivalved short leg plaster cast. They are then begun on non–weight-bearing ambulation on postoperative day 1. When the patients are comfortable and able to walk safely on crutches, they are discharged from the hospital. Sutures are removed at 2 weeks. If the indication for surgery was a Charcot joint, a short leg non–weight-bearing cast is applied. This technique is also used if the surgery was done for other reasons but the fixation was less than satisfactory. If surgical fixation was satisfactory, the patients are placed in a removable splint, and ankle and toe motion are begun at this time. Radiographs are performed 6 weeks postoperatively. If the healing appears to be progressing satisfactorily, the patients are continued non–weightbearing with no immobilization when placed in a short leg weight-bearing cast. Generally speaking, those fusions performed for Charcot midfoot collapse are casted for approximately 16 weeks. Those done for degenerative or posttraumatic changes are not casted beyond 6 to 8 weeks unless evidence of delayed union is present.

Roughly 80% of the patients will heal a solid arthrodesis within 3 months. All patients are told that although the healing of the arthrodesis takes 3 months, it will be 6 months before they are comfortable walking on their foot. This is a major reconstructive procedure. Though some patients will respond much faster, it is far easier to let them know ahead of time that 6 months is not an unreasonable expectation for recovery. The patient should be warned ahead of time that the procedure results in a stiff foot and that they will need to wear comfortable supportive shoes after the operation. This can range anywhere from a comfortable athletic shoe to a prescription type shoe. In most cases, standard lace-up shoes are acceptable shoe-wear after this operation. Routinely, we provide a custom molded insole for the patient to use after casting for as long as the patient feels the need.

COMPLICATIONS

1. *Injury to the superficial peroneal nerves:* The incision crosses the superficial peroneal nerve at many points during this operative procedure. The anatomy is also distorted. Care is taken to avoid cutting the nerve primarily by cutting sharply through the skin, then finding the nerve, and then completing the dissection. Patients are counseled preoperatively that they may be left with sensory deficits.
2. *Incomplete reduction:* Because of the long-standing nature of the deformity and the obscured anatomy, incomplete reduction is common. Paying attention

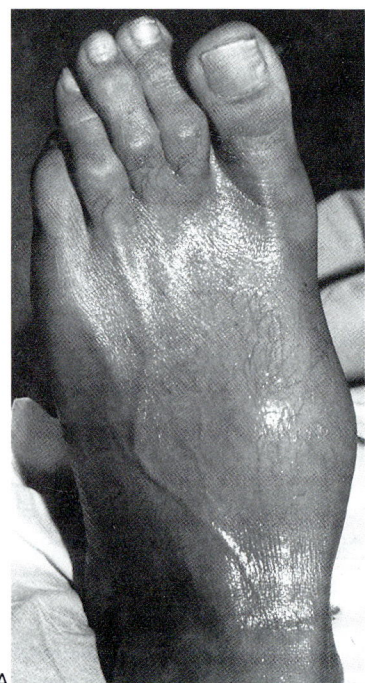
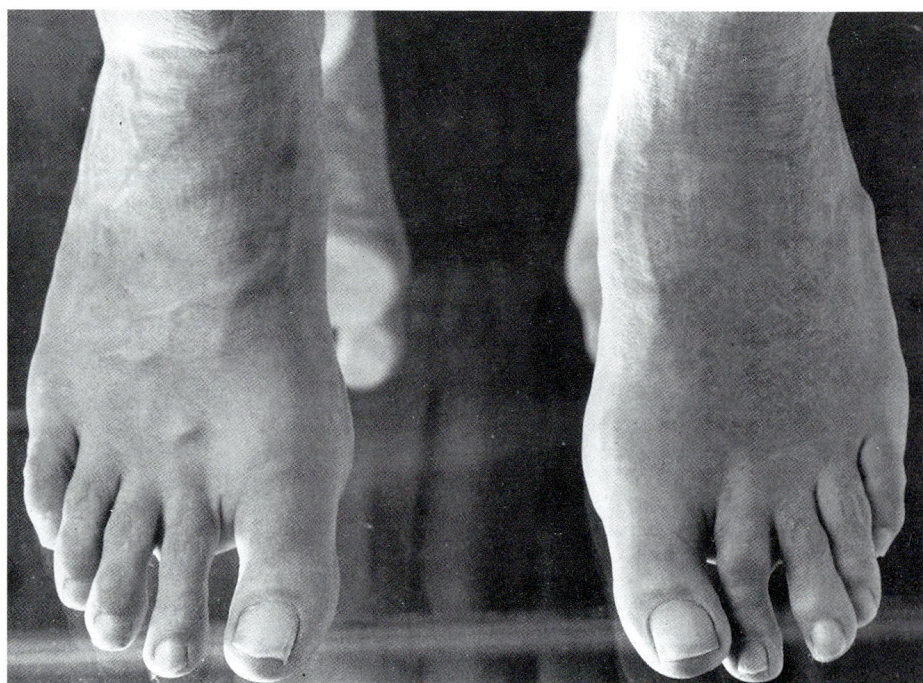

Figure 11. A: A photograph of a left foot with a typical abducted position of the forefoot. Note the convex medial border of the foot. This deformity is actually exaggerated during weight bearing. **B:** A clinical photograph of the same patient after reduction and fusion. Note that the foot is moderately swollen but its contours have been largely restored.

to the shape of the foot rather than the appearance of the radiographs is often helpful in establishing a functional position for the foot. Position of the foot is what patients see and what allows them to fit into shoes. It is helpful to grasp the forefoot across the metatarsal head and the hindfoot and reduce the midfoot position by making sure that the hindfoot and the forefoot are in the

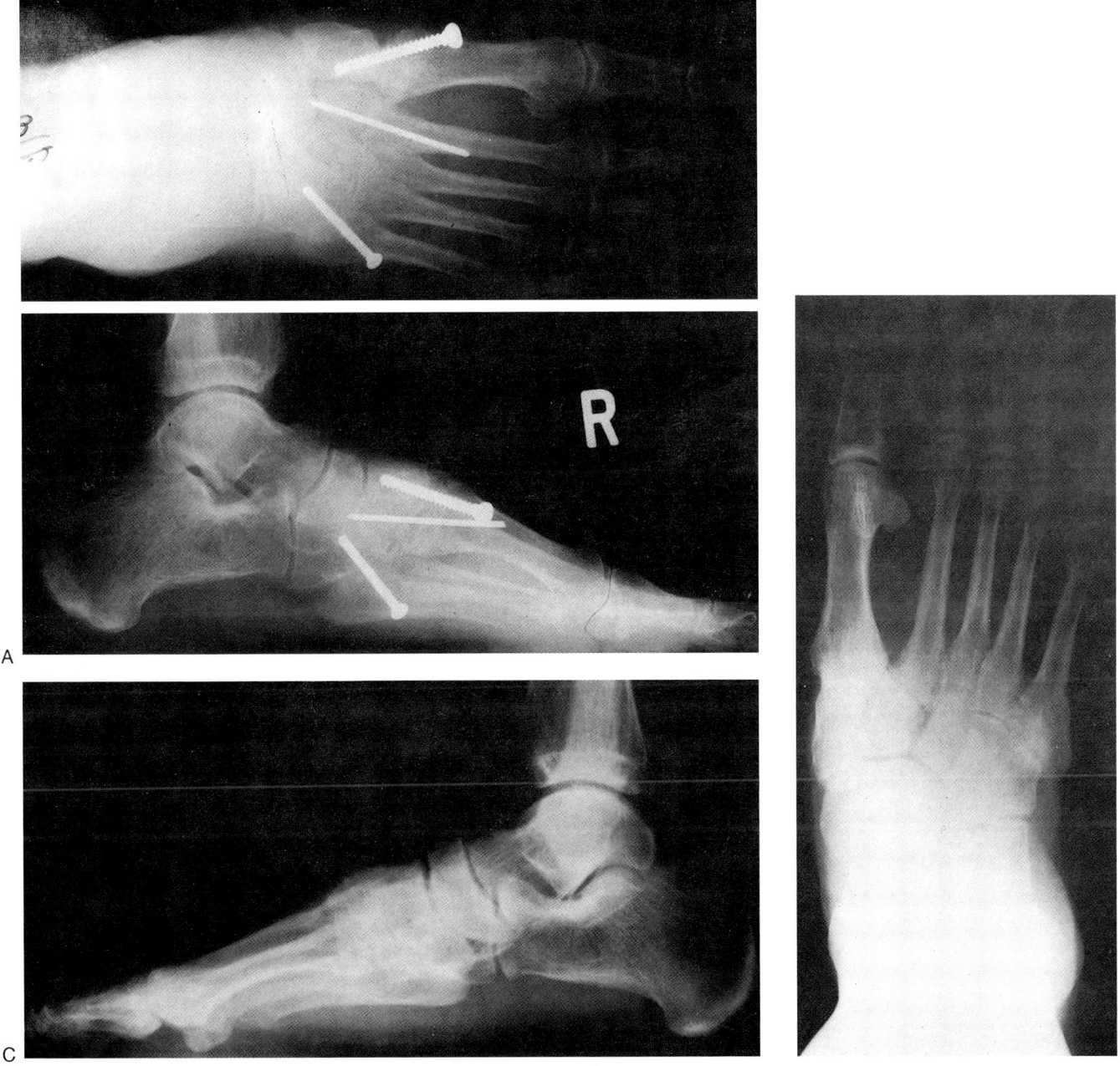

Figure 12. A: An AP and lateral view of a patient who underwent a tarsometatarsal fusion in 1986 following failed treatment of a Lisfranc injury with Schanz pins. It improved from his initial position. The first metatarsal is not medialized enough. A screw should have been placed on the lateral side of the first metatarsal to bring it over and down onto the cuneiform. Alternatively a plate should have been placed medially. The second metatarsal is incompletely reduced as well. **B:** Five years later the patient is having pain in his talonavicular, and clinically the forefoot is abducted. **C:** The lateral view shows no abnormality because the first metatarsal has been adequately plantar flexed. The metatarsals appear to have a normal relationship with the foot and are solidly fused to the cuneiforms. However, there is a slight talonavicular sag and some narrowing of the talonavicular joint.

same plane. Provisional fixation can then be performed to maintain that position and definitive fixation performed after this position is confirmed radiographically.

3. *Nonunion:* Nonunion is common in neuropathic feet. The changes that are made when operating on neuropathic feet include the use of generous amounts of fixation. At least two screws across the first tarsometatarsal joint as well as screws across the second and third tarsometatarsal joint are needed; often additional oblique screws are added to maintain this position. In these circumstances casting is performed until evidence of solid healing is underway (Fig. 11).

4. *Malunion:* Because the most common position of deformity of the first metatarsal is dorsiflexed and abducted, specific attention should be directed toward making this joint plantar flexed and adducted at the time of surgery (Fig. 12). In hallux valgus correction, the goal is to place the first metatarsal parallel to the second. This is not the desired position in midfoot fusion. Again, the position should be established by placing the first metatarsal head in an appropriate position and not worrying quite so much about the radiographic appearance. If the first metatarsal appears too short relative to the second and third, a corticocancellous bone graft is placed across the tarsometatarsal joint. This can be inserted by placing a 0.062-inch Kirschner wire into the first metatarsal and into the intermediate cuneiform and distracting the first tarsometatarsal joint. Corticocancellous graft is placed in with the cortical surface positioned dorsally. It should be shaped to provide plantar flexion and adduction of the first metatarsal.

ILLUSTRATIVE CASE FOR TECHNIQUE

A 50-year-old woman, a college professor, active athlete, and hiker, presents with a 1-year history of increasing foot pain. The pain is exacerbated by walking up hill and mitigated to some extent by stiff-soled shoes. She notes that her shoes are now wearing out and breaking through the midfoot. She has no history of diabetes or significant trauma. The pain has gotten to the point of not only restricting athletic activities but making it difficult for her to walk around campus.

Clinical examination demonstrates an intact pulse, normal sensation to Semmes Wienstein filament testing, and no ulceration. There is clinical instability across the tarsometatarsal joint in the sagittal and coronal planes. The heel cord was tight and the foot clinically flat. There is an area of erythema on the plantar medial aspect of the medial cuneiform from excessive pressure in her shoes where it collapsed over the arch of the shoe.

Radiographs (Fig. 13A, B) show an abducted forefoot with significant erosion at the tarsometatarsal joint. There is a tarsometatarsal sag on the lateral view. Intraoperatively, when the forefoot position has been reduced to a clinically satisfactory position, a large defect exists in the tarsometatarsal region (Fig. 13B). The bone graft helps to maintain the plantar flexed and abducted position of the

Figure 13. A: An AP and lateral view of a foot of a 50-year-old woman with midfoot aching and foot fatigue. Although she has no history of injury, the forefoot is subluxed laterally, there is significant erosion of the tarsal metatarsal joint, and a midfoot planus. **B:** A lateral intraoperative view as the forefoot is placed in what appears to be a reduced position. A large dorsal defect exists. This will be filled with bone graft after the foot has been stabilized with screws. **C:** A lateral view postoperatively showing that defect filled in with bone graft and multiple screws maintaining the plantigrade position of the forefoot. **D:** An AP view of the same patient showing a solid fusion with a reduced forefoot—approximately 10 weeks postoperative.

18 CUNEIFORM-METATARSAL ARTHRODESIS (Lisfranc) 245

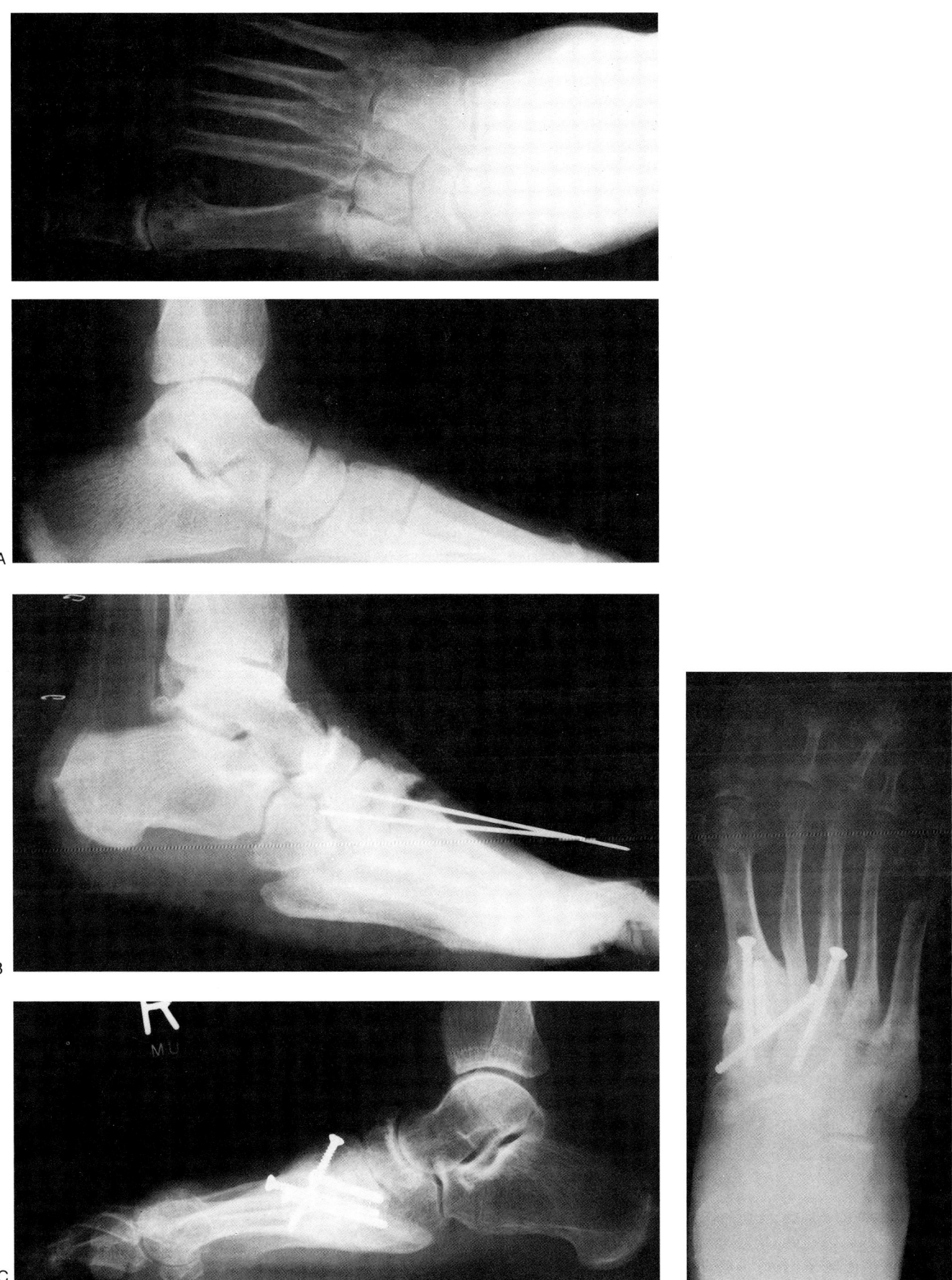

metatarsal (Fig. 13C). Postoperatively, she returned to full-time work at approximately 6 weeks in a walking cast and returned to her athletic activities in approximately 4 months. Clinically, the foot is in a neutral position and symmetrical when compared to her uninvolved foot (Fig. 13D).

RECOMMENDED READING

1. Graham, H. K., and Fixsen, J. A.: Lengthening of the calcaneal tendon in spastic hemiplegia by the White slide technique. A long term review. *J Bone Joint Surg.*, 70B: 742–745, 1988.
2. Johnson, J. E., and Johnson, K. A.: Dowel arthrodesis for degenerative arthrodesis of the tarsometatarsal (Lisfranc) joints. *Foot Ankle*, 5: 243–253, 1986.
3. Sangeorzan, B. J., Veith, R., and Hansen, S. T.: Fusion of Lisfranc's joint for salvage of tarsometatarsal injuries. *Foot Ankle*, 10(4): 193–200, 1989.

PART V

Midtarsal

19

Talonavicular Arthrodesis

G. James Sammarco

INDICATIONS/CONTRAINDICATIONS

The talonavicular joint is a modified ball and socket joint, functioning in dorsiflexion, plantar flexion, medial and lateral rotation, supination, and pronation. It works in concert with the subtalar joint and the calcaneocuboid joints to achieve combined motion that allows the foot to accommodate to a variety of surfaces. Arthrodesis of this joint, therefore, affects motion in the other two hindfoot joints, the subtalar joint and the calcaneocuboid joint. The talonavicular joint is continuous with the anterior facet of the subtalar joint. Talonavicular arthrodesis is indicated when disease causes pain, deformity, and alteration of motion, limiting function of the foot. Such indications include infection, arthritis, tumor, and tuberculosis, all of which have been reported to affect this joint. Tibialis posterior dysfunction includes attritional tears of the tendon, resulting in collapse of the medial longitudinal arch, and has been described as an indication, as well as fracture, of the navicular or talar head, which results in traumatic arthritis.

If multiple joints are involved in arthritis and are symptomatic, this is a contraindication to surgery. Likewise, collapse of the foot in pronation due to hyperflexion or from tarsometatarsal arthritis will not be improved by this arthrodesis.

Age is not a factor in the adult since symptoms can occur at any time due to the variety of conditions that cause pain and deformity at the talonavicular joint.

PREOPERATIVE PLANNING

Discussion of the indications, technical aspects of the procedure, and realistic expectations including some limited motion in the hindfoot and midfoot are presented to the patient. Alternative treatment such as orthotics, antiinflammatory medications and shoe modifications should be mentioned as well as the consequences of not having surgery.

G. J. Sammarco, M.D.: The Center for Orthopaedic Care, Inc., Cincinnati, OH 45219.

The foot is examined to determine that localized tenderness is present at the talonavicular joint. Injection with 1% lidocaine 2 cc into the joint confirms the diagnosis when pain is relieved. Collapse of the longitudinal arch of the foot with a prominant head of the talus may be palpable medially. Radiographic evaluation including weight-bearing anterior, posterior, and lateral views of the foot and an oblique view of the foot is done to confirm the presence of talonavicular arthritis and the presence of other bony lesions that might contribute to the patient's symptoms.

Symptoms of pain and clinical deformity are more important than "anatomic alignment." The actual measured degrees of alignment on radiographs are of less importance than the clinical change noted by the patient and joint destruction on the radiographs.

SURGERY

This surgery is performed on an outpatient basis under general or spinal anesthesia. This should be done in an operating room equipped to treat emergencies encountered during anesthesia. Instrumentation should include those instruments used in foot surgery such as a set of small osteotomes (2 to 15 mm in size), small surgical scapels (Bard-Parker #15 blades), small scissors (Converse), and a mini C-arm image intensifier x-ray machine (Xitek). The author prefers to use the protection of a lead apron and protective lead operative rubber gloves as well as a face shield. A tourniquet set at 300 mm Hg is used on the thigh. Cast material should be available to immobilize the foot following surgery.

The patient is positioned supine on the operating table. Under general or spinal anesthesia and thigh tourniquet control, the lower extremity is prepped and draped to insure asepsis. In selected high-risk patients, an ankle block may be used.

A 5-cm long linear incision is made over the medial aspect of the navicular tuberosity and head of the talus just above the insertion of the tibialis posterior tendon (Fig. 1). The soft tissues are dissected down to the joint capsule.

Technique. The tibialis posterior tendon is identified at its superior border and examined to insure that no gross evidence of disruption is present (Fig. 2). The dorsal attachment of the capsule overlying the talonavicular joint is stripped from its attachments on the navicular body. The head of the talus is then exposed, using a metatarsal head retractor. Following this, a 10-mm osteotome is used to remove the articular surface of the navicular and talar head opposing articular surfaces (Fig. 3). As dissection proceeds, starting from the medial side, the articu-

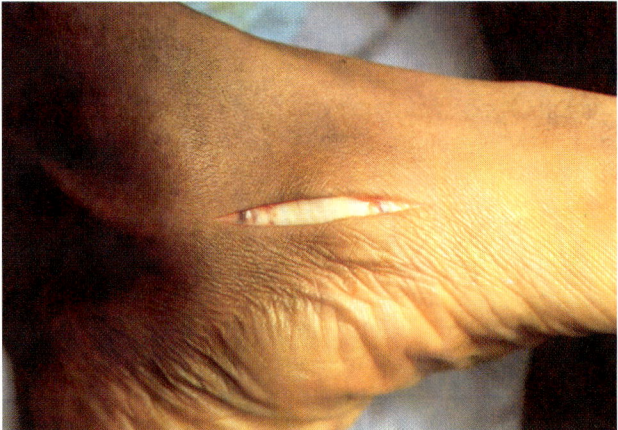

Figure 1. Surgical incision 5 cm long centered over the navicular tuberosity. Toes are to the right.

19 TALONAVICULAR ARTHRODESIS

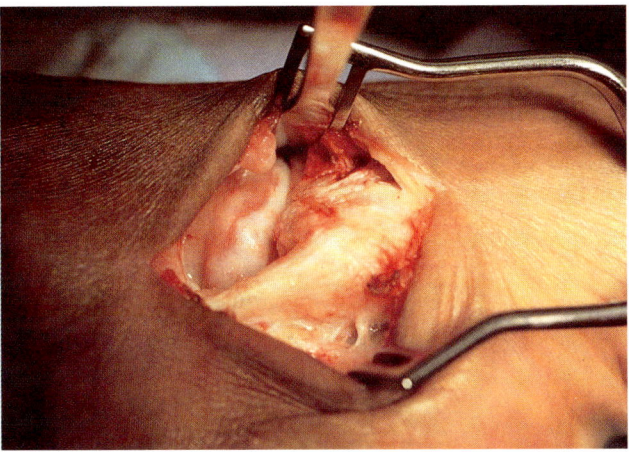

Figure 2. Soft tissue dissection is performed to expose the talonavicular joint *(center)*. The posterior tibial tendon is in the lower half of the operative field.

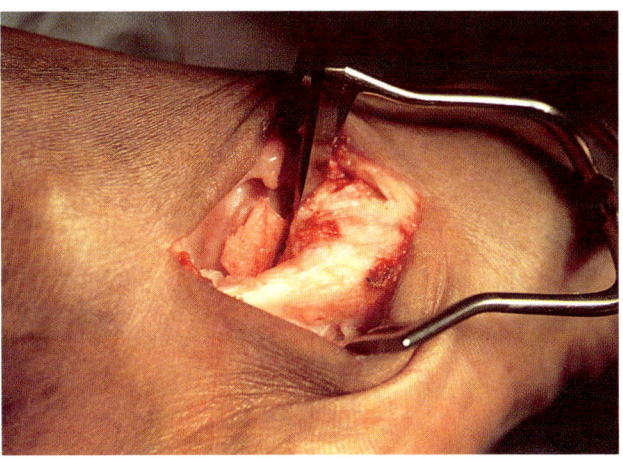

Figure 3. The articular surfaces of the joint are removed with an osteotome *(upper center)* down to subchondral bone.

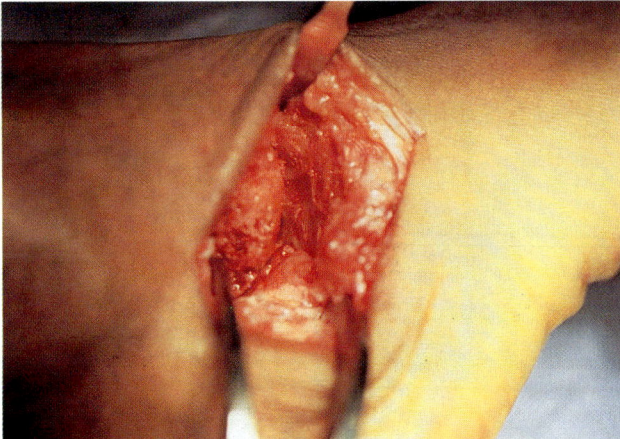
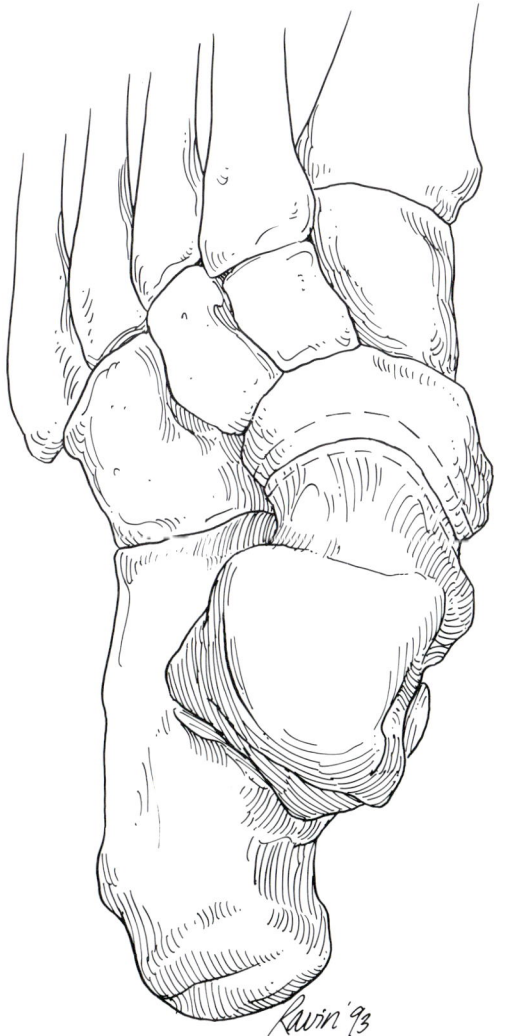

Figure 4. A: As the deeper portions of the joint become visible, curettes and a rongeur are used to remove the cartilaginous debris. The deep articular surface is visible on both the talar head and navicular. An Inge retractor (in interior part of wound) is used to distract the talonavicular joint. **B:** The approximate site of bone resection is shown.

lar surface including subchondral bone is excised. An Inge retractor (self-retaining cervical lamina spreader) is inserted to expose the depths of the wound including the lateral portions of the navicular and talar head (Fig. 4). Curved and straight curettes are used to remove additional articular cartilage and subchondral bone.

A 3-cm longitudinal incision then is made over the distal medial aspect of the tibial metaphysis. The incision is carried down through the soft tissues to the periosteum, which is split, and a 1 × 2 cm cortical bone window is removed. Osteotomes and curettes are used to harvest cancellous bone graft (Fig. 5). The bone window is then replaced and a closure made with absorbable 3-0 suture in the subcutaneous tissue and with a subcuticular 4-0 absorbable suture on the skin. The bone graft is placed into the talonavicular articulation and packed with 2- and 4-mm impactors. When this is complete, a 2-mm guide pin is inserted from the medial inferior aspect of the navicular body, across the joint and into the talar neck (Fig. 6). The position of the pin is checked with an image intensifier. A countersink is used to allow the screw head and washer to be seated in the navicular. A cannulated 45-mm long, 4.5-mm diameter cancellous self-tapping titanium lag screw with washer (Ace) is then inserted. This is checked with an image intensifier again for position and to ensure compression is achieved at the joint surface (Figs. 7 and 8).

The deep tissues are reapproximated with 3-0 absorbable suture and the skin is closed with 4-0 subcuticular absorbable suture. Steri-strips and a dressing of a 4" × 4" sponge folded once are placed over the wound. A compression dressing and a short leg cast are applied following which the tourniquet is released and the patient is awakened and transferred to the recovery room.

POSTOPERATIVE MANAGEMENT

This procedure is performed as outpatient surgery. The patient ambulates with crutches. Follow-up includes an office visit 3 days postoperatively. The cast and dressing are changed and radiographs obtained to check bony alignment. A removable cast boot is prescribed. This is locked at 0° motion for the first month. The cast boot (Air Cast) is removed for bathing only. After 4 weeks, 10° of plantar flexion and 10° of dorsiflexion are programmed into the cast boot. At 8 weeks postoperatively, an isometric exercise program also is instituted and 40% weight bearing is permitted. After 10 weeks, full weight bearing is permitted if healing is complete. The patient is usually permitted to wear the shoes of choice 12 weeks postoperatively.

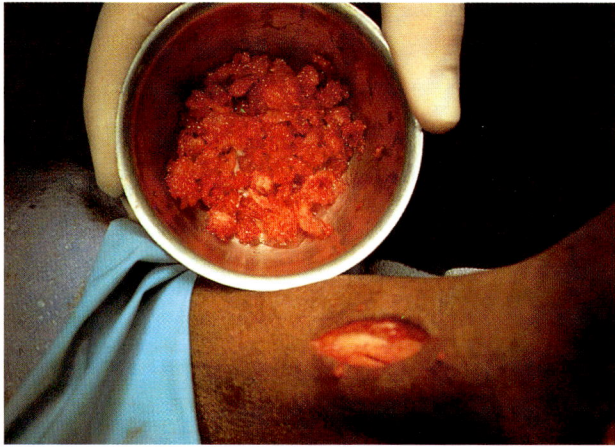

Figure 5. Through a 3-cm incision above the ankle, a bone window is removed and cancellous bone harvested.

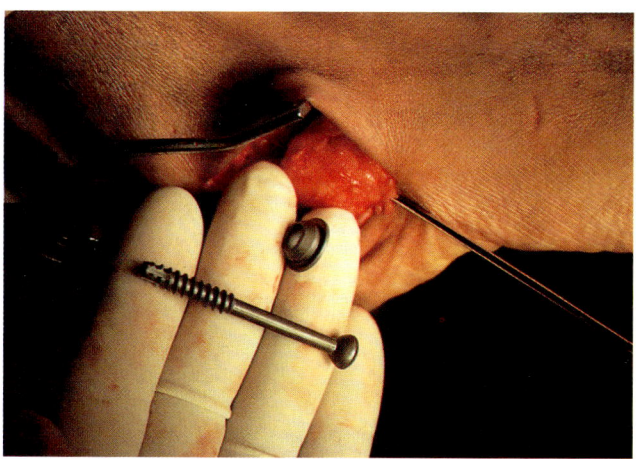

Figure 6. A guide pin is inserted axially through the navicular into the talar head and neck. A 45-mm long, 4.5-mm diameter self-tapping titanium compression cannulated lag screw (Ace) with a washer are chosen. The position of the guide pin is checked with radiography.

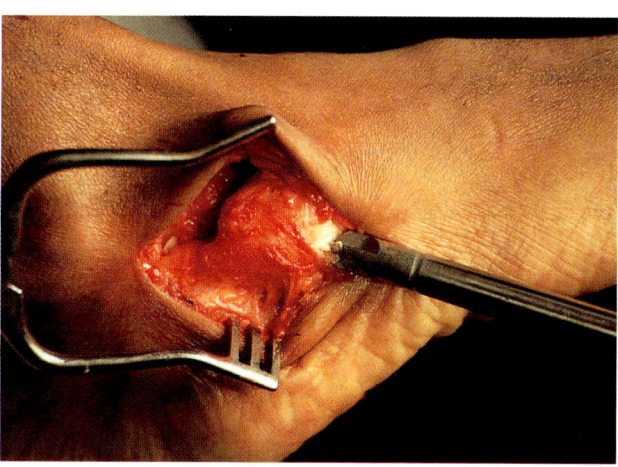

Figure 7. A cannulated countersink (Ace) inserted over the guide pin is used to prepare the navicular to receive the head of the screw and washer.

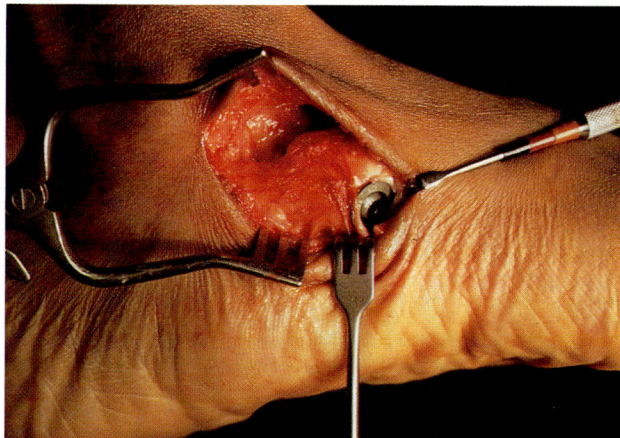
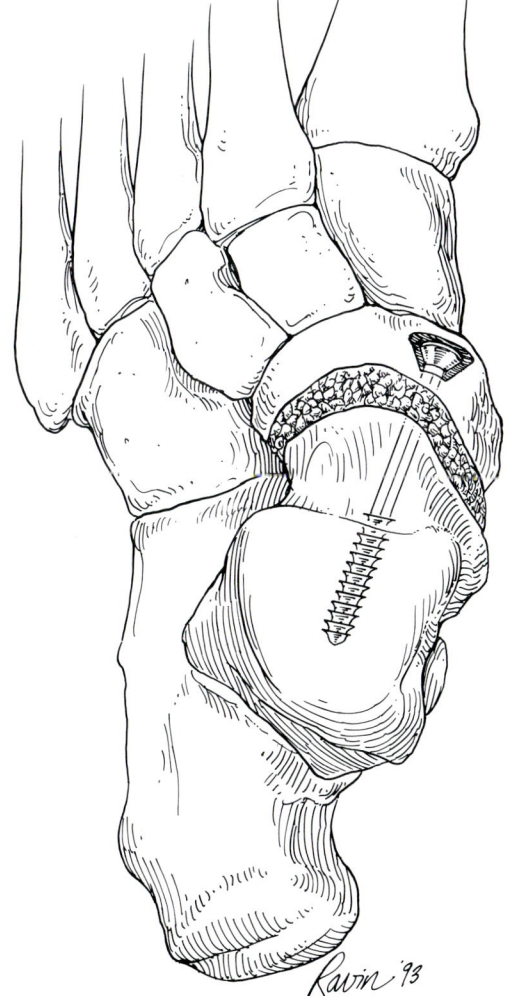

Figure 8. A: The compression screw and washer in place after bone graft has been inserted into the joint. **B:** The morcellated bone graft maintains medial column length and conforms to the irregular arthrodesis site.

COMPLICATIONS

1. *Nonunion.* The most common complication of talonavicular arthrodesis is nonunion, which can occur in up to 10% of cases. The relatively small tarsal navicular with rather dense bone contributes to the delay in healing. The high stresses that are produced across the joint and a noncompliant patient can contribute to this. Screw breakage, although uncommon, can occur. A titanium screw has the ability to bend more than a stainless steel one does and is the material of choice. These screws, however, have been known to break also, usually at the screw/shaft junction. If nonunion exists, collapse of the arch may develop with a resultant flatfoot deformity. This may require revision surgery combining subtalar arthrodesis with the talonavicular revision arthrodesis. The most common symptom in a patient with a nonunion is pain at the site of failed fusion. If no loss of position has occurred, and this is associated on radiography only with loosening of the screw fixation, the screw may be advanced to increase compression at the joint line. If necessary, additional bone graft may be harvested from the proximal tibia to be added in the nonunion site. Staple fixation also may be used to supplement screw fixation.

    In some conditions, such as chronic tear of the tibialis posterior tendon, the longitudinal arch may collapse in spite of a successful arthrodesis. It is then necessary to perform an additional subtalar arthrodesis in order to stabilize the hindfoot. The resulting double arthrodesis is quite functional.

2. *Malunion.* Malunion is usually the result of improper alignment in performing the initial surgery or the consequence of a collapsing joint following infection, or the ultimate position of a delayed union after it has healed. Treatment options include osteotomy of the malunion with or without extension of the arthrodesis to include the subtalar and/or calcaneocuboid joints. The decision as to the extent of the arthrodesis depends on the clinical alignment of the foot preoperatively and the ability to achieve a plantar-grade foot during revision surgery.

3. *Neuroma/Infection.* Another problem is incisional neuroma caused by excessive traction on the cutaneus branches of the superficial peroneal nerve. Injection with cortisone into the neuroma may be of benefit. However, care should be exercised so as not to create subcutaneous tissue atrophy and loss of skin pigmentation. The patient should be counseled prior to injection. If this fails, simple excision of the neuroma is suggested. Infection is treated with appropriate antibiotics chosen after aerobic and anaerobic cultures are obtained. If osteomyelitis occurs, prolonged immobilization and antibiotics with or without surgical debridement is indicated. Antibiotics are continued until clinical and radiographic evidence of healing is present.

ILLUSTRATIVE CASE FOR TECHNIQUE

A 45-year-old man described pain over the medial aspect of his foot anterior to the ankle on the left. As a teenager, he played sports but could not remember specific injuries to his foot. Over the ensuing years, a hard knot appeared in front of his ankle above the arch of the foot. Until the last year, the deformity was of no consequence and did not affect fitting shoes but the pain gradually increased, making it difficult for him to stand for longer than 2 hours.

Examination of the left foot revealed tenderness over the talonavicular joint with bony osteophytes palpable superiorly and a slight sagging of the longitudinal arch of the foot when weight bearing.

Weight-bearing radiographs revealed osteophytes on the talus and navicular with some increased bone density noted in the navicular (Fig. 9).

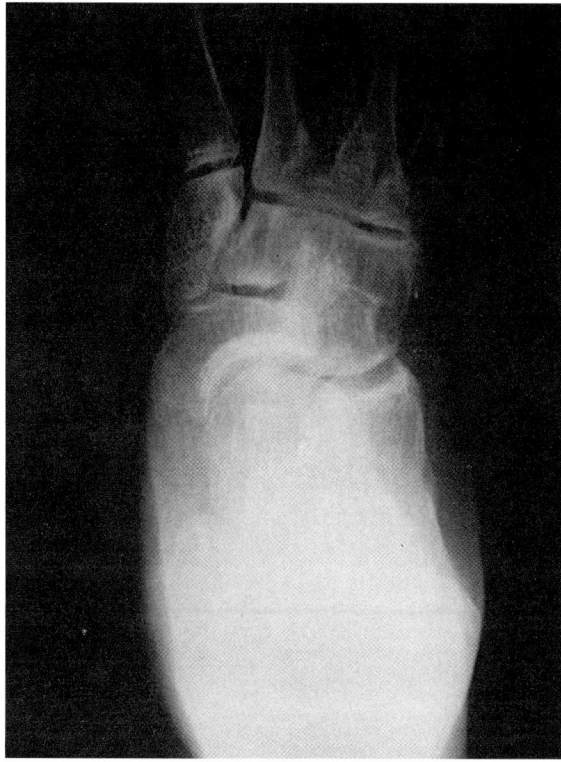
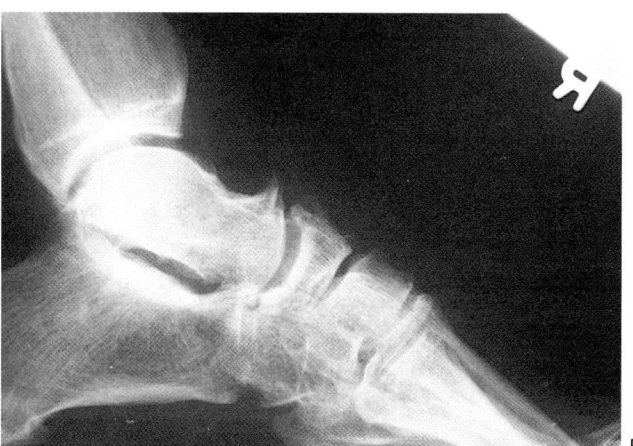

Figure 9. Preoperative AP **(A)** and lateral **(B)** radiographs of a 45-year-old man with pain in the medial midfoot. Decreased joint space, sclerosis, and osteophytes are present in the talonavicular joint. Arthritic changes in the other joints were present but asymptomatic. Local anesthetic injected into the talonavicular joint gave almost complete relief of pain.

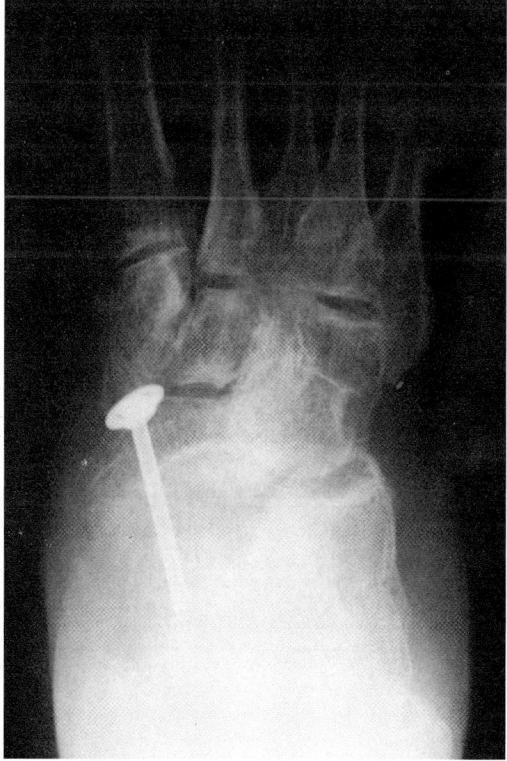
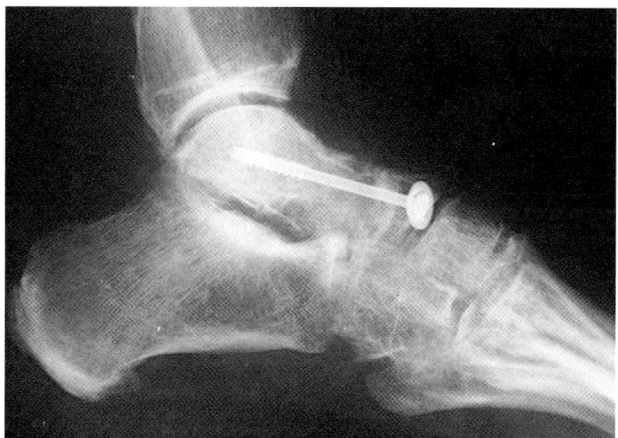

Figure 10. Postoperative AP **(A)** and lateral **(B)** radiographs of the patient in Fig. 9 after successful arthrodesis. The patient was asymptomatic 1 year later.

An injection of 2 cc of lidocaine into the talonavicular joint dramatically relieved the symptoms of pain. A talonavicular arthrodesis with screw fixation was performed as an outpatient surgical procedure under general anesthesia. He was discharged the same day in a cast.

The cast was changed on the first postoperative visit 3 days later. The wound was examined and a new cast applied. The patient was seen regularly on subsequent visits and by 12 weeks postoperatively the arthrodesis was complete and the patient was allowed full weight bearing. At 16 weeks postoperatively, the patient was wearing the shoe of his choice and able to tolerate full weight bearing during the entire day.

At follow-up 1 year following surgery, he was asymptomatic. Radiographs revealed arthrodesis of the talonavicular joint to be complete and no motion or tenderness at the operative site (Fig. 10). He was satisfied and without limitation on activity or shoe selection.

RECOMMENDED READING

1. Adam, W., and Ranawat, C.: Arthrodesis of the hindfoot in rheumatoid arthritis. *Orthop. Clin. North Am.,* 7: 827–840, 1976.
2. Cracchiolo, A.: Surgical arthrodesis techniques for foot and ankle pathology. *Instr. Course Lect.,* 39: 49–63, 1990.
3. Dalziel, R., Thornhill, T. S., and Thomas, W. H.: Isolated talonavicular fusion for hindfoot arthritis. *Orthop. Trans.,* 6: 341, 1982.
4. Elbaor, J. E., Thomas, W. H., Weinfeld, M. S., and Potter, T. A.: Talonavicular arthrodesis for rheumatoid arthritis of the hindfoot. *Orthop. Clin. North Am.,* 7: 821–826, 1976.
5. Gellman, H., Lenihan, M., Halikis, N., Botte, M. J., Giordani, M., and Perry, J.: Selective tarsal arthrodesis: an in vitro analysis of the effect on foot motion. *Foot Ankle,* 8(3): 127–133, 1987.
6. Ljung, P., Kaij, J., Knutson, K., Pettersson, H., and Rydholm, U.: Talonavicular arthrodesis in the rheumatoid foot. *Foot Ankle,* 13(6): 313–316, 1992.
7. Ruff, M. E., and Turner, R. H.: Selective hindfoot arthrodesis in rheumatoid arthritis. *Orthopedics,* 7: 49–54, 1984.

20

Compartment Releases of the Foot

Arthur Manoli II

INDICATIONS/CONTRAINDICATIONS

Many traumatic injuries of the foot result in severe pain and swelling. Multiple fractures and/or dislocations and fractures as a result of high-energy injuries (calcaneal fractures) may produce blood and interstitial fluid accumulation within the rigid, fascial confines of the compartments of the foot. As seen in compartment syndromes elsewhere in the body, the pressure built up in the compartments may result in muscle necrosis with subsequent scar formation and the formation of contractures of the soft tissues and nerve dysfunction. Early fasciotomy, performed soon after the diagnosis of foot compartment syndrome is made, minimizes the chance of developing late contracture and nerve dysfunction.

Severe injuries of the foot, particularly those with multiple fractures or an element of crushing, are prone to develop foot compartment syndrome. Tense foot swelling that develops after an injury should alert the practitioner to the possibility of a compartment syndrome. Severe pain, pain with passive stretch of the foot muscles (toe dorsiflexion stretches the plantar muscles), and nerve dysfunction (paresthesias, muscle paralysis) may be seen, but are thought to be less diagnostic in the foot than elsewhere. The direct measurement of compartmental pressures is suggested in suspicious instances to confirm the diagnosis of foot compartment syndrome. The presence or absence of the peripheral pulses is of no use in diagnosing foot compartment syndrome.

A. Manoli II, M.D.: Department of Orthopedic Surgery, Wayne State University, Detroit, MI 48202; and Department of Orthopedic Surgery, Hutzel Hospital, Detroit, MI 48201.

PREOPERATIVE PLANNING

Catheterization of the compartments of the foot can be done using any of the well-known established apparatuses. In recent years, the development of portable pressure monitors (PressureSense Monitor, Ace Medical Co., Los Angeles, CA, or Digital Quickset, Stryker Corp., Kalamazoo, MI) has made the measurement of pressures much easier. They may be performed almost anywhere with ease and accuracy.

The pressures within the compartments of the foot may be measured using local, infiltrative anesthesia (Fig. 1). In the hindfoot, the medial compartmental pressure is measured with a stick approximately 4 cm inferior to the medial malleolus, over the abductor hallucis muscle (Fig. 2). After the pressure in the medial compartment is taken, the needle is advanced throughout the medial intermuscular septum of the foot into the deep hindfoot compartment, the calcaneal. Here, the pressure is often found to be the highest.

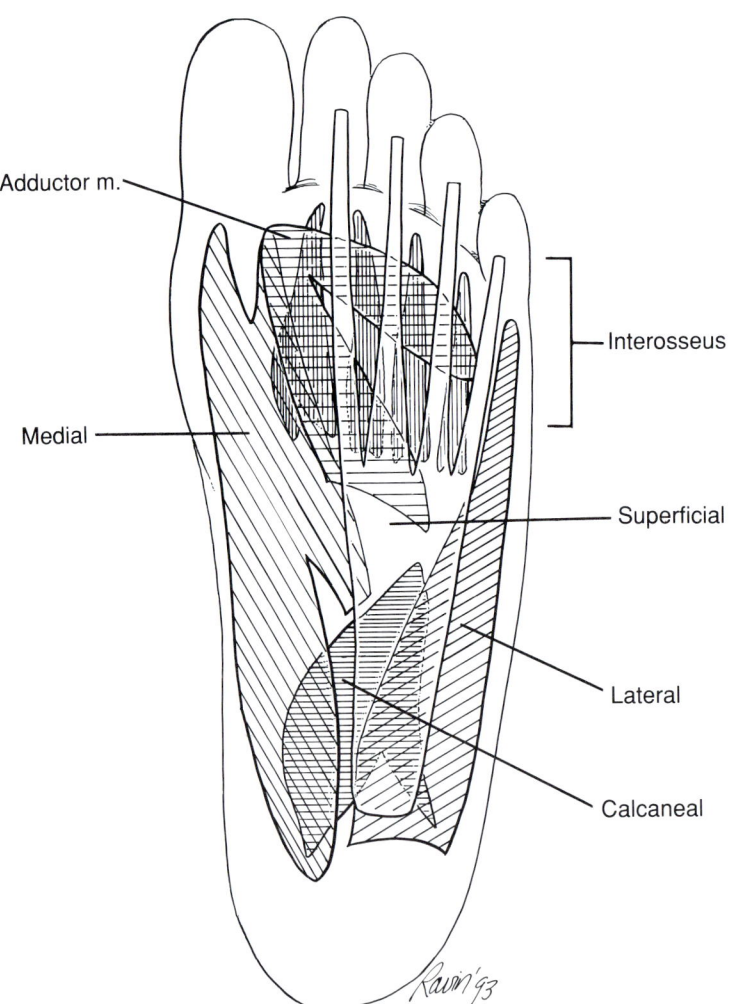

Figure 1. A plantar view of the compartments of the foot. The medial superficial and lateral run the entire length of the foot. The adductor and four interosseous compartments are located in the forefoot only. The calcaneal compartment is situated in the hindfoot. (Redrawn and reprinted from ref. 6, with permission. Copyright by W. B. Saunders Company.)

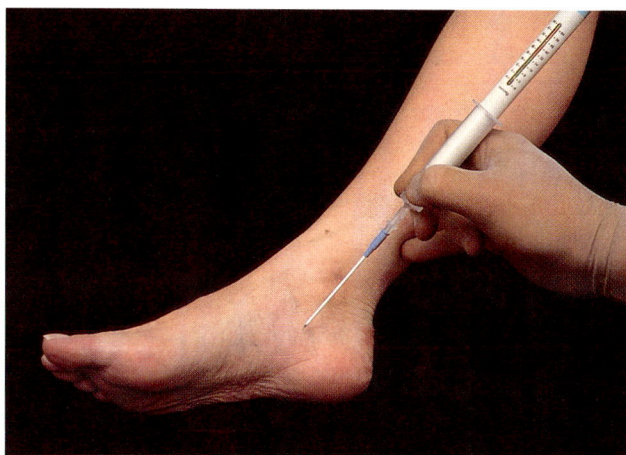

Figure 2. The medial stick, 4 cm below the medial malleolus, measures the pressure in the medial and calcaneal compartments.

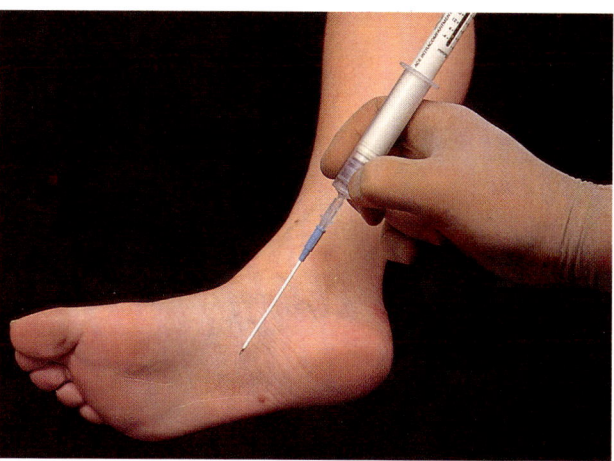

Figure 3. On the plantar surface of the foot, in the arch area, the superficial compartmental pressure is measured. This compartment contains the flexor digitorum brevis muscle.

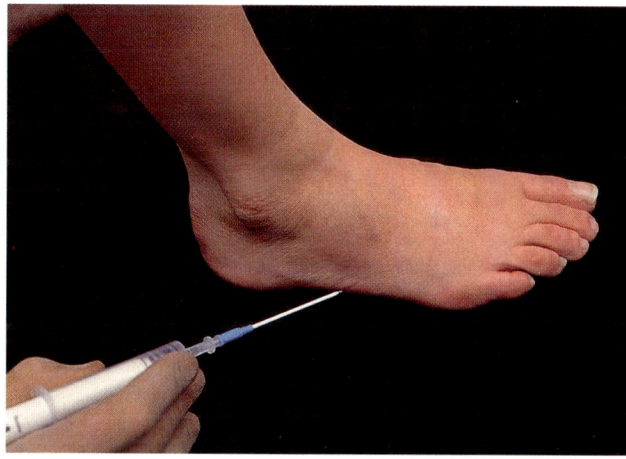

Figure 4. The lateral stick is just below the fifth metatarsal base. It measures the pressure in the lateral compartment.

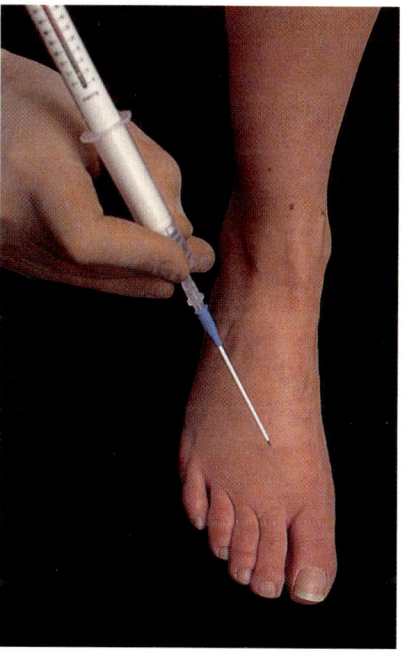

Figure 5. A stick in the first or second interspace measures the pressure in that space. Advancement of the needle deeper into the forefoot measures the pressure in the adductor compartment.

The needle is removed and reinserted into the flexor digitorum brevis muscle in the arch, measuring the superficial compartment (Fig. 3).

A third stick, on the lateral aspect of the foot, just below the fifth metatarsal, measures the pressure in the lateral compartment (Fig. 4).

Any or all of the separate interosseous compartments can be sampled in the forefoot. It is recommended that at least one of the first and second interosseous compartments be measured (Fig. 5). Here, if the needle is advanced deeply between the respective metatarsals, the pressure in the adductor compartment can also be measured.

Although the absolute pressure at which fasciotomy should be performed continues to be an unknown, certain guidelines have been developed. Some authors recommend performing a fasciotomy for pressures exceeding 30 mm Hg. Whitesides et al. (12) suggest that they be performed for pressures greater than 10 to 30 mm Hg below diastolic blood pressure. Schneck et al.'s (11) recent study has indicated that metabolic dysfunction is severe when the pressure exceeds 30 to 40 mm Hg below mean arterial pressure. Certainly the patient's overall metabolic status, circulatory status (blood pressure and pulse), and the clinical evaluation must also be considered. Hypotensive patients, usually from polytrauma, generally have a greater risk of developing compartmental syndromes at lower pressures. The duration of increased pressure and pressure trends may also be helpful.

The antiquated notions that "foot compartment syndromes don't exist," that "the foot can tolerate higher pressures than other parts of the body," and that

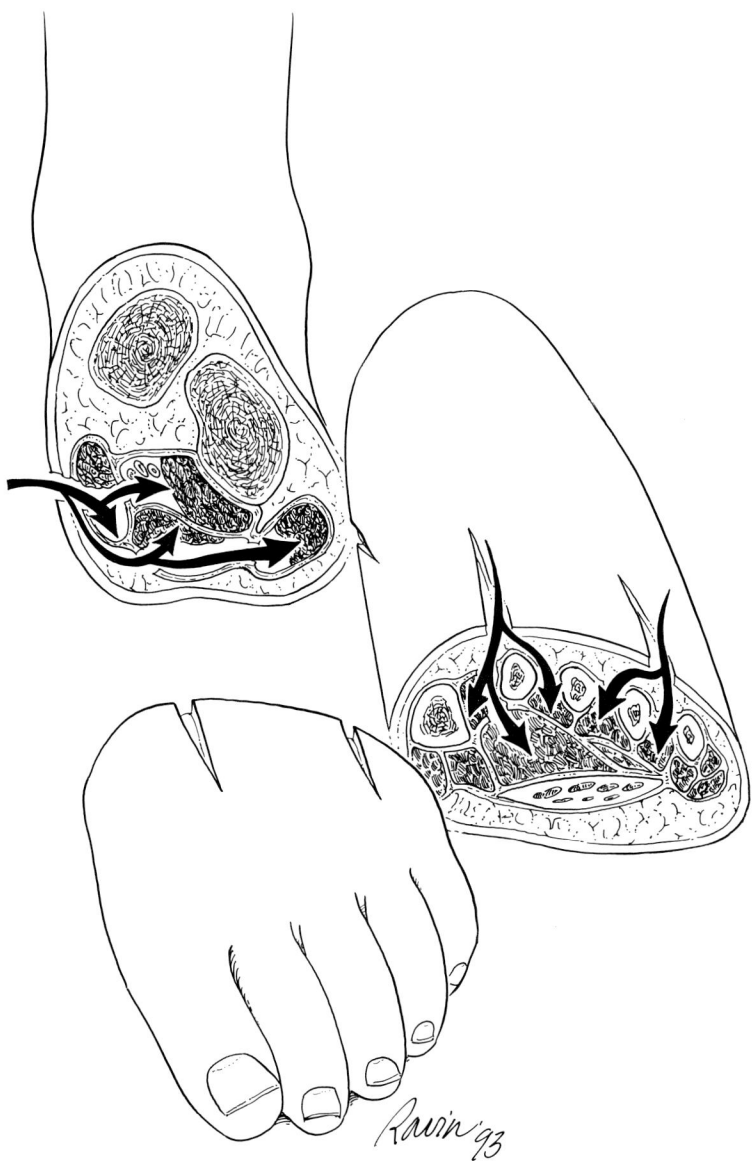

Figure 6. Summary of the surgical approach. Two dorsal forefoot incisions and one medial hindfoot incision are used to decompress the foot compartments. (Redrawn and reprinted from ref. 7, with permission. Copyright by American Orthopaedic Foot and Ankle Society.)

the late sequelae are "not too bad," should be abandoned. In a recent study, Mittlmeier et al. (9) have shown that 11 of 16 feet that had measured pressures greater than 30 mm Hg after calcaneal fractures developed rigid toe clawing, plantar scarring, cavus, sensory disturbances, and significant disability.

SURGERY

Foot fasciotomy may be performed under regional or general anesthesia. The patient is positioned supine on the operating table. A tourniquet is used to insure a bloodless field. Either a thigh or a lower leg tourniquet may be used.

Technique. A three-incision fasciotomy is used to decompress the compartments of the foot (Fig. 6). A medial hindfoot incision is used to decompress the deeply situated calcaneal compartment, and the compartments that run the entire length of the foot (medial, lateral, and superficial). This incision begins approximately 4 cm from the back of the heel and 3 cm from the plantar surface (Fig. 7). It extends distally over the abductor hallucis muscle for a distance of approximately 6 cm. After the skin and subcutaneous tissue are divided, the very thin fascia over the abductor hallucis muscle is encountered and opened the length of the incision (Fig. 8). Undermining the skin slightly in the distal portion of the incision allows for the majority of the medial compartment to be released. Following this, the inferior portion of the abductor hallucis muscle is defined. A small elevator is

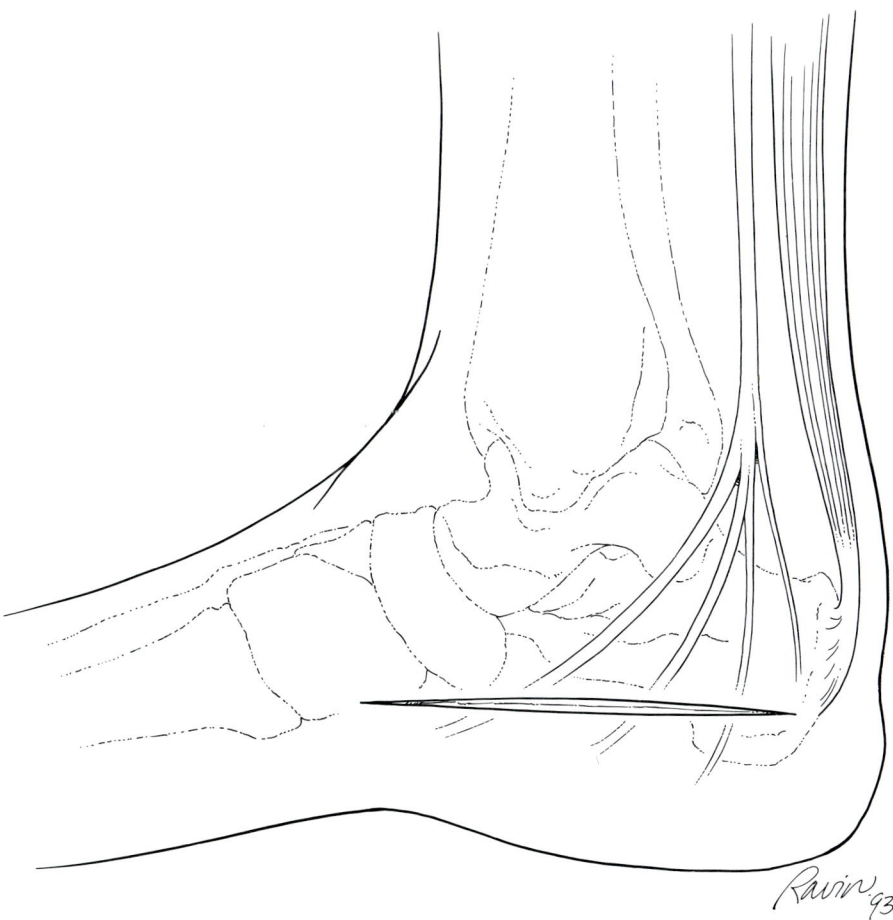

Figure 7. The hindfoot incision starts approximately 4 cm from the back of the heel, and 3 cm from the plantar surface of the foot. It extends for a distance of about 6 cm distally. (Redrawn and reprinted from ref. 6, with permission. Copyright by W. B. Saunders Company.)

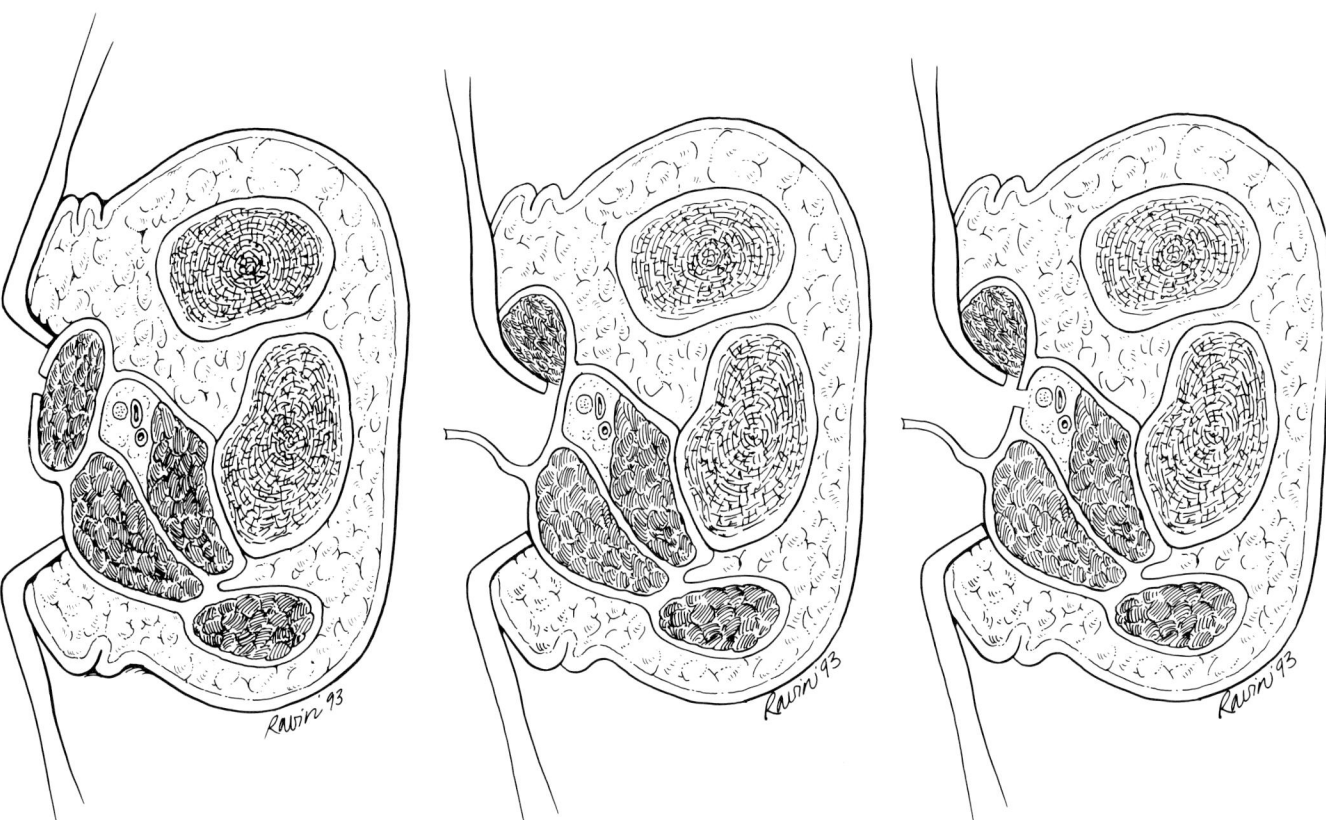

Figure 8. This hindfoot section illustrates the release of the medial compartment (see text). (Redrawn and reprinted from ref. 6, with permission. Copyright by W. B. Saunders Company.)

Figure 9. The abductor hallucis muscle is retracted superiorly. The medial intermuscular septum of the foot is then observed. (Redrawn and reprinted from ref. 6, with permission. Copyright by W. B. Saunders Company.)

Figure 10. The medial intermuscular septum is opened. The lateral plantar neurovascular bundle lies just deep to the septum in the calcaneal compartment. The quadratus plantae muscle may bulge considerably around these vessels as the calcaneal compartment is released (see Fig. 11). (Redrawn and reprinted from ref. 6, with permission. Copyright by W. B. Saunders Company.)

useful and the muscle is lifted dorsally from the inferior portion of its investing fascia. Retracting the muscle upward, one encounters the thick, glistening white, intermuscular septum of the foot (Fig. 9). This is the medial border of the deeper, calcaneal compartment. Occasionally a headlamp may be useful during this part of the procedure.

The calcaneal compartment is released by opening the intermuscular septum (Fig. 10). This is done by first poking a small hole through the septum and carefully opening it with either a small dissecting scissors or a knife. Great care is necessary at this point to avoid any injury to the lateral plantar nerve or blood vessels that lie immediately under the septum. The septum should be opened for the length of the skin incision. If one wishes to open the septum more distally in the foot, it is suggested to use the gloved finger to "push" it open, separating the fibers. As the medial plantar nerve and vessels run either in the calcaneal compartment, superficial compartment, or actually in the septum itself in the middle of the foot, a blunt technique is suggested here to avoid injury to these structures. Considerable bulging of the quadratus plantae muscle may occur when this fascia is opened. The muscle may bulge considerably around the lateral plantar nerve and artery (Fig. 11). If encountered, this bulging is suggestive of an adequate release of the

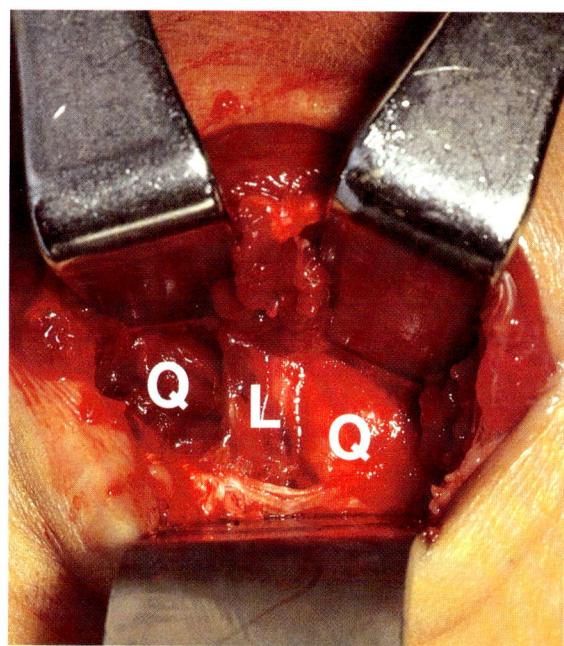

Figure 11. The quadratus plantae muscle (Q) is seen bulging proximally and distally to the lateral plantar neurovascular bundle (L).

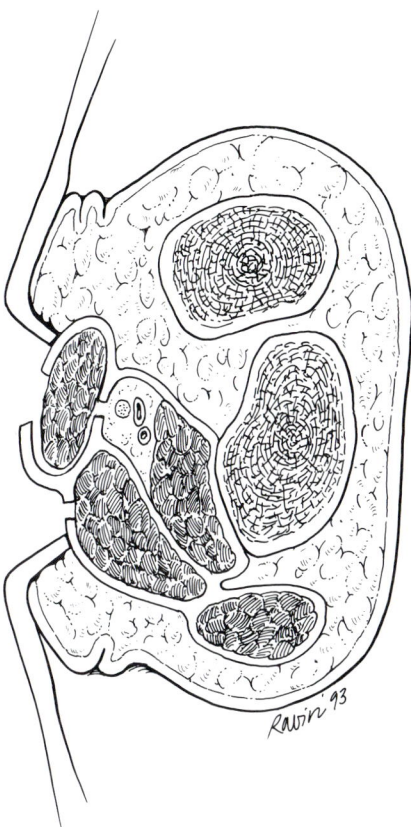

Figure 12. The superficial compartment is identified on the plantar surface of the foot and is opened longitudinally. The flexor digitorum brevis muscle is then seen. (Redrawn and reprinted from ref. 6, with permission. Copyright by W. B. Saunders Company.)

calcaneal compartment. The retractors are removed from this portion of the approach and the abductor muscle is allowed to return to its usual position.

Dissection then continues outside of the medial compartment in the plantarward direction. The investing fascia of the abductor hallucis muscle is followed plantarward retracting the fat from the medial side of the heel medially. On the plantar aspect of the foot the superficial compartment is then encountered. This compartment is opened longitudinally, releasing the flexor digitorum brevis muscle (Fig. 12). The soft tissues may be undermined distally to insure that the superficial compartment is opened completely.

The flexor digitorum brevis muscle is then separated from the fascia overlying the dorsum of the compartment (the transverse septum of the hindfoot) and the flexor digitorum brevis muscle is retracted plantarward (Fig. 13). As the flexor digitorum brevis muscle is retracted, the medical aspect of the lateral compartment is identified. This medial border of the lateral compartment is the lateral intermuscular septum of the foot. As one follows this septum posteriorly, it is noted that the lateral compartment actually sweeps medially in the posterior aspect of the heel.

The lateral compartment is best opened by using either a small dissecting scissors or a sharp elevator beginning in the posterior aspect of the compartment and extending anteriorly to the middle of the foot (Fig. 14). When the lateral compartment is released the abductor digiti quinti muscle and flexor digiti minimi muscle are visible.

The muscular compartments of the forefoot are then released. Generally this is done through two separate longitudinal incisions located slightly medial to the second metatarsal and slightly lateral to the fourth metatarsal, to insure as wide a skin bridge as possible. Although theoretically these incisions may compromise the skin on the dorsum of the foot, sloughing in this area has only been seen when the skin was already injured, as in a crush injury. If one is concerned about the viability of the skin bridge in cases of crush injury of the forefoot, an alternate lateral skin incision may be made. This is a small transverse incision over the distal one-third of the fourth metatarsal. Undermining the skin proximally allows one to release the interosseous compartments in the third and fourth interspace without compromising the skin viability.

Through the medial incision the dorsal interosseous muscles that lie in the first and second interspaces are identified (Fig. 15A). The thin dorsal fascia is opened using either a small scissors or a sharp elevator. Next the muscles of the first interspace are stripped off of the medial portion of the second metatarsal, along the length of the metatarsal (Fig. 15B,C). As the interosseous muscles are retracted medially, the fascia of the adductor musculature is identified deep in the interspace. This fascia is then opened longitudinally, preferably with an elevator (Fig. 15B,C). Through the lateral forefoot incision the dorsal fascia of the third and fourth interosseous muscles are identified and these interosseous compartments are opened longitudinally (Fig. 15A).

After the fasciotomy is completed, any fractures of the forefoot or midfoot can

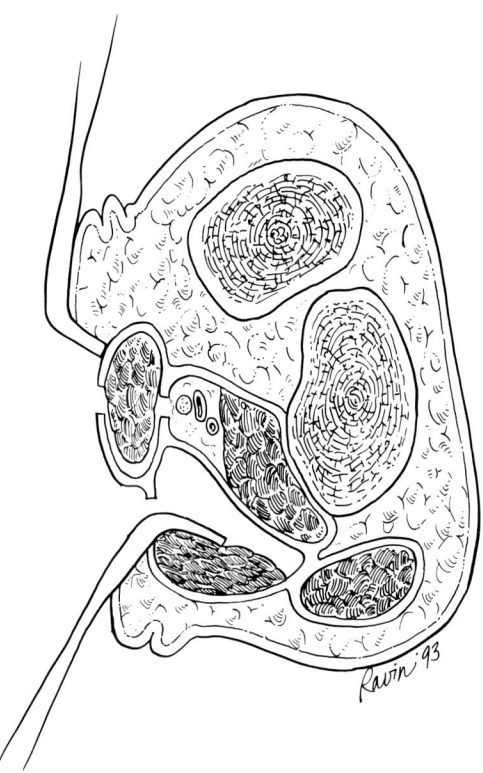

Figure 13. The flexor digitorum brevis muscle is retracted plantarward. The lateral intermuscular septum is identified, overlying the lateral compartment. (Redrawn and reprinted from ref. 6, with permission. Copyright by W. B. Saunders Company.)

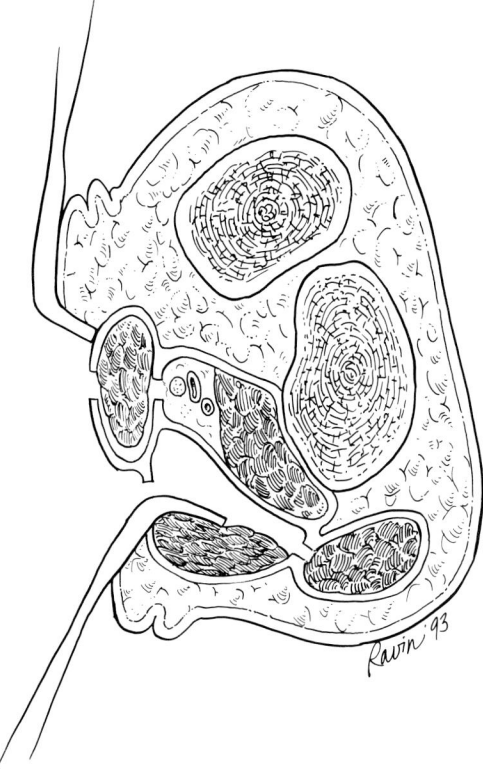

Figure 14. The lateral compartment is released longitudinally.

20 COMPARTMENT RELEASES OF THE FOOT

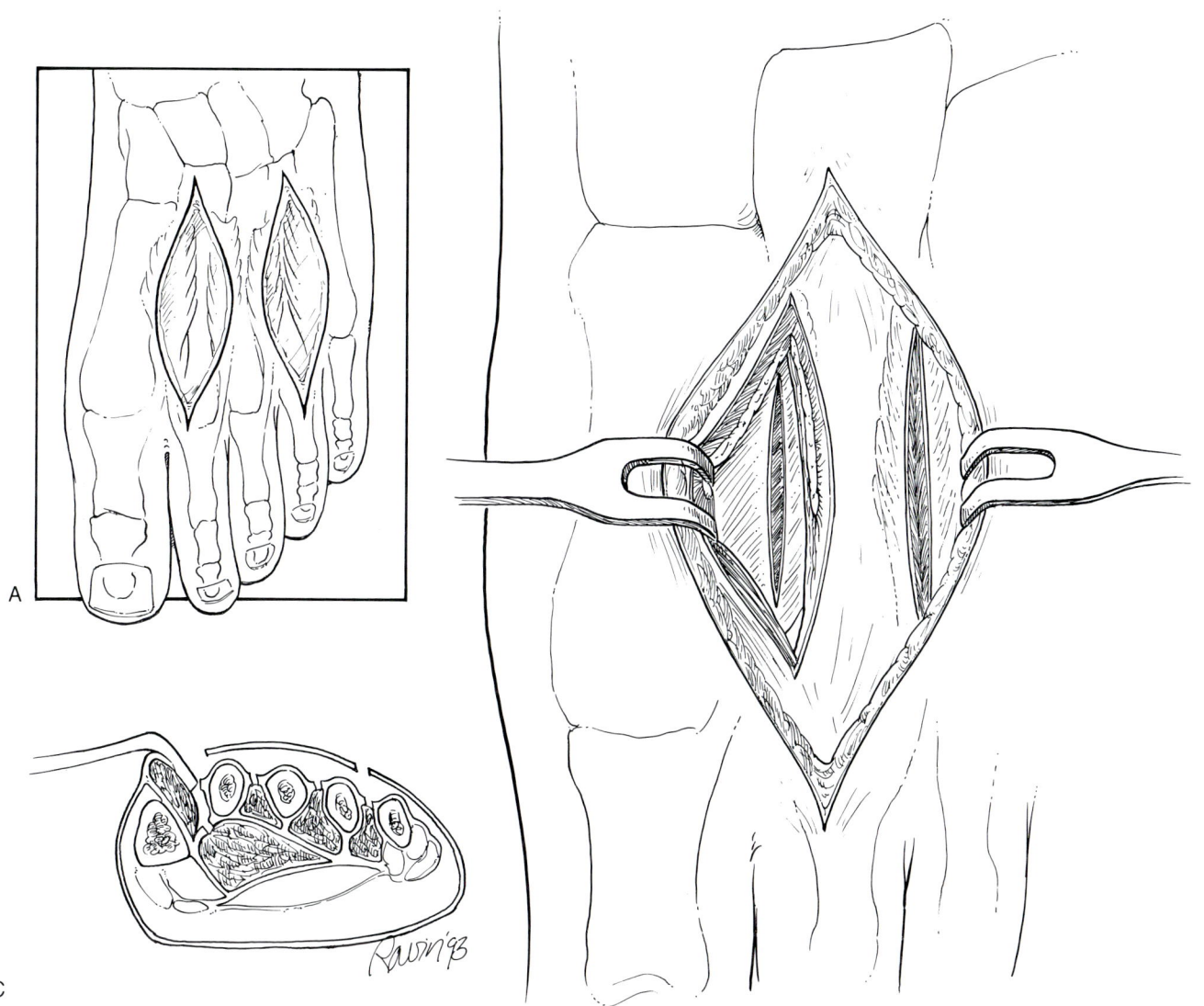

Figure 15. A: Two incisions are made approximately over the second and fourth metatarsal shafts. This allows for the individual interosseous compartments to be opened. **B:** The interosseous muscles are stripped from the medial surface of the second metatarsal shaft and the fascia overlying the adductor muscle is seen. The adductor fascia is then opened longitudinally. **C:** Cross section of A and B.

be treated through the forefoot incisions. It may be necessary to extend them proximally or distally. Fractures of the talus of ankle may be approached through additional standard incisions. It is suggested, however, that a comminuted fracture of the calcaneus not be repaired at the time of fasciotomy. Although Rorabeck recommends that the skeleton be fixed at the time of fasciotomy in other locations to provide stability, this is probably not necessary when dealing with a calcaneal fracture. Here, stability is not generally a problem but restoration of the architecture of the calcaneus is usually the goal. Therefore, we recommend repairing a calcaneal fracture, if desired, later, through an additional lateral incision after the fasciotomy wounds are healed.

POSTOPERATIVE MANAGEMENT

The fasciotomy wounds are left open and dressed with a sterile dressing. The patients are generally returned to the operating room on the third through the fifth day postoperatively. The wounds are all irrigated and debrided as necessary. The skin may be closed at that time if the wound conditions permit. Otherwise it may be done at a later date. Split-thickness skin grafting should be used if the wound edges cannot be approximated without excessive tension. We have found it necessary to skin graft approximately one-third of the cases. These grafts are generally needed over the forefoot incisions.

COMPLICATIONS

The complications from the procedure of foot fasciotomy by themselves are minimal. The major complications tend to be from either not performing a fasciotomy or performing it too late. Clawing of the lesser toes and paresthesias in either the medial or lateral plantar nerve distribution, cavus deformity, stiffness, and residual pain are primarily seen after foot compartment syndrome without release.

The nerve damage can usually be avoided. There are three areas where nerves may be encountered and should be avoided. When making the initial skin incision, one should begin the incision at least 4 cm from the posterior aspect of the heel, to avoid the medial calcaneal branches of the tibial nerve. When opening the medial intermuscular septum of the foot, the lateral plantar vessels and nerve lie *immediately* under this fascia. Care must be taken to avoid these structures here. Finally, the medial plantar nerve and vessels lie just distal to the skin incision, either in the calcaneal or superficial compartments, or in the medial intermuscular septum itself. It has been useful to use the gloved finger to open the most distal part of the medial intermuscular septum, avoiding nerve damage here.

Although these nerves are nearby during this dissection, they appear to be consistently located and can be avoided or protected. With this approach one can actually release the lateral side of the foot (lateral compartment) from the medial side. Utilizing an approach through the superficial compartment, the medial and lateral plantar nerves are protected from the plane of dissection by the transverse hindfoot septum described by Martin (8).

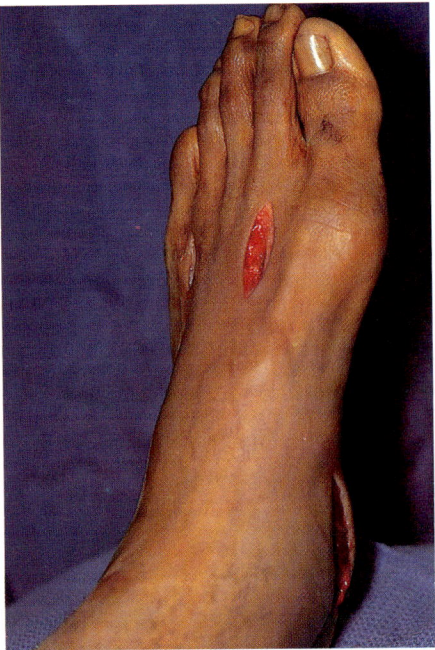

Figure 16. The incisions used to decompress this foot after a compartment syndrome developed following a calcaneal fracture.

ILLUSTRATIVE CASE FOR TECHNIQUE

A 28-year-old man jumped off a fence, sustaining a comminuted fracture of the calcaneus. After being admitted to the hospital, the patient developed severe pain in the plantar aspect of his foot. He had numbness in both the medial and lateral plantar nerve distribution on the bottom of the foot. The patient had severe pain in the hindfoot with dorsiflexion of the toes. Catheterization of the foot revealed elevated pressures in the calcaneal compartment (80 mm Hg), the medial compartment (45 mm Hg), and the lateral compartment (65 mm Hg). Six hours after his injury he was taken to the operating room where he underwent a three-incision fasciotomy of the foot (Fig. 16). There was severe bulging of the quadratus plantae muscle in the calcaneal compartment (Fig. 11).

On awakening from his anesthetic the patient had relief of this severe pain in his foot. The wounds were closed with a delayed primary closure 4 days after his injury. Fourteen days after his injury, he underwent open reduction and internal fixation with iliac crest bone grafting of the comminuted fracture of the calcaneus through a lateral incision.

RECOMMENDED READING

1. Bonutti, P. M., and Bell, G. R.: Compartment syndrome of the foot. *J. Bone Joint Surg.*, 68A: 1449–1451, 1986.
2. Bourne, R. B., and Rorabeck, C. H.: Compartment syndromes of the lower leg. *Clin. Orthop.*, 240: 97–104, 1989.
3. Fakhouri, A. J., and Manoli, A., II: Acute foot compartment syndromes. *J. Orthop. Trauma*, 6: 223–228, 1992.
4. Hargens, A. R., Akeson, W. H., Mubarak, S. J., et al.: Tissue fluid pressures: from basic research tools to clinical applications. *J. Orthop. Res.* 7: 902–909, 1989.
5. Manoli, A., II: Compartment syndromes of the foot: current concepts. *Foot Ankle*, 10: 340–344, 1990.
6. Manoli, A., II, Fakhouri, A. J., and Weber, T. G.: Compartment catheterization and fasciotomy of the foot. *Operative Tech. Orthop.*, 2: 203–210, 1992.
7. Manoli, A., II, and Weber, T. G.: Fasciotomy of the foot: an anatomical study with special reference to release of the calcaneal compartment. *Foot Ankle*, 10: 267–275, 1990.
8. Martin, B. F.: Observations on the muscles and tendons of the medial aspect of the sole of the foot. *J. Anat.*, 98: 437–453, 1964.
9. Mittlmeier, T., Machler, G., Lob, G., Mutschler, W., Bauer, G., and Vogl, T.: Compartment syndrome of the foot after intra-articular calcaneal fracture. *Clin. Orthop.*, 269: 241–248, 1991.
10. Myerson, M. S.: Diagnosis and treatment of compartment syndrome of the foot. *Orthopedics*, 13: 711–717, 1990.
11. Schneck, S., Sapega, A., Dobrasz, J., et al.: The metabolic stages in an evolving compartment syndrome. Transactions of the annual meeting. *Orthop. Res. Soc.*, 15: 261, 1990.
12. Whitesides, T. E., Henry, T. C., Morimoto, R., et al.: Tissue pressure measurements as a determinant for the need of fasciotomy. *Clin. Orthop.*, 113: 43–51, 1975.
13. Ziv, I., Mosheiff, R., Zeligowski, A., et al.: Crush injuries of the foot with compartment syndrome: immediate one-stage management. *Foot Ankle*, 9: 185–189, 1989.

PART VI

Hindfoot

21

Tibialis Posterior Tendon Release-Substitution

Kenneth A. Johnson

INDICATIONS/CONTRAINDICATIONS

Abnormalities of the tibialis posterior (TP) tendon have been classified into three stages (Table 1). Stage I denotes a tendon that is afflicted with a peritendinitis or tendinosus but that remains at its normal length. In stage II the TP tendon is elongated as a result of the inflammation/degeneration process. The hindfoot articulations in this second stage are still supple with no fixed hindfoot deformity. With weight bearing the arch of the foot may be flattened, but in a non–weight-bearing situation the normal motions in the hindfoot are present. Stage III indicates the later development of a fixed hindfoot deformity where the hindfoot is in eversion and forefoot in abduction as a result of loss of the TP tendon function.

Staging of the changes associated with dysfunction of the TP tendon is important in selecting the proper treatment. For the initial symptoms of TP inflammation conservative measures such as rest, soft arch supports, physical therapy, and oral antiinflammatory agents may be utilized. If the TP inflammation continues in spite of adequate conservative care over a period of a few months, then the stage I situation should be treated with the TP tendon release, tenosynovectomy, and debridement. It is important to realize that a persistent tenosynovitis will progress to the later stage II and III changes unless the inflammatory process is interrupted by either the nonoperative or operative measures. Because of this, surgical release should be utilized early rather than late. Recalcitrant TP tenosynovitis is a problem that should be treated surgically early even if pain is at a tolerable level.

When the tendon has elongated and a flexible secondary deformity (stage II) has developed, then in addition to the tendon release and tenosynovectomy, a transfer of the flexor digitorum longus (FDL) tendon is suggested. This tendon

---

K. A. Johnson, M.D.: Division of Foot and Ankle Surgery, Mayo Clinic Scottsdale, Scottsdale, AZ 85259.

TABLE 1. *Stages of posterior tibial tendon disease and treatment*

	Abnormality	Tendon length	Hindfoot deformity	Treatment
Stage I	Tenosynovitis tendinosis—mild	Normal	No	Release—synovectomy debridement
Stage II	Tenosynovitis and tendinosis—moderate	Elongated	Yes—supple	Release—synovectomy debridement—FDL transfer
Stage III	Tendinosis—marked	Elongated	Yes—fixed	Subtalar arthrodesis

FDL, flexor digitorum longus tendon.

transfer will substitute partially for the loss of the TP tendon function. This "window" of opportunity for the tendon transfer is probably relatively brief since after tendon elongation the development of fixed stage III changes may occur within several months.

For a stage III fixed foot deformity, an arthrodesis procedure of the hindfoot is suggested. Various combinations of arthrodesis for the talonavicular, calcaneocuboid, and talocalcaneal joints have been utilized. Most frequently, a moldable arthrodesis of the talocalcaneal joint is the preferred procedure. This surgical technique of subtalar arthrodesis is described in detail elsewhere in this volume.

Contraindications to the surgical care of the TP tendon difficulties center about the patient and the diagnosis. A physiologically old patient with not much pain could be treated with nonoperative measures. The use of cortisone and antimetabolic agents such as methotrexate by the patient are partial contraindications to surgical treatment since tissue healing may be delayed with such medications. Diabetes mellitus patients may have a predilection for TP difficulties and should be treated cautiously. The presence of marked obesity may place excessive stress on the transferred FDL tendon for stage II disease.

The correct diagnosis is also important. Excluding other causes of foot swelling and deformity such as neuropathic arthropathy, tarsometatarsal degenerative arthritis (Lisfranc), or just relaxed pes planus deformity by appropriate history, physical examination, and radiologic evaluation is necessary.

PREOPERATIVE PLANNING

Anticipating the correct surgical procedure before surgery is aided by the staging of the patient's foot deformity. In general, the degree of tendon degeneration and tenosynovitis viewed at surgery will be worse than would be suggested by the physical examination. That is, the swelling and pain may be mild and yet the tendon will show thickening, yellowish discoloration, longitudinal split tears, and a significant synovial proliferation. Usually for an apparent stage I or early stage II type of TP tendon involvement, the patient will be counseled that a FDL tendon transfer may be necessary in addition to the tendon release and debridement.

The physical examination involves assessment of the location of pain symptoms, the associated swelling and hindfoot deformity, as well as the strength of the posterior tibialis tendon. With involvement of the posterior tibialis tendon the tenderness will be along the course of this tendon just posterior to the medial crest of the distal tibia. It will then extend around the tip of the medial malleolus to the insertion of the tendon on the undersurface of the navicular. Swelling is most evident by viewing the patient from a posterior aspect while standing. A fullness in the inframedial malleolar region is then easily evident. The deformity of the foot is also assessed from viewing the patient standing from a posterior view. Increased hindfoot valgus will be seen and the lateral rotation of the forefoot made evident by the "too many toes" sign, i.e., with loss of the tibial posterior tendon function more toes will be evident as seen lateralward to the hindfoot than the unaffected side. Finally, strength of the tendon is assessed by a single heel rise test. This is done by asking the patient to rest his or her hands on the wall while the physician view the feet posteriorly. While one foot is raised in the air, the patient is first asked to go up on the normal foot, which should be easily accomplished. The heel will go into inversion, following which the heel will come off the ground strongly. When the same test is used on the affected foot with loss of the tibialis posterior tendon, the ability to invert the foot is absent and the patient describes weakness. Although the patient may, with a great deal of effort, rise up on the ball of the affected foot, this will be reported as a weaker foot and the heel will not have the capacity to invert.

When secondary deformity has occurred, there may be tenderness over the sinus tarsi region laterally as the anterior portion of the talar posterior facet impinges on the dorsal aspect of the calcaneus just anterior to the calcaneal posterior facet.

Routine preoperative radiographs should include weight-bearing lateral and anteroposterior views of the feet. The deformity of the foot that develops if the tendon lengthens or ruptures is a rotation outward of the calcaneus from beneath the talus about a vertical axis approximately through the posterior calcaneal facet. As the head and neck of the talus is left unsupported, the talus goes into a plantarflexed position when viewed laterally. These changes can then be seen on the routine radiographs. On the anteroposterior view, an increase in the angle between the longitudinal axis of the talus and calcaneus will be seen. Also on this view the displacement of the forefoot into abduction with the calcaneus can be assessed. A subluxation at the talonavicular joint correlates with the amount of deformity. From a lateral view with plantar flexion of the talus an increased angle between the longitudinal axis of the talus and calcaneus will be seen (see Fig. 5). Close evaluation of the radiographs will show early changes that might not be detected on physical examination.

By the physical examination and routine radiographs, staging of the tendon involvement is usually evident. Occasionally a magnetic resonance (MR) type of radiologic examination will be necessary. Such a radiologic technique is most helpful early when the cause of the medial ankle pain is uncertain and the possibility of TP tendon involvement is being considered (see Fig. 6).

SURGERY

The procedure is carried out with the patient supine, under general or spinal anesthetic. A pneumatic thigh tourniquet is utilized.

Technique. The incision starts about 10 cm proximal to the tip of the medial malleolus about 1 cm posterior to the medial border of the tibia (Fig. 1). The incision is then extended distally along the tibia margin to just behind the tip of the medial malleolus (Fig. 2). From the tip of the medial malleolus the incision gently curves along the medial aspect of the foot to the TP insertion at the lower aspect of the navicular tuberosity.

The deep fascia is exposed and the medial tendons can usually be seen through the partially translucent fascia (Fig. 3). At the upper end of the skin incision the deep fascia is incised and the TP exposed. The large TP tendon lies very close to the posterior margin of the tibia. The tendon is then traced distally to its insertion while leaving a 2-cm wide pulley just posterior to the medial malleolus at the level of the tibial plafond. At this juncture a decision is made as to whether the tendon is of a normal length or elongated. This decision dictates the subsequent operative treatment. If the tendon is of normal length (stage I) then tendon debridement, tenosynovectomy, and sheath resection will be done and the wound closed. If the tendon is elongated (stage II), a tendon transfer of the flexor digitorum longus (FDL) will be added to the procedure.

The debridement of the tendon varies depending on the surgical findings. If there is some fraying of the tendon, the tags of tendon tissue are smoothly excised leaving the major portion of the tendon intact. In some instances, there will be a bulbous enlargement of the tendon just distal to the tip of the medial malleolus. With such an abnormality an ellipse is removed from the bulb and the tendon sutured burying the knots to leave the tendon a normal size. Occasionally a prominent longitudinal split of the tendon will be present, in which case the inner sides of the tear will be cleared of scar tissue and the sides apposed with a buried knot technique.

A tenosynovectomy will vary from removing a minimal amount of tissue for mild involvement to a large amount of tissue when the synovium is luxuriant.

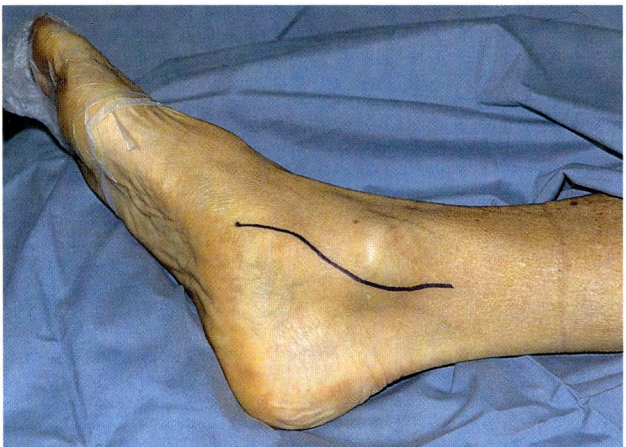

Figure 1. Position of the foot at the time of surgery is seen with the skin incision marked.

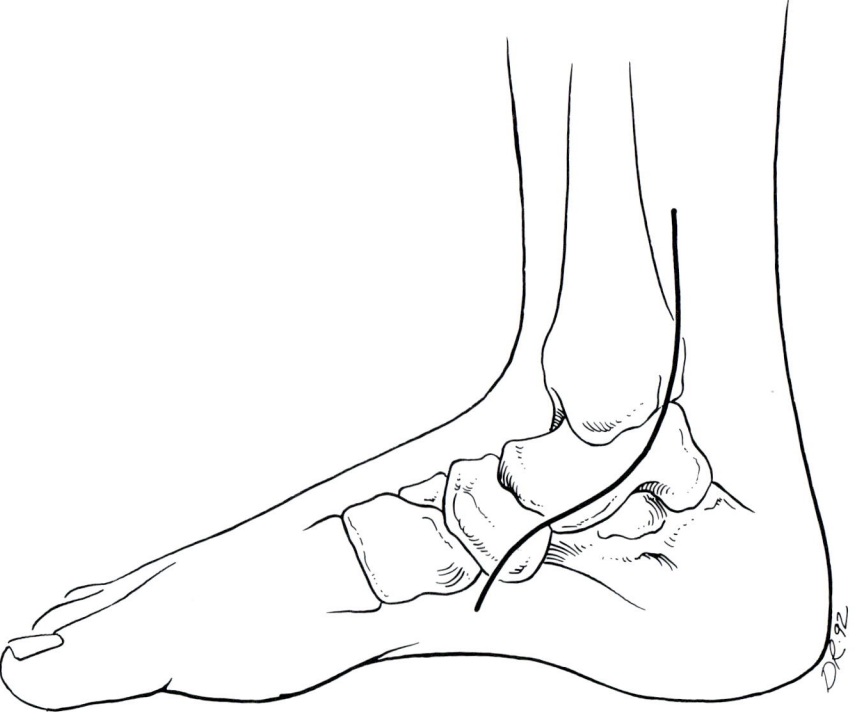

Figure 2. Relationship of the skin incision to the underlying bone structure.

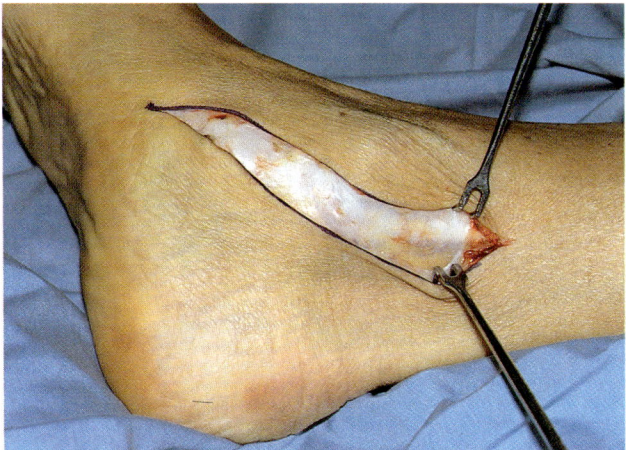

Figure 3. The tibialis posterior tendon beneath the superior flexor retinaculum is seen.

Finally the outer portion of the tendon sheath distal to the pulley is removed to prevent possible reformation of a stenotic tendon sheath.

If on close inspection of the TP tendon there is evidence of elongation, then a transfer of the FDL into the undersurface of the navicular tuberosity will be done in addition to the debridement, tenosynovectomy, and partial tendon sheath resection.

The tendon may show degeneration over several centimeters with enlargement, multiple longitudinal tears, and adhesions to the tendon sheath (Fig. 4). Proximal to the directly involved region, the tendon will have a white fish-flesh appearance if the tear is old and tension has not been transmitted through the tendon for some time (Fig. 5). In other cases, there will be a single complete transverse tear with rounding off of the tendon ends.

The transfer of the FDL entails detaching the FDL distally and reinserting it into the undersurface of the navicular through a drill hole (see Fig. 8). The skin incision is the same as for a stage I TP problem. When it is evident that an FDL transfer will be necessary, the incision is extended distally to the crossover area of the FDL and flexor hallucis longus (Fig. 6). The FDL is cut under direct vision giving as much length as possible for transfer. The distal portion of the FDL does not need to be tenodesed to the adjacent flexor hallucis longus tendon. The intrin-

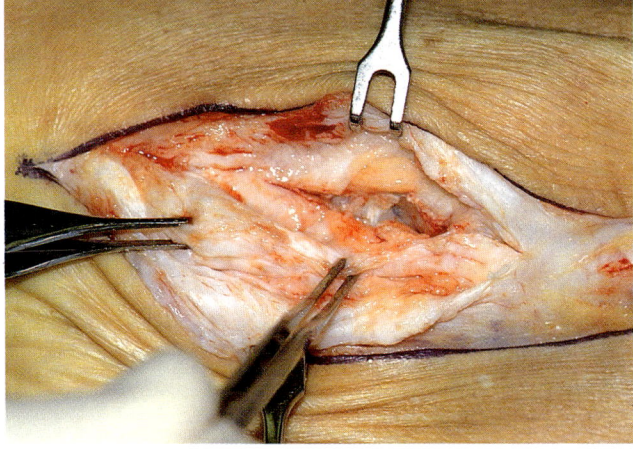

Figure 4. This tendon shows marked degeneration with loss of the tendon architecture.

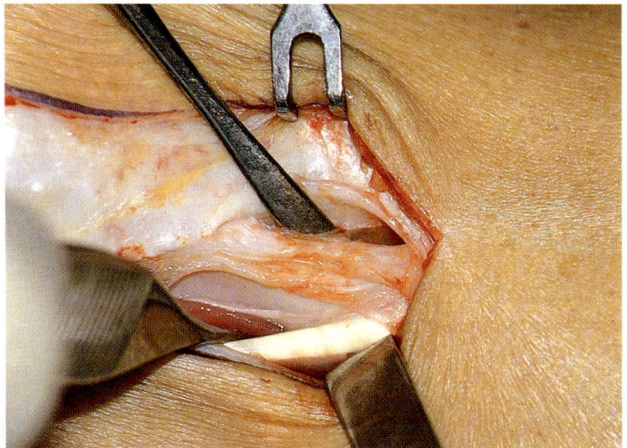

Figure 5. Tibialis posterior tendon proximal from its distal tear. This has the appearance of fish flesh.

sic toe flexors are so strong that leaving the distal portion of the FDL alone will cause no functional loss of lesser toe function later. Avoiding the tenodesis to the flexor hallucis longus allows a greater length of FDL to be used for transfer. A zigzag suture of a strong nonabsorbable material is then placed through the end of the FDL and the tendon elevated from its sheath (Fig. 7).

The tuberosity of the navicular is identified by moving the forefoot back and forth from abduction-adduction and feeling the joint movement. A longitudinal incision is made in the joint capsule at the inferior surface of the navicular and in the superior surface (Fig. 8). Usually a ¼" or ⅜" drill bit is passed through the tuberosity from superior to inferior (Fig. 9). This drill hole should come out inferior to the main insertion of the TP (Fig. 10).

The FDL is left in its own sheath and is not rerouted through the diseased TP sheath. Using a bent wire or suture passer, the FDL is brought through the drill hole from inferior to the superior (Fig. 11). It is pulled as tight as reasonably possible with the ankle in equinus and the forefoot in varus (Fig. 12). The zigzag suture can be placed through soft tissue capsule dorsally to hold the tendon in place. A line of nonabsorbable sutures is also placed along the transferred FDL tendon to the TP distal portion before the tendon enters the drill hole (Fig. 13). This provides a secure soft tissue and bony attachment for the transferred FDL.

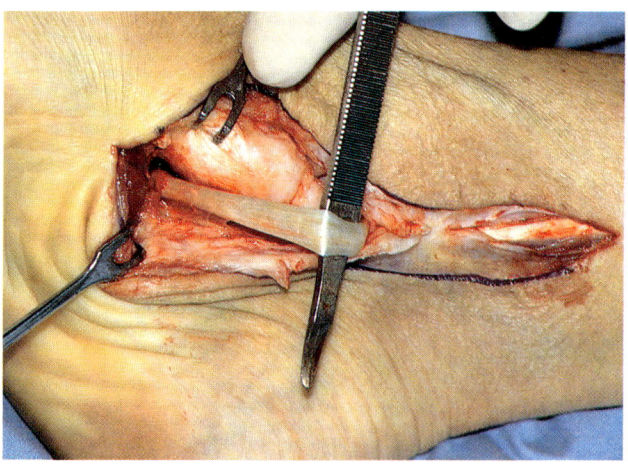

Figure 6. The flexor digitorum longus tendon is exposed leaving the pulley of flexor retinaculum just posterior to the medial malleolus.

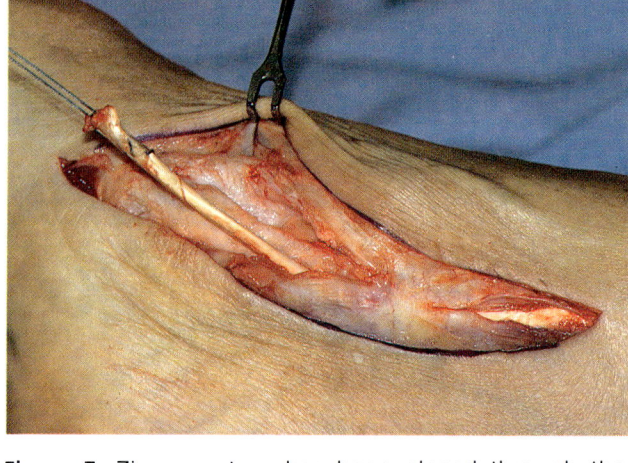

Figure 7. Zigzag suture has been placed through the flexor digitorum longus tendon after it has been cut distally at the "knot of Henry" area.

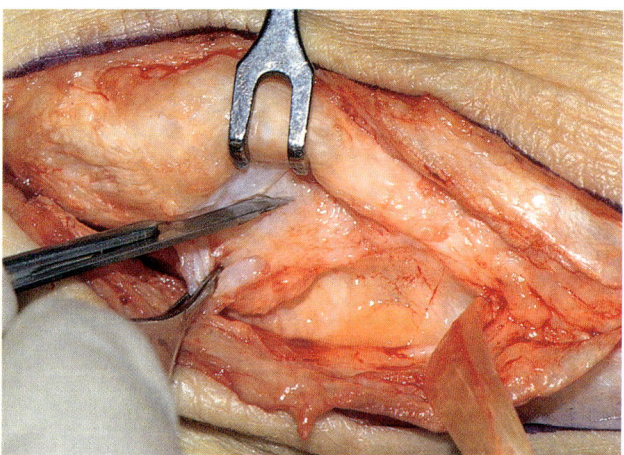

Figure 8. Locating the tuberosity of the navicular is done by retracting dorsalward the insertion of the tibialis posterior tendon.

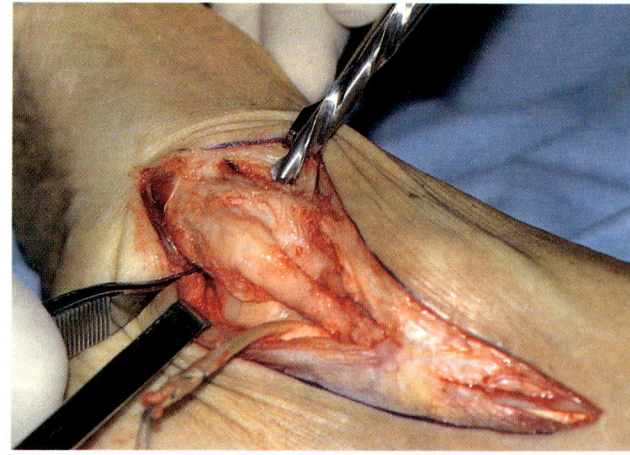

Figure 9. Drill entering superior aspect of navicular tuberosity.

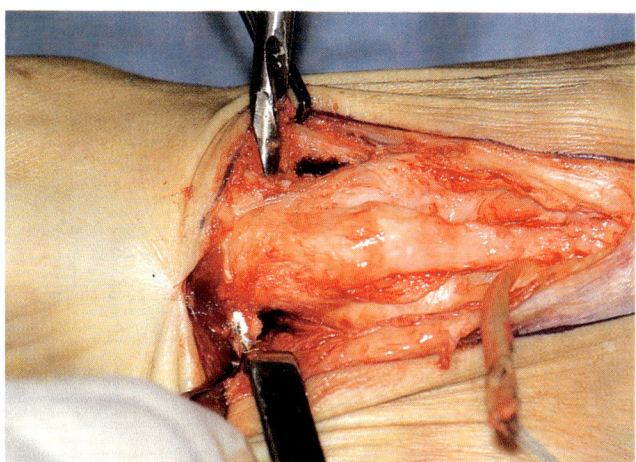

Figure 10. Drill protruding out through the inferior aspect of the tuberosity of the navicular.

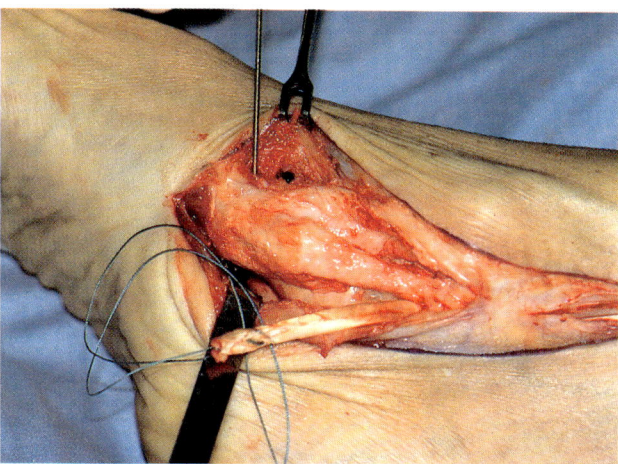

Figure 11. A folded wire is placed through the drill hole, which then catches the suture through the tibialis posterior tendon.

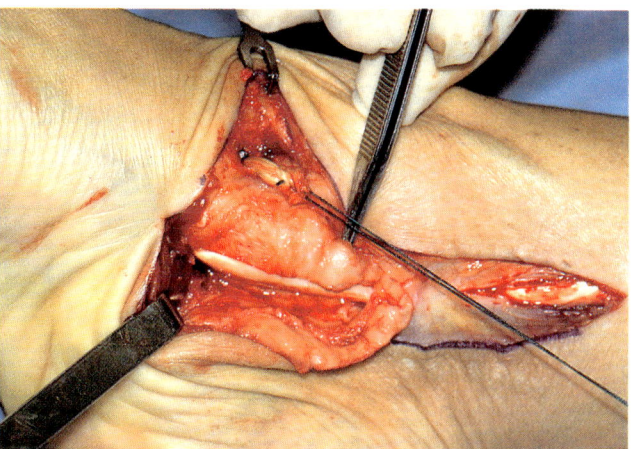

Figure 12. The flexor digitorum longus tendon has been pulled through the drill hole in the tuberosity of the navicular and will be sutured to the surrounding soft tissues.

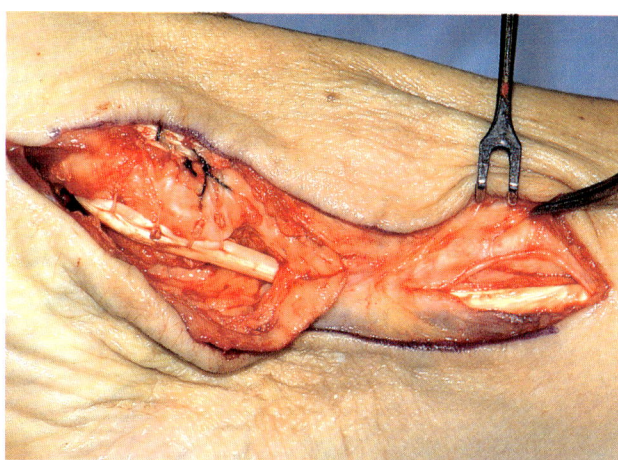

Figure 13. The tendon has been attached both dorsally to the soft tissues and to the remaining portion of tibialis posterior tendon where the flexor digitorum longus passes below it.

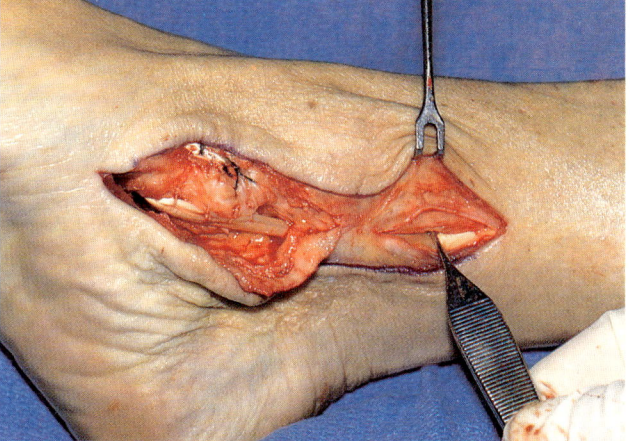

Figure 14. The fibrotic muscle tendon unit of the tibialis posterior. Because it is nonfunctional it will not be tenodesed to the transferred flexor digitorum longus tendon.

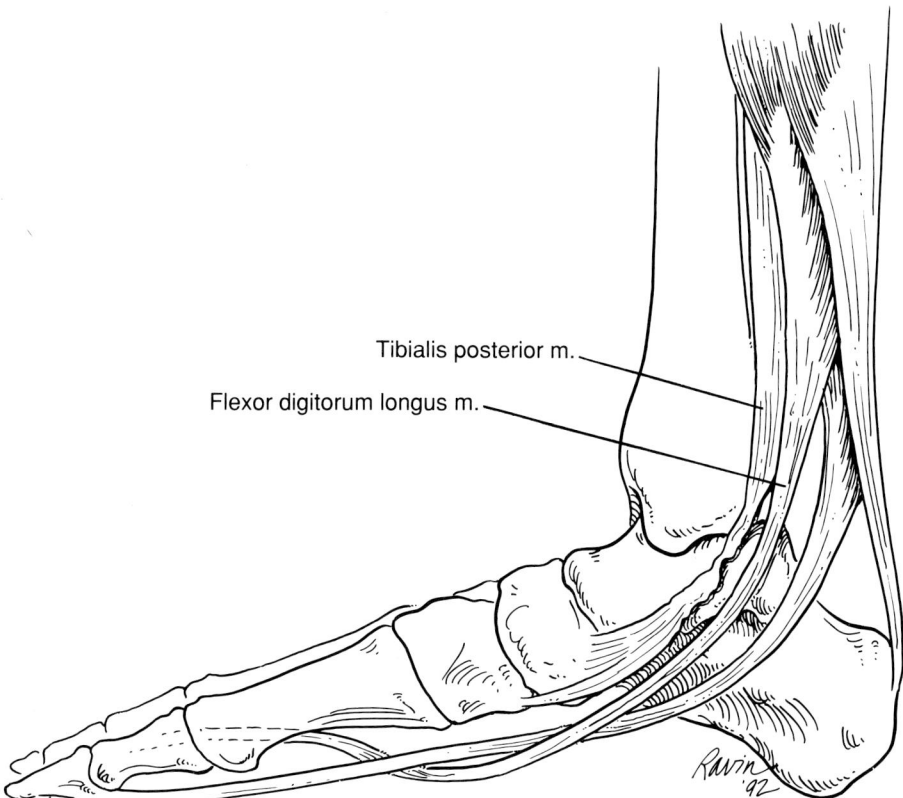

Figure 15. The preoperative situation with degeneration of the tibialis posterior tendon shown distal to the medial malleolus.

Next, the advisability of doing a proximal tenodesis of the TP muscle power to the FDL is assessed (Fig. 14). With disuse the muscle will become fibrotic and stiff. By pulling on the proximal portion of the TP tendon the pliability of the muscle can be determined. If there is some elasticity suggesting a functional muscle, then a tenodesis of the TP to the transferred FDL is completed with side to side technique using multiple buried sutures. Otherwise with a fibrotic stiff muscle, the TP is left unattached proximally. A substitution for the TP has been accomplished by the FDL transfer (Figs. 15 and 16).

It has been suggested that a reefing of the talonavicular capsule and calcaneonavicular (spring) ligament should be a part of this procedure to provide static stability. Suturing of the FDL to the undersurface of the talonavicular joint may accomplish this to some degree. Static transfers alone, historically, have not been successful in maintaining the arch of the foot.

A negative exploration for a TP disruption has become infrequent. Usually what is found at operation is more extensive than what was suspected clinically. It is necessary to carry the surgical exploration all the way to the TP insertion where the tearing and elongation may be located.

There is a tendency to try suturing the FDL to the distal portion of the TP and avoid the extra surgical tasks of making a drill hole and inserting the FDL into bone. This limited procedure has not been satisfactory, however. When doing the FDL transfer, it is necessary to do the whole procedure including insertion of the tendon into bone for a secure attachment. Closure is secured with absorbable subcutaneous suture and nylon 2-0 mattress suture for the skin.

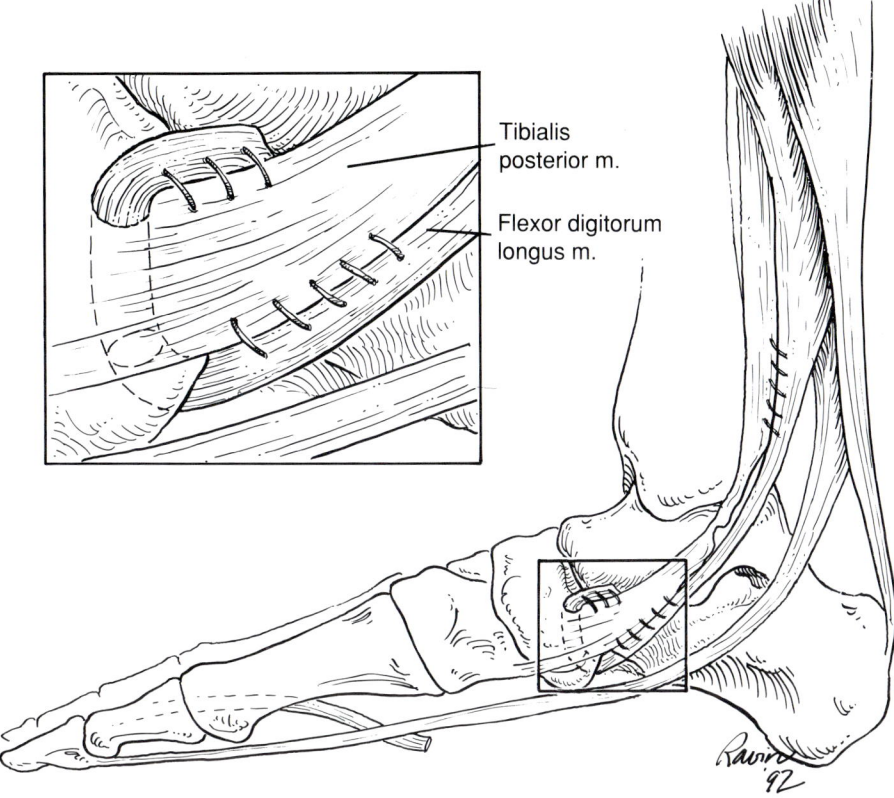

Figure 16. The transection of the flexor digitorum longus at the crossover with the flexor hallucis longus and subsequent transfer to the tuberosity of the navicular with suturing. A proximal tenodesis of the muscle of the tibialis posterior to the flexor digitorum longus is also shown.

POSTOPERATIVE MANAGEMENT

When the TP tendon sheath release, debridement, and tenosynovectomy are done with or without an FDL transfer, a compressive dressing with plaster splints is applied immediately postoperative holding the ankle in plantar flexion and inversion. After about 1 or 2 days, a short leg cast is applied.

Without the FDL transfer, it is a walking cast that holds the hindfoot in a neutral right angle position for about 3 weeks. The cast is then removed and walking is encouraged, initially, in a postoperative shoe. A gradual progression is advised from the postoperative shoe to a spacious lace-up low-heeled shoe to usual footwear. Resolution of pain and postoperative swelling is gradual over a few months' period.

With the FDL transfer, the postoperative recuperation is more prolonged. The initial cast, 1 to 2 days after surgery, is a non–weight-bearing cast that holds the foot in adduction and hindfoot in inversion. After 3 weeks, sutures are removed and the foot and ankle are brought to neutral positions and a second short leg non–weight-bearing cast applied for an additional 3 weeks. At 6 weeks postoperative immobilization is stopped and the patient instructed to begin weight bearing as tolerated. Over a 3- to 6-week period, shoe and weight-bearing progression should evolve.

Formal physical therapy to facilitate weight bearing and strength development are occasionally necessary. Crutches or a walker are necessary of course for non–weight-bearing status. A compression stocking after cast removal helps control postoperative swelling. The patient is instructed to use the compression stocking during the waking hours only and as long as necessary for swelling. Usually the duration of appreciable swelling will be about as long as the period of cast immobilization.

The expectations for recovery depend on the tendon changes seen at surgery and the specific surgical procedure. When the procedure just involves sheath release, debridement, and tenosynovectomy without FDL transfer, the outlook is excellent. Usually the sequence of inflammation and tendon degeneration is halted and pain relief is obtained. These patients have not had recurrence of their tendon disease at a later time.

With transfer of the FDL the patient can expect pain relief. Restitution, however, of TP function by the transferred FDL does not usually occur. The patient will still have a pes planus deformity and the single heel rise test will indicate loss of heel inversion. On a more positive note, the hindfoot deformity will not progress and recurrent pain has not been a problem after FDL transfer.

COMPLICATIONS

The difficulties associated with surgery for TP tendon inflammation include wound healing, stiffness, persistent deformity, pain, and a long recuperation.

Wound healing can be a problem if wound closure is not secure and if steroid is used either locally or systemically. In early cases, it was felt that in surgery for stage I TP disease, leaving some steroid bathing the tendon would help decrease inflammation. Wound healing, however, was significantly impaired and in a few instances led to wide dehiscence. The incision used for the tendon surgery is under tension with swelling and ankle motion. Utilizing multiple mattress sutures with 2-0 nylon for the skin closure and leaving them in place for 3 weeks has improved wound healing.

Stiffness may occur after the FDL transfer procedure. Instead of holding the ankle and foot in equinus and adduction for a full 6 weeks, the postoperative plan advised is to bring the ankle and foot to neutral position after 3 weeks at the time of first cast change. This practice has decreased the stiffness that otherwise was a problem.

Continued pes planus deformity is a common result after FDL transfer. If the patients are advised before treatment of such an expectation, they can adjust to the abnormal foot position. If a normal alignment of the foot is very important, then a subtalar arthrodesis would insure proper realignment of the foot at the expense of subtalar motion.

Pain that persists after FDL transfer is probably related to the abnormal subtalar position. If the deformity preoperative is moderate to severe, there may be impingement of the anterior wedge of the posterior subtalar facet on the superior aspect of the calcaneus. This problem can be anticipated if the deformity is significant and preoperative pain is located laterally over the sinus tarsi. In such a situation subtalar arthrodesis rather than FDL transfer is suggested.

Prolonged recovery after a TP release with or without FDL transfer is not unusual. Swelling in the incision area and about the ankle can be controlled with compressive stockings. If the patients understand that they will not be going back to dancing the night after the final cast is removed, it is easier for them as well as for the surgeon. Allowing a few months for recuperating is appropriate.

ILLUSTRATIVE CASE FOR TECHNIQUE

This 61-year-old woman described progressive weakness of her left hindfoot region without any history of prior trauma. She had mild pain on the medial aspect of the ankle with some swelling toward the end of the day.

While standing (Fig. 17) she demonstrated increased forefoot abduction and some subtle swelling in the medial malleolar region. When viewed posteriorly (Fig. 18) the intramalleolar swelling medially was more evident and she showed three toes lateral to the ankle on the left, while only 1½ on the right. A single heel rise test was done and the patient was unable to invert the left hindfoot and rise up on the ball of her foot (Fig. 19).

A radiograph of her foot from a lateral view demonstrated a sag at the talonavicular joint and an increased angle of the longitudinal axis of the talus with longitudinal axis of the calcaneus (Fig. 20A). Her AP views (Fig. 20B) demonstrated a dissociation between the head of the talus and the calcaneus and a widening of the longitudinal axis of the talus with the longitudinal axis of the calcaneus. The line along

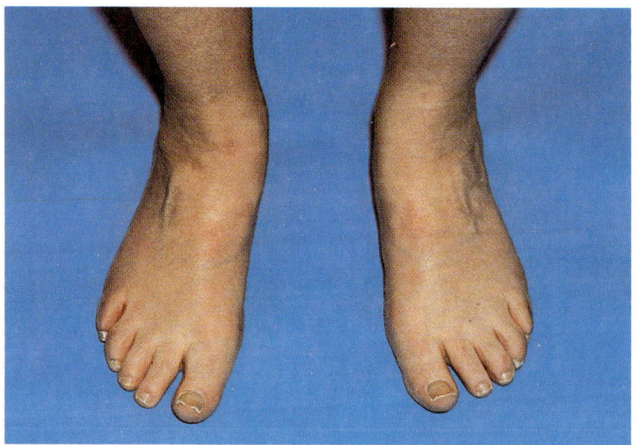

Figure 17. View of the patient while standing in a dorsoplantar direction. Patient has loss of left tibialis posterior tendon function.

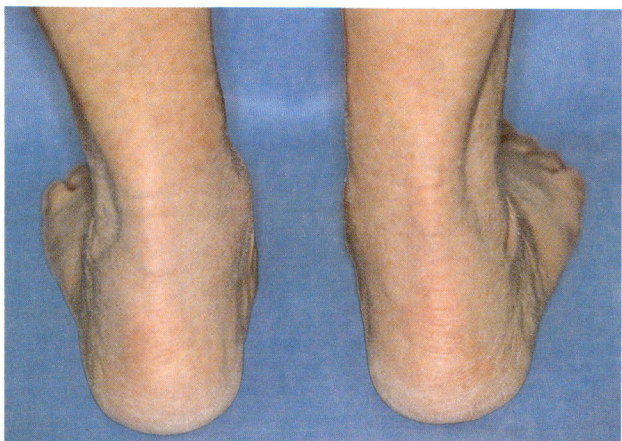

Figure 18. Posterior view of same patient showing more toes on the affected left side than on the right.

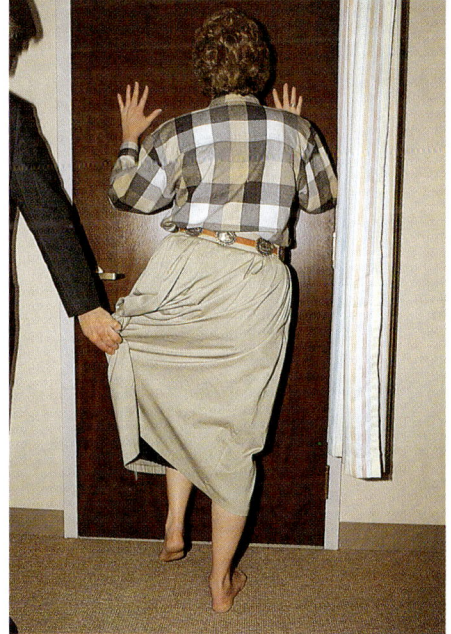

Figure 19. The patient is being tested for strength of the posterior tibial tendon with a single heel rise test. She is unable to go up on the ball of the left foot.

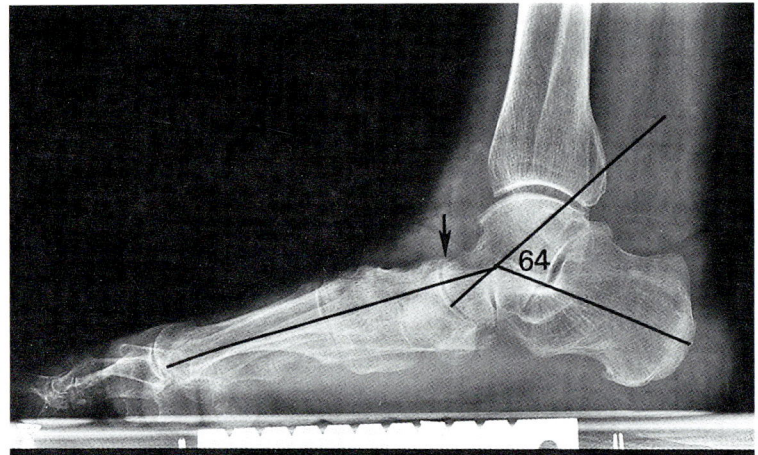

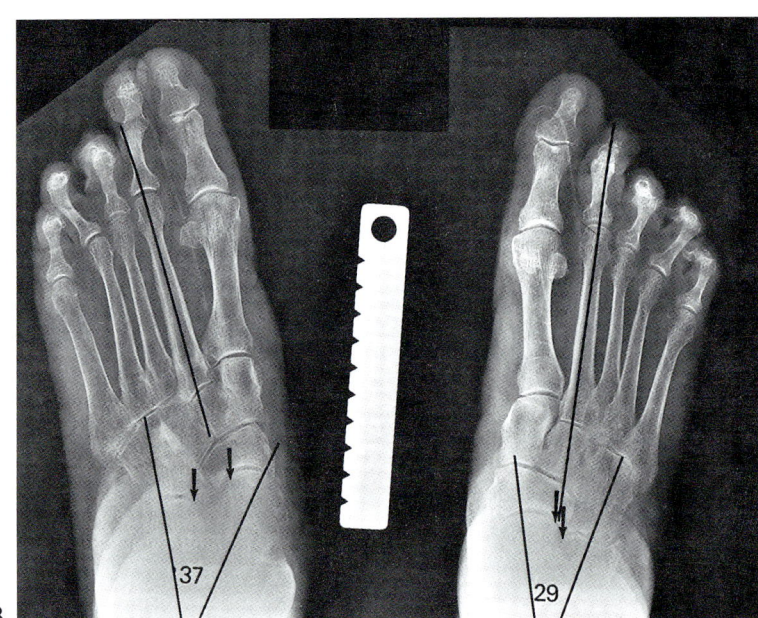

Figure 20. A: Lateral radiograph shows secondary changes of tibialis posterior tendon loss. **B:** AP radiograph shows the abnormal relationship of the talus to the rest of the hindfoot secondary to tibialis posterior tendon loss.

the second metatarsal did not bisect the hindfoot angle indicating lateral rotation of the forefoot along with the calcaneus.

She was treated by a debridement of the tibialis posterior tendon, release of the tendon sheath, and a transfer of her flexor digitorum longus. One year later the patient described relief of her pain symptoms, but persistent weakness when trying to do a single heel rise test. She has not had increased secondary deformity although some of her preoperative deformity persists.

RECOMMENDED READING

1. Alexander, I. J., Johnson, K. A., and Berquist, T. H.: Magnetic resonance imaging in the diagnosis of disruption of the posterior tibial tendon. *Foot Ankle*, 8: 144, 1987.
2. Funk, D. A., Cass, J. R., and Johnson, K. A.: Acquired flat foot secondary to posterior tibial tendon pathology. *J. Bone Joint Surg.*, 68A: 95, 1986.

3. Jahss, M. H.: Spontaneous rupture of the tibialis posterior tendon: clinical findings, tenographic studies, and a new technique of repair. *Foot Ankle*, 3: 158, 1982.
4. Johnson, K. A.: Tibialis posterior tendon rupture. *Clin. Orthop.*, 177: 140, 1983.
5. Johnson, K. A., and Strom, D. E.: Tibialis posterior tendon dysfunction. *Clin. Orthop.*, 229: 196, 1989.
6. Kaye, R. A., and Jahss, M. H.: Tibialis posterior: a review of anatomy and biomechanics in relation to support of the medial longitudinal arch. *Foot Ankle*, 11(4): 244–247, 1991.
7. Mann, R. A., and Thompson, F. M.: Rupture of the posterior tibial tendon causing flat foot. *J. Bone Joint Surg.*, 67A: 556, 1985.

22

Peroneal Tendon Repair-Reconstruction

Mark Sobel and Walther H. O. Bohne

INDICATIONS/CONTRAINDICATIONS

Ankle inversion injury can result in lateral retromalleolar pain and plantar-lateral foot pain. This pain may be from injury to the peroneal tendons, usually at or near the posterior ridge of the fibula in the fibular groove (8) (Figs. 1 and 2). Acute traumatic subluxation of the peroneal tendons can affect both tendons as well as the superior peroneal retinaculum at the level of the fibular groove. These injuries are the result of acute traumatic dorsiflexion eversion. Injury to the peroneus longus tendon usually occurs distal to the fibular groove along the lateral wall of the calcaneus, or within the cuboid tunnel.

The role of the superior peroneal retinaculum (SPR) as the primary restraint to peroneal subluxation is well recognized. We believe that incompetence of the SPR also plays a major etiologic role in the dynamics of peroneus brevis splits.

A trial of cast or CAM walker immobilization of the foot and ankle in neutral position can together with nonsteroidal antiinflammatory medication diminish the pain. Persistent pain along the course of the peroneal tendons (either retromalleolar, or more distally along the lateral wall of the calcaneus or at the cuboid tunnel) that has not responded to conservative treatment is an indication to peroneal tendon exploration and repair.

Contraindications to surgical exploration and peroneal tendon repair are absence of pain, chronic infection, and presence of skin breakdown. An inadequate

---

M. Sobel, M.D.: Orthopaedic Foot and Ankle Service, Beth Israel Medical Center, North Division, New York, NY 10021; Beth Israel Medical Center, Petrie Campus, New York, NY 10003; private practice: 755 Park Avenue, New York, NY 10021.

W. H. O. Bohne, M.D.: Department of Orthopaedic Surgery, New York Hospital-Cornell University Medical Center, New York, NY 10021; Department of Orthopaedic Surgery, The Hospital of Special Surgery, New York, NY 10021.

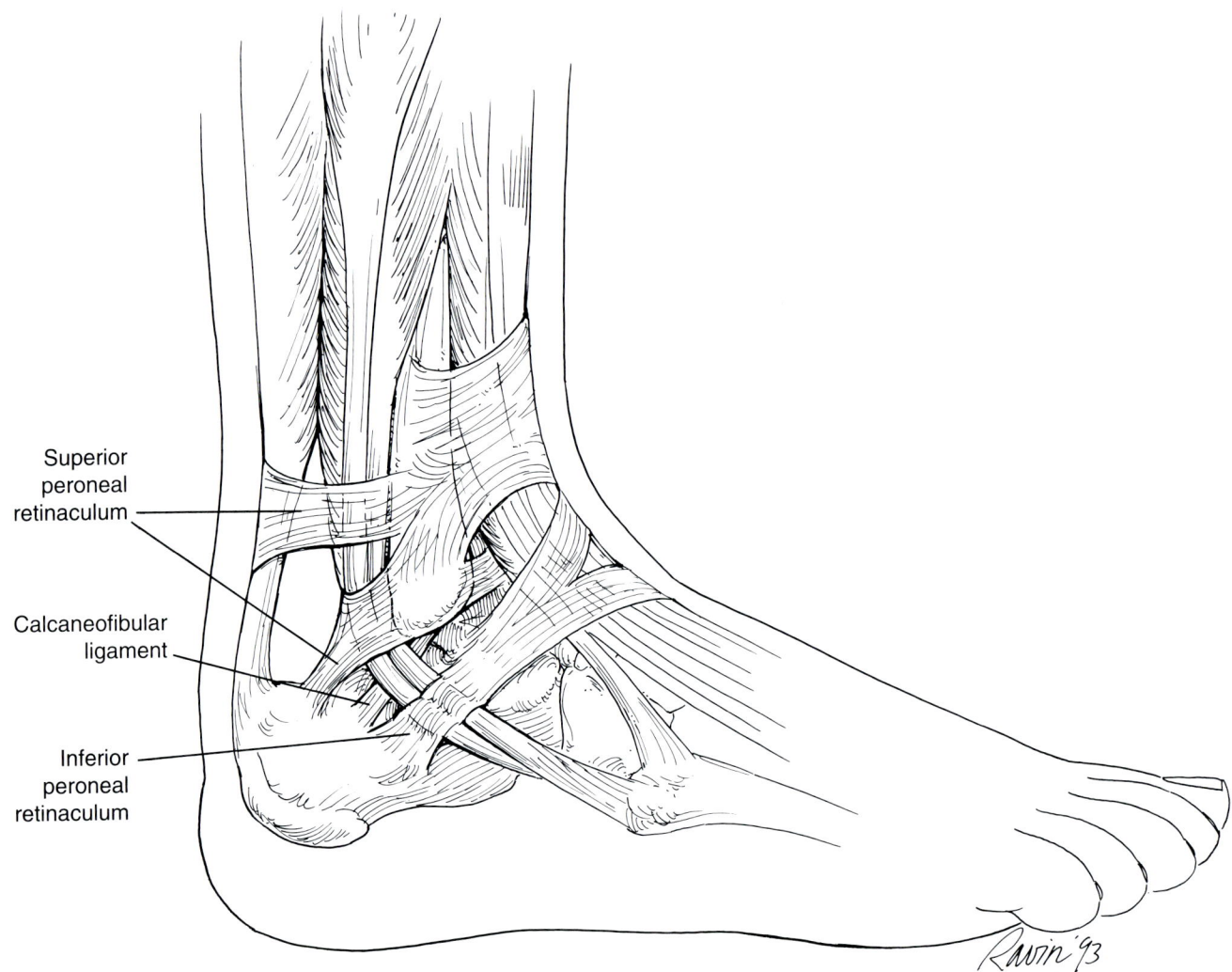

Figure 1. Normal anatomy of the tendons and ligaments at the lateral side of the ankle and hind foot.

vascular supply and severe vasculitis are also contraindications to hindfoot and ankle surgery.

PREOPERATIVE PLANNING

The patient generally presents with retromalleolar pain that is located over the posterior ridge of the fibula radiating proximally along the course of the peroneal tendons and distally along the fibular groove. In most instances, a history of ankle inversion supination sprain can be elicited. In some patients, the history is consistent with chronic ankle instability and repeated inversion sprains. The ages of the patients in this group vary; however, many are in the young adult athletic population.

In patients with peroneus brevis splits, tenderness is well localized at the retromalleolar region just at the posterior ridge of the fibula. This ridge is usually located 1 cm proximal to the distal extent of the fibula. The peroneal tunnel at this region may have a sensation of fullness compared to the opposite side (Fig. 3).

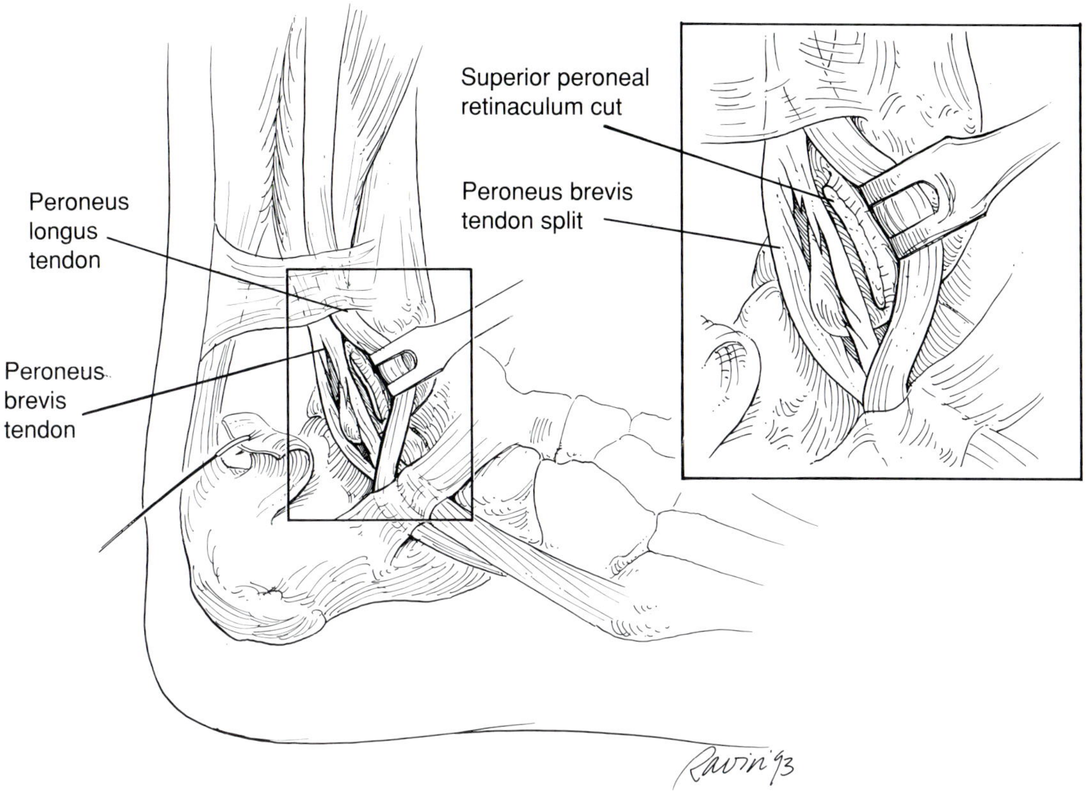

Figure 2. Course of the peroneal tendons along the lateral aspect of the ankle and foot. Retraction of the peroneus longus shows the split tear of the peroneus brevis tendon.

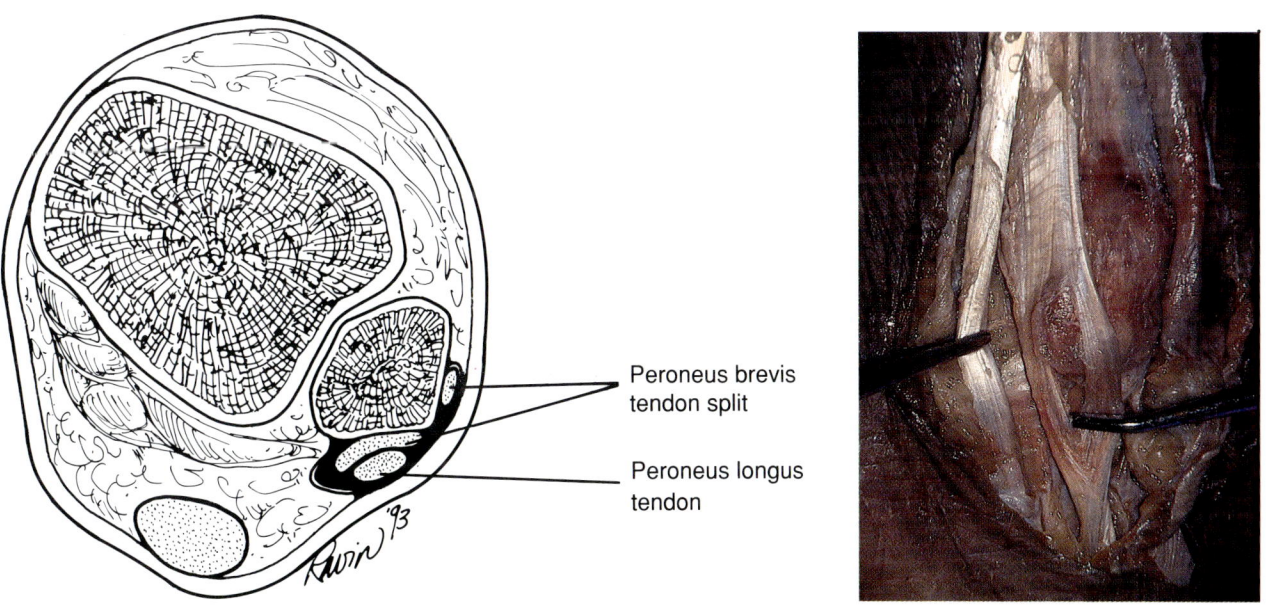

Figure 3. A: Cross-section view at the level of the fibular groove shows the lateral part of the split peroneus brevis tendon has dislocated over the posterior ridge of the fibula. **B:** This cadaver specimen had a tear of the peroneus brevis with a "buttonholing" over the posterior ridge of the fibula.

Longitudinal splits in the peroneus brevis tendon do not necessarily affect the strength of the tendon. Therefore, dorsiflexion eversion muscle testing elicits little or no weakness. In many instances, the peroneus brevis pathology may be associated with ankle instability. If lateral ankle ligament instability is present with a presumed peroneus brevis split, a modification of the Brostrom-Gould procedure is recommended.

Careful palpation of the posterior border of the fibula at the region of the SPR, while the patient everts the involved ankle against resistance, allows detection of a snapping, popping, or partial tendon subluxation (3). These findings are accompanied by pain in patients with symptomatic longitudinal splits of the peroneus brevis tendon (7). Examination for lateral ankle instability should be performed to rule out the coexistence of lateral ankle ligament injury and peroneus brevis splits. In the radiograph one may see telltale signs of ankle inversion injury including bony SPR pull-off, lateral process of talus fracture, cuboid avulsion fractures, and fifth metatarsal base fractures.

Magnetic resonance imaging (MRI) visualizes the contents of the peroneal tunnel very well. If the diagnosis is uncertain, the magnetic resonance (MR) examination can be helpful. MRI may demonstrate the presence of an extra anomalous tendon such as the peroneus quartus but also the irregularities of a splayed-out peroneus brevis tendon next to the more normal-appearing peroneus longus tendon. Longitudinal attrition of the peroneus brevis tendon is confirmed by a thinned-out wavy tendon with interruptions in the normal smooth contour and by irregularity within the tendon itself. In addition, the superior peroneal retinaculum is well visualized in the axial cuts at the level of the fibular groove. MRI utilizing perpendicular axial cuts at the level of the fibular groove should not normally show the peroneus brevis muscle belly at this level.

The role of ultrasound or needle arthroscopy in the diagnosis of peroneus brevis tendon pathology is undetermined at present but shows promise.

SURGERY

Either spinal or general anesthesia is used. The patient is positioned supine on the operating table with a sandbag elevation under the ipsilateral greater trochanteric.

Technique. A curved 7-cm incision is made through the skin and subcutaneous tissue along the posterior one-third of the fibula, off its central prominence (Fig. 4). Full-thickness flaps are elevated with exposure of the superior peroneal retinaculum. Subluxation of the anterior portion of the peroneus brevis tendon can sometimes be demonstrated with the superior peroneal retinaculum exposed. The competence of the superior peroneal retinaculum is determined.

The peroneal sheath is then sharply incised near its anterior attachment to the fibula (Fig. 5). Proximal traction of the peroneus longus tendon can cause subluxation of the anterior portion of a split peroneus brevis tendon (Fig. 6). The peroneus brevis tendon is inspected and if attrition or a split is evident, the attenuated or degenerated tissue can be debrided, and the tendon repaired and then tubulated (Fig. 7). If the peroneus brevis muscle belly is found to be low-lying and thus creating an encroachment phenomenon within the peroneal tunnel, this low-lying muscle belly can be removed (Fig. 8) to create more space for the peroneal tendons within the fibular groove. If there is an anomalous peroneus quartus tendon present in the groove creating an encroachment phenomenon, this tendon may also be removed (Fig. 9).

Other surgical treatment options include (a) excision of the diseased peroneus brevis segment and suturing of the proximal and distal stumps to the peroneus longus tendon (this option should be reserved for cases where the peroneus brevis

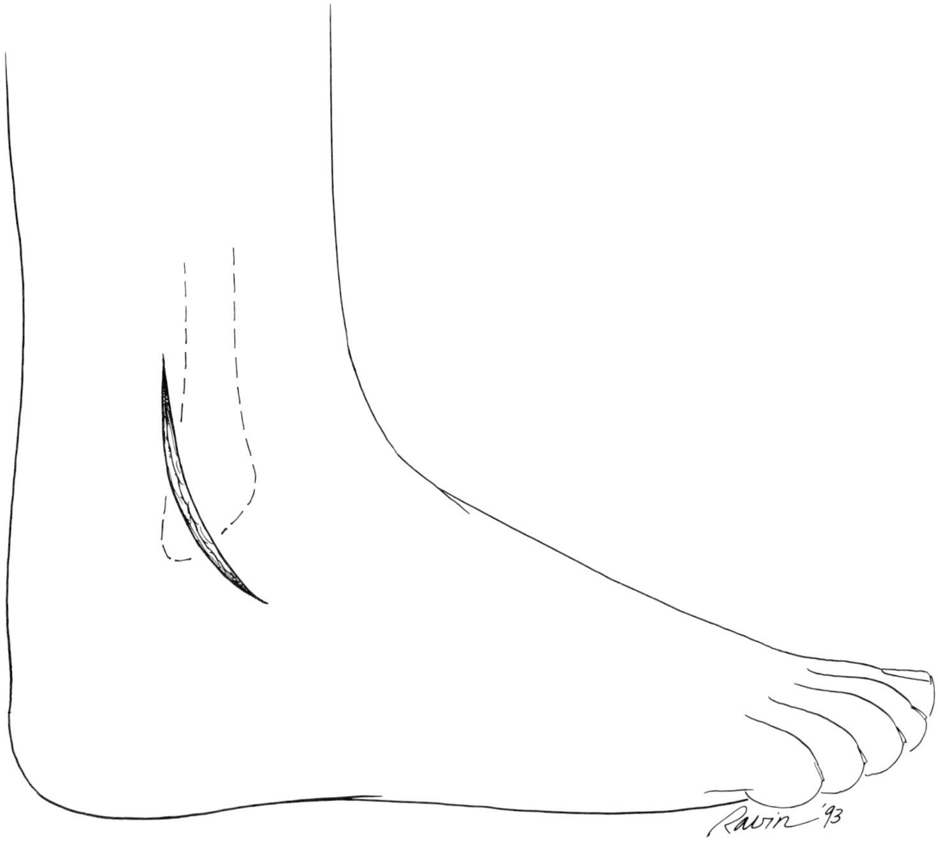

Figure 4. The lateral skin incision location is seen.

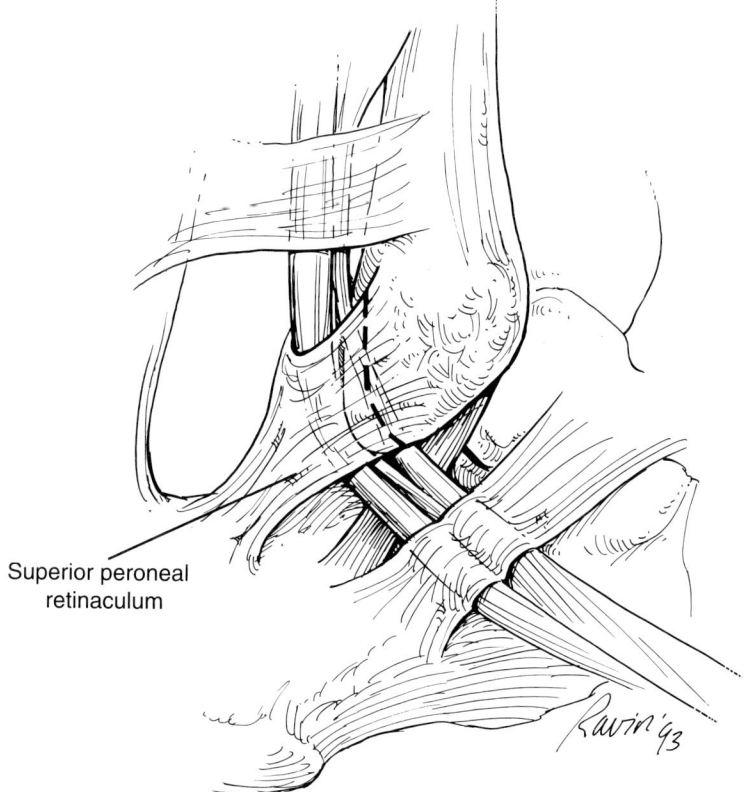

Figure 5. The peroneal sheath is incised close to the border of the fibula.

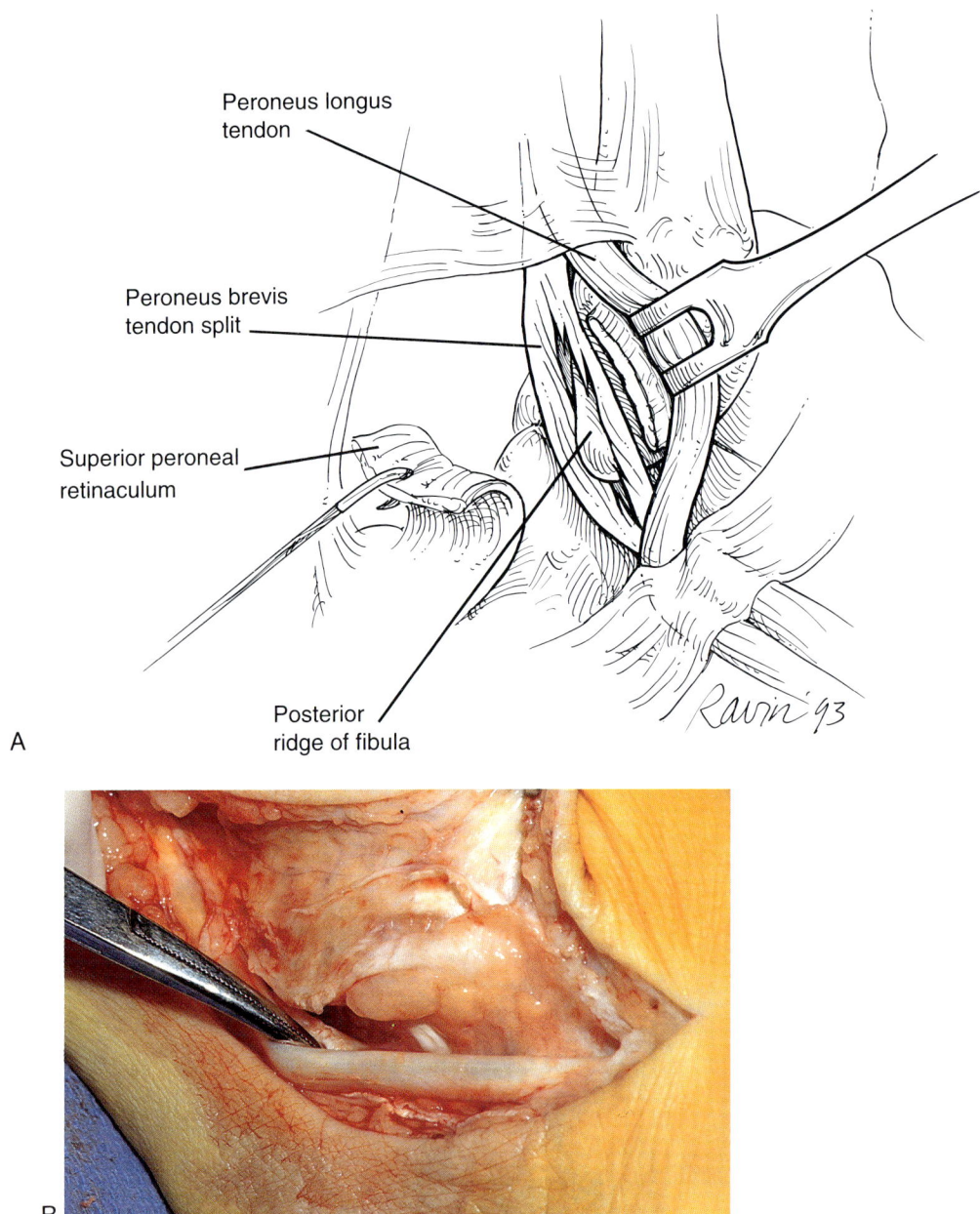

Figure 6. A: Exposure of the peroneus brevis tendon split by retraction of the superior peroneal retinaculum posteriorly, and the peroneus longus tendon anteriorly. **B:** Intraoperative exposure of the peroneal tendons reveals tenosynovitis involving the peroneal tendons along the lateral wall of the calcaneus.

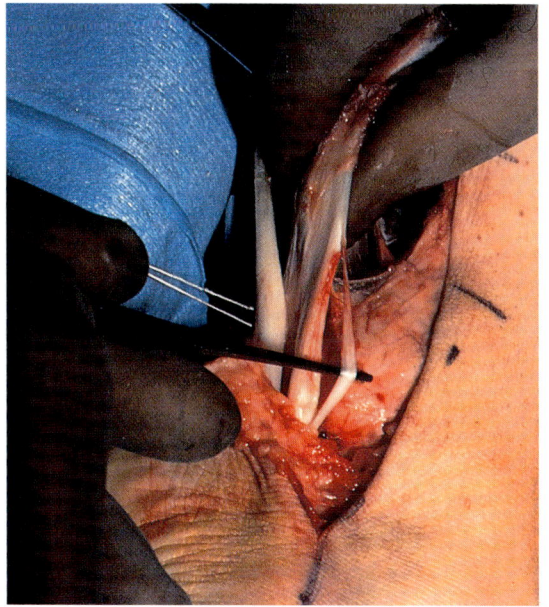

Figure 7. A: Debridement—repair of the peroneus brevis tendon and tubulation. Up to one-third of the anterior portion of the peroneus brevis tendon can be resected. **B:** Intraoperative photograph showing a split in the anterior third of the peroneus brevis tendon, which was resected. After adequate reefing and repair of the superior peroneal retinaculum, this young athlete went back to full activity without any pain at 1 year follow-up.

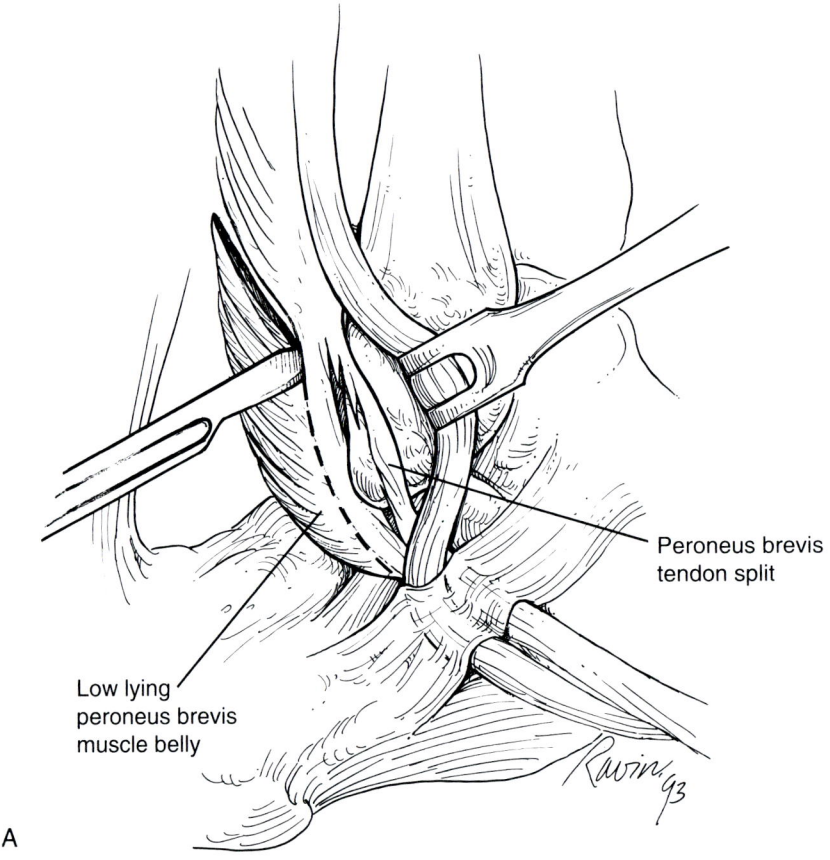

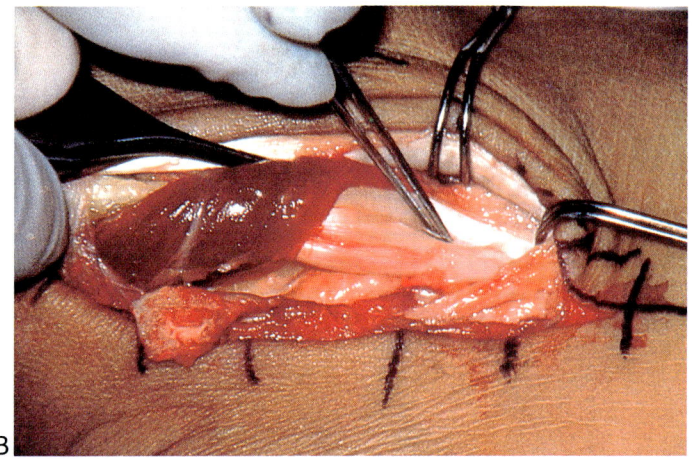

Figure 8. A: An abnormally low-lying portion of the muscle belly of the peroneus brevis should be resected. **B:** At surgery, the muscle belly of the peroneus brevis extended behind the fibula in the peroneal groove region.

Figure 10. A: If a severely frayed peroneus brevis tendon is found, the degenerated area may be resected and the proximal and distal ends of the tendon sutured to the peroneus longus tendon. **B:** Intraoperative photographs of a 30-year-old male athlete with chronic peroneal tendon attrition. Note retrofibular thickening in the involved ankle.

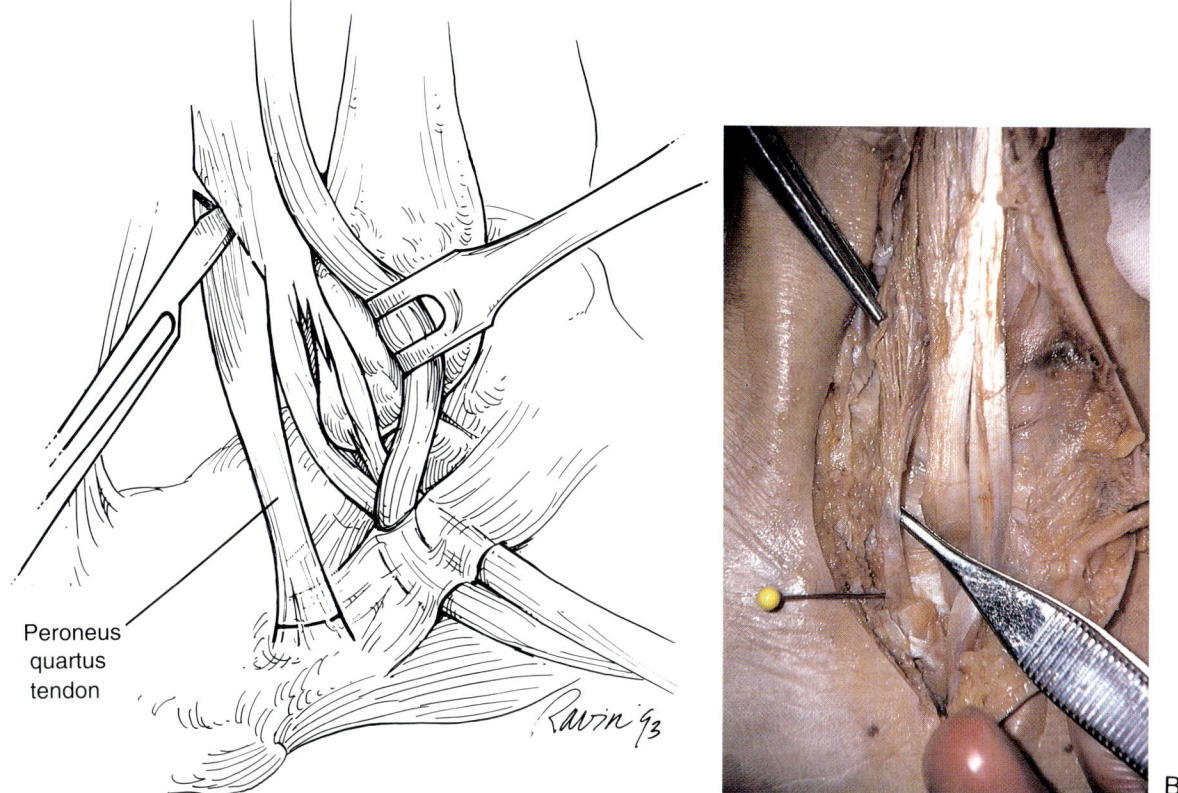

Figure 9. A: An anomalous peroneus quartus tendon in the peroneal tendon sheath should be removed. **B:** At surgery this tendon can be quite prominent.

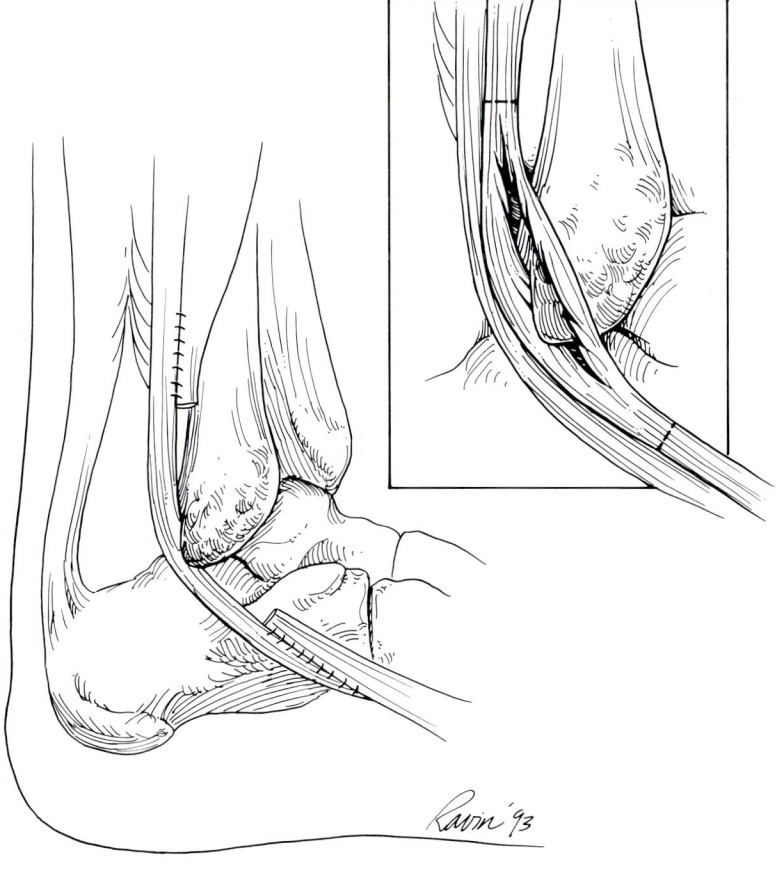
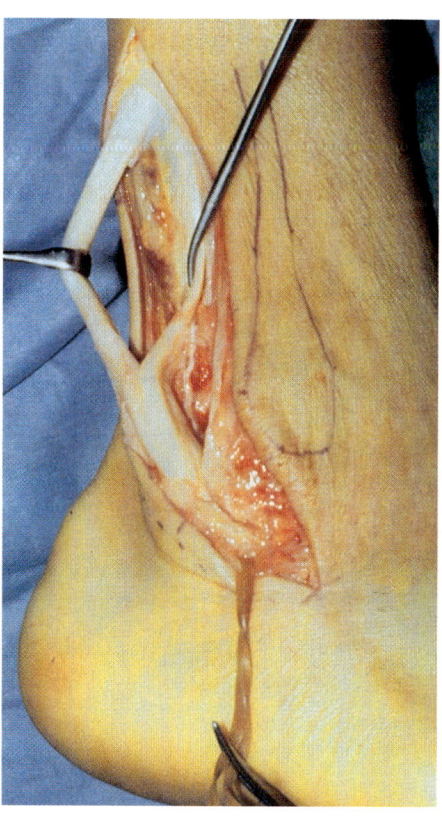

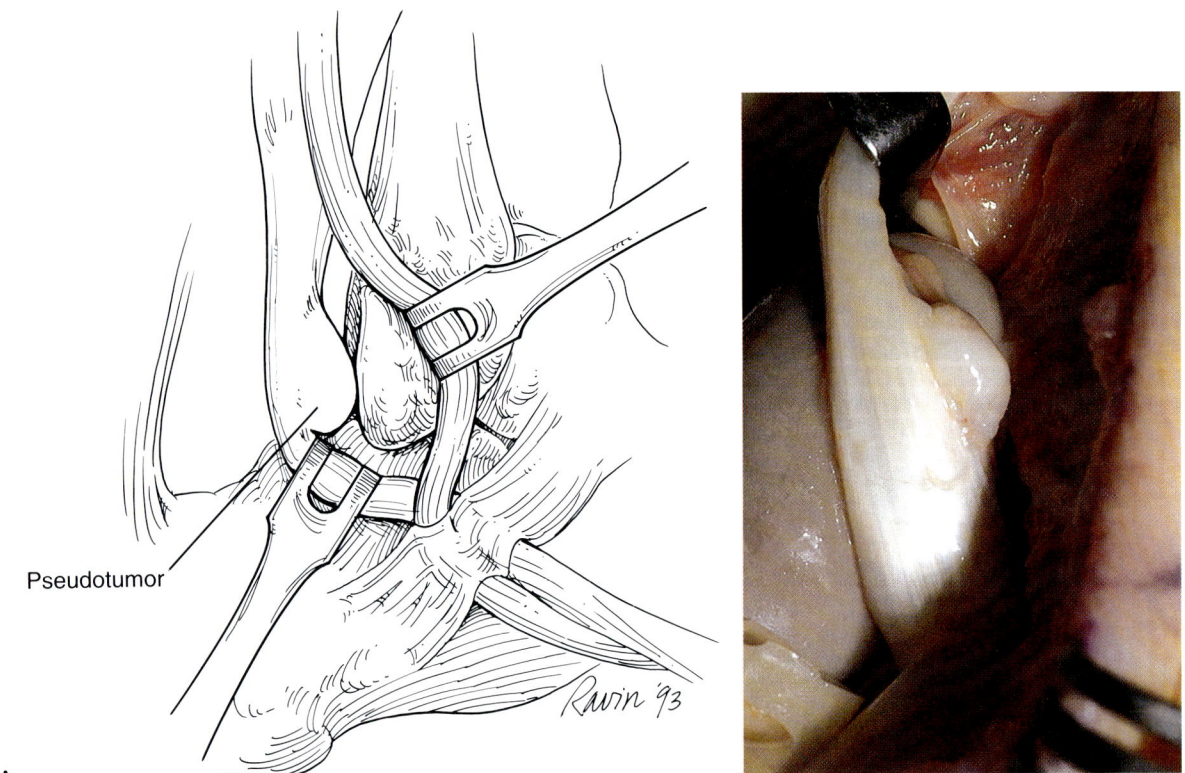

Figure 11. A: A thickened area of the peroneus brevis tendon is resected, leaving the tendon in continuity. **B:** Photograph of this thickened "pseudotumor" (within the peroneus brevis tendon at the level of the fibular groove).

tendon is severely degenerated) (Fig. 10); (b) resection of a thickened area of peroneus brevis tendon, leaving the tendon in continuity (Fig. 11); (c) utilizing the anterior one-half of the split peroneus brevis tendon for a modification of the Chrisman-Snook, or other tendon weaving procedures (Fig. 12); it is important to note that significant fraying of the peroneus brevis tendon at the site of the split may preclude weave-type reconstruction; and (d) transfer of the flexor hallucis longus tendon to repair combined tears of the peroneus brevis and peroneus longus tendon; attempts have been made to create a proper gliding tunnel for such a free tendon transfer by inserting a Hunter rod in a first procedure in the area of the peroneal tendons and in a second procedure performing a tendon transfer.

The sharp posterior ridge of the fibula can be removed with a rongeur and filed smooth, thus creating a fresh bony bed for the SPR repair. The superior peroneal retinaculum is then advanced and inserted onto the fresh bony bed on the posterior aspect of the fibula (Fig. 13). The SPR can be firmly secured to the fibula with an acuflex anchor or sutured to the periosteum as advocated by Gould. A posteriorly based trapdoor is then created using the periosteum anteriorly to the repaired SPR. This trapdoor is turned back and sutured on top of the SPR, thus reinforcing it.

Distal extension of the incision with anterior retraction of full-thickness flaps allows the primary repair of the attenuated anterior talofibular and calcaneofibular ligaments (4,9). After the repair, eversion stress and tension on the peroneus longus tendon tests for peroneal tendon subluxation. A gentle anterior drawer tests the tightness of the lateral ankle ligament repair and is compared to the preoperative laxity under anesthesia. Standard closure with a compressive soft tissue dressing and a posterior splint or cast is applied.

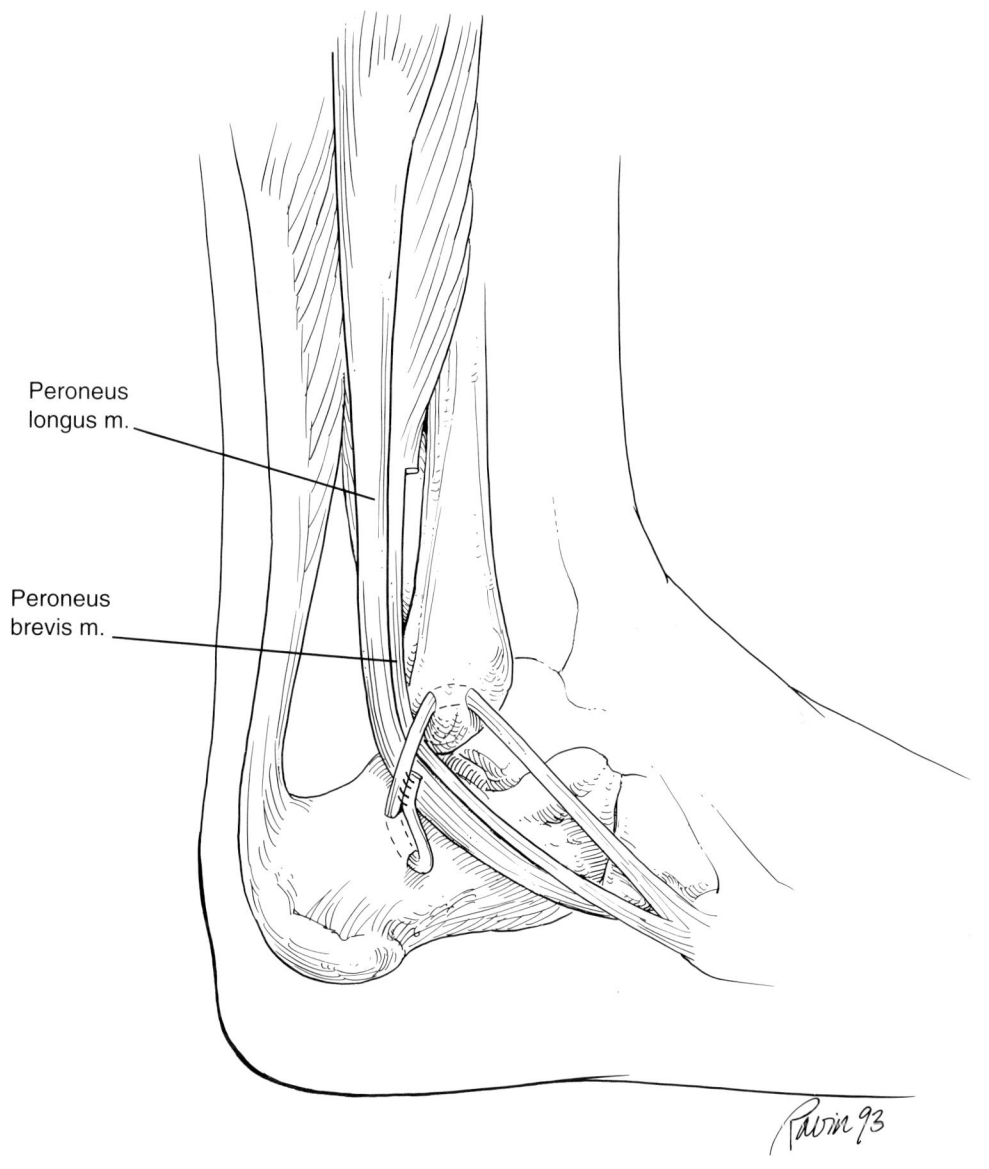

Figure 12. In the patient with lateral instability of the ankle, the lateral part of the split peroneus brevis tendon may be used for a reconstruction of the lateral collateral ligaments of the ankle in a tenodesis-type repair.

There are some pitfalls associated with surgical treatment of peroneal tendon injury since the blood supply to both peroneal tendons enters through posterolateral vincula. These synovial and vascular attachments to the peroneal tendons should not be violated. After repair or debridement of the peroneus brevis split, careful anatomic reconstruction of the SPR may have to be done to insure stability of the tendons within the groove.

Failure to identify and remove anomalous tissue within the groove (low-lying peroneus brevis muscle belly or peroneus quartus tendon) will allow an overpacking phenomenon and place the SPR under excess stress. Failure to recognize concurrent lateral ankle instability can lead to recurrent laxity and subsequent peroneal tendon injury.

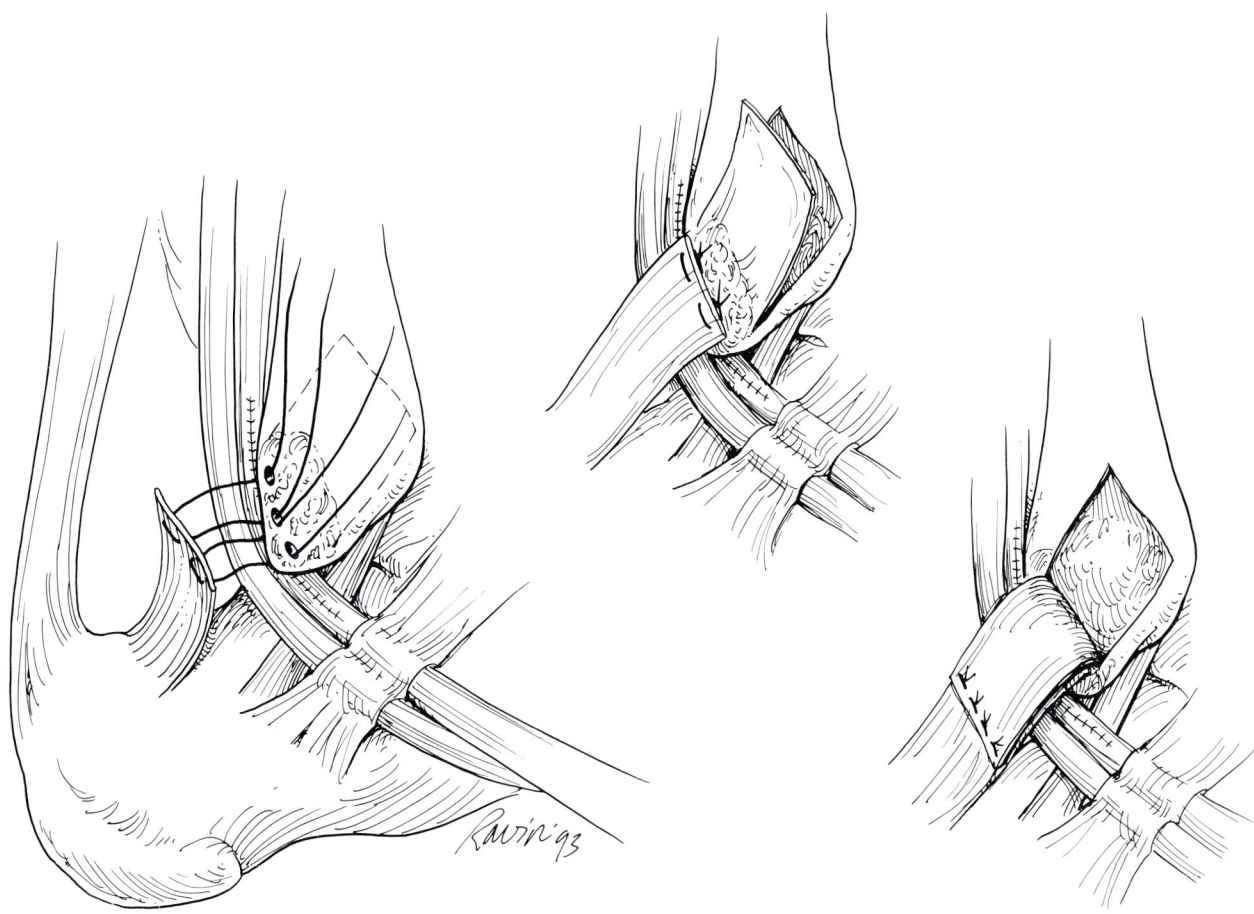

Figure 13. Illustration of the reefing and advancement of the superior peroneal retinaculum into the freshened bony bed on the posterior ridge of the lateral malleolus. A periosteal flap may be used to reinforce the retinacular repair.

POSTOPERATIVE MANAGEMENT

The patient is kept from weight bearing for 2 weeks. A short leg walking cast is used for a month and an air splint for another month, at which time peroneal strengthening exercises are begun.

COMPLICATIONS

Sural nerve injury and superficial peroneal nerve injury may be caused by improper placement of the incision proximally, or lack of appreciation of the branching and course of the sural nerve distally in the foot. Failure to perform anatomic reconstruction and advance of the stretched SPR can allow partial subluxation and recurrent peroneal tendon injury. It is important to appreciate and correct concurrent lateral ankle instability, otherwise SPR injury and peroneal tendon injury may occur. The posterolateral vincula of the peroneal tendons must be preserved during exploration to insure the tendon's ability for repair. The peroneus longus to brevis tenodesis presents theoretical disadvantages as this procedure sacrifices the function of the peroneus longus tendon insertion onto the first metatarsal. A dorsal bunion may develop secondary to loss of peroneus longus tendon function; additionally, loss of the plantar flexion of the first ray may occur.

ILLUSTRATIVE CASE FOR TECHNIQUE

A 30-year-old woman, a competitive soccer and tennis player since childhood, presented with a 4-year history of chronic pain in the lateral aspect of the right ankle and instability excluding her from sports. She recalled an initial twisting injury to the ankle approximately 4 years prior to presentation while playing tennis.

On active dorsiflexion and eversion of the ankle, the peroneal tendons subluxated from behind the lateral malleolus and this motion was painful through the entire distal course of the peroneal tendons in their sheath. A boggy swelling was noted in the peroneal sheath at the fibular groove.

Routine radiographs were normal. Upon exploration of the peroneal tendons, a posteriorly based osteoperiosteal flap was raised from the lateral aspect of the fibula. An abnormally low peroneus brevis muscle belly was noted to fill the fibular groove creating an overpacking phenomenon within the groove. There was a partial-thickness longitudinal split in the peroneus brevis tendon measuring 1 cm in length that was centered on the posterior edge of the fibula. In addition, an inflamed, thick, tenosynovium was present around the peroneal tendons at the fibular groove.

After a synovectomy, repair of the peroneus brevis, and excision of encroaching portion of the peroneus brevis muscle (approximately 3 cm proximal to the fibular groove), the peroneal tendons fell into their anatomic position. The attenuated superior peroneal retinaculum was then advanced anteriorly on the fibula and attached to a newly freshened bony surface as described above. The peroneal tendons no longer subluxated on dorsiflexion of the ankle and with the decompression and debulking, there was ample room for gliding of both peroneal tendons in their groove.

After the operation the leg was immobilized in a short leg cast for 4 weeks with the ankle in slight plantar flexion and eversion. Two months after removal of the cast the patient returned to full activity. At 1 year follow-up the patient had no symptoms of pain or instability in the ankle and no evidence of dislocation of the peroneal tendons.

RECOMMENDED READING

1. Burman, M.: Stenosing tendovaginitis of the foot and ankle: studies with special reference to the stenosing tendovaginitis of the peroneal tubercle. *Arch Surg.*, 67: 686–698, 1953.
2. Burman, M.: Subcutaneous tear of the tenon of the peroneus longus: its relationship to the giant peroneal tubercle. *Arch Surg.*, 73: 216–219, 1956.
3. Geppert, M. J., and Sobel, M.: The mechanism of the superior peroneal retinaculum laxity secondary to lateral ankle instability: an anatomic study. Presented at the AOA Residents and Fellows Meeting, March 14, 1992. *Foot Ankle*, in press Dec. 1992.
4. Gould, N., Seligson, D., and Gassman, J.: Early and late repair of lateral ligament of the ankle. *Foot Ankle*, 1: 84–89, 1980.
5. Sammarco, G. J., and DiRaimondo, C. V.: Chronic peroneus brevis tendon lesions. *Foot Ankle*, 9: 163–170, 1989.
6. Sobel, M., DiCarlo, E., Bohne, W. H. O., and Collins, L.: Longitudinal splitting of the peroneus brevis tendon: an anatomic and histologic study in cadaveric material. *Foot Ankle*, 12(3): 165–170, 1991.
7. Sobel, M., and Geppert, M. J.: Repair of concomitant lateral ankle ligament instability and peroneus brevis splits through a posteriorly modified Brostrom-Gould: technique tips. *Foot Ankle*, 13(4): 224–225, 1992.
8. Sobel, M., Geppert, M. J., Olson, E. J., Bohne, W. H. O., and Arnoczky, S. P.: The dynamics of peroneus brevis splits (PBS): a proposed mechanism, technique of diagnosis, and classification of injury. *Foot Ankle*, 13(7): 413–422, 1992.
9. Thompson, F. M., and Patterson, A. H.: Rupture of the peroneus longus tendon: a report of three cases. *J. Bone Joint Surg.*, 71A: 293–295, 1989.

23

Acute Repair of the Achilles Tendon

Keith L. Wapner

INDICATIONS/CONTRAINDICATIONS

Acute Achilles tendon ruptures most commonly occur in male patients aged 30 to 50 engaged in occasional sporting activities (1). Many etiologies have been suggested as predisposing factors, most of which suggest decreased vascularity of the tendon, placing it at risk (7). Relatively minor injury from an abrupt push-off or sudden falls causing acute contracture of the powerful tricep surae muscle complex or forced dorsiflexion of the ankle may produce rupture. Rupture may also occur in "weekend" athletes during high-demand sporting activities such as tennis or basketball. Some authors believe that acute rupture is proceeded by peritendinitis or tendinosis and is caused by a combination of mechanical and degenerative injury (6).

The diagnosis of an acute rupture of the Achilles tendon is made by a history of a pop or snap in the posterior aspect of the ankle with the acute onset of pain. Physical examination will reveal a swollen, painful ankle with ecchymosis often posteriorly. Swelling and hematoma within the paratenon may obscure a palpable gap within the tendon itself, but tenderness is generally present on examination. Many patients can still actively plantar flex the ankle against mild resistance because of the pull of the posterior tibial tendon and the long flexor tendons (1,17). A heel resistance test, performed by grasping the heel and resisting plantar flexion will demonstrate absence of plantar flexion power consistent with an Achilles tendon rupture. The Thompson test (3) has proved to be the most reliable indicator of Achilles tendon rupture (Fig. 1). With the patient prone and the feet extending over the end of the examination table the calf muscle is squeezed. If the tendon

---

K. L. Wapner, M.D.: Division of Foot and Ankle Surgery, Department of Orthopaedic Surgery, Thomas Jefferson University, Philadelphia, PA 19107.

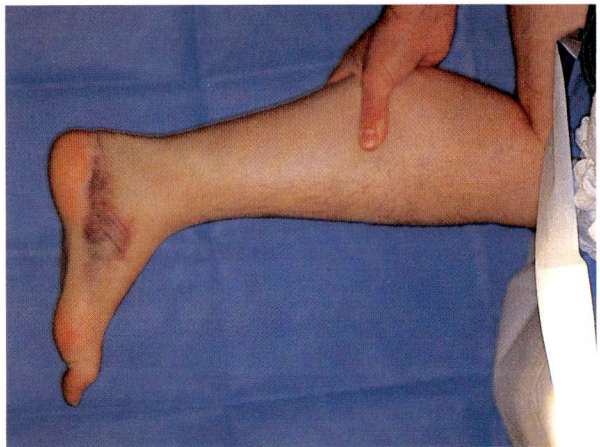

Figure 1. Demonstration of the Thompson test. As the calf is squeezed the foot does not plantar flex.

is intact the foot will plantar flex. If it is ruptured the foot will not move. This is diagnostic of Achilles tendon rupture.

Controversy exists regarding indications for open versus closed treatment of acute tendon ruptures. Proponents of open treatment cite many factors such as the ability to use a short leg cast postoperatively, lower re-rupture rates, greater strength, and greater endurance following open treatment (4,5,8,11,15,18). In the older or lower-demand patients nonoperative treatment may be adequate. In the younger or higher-demand patients I recommend open surgical treatment.

The general health of the patient and any associated system systemic diseases may influence the decision process regarding open versus closed treatment. Frank discussion of the risk and benefits of closed versus open treatment should be undertaken with the patient, and an informed mutual decision of treatment should be reached.

Contraindications to surgical care in addition to a low demand older patient are many and revolve about wound healing. The use of systemic cortisone and methotrexate, the presence of insulin-dependent diabetes mellitus, and vascular compromise of the lower extremity are relative contraindications to open surgical treatment.

PREOPERATIVE PLANNING

If operative treatment is planned, the foot should be maintained in a compressive Jones type dressing in mild plantar flexion prior to surgery. This will prevent the formation of fracture blisters and diminished swelling, which could compromise wound healing.

Plain lateral radiographs may reveal a defect in the shadow of the Achilles tendon, and the triangular lucency of the fat pad anterior to the Achilles tendon is generally obliterated. Magnetic resonance imaging (MRI) can also confirm the level and the extent of rupture. The diagnosis of rupture, however, is generally made clinically and the MRI, although instructional for educational purposes should generally be reserved for cases where the diagnosis is in doubt.

Ruptures may occur at the myotendinous junction but more commonly occur in the midsubstance of the tendon. Avulsion off of the calcaneal insertion may also occur. The level of rupture can usually be determined by physical examination, and identification of the level of the gap within the substance of the hindtendon.

SURGERY

The patient is placed in a prone position with axillary rolls under the chest and adequate padding of the upper extremities to avoid any possible neurovascular injury during surgery. Either general or spinal anesthesia is satisfactory. A pneumatic tourniquet is applied at the level of the thigh of the affected extremity, which is then prepped and draped in sterile fashion. After inflation of the tourniquet an incision is made along the posteromedial aspect of the leg starting just above the level of the myotendinous junction and extending to the level of the tendinous insertion on the calcaneus (14) (Fig. 2). In instances where avulsion of the tendon from its calcaneal insertion is suspected the incision may be lengthened distally to give better exposure. The incision should be deepened to the level of the paratenon. The paratenon is then opened to give exposure to the Achilles tendon (Fig. 3). It is critical that no flaps be raised until this level is reached so that the blood supply to the overlying skin can be protected.

A careful review and understanding of the anatomy of the Achilles tendon and its surrounding paratenon is essential to avoid postoperative wound complications. The sural nerve perforates the crural fascia at the myotendinous junction and

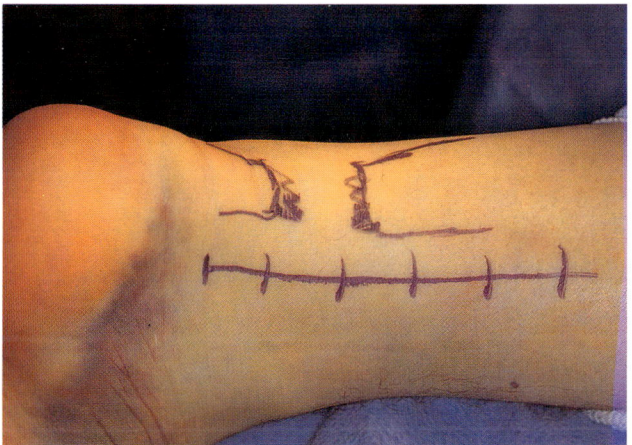

Figure 2. Demonstration of the site of the incision for posterior medial approach.

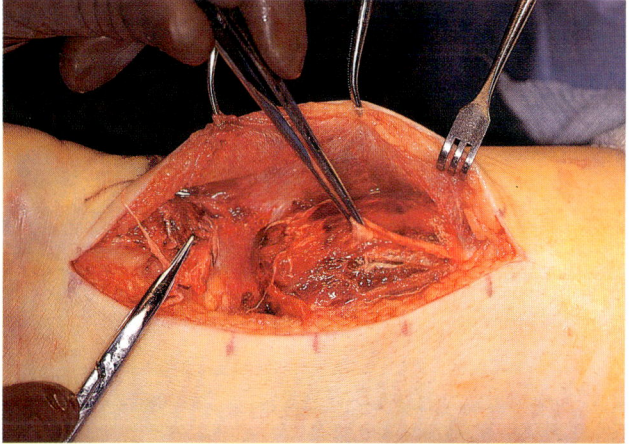

Figure 3. The paratenon is opened giving exposure to the Achilles tendon. The paratenon can be seen grasped by the hemostats. The posterior flap of skin should be a full-thickness flap including skin, subcutaneous fat, extending down to this level of the paratenon.

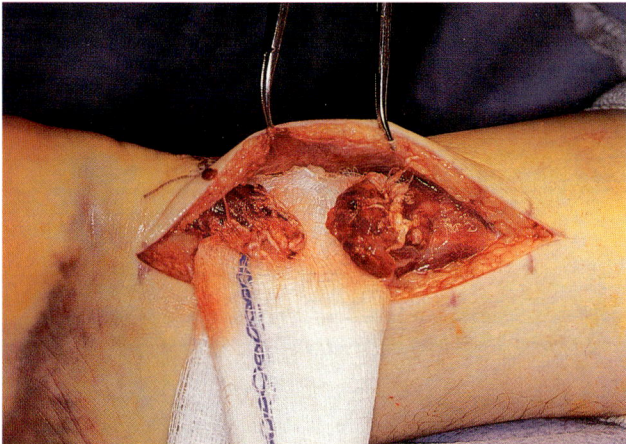

Figure 4. Demonstration of the mop-handled tear of the midsubstance of the Achilles tendon.

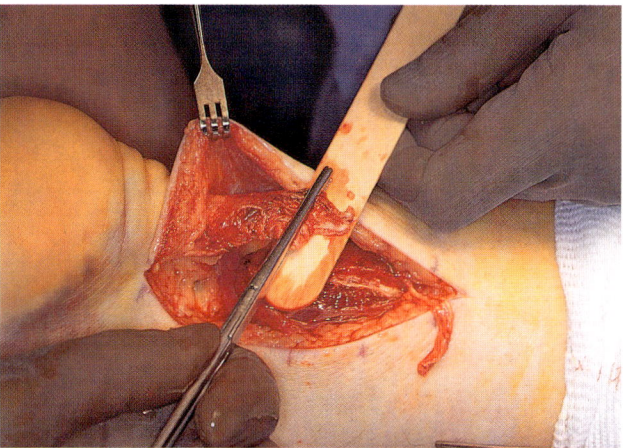

Figure 5. Debridement of the torn end of the tendon using a tongue depressor and a wide blade.

passes subcutaneously distally on the lateral aspect of the Achilles tendon. A medial incision avoids injury to this nerve. It also allows easier access to the plantaris tendon, which, if present, passes deep to the crural fascia along the medial aspect of the Achilles tendon. The plantaris may be used to augment primary surgical repair of the tendon.

The Achilles tendon itself is not covered by a tendon sheath, but rather a paratenon composed of areolar connective tissue and elastic fibers (6). In any surgical repair the tendon should be exposed deep to the layer of the paratenon. The paratenon should be reflected as part of the full-thickness flap with the overlying subcutaneous tissue and skin to avoid disruption of the vascular supply to the skin.

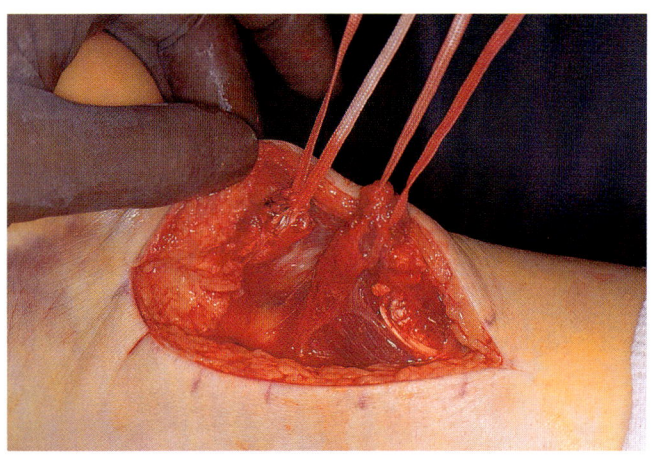

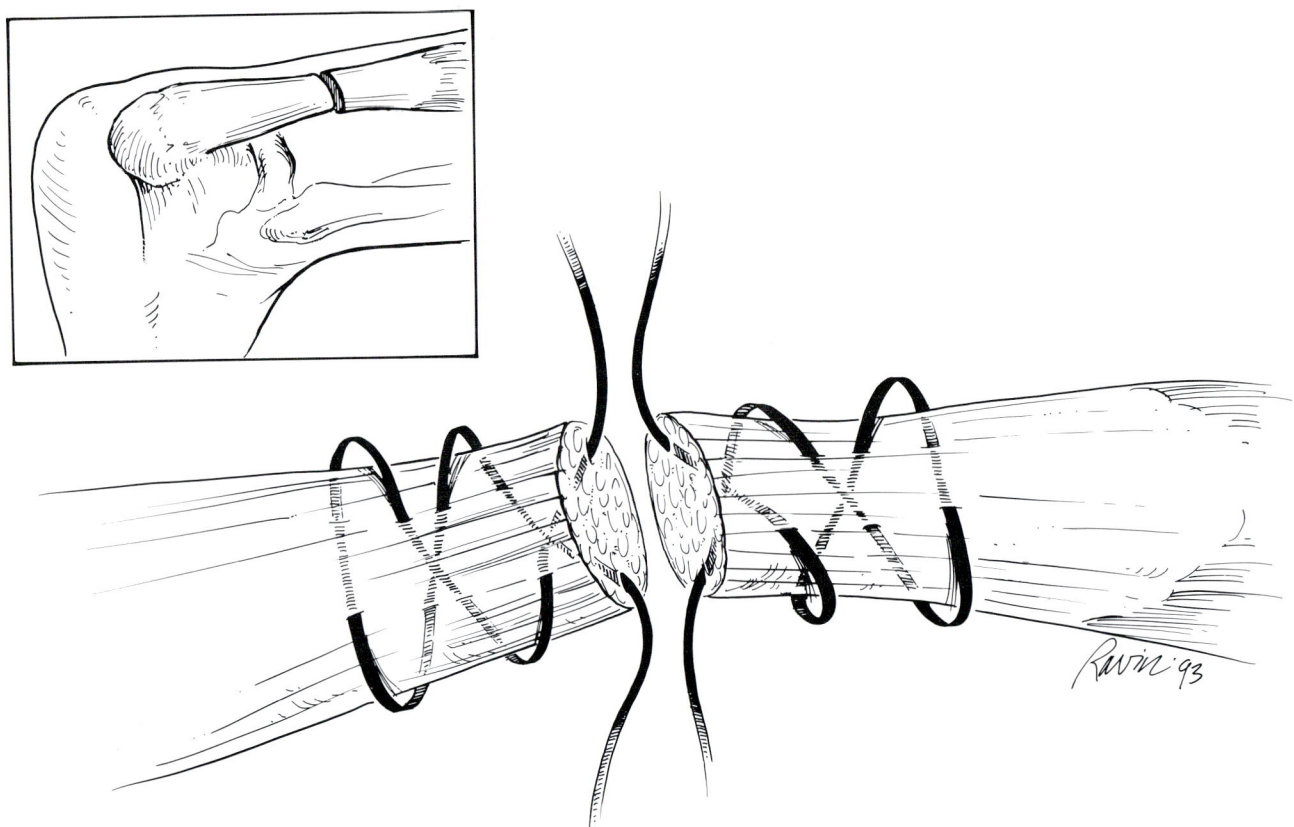

Figure 6. A: A heavy suture such as #3 cottony Dacron is placed in the proximal and distal stumps using a Kessler type stitch. **B:** Suture placement.

If the plantaris tendon is present it will be easily identified within the substance of the wound. The paratenon can then be elevated as part of a full-thickness flap off of the Achilles tendon, and inspection of the level of the rupture can be performed. Any intervening hematoma at this time should be evacuated with lavage. The ruptures are generally mop-handle type tears (Fig. 4), and the frayed ends of the tendon can be debrided at this time. This is best accomplished by placing the torn end of the tendon over a tongue depressor and using a wide blade to trim the cut ends of the tendon (Fig. 5).

A tear at the level of the myotendinous junction is often difficult to repair because of inadequate purchase of suture material into the proximal tissues. A modification of the Lindholm (12) technique can be useful in this instance. Rather than inverted tendon strips being raised from proximal and reflected distally, the tendon strips are raised from the long distal portion of the tendon and inverted proximally. These strips can be woven into place to allow continuity of tendon material to augment the repair. Primary suturing of the tendon is carried out in an identical fashion to midsubstance tendon ruptures as described below.

For a midsubstance tear of the Achilles tendon, after debridement of the tendon edges, a heavy suture such as #3 cottony Dacron is placed using a Kessler technique in the proximal stump. A second suture is then placed in the distal stump (Fig. 6). The knee is then flexed and the foot is plantar flexed and the ends of the suture can then be tied without tension (Figs. 7 and 8). The repair is then aug-

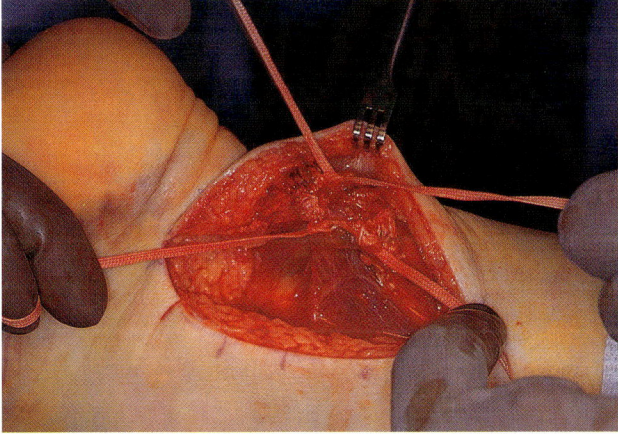

Figure 7. With the knee flexed and the foot plantar flexed the torn end of the tendon can be opposed without tension.

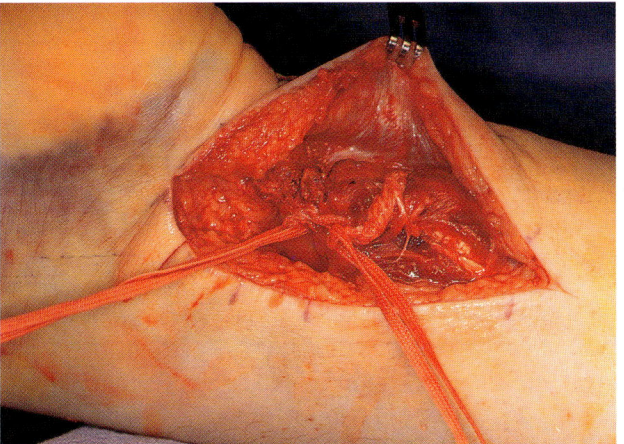

Figure 8. The ends of the suture are then tied to secure repair and opposition of the tendon ends.

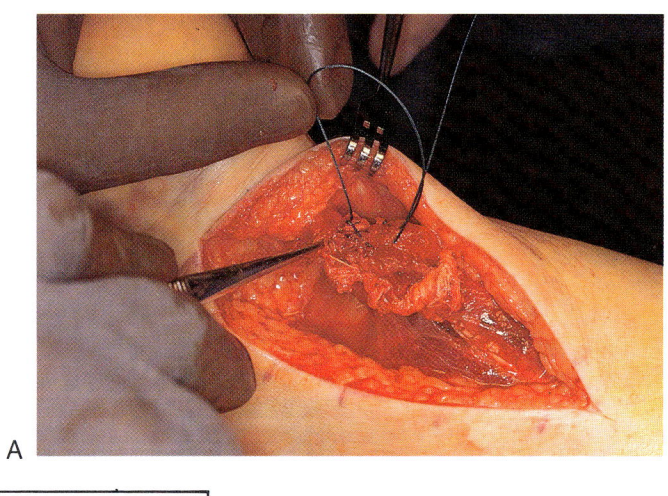

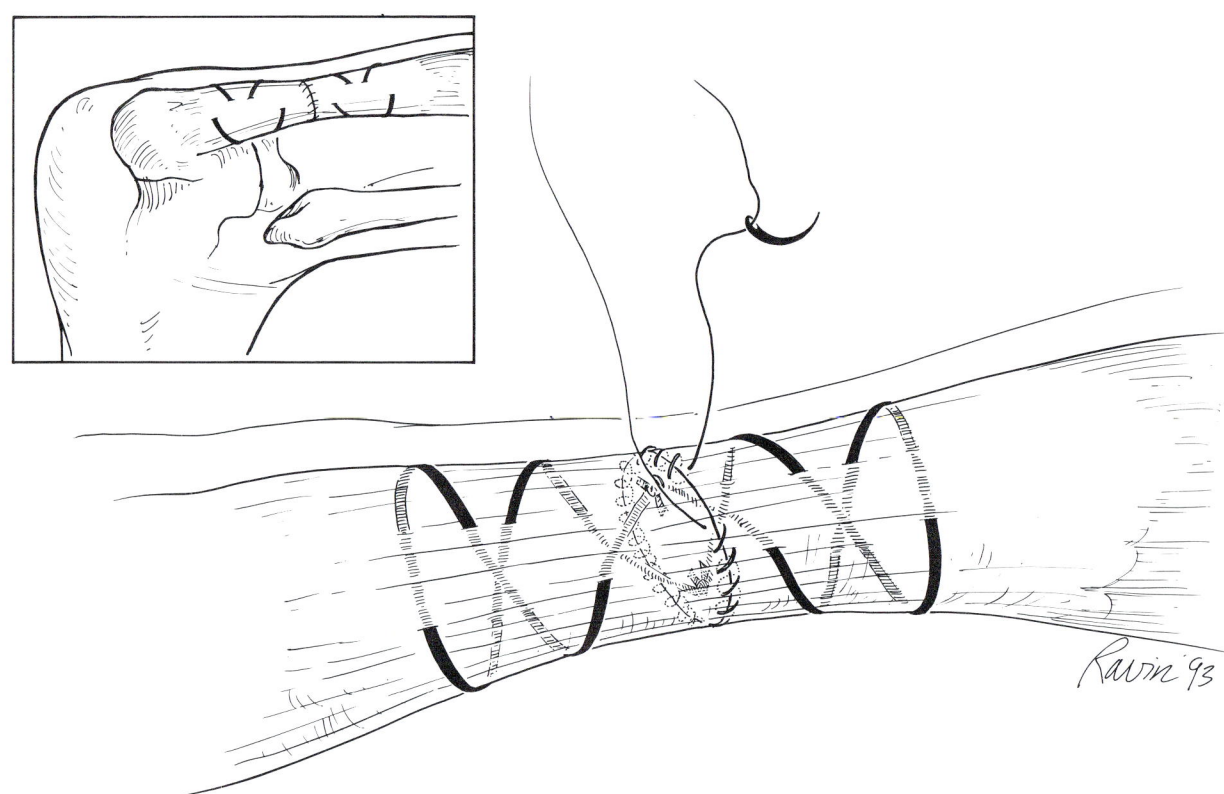

Figure 9. A: Repairs augmented using a #1 cottony Dacron vertical locking circumferential suture. **B:** Suture placement.

mented using a #1 cottony Dacron vertical locking circumferential suture (Fig. 9).

When the tendon has been avulsed off of the insertion of the calcaneus, repair is accomplished by placing drill holes through the area of insertion of the tendon and the area of the avulsion is curetted of its overlying fibrous tissue down to cancellous bone. A #3 cottony Dacron suture is placed through the stump of the tendon as described above and the ends of the suture are then brought through these drill holes within the substance of the bone. They are then tied over the bony bridge to secure fixation of the portion of the tendon to the underlying bone.

When the plantaris tendon is present, it may be useful to weave this tendon through this area of repair to augment the ultimate strength (13,16). At this point the wound is copiously irrigated and care is taken to approximate the edges of

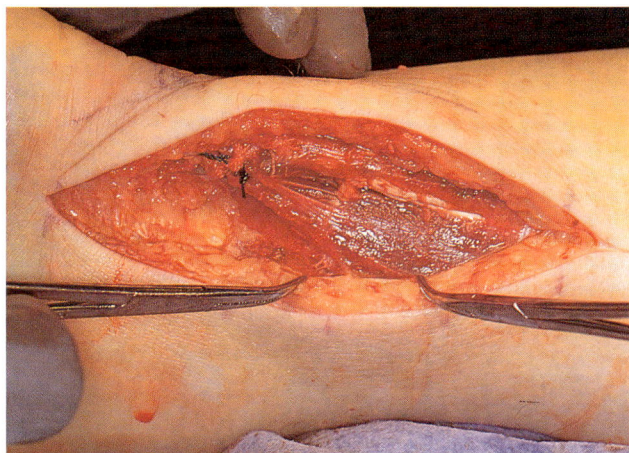

Figure 10. Demonstration of the anterior margin of the paratenon. The anterior/posterior margins should be closed prior to skin closure.

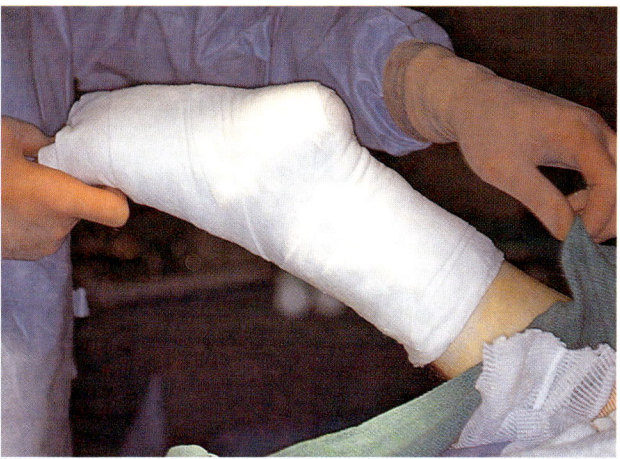

Figure 11. The foot is maintained in 20° of plantar flexion. The initial soft dressing seen here is covered with a bulky compressive dressing and plaster splints to maintain the foot in this plantar flexed position.

the paratenon. Closure of this will help prevent scarring of the tendon to the overlying soft tissues and skin. Closure of the paratenon (Fig. 10) and closure of the overlying skin should be accomplished with the foot maintained in plantar flexed position to keep tension off of the area of repair. The foot is placed in a below-knee bulky compressive dressing with plaster splints holding the foot in 20° of equinus (Fig. 11). In the instances of a very proximal rupture at the level of the myotendinous junction, if the sutures are felt to be at risk of pull-out, the patient will be placed in a long leg splint with the knee maintained in 30° of plantar flexion and the foot at 20° of the equinus.

POSTOPERATIVE MANAGEMENT

The patient is maintained in a bulky compressive dressing for the initial 10 days postoperatively, at which time he or she is seen in the office. The dressings are removed and the wound inspected. Sutures are generally removed at this point and Steri-strips applied to the wound. Care must be taken to maintain the foot in its plantar flexed position during the cast change. The patient is then recast, maintained in 20° of plantar flexion, and continued non-weight bearing for an additional 2½ weeks.

At 4 weeks the patient is taken out of the cast and placed in a sitting position on the side of an examination table. A foot rest is then placed under the ball of the foot elevated so that the hip is flexed and the knee is flexed (Fig. 12). The patient is placed in this position and allowed to sit for approximately 15 to 20 minutes. This allows gradual reduction of the foot to a more neutral posture through the effects of gravity rather than active motor or passive manipulation. Most patients at this juncture can reach a neutral position and are then recast in a short leg walking cast for an additional 4 weeks. If a neutral posture is not obtained the patient is brought back to the office in 1 week and again sits in the same position to allow achievement of neutral position.

At 8 weeks the patient is taken out of the cast and placed into a shoe with a 1-inch heel lift. Active physical therapy is then started. The instance of re-rupture of the Achilles tendon in most reports is lower following surgical repair than nonoperative repair (2,9,10). One of the contributing factors to preventing re-rupture is a very gradual but continued program of stretching. Attempts should be made to regain full dorsiflexion of the involved ankle but patients should be cautioned that

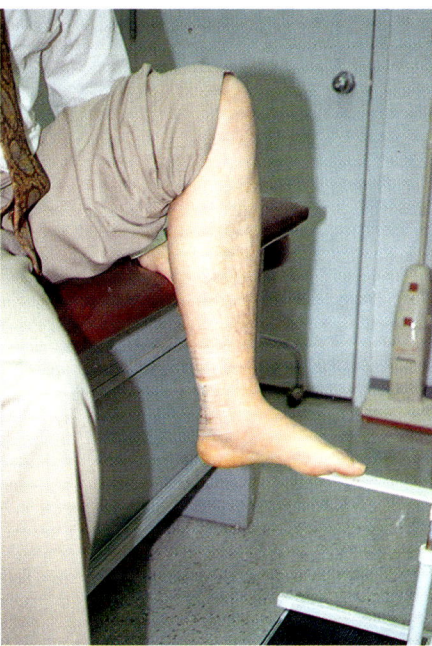

Figure 12. The patient is placed sitting with the hip and knee flexed and the forefoot resting on a foot rest. The patient stays in this position until gravity allows the foot to achieve a plantar grade posture. At this point a short leg walking cast is applied.

this is a very slow process. Similarly, physical therapists should be cautioned about their enthusiasm regarding passive stretching of the repaired tendon. Instructing patients in the importance of compliance of long-term stretching, especially prior to engaging in any sporting events, will also diminish the incidence of re-rupture of the tendon.

REHABILITATION

Initial therapy involves general passive stretching and active use of Theraband to return strength to not only the gastrosoleus complex but the other muscles about the foot and ankle. The heel lift is continued until 10° of dorsiflexion is obtained. A physical therapy program should incorporate retraining of all the muscles about the foot and ankle as well as proprioceptive training. This is critical in order to avoid further injury to the ankle. Most of the therapy can be done as a home program if the patient is well motivated. The patient is allowed to resume normal activities once he has achieved full motor strength equal to the uninvolved extremity. Patients are instructed to continue on a long-term stretching program for at least 1 year postoperatively. They are also instructed to perform stretching exercises prior to commencing any type of sporting activity on a permanent basis.

COMPLICATIONS

Most complications of operative Achilles tendon repair can be avoided by meticulous technique. The most significant complication is one of skin slough. By taking care to carry out the dissection to the level of the paratenon and avoid separating the paratenon from the overlying subcutaneous tissues and skin, this complication can generally be avoided. Adequate immobilization with compressive dressings prior to the time of surgery also significantly contributes to the avoidance of this complication. When skin slough occurs, the size of the slough will determine what options are available. For small slough, local myocutaneous gastroc Y-V slides or medial plantar artery flaps may be adequate to close the area of slough. If the slough is larger it may be necessary to incorporate a free flap using either radial forearm or scapular flap.

Painful scar may be a long-term complication of surgical repair. The location of the incision may contribute to this problem. Avoidance of the sural nerve by placing the incision posteromedially and avoidance of direct posterior incision, which would be irritated by common shoe wear, are recommended.

ILLUSTRATIVE CASE FOR TECHNIQUE

A 46-year-old man was playing handball and made a sudden uncoordinated move. He had immediate pain and swelling in the posterior aspect of his ankle. In the emergency room, a radiograph (Fig. 13) shows a bone avulsion fracture off the posterior aspect of the calcaneal tuberosity. A compression dressing was applied and the patient was treated surgically the following day.

At the time of surgery, the bone fragment, which had been avulsed from the posterior aspect of the tuberosity, was located at the distal end of the Achilles tendon (Fig. 14). This bone fragment was removed and then an O-Ethibond suture

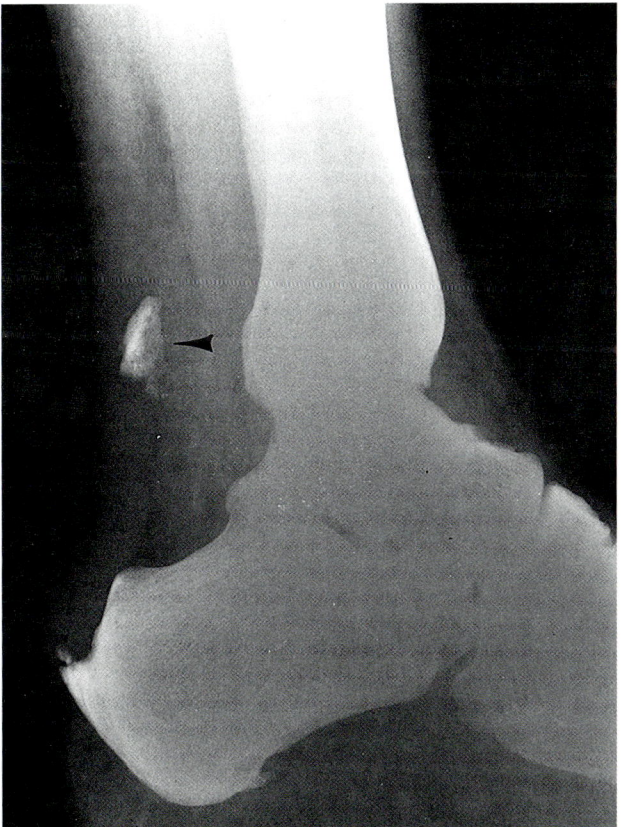

Figure 13. A portion of the calcaneal tuberosity, which is attached to the distal end of the Achilles tendon *(arrow)*, is seen riding well above the tuberosity of the calcaneus.

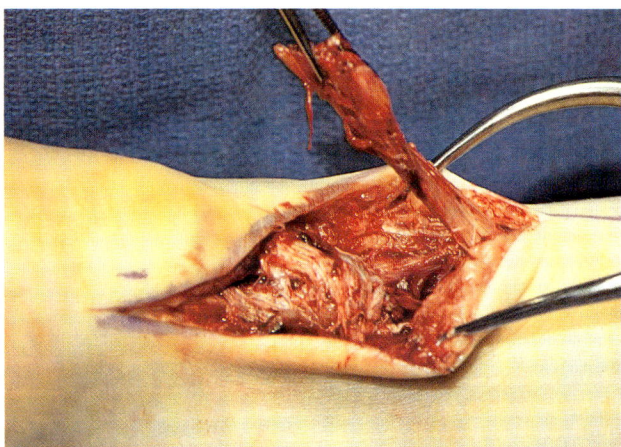

Figure 14. The thumb forceps holds the bony fragment that had been avulsed from the calcaneal tuberosity.

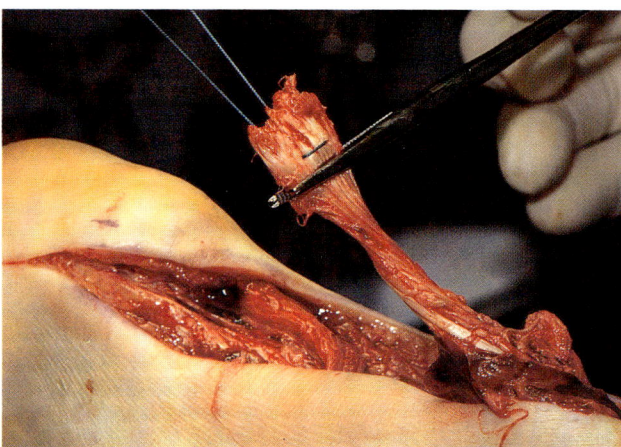

Figure 15. An O-Ethibond suture is woven through the distal end of the Achilles tendon.

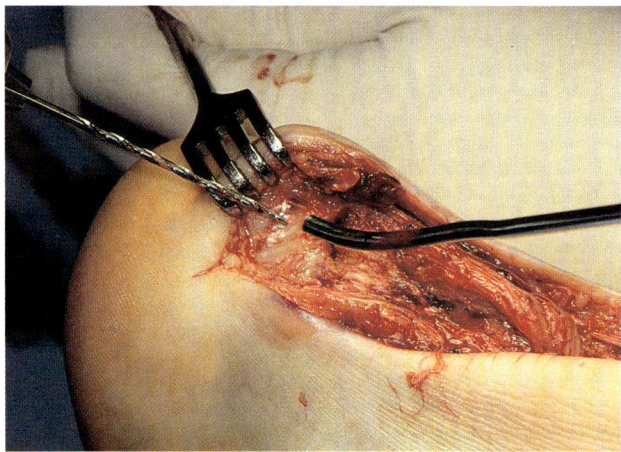

Figure 16. A $\frac{1}{8}''$ drill is placed through the tuberosity of the os calcis up to the defect where the bone fragment was avulsed. Two drill holes are placed.

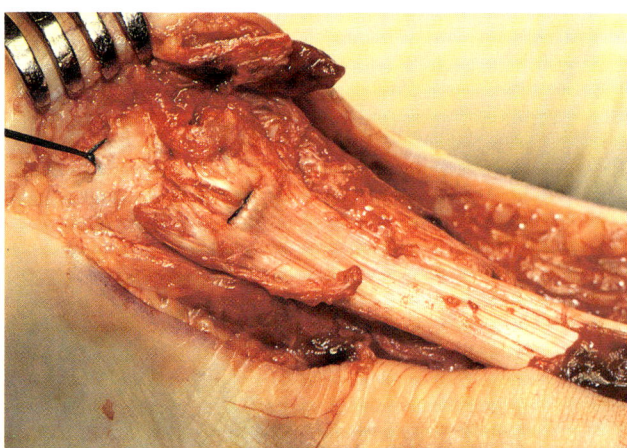

Figure 17. The end of the Achilles tendon is brought down into the cancellous area of the calcaneal tuberosity and the suture is tied over the bone island between the drill holes distally.

was woven through the distal end of the Achilles tendon (Fig. 15). Drill holes were placed in the Achilles tendon so that the tendon would be brought down to a denuded calcaneus area of bone where the tendon had avulsed off the bony fragment (Fig. 16). The tendon was then pulled down into the proper position over the denuded area of bone (Fig. 17).

The patient's ankle was kept in an equinus position for a period of 10 weeks, as it was anticipated it would take a longer period of time for the tendon to heal to the bone and also because the intrinsic strength of the repair was less than would be present if it was a midsubstance tendon repair. The patient's ankle was then gradually brought up into a neutral position and active and passive range of motion exercises as well as strengthening exercises were begun. At 1 year he had excellent function and was beginning to return to active sports activities.

RECOMMENDED READING

1. Arner, O., and Lindholm, A.: Subcutaneous rupture of the Achilles tendon. *Acta Chir. Scand. [Suppl.]*, 239: 1–51, 1959.

2. Beskin, J. L., Sanders, R. A., Hunter, S. C., and Hugitston, J. C.: Surgical repair of Achilles tendon ruptures. *Am. J. Sports Med.*, 15: 1, 1987.
3. Elstrom, P. A.: In: *Surgery of Musculoskeletal System*, vol 8, C. McC. Evarts, editor, pp. 172–179. Churchill Livingstone, New York, 1983.
4. Gillies, H., and Chalmers, J.: The management of fresh ruptures of the tendoachilles. *J. Bone Joint Surg.*, 52A: 337, 1970.
5. Haggmark, T., Liedberg, H., Eriksson, E., Wredmark, T.: Calf muscle atrophy and muscle function after non-operative vs. operative treatment of Achilles tendon ruptures. *Orthopedics*, 9: 160: 1986.
6. Hansen, S. T.: Trauma to the calcaneus and its tendon: trauma to the heel cord. In: *Disorders of the Foot and Ankle: Medical and Surgical Management*, edited by M. H. Jahss. Saunders, Philadelphia, 1991.
7. Hatrup, S. J., and Johnson, K. A.: A review of ruptures of the Achilles tendon. *Foot Ankle*, 6: 34, 1985.
8. Inglis, A. E., Scott, W. N., Sculco, T. P., and Patterson, A. H.: Ruptures of the tendoachilles. *J. Bone Joint Surg.*, 58A: 990, 1976.
9. Inglis, A. E., and Sculco, T. P.: Surgical repair of ruptures of the tendoachilles. *Clin. Orthop.*, 156: 160, 1981.
10. Jacobs, D., Marteus, M., and Van Audekercke, R.: Comparison of conservative and operative treatment of Achilles tendon rupture. *Am. J. Sports Med.*, 6: 107, 1978.
11. Lea, R. B., and Smith, L.: Non-surgical treatment of tendoachilles rupture. *J. Bone Joint Surg.*, 54A: 1398, 1972.
12. Lindholm, A.: A new method of operation in subcutaneous rupture of the Achilles tendon. *Acta Chir. Scand.*, 117: 261, 1959.
13. Lynn, T. A.: Repair of the torn Achilles tendon, using plantaris tendon as a reinforcing membrane. *J. Bone Joint Surg.*, 48A: 268, 1966.
14. Mann, R. A.: Traumatic injuries to the soft tissues of the foot and ankle. In: *Surgery of the Foot*, 5th ed., edited by R. A. Mann, C. V. Mosby, St. Louis, p. 480. 1985.
15. Nistor, L.: Surgical and non-surgical treatment of Achilles tendon rupture. *J. Bone Joint Surg.*, 63A: 394, 1981.
16. Phillips, B. B.: Traumatic disorders. In: *Campbell's Operative Orthopedics*, 8th ed., edited by A. H. Crenshaw, C. V. Mosby, St. Louis, p. 1905. 1991.
17. Ralston, E. L., and Schmidt, E. R.: Repair of the ruptured Achilles tendon. *J. Trauma*, 11: 15, 1971.
18. Stein, S. R., and Leukens, C. A.: Closed treatment of Achilles tendon ruptures. *Orthop. Clin. North Am.*, 5: 89, 1974.
19. Thompson, T. C., and Doherty, J. H.: Spontaneous rupture of tendon of Achilles: a new clinical diagnostic test. *J. Trauma*, 2: 126, 1962.

24

Delayed Repair of the Achilles Tendon

Jason H. Calhoun

INDICATIONS/CONTRAINDICATIONS

The indications for repairing delayed Achilles tendon ruptures are complaints of plantar flexion weakness of the ankle during ambulation, climbing, or carrying objects (4). Patients with an old rupture will usually seek help only if they have such a disability and would benefit from a repair (4).

Nonsurgical management is directed toward shoe-wear modifications including heel lifts and lace-up high-top shoes, boots, or braces that hold the foot in plantar flexion during gait. Work or activity modifications may also be tried to decrease the need to plantar flex the foot.

The decision to operate is based on host factors such as systemic disease and the quality of the tissue. If the etiology is a laceration and the duration fairly recent, then the tendon will be easier to repair than if the time from rupture is longer or due to a connective tissue disease such as rheumatoid arthritis. Other systemic factors that make the repair weaker include advanced age, diabetes mellitus, obesity, autoimmune disorders, and malnutrition. Local factors that make the repair weaker or cause postoperative wound problems include ischemia due to peripheral vascular disease, scars, and infections about the foot. The patient must also be able to tolerate a cast for at least 8 weeks and then be active in rehabilitation to obtain a functional range of motion. In general, healthy, young, active patients will do well, whereas older, debilitated, inactive patients will have more problems with a surgical repair.

J. H. Calhoun, M.D., M.Eng.: Department of Orthopaedic Surgery, University of Texas Medical Branch, Galveston, TX 77555-0792.

PREOPERATIVE PLANNING

The diagnosis is made by reviewing the patient's history and performing a physical examination. The usual history of an acute rupture is pain and inability to rise onto the toes. At the time of rupture, patients often report the sensation of being hit in the calf from behind but have minimal pain until hematoma formation occurs. Patients with systemic connective tissue disorders such as rheumatoid arthritis may relate a more gradual onset with Achilles tendinitis pain and eventual loss

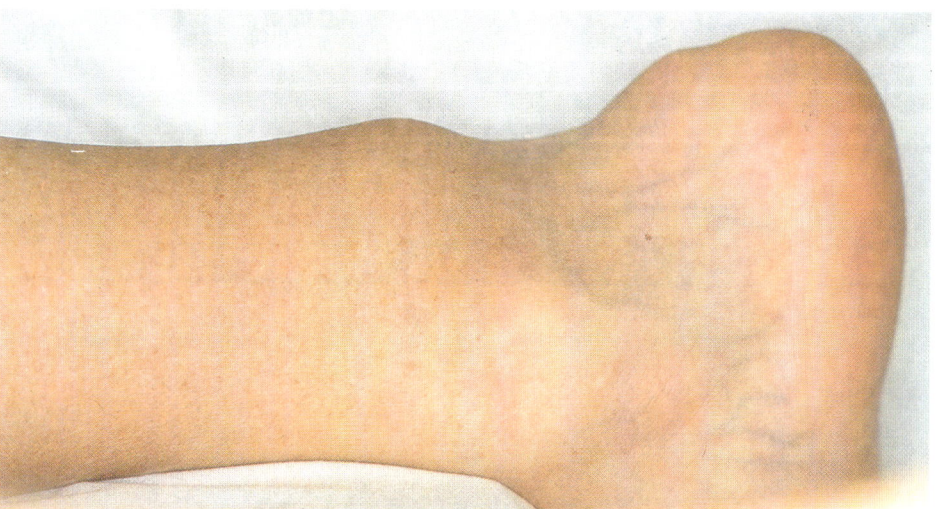

Figure 1. Appearance of the depression in the Achilles tendon with an untreated rupture.

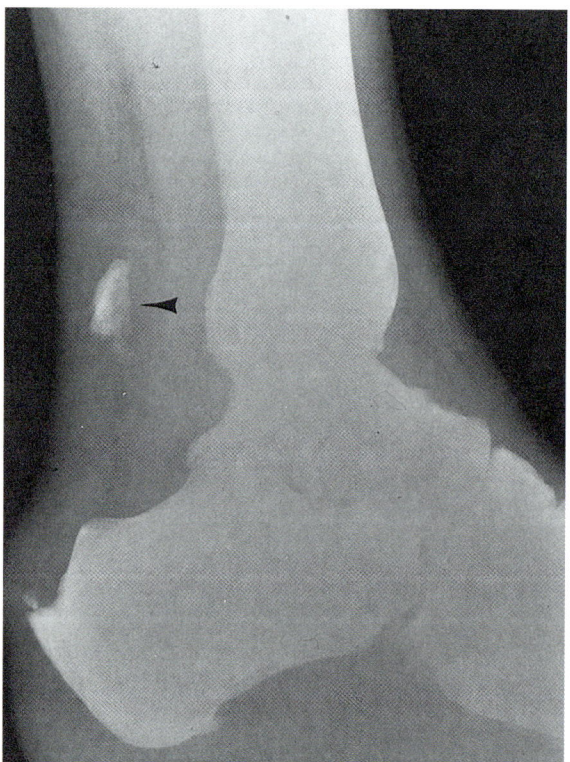

Figure 2. Proximal migration of an avulsion fracture fragment (*arrow*) from the Achilles tendon insertion.

of the ability to rise onto the toes. In either case, some active plantar flexion is maintained due to the extrinsic toe flexors, posterior tibial, and peroneal tendons. Misdiagnosis of the time of the rupture is quite high at 20%. Initially, there may not be an obvious defect but with time the ends of the rupture separate and the overlying skin shrinks to conform with the back of the ankle. In fact, it may appear that there is an overgrowth of the posterior calcaneus (Fig. 1). The Thompson, or calf squeeze, test will be positive but will not cause much pain in an old injury. Radiographs should be obtained to rule out avulsion of the posterior tuberosity of the calcaneus (Fig. 2), bony deformities, and calcification of the tendon. Magnetic resonance imaging (MRI) may be helpful in the uncertain diagnosis of an Achilles tendon rupture. It is most helpful in a sagittal plane to determine the length of tendon injured and to anticipate the type of surgical procedure needed.

The rupture usually occurs 2 to 6 cm from the calcaneal insertion, which is the most avascular region of the tendon. If the defect, by clinical examination or MRI, is less than about 4 cm, then local tissue may be used. If the gap is greater than 4 cm after scar tissue debridement, then a V-Y lengthening to close the gap will be necessary. These will be described individually.

SURGERY

Technique. After general anesthesia, the patient is placed in the prone position. Under tourniquet control, the skin incision is made lateral to the tendon. An incision made straight posterior will produce an unsightly scar that will be adherent to the repaired tendon. The sural nerve needs to be protected when making the lateral incision. It is quite variable in location and prone to neuroma formation. I identify the sural nerve by palpation in the incision and with minimal dissection. The sural nerve is then protected by leaving a wide margin of fat around it and by not exposing it after identification. The skin flap posterior to the tendon is kept as thick as possible to avoid later wound edge necrosis. Intraoperative and postoperative antibiotics are used.

The surgical technique utilizing local tissue is applicable when the gap to be closed can be bridged by local tissue along with placing the ankle in plantar flexion. This usually involves a suturing of the Achilles tendon along with one or more local tissue transfers. Besides the end-to-end suturing, transfer of the plantaris tendon, flexor digitorum longus tendon, and a turndown of fascia may also be reasonable, depending on the surgeon's preference and tissue available.

My own practice, after suturing the tendon in an end-to-end manner, is to splay out the plantaris tendon if it is present and suture it across the repair. If no plantaris is present, I will instead utilize the flexor digitorum longus across the tendon repair. If after the tendon transfer the repair is still tenuous, I will then turn down a proximal length of the gastrocsoleus fascia.

End-to-end repair alone is seldom successful in the delayed Achilles tendon rupture, but it is usually included in all repairs. The ruptured ends are trimmed of scar tissue to encourage healing after repair. The foot is plantar flexed and the knee bent to relax the gastrocnemius and soleus muscle and the ends are repaired with a heavy (#5) nonabsorbable braided suture (Fig. 3). Then the tendon edges are completely closed with interrupted (2–0 to 4–0) nylon sutures. Usually the end-to-end repair will need to be augmented with tissue transfers.

The plantaris tendon is located medial to the Achilles tendon. The tendon may be weaved through the Achilles tendon or be thinned and splayed out to cover the Achilles tendon (Fig. 4). Although the plantaris tendon is present in over 90% of cadaveric dissections, it may be absent in 60% of patients with a ruptured Achilles tendon or it may be ruptured along with the Achilles in many patients.

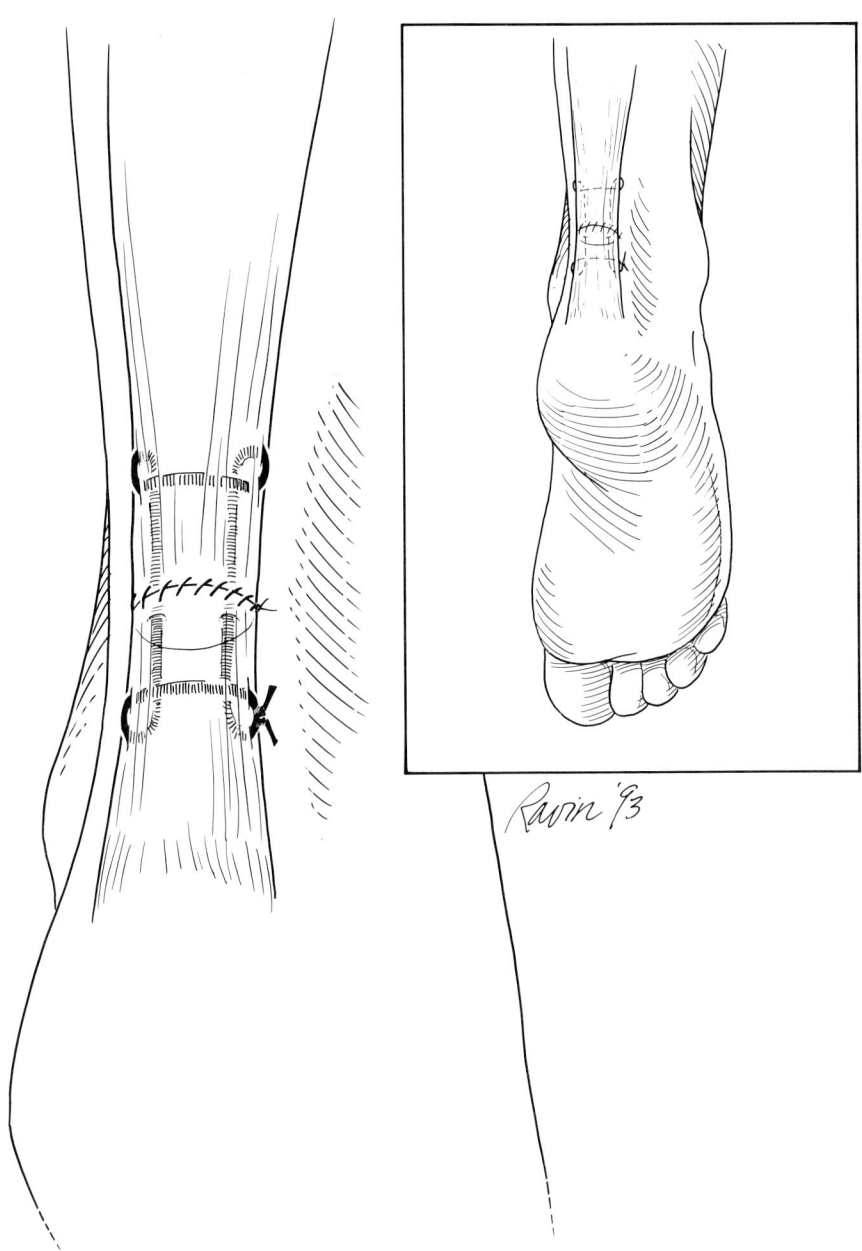

Figure 3. A technique of end-to-end suture of the Achilles tendon.

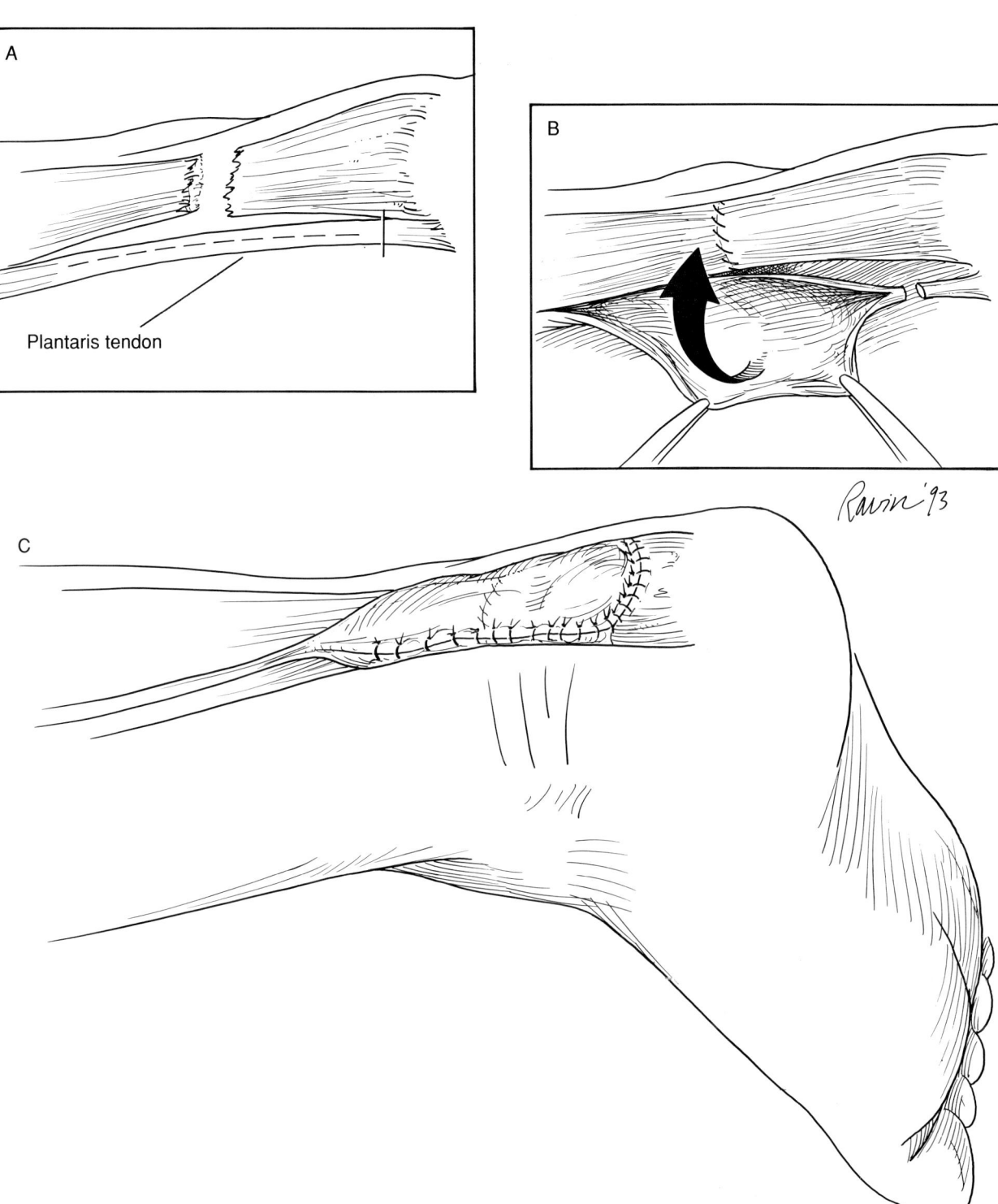

Figure 4. Plantaris tendon repair. **A:** Lynn technique of the use of plantaris tendon for augmentation. The Achilles tendon ruptured ends are identified with the plantaris tendon medial to the Achilles tendon. **B:** The Achilles tendon is repaired by end-to-end technique and the plantaris tendon is "fanned-out." **C:** Plantaris tendon is wrapped around the repaired Achilles tendon and sutured into place.

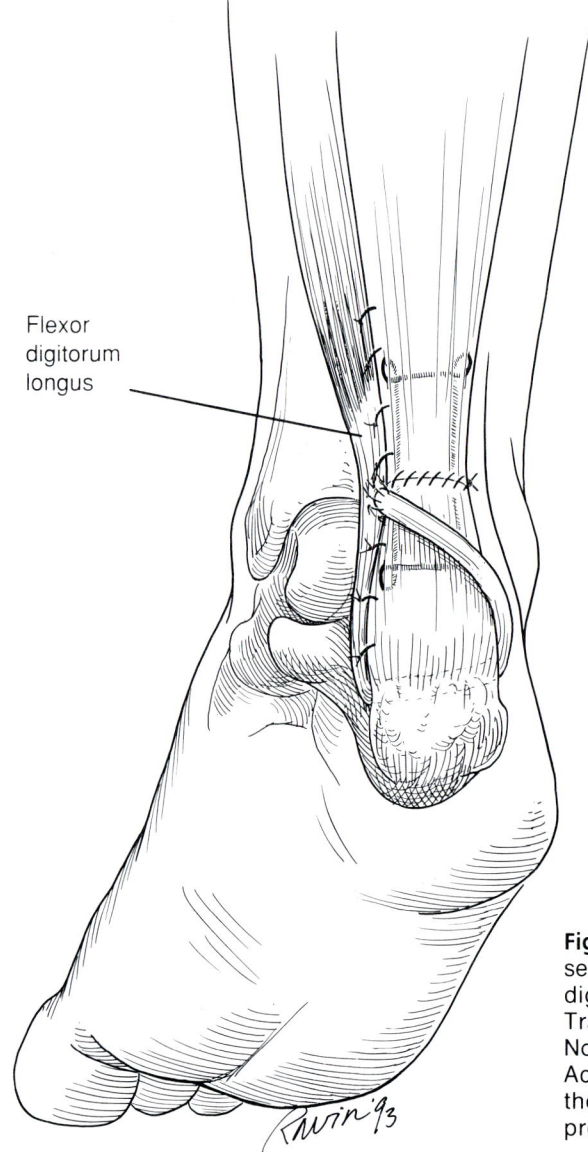

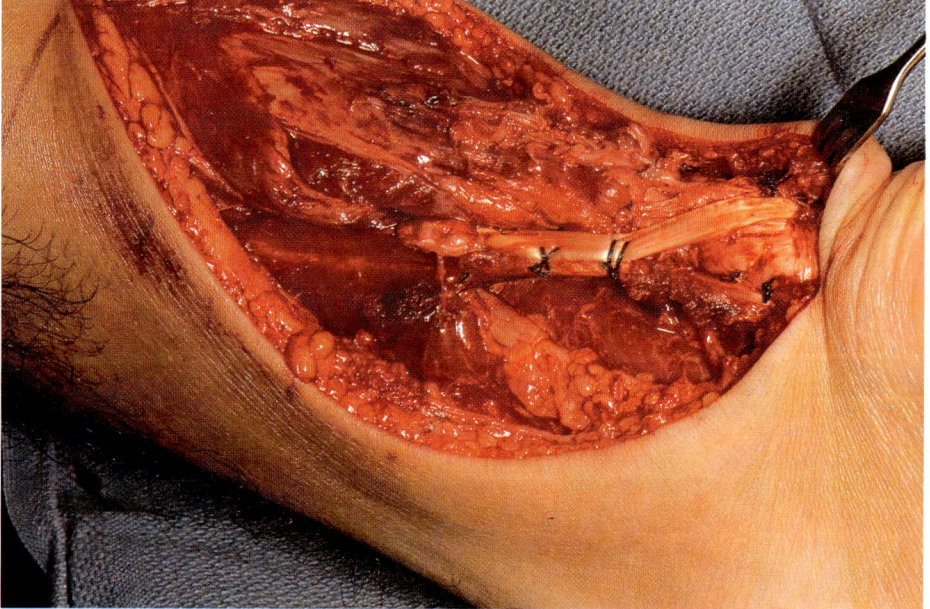

Figure 5. A: Diagrammatic representation of a transfer of the flexor digitorum longus (FDL) tendon. **B:** Transfer of the FDL at surgery. Note that an incision medial to the Achilles tendon was used, although a lateral incision is also appropriate.

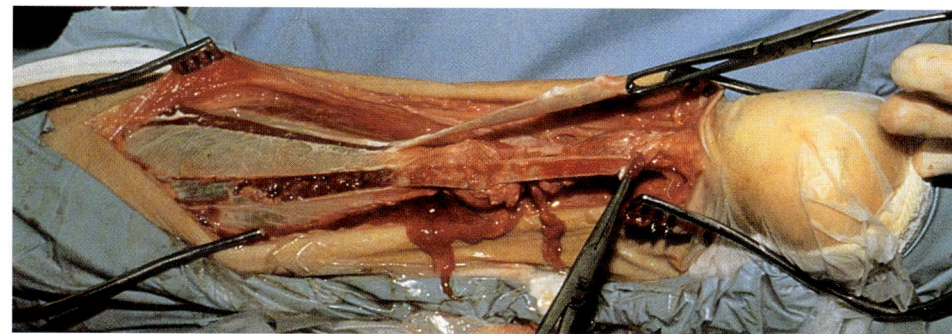
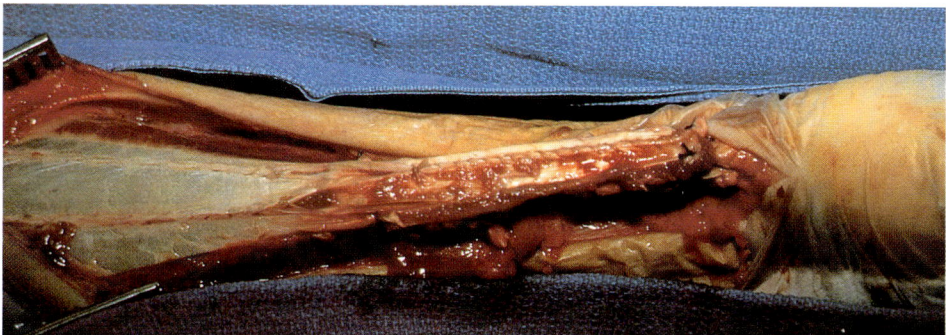

Figure 6. A: Two flaps from the fascia overlying the gastrocsoleus are "turned down." Note defects in aponeurotic fascia. **B:** Flaps sutured in place across the Achilles tendon repair and proximal defects closed.

If the plantaris tendon is not present then the flexor digitorum longus (FDL) can be used. A midfoot incision is made between the navicular and the abductor hallucis. The knot of Henry is released and the tendons identified. Passing a loop of 5–0 suture around the FDL proximally and pulling it into the midfoot incision also helps to identify all branches of the FDL. The FDL is released just before it bifurcates in the midfoot. The distal portion of the FDL is sutured to the flexor hallucis longus and the proximal portion of the FDL is pulled out proximally. The FDL is then forced through the calcaneus or the Achilles insertion and sutured back onto itself (Fig. 5).

The Achilles tendon can be "turned down" as either one central piece (3) or two pieces, one medially and one laterally (Fig. 6). This requires a longer incision proximally and increases the chance of wound problems. The turndown technique, however, is very effective for ruptures that have a small segmental gap. When the augmentation by either the plantaris or the flexor digitorum longus tendons seems inadequate, this turndown procedure is very useful.

An inverted V-Y sliding tendinous flap can be used to lengthen the Achilles tendon for end-to-end repair (Fig. 7). The lateral incision is extended proximally to expose the paretenon of the gastrocnemius. An inverted V incision is made, leaving the underlying muscle attached to the anterior paratenon. The flap is then advanced distally and the rupture repaired as described above for an end-to-end repair. This V-Y technique is the most helpful when a defect of more than 4 cm is present after the Achilles tendon is debrided to healthy tissue. If the gap is large, then a very long V with an acute angle is necessary to provide the proper length of tendon advancement. Up to about 7 cm can be spanned in some instances. If the tendon does not advance with moderate pulling on the tendon end, then release of the centrally lacerated tendon raphe on the deep surface of the soleus may be helpful. By turning up the Achilles tendon this central raphe is seen and judiciously released in increments.

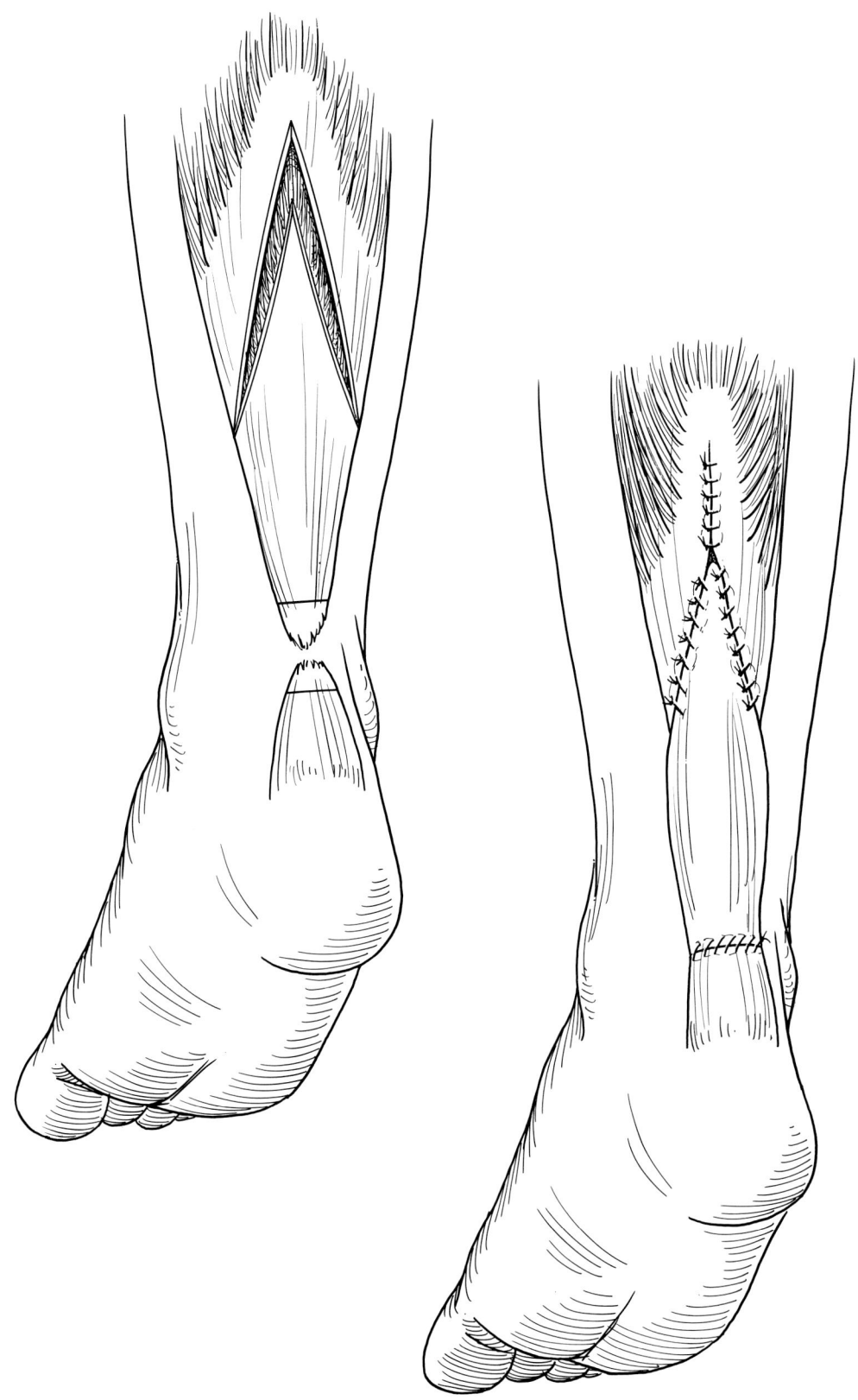

Figure 7. Diagrammatic representation of V-Y lengthening to close a gap in the Achilles tendon.

The wound closure after an Achilles tendon incision needs meticulous attention. Absorbable sutures in the subcutaneous tissue followed by nonstrangulating interrupted nylon mattress sutures in the skin will preserve the skin envelope over the Achilles tendon repair.

POSTOPERATIVE MANAGEMENT

Most delayed repairs of the Achilles tendon are achieved only with a fair amount of tension on the repair. For this reason, a long leg cast with the knee bent and 20° to 30° of plantar flexion is usually needed. This is usually obvious at surgery by extending the knee after the repair and seeing how much tension is possible. The cast is usually changed within the first few weeks or as swelling subsides, and the knee is extended out some more. After 4 to 6 weeks the knee is removed from the cast and knee motion exercises begun. At this point, a short leg cast or locked hinge ankle brace is used. Six weeks after the surgery the cast or hinge is changed every 2 weeks and the foot brought to neutral. Depending on the patient's healing capacity and the strength and type of repair, the cast is discontinued and ankle motion exercises and weight bearing are begun. In our experience it will take 3 months for young patients and 6 months for older patients to be fully weight bearing. Full return to activities may take an additional 6 months.

COMPLICATIONS

The main complications are wound necrosis, infection, rerupture, ankle stiffness, and sural neuroma formation.

Wound edge necrosis is prevented by keeping the posterior flap as thick as possible, avoiding excessive flap retraction, very careful wound closure, and an adequate postoperative period of wound compression and immobilization. If skin necrosis occurs, debridement, soaks, and antibiotics should allow healing by secondary intention.

Infection is closely related to wound necrosis. If the infection occurs deep to a wound that was closed by primary intention, it would need to be drained and treated by parenteral antibiotics and suction tubes or left open to heal by secondary intention.

Rerupture is unusual if the rehabilitation is gradual and allows hypertrophy of the repaired tendon. It is important that healthy tissue be used to span the site of repair.

Sural nerve neuroma formation is possible. Leaving the fatty tissue around the nerve after identification is important. If inadvertently the nerve is injured, then a more proximal nerve transection in a relatively undisturbed subcutaneous site will decrease the sensitivity of the resulting end-bulb neuroma.

ILLUSTRATIVE CASE FOR TECHNIQUE

A 32-year-old woman was playing tennis when she attempted to push off from a dorsiflexed ankle. She suffered a complete tear of her Achilles tendon. It was elected to treat her in an equinus cast for 6 weeks instead of utilizing primary repair.

Two years after her injury, she had weakness of ankle plantar flexion that was disabling for even mild sports activities. She was treated by a V-Y lengthening procedure (Fig. 8). One year after this procedure she had returned to her normal activities with no functional impairment.

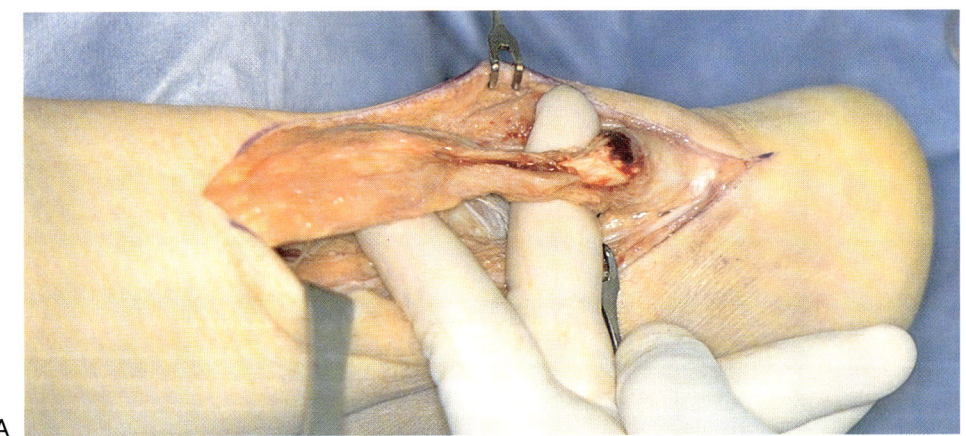

A

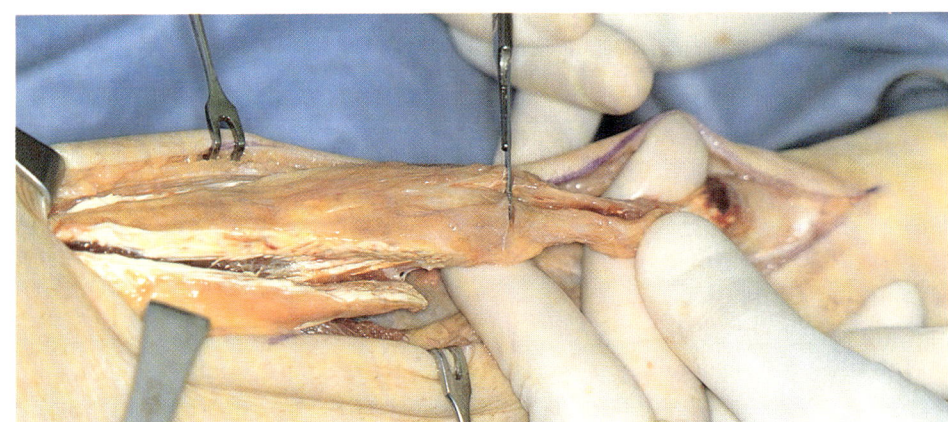

B

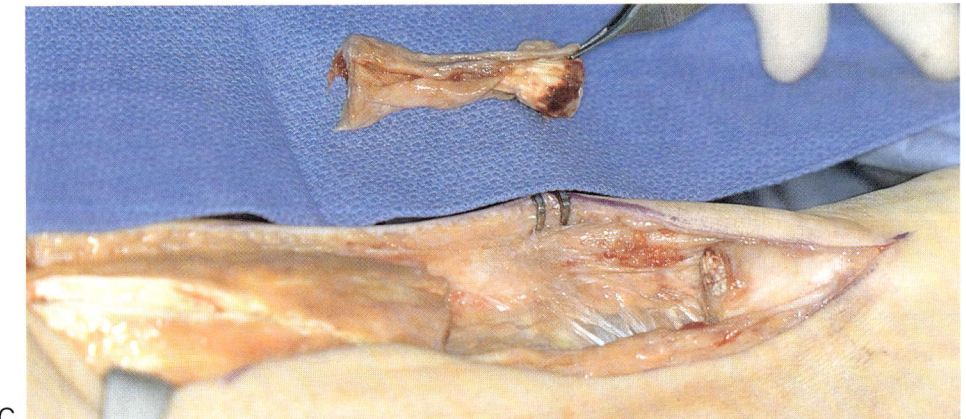

C

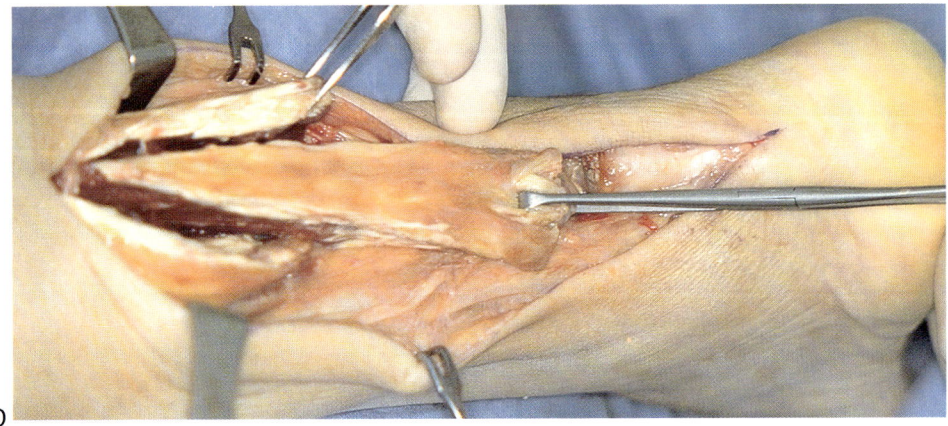

D

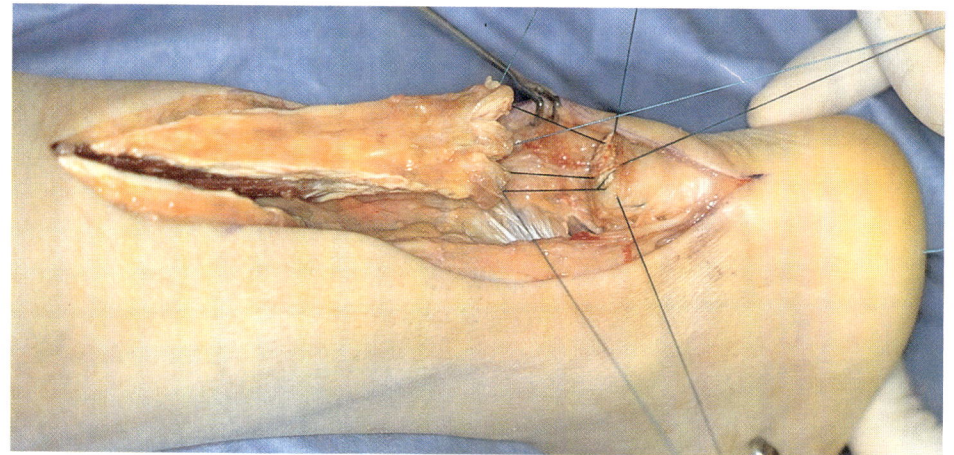

E

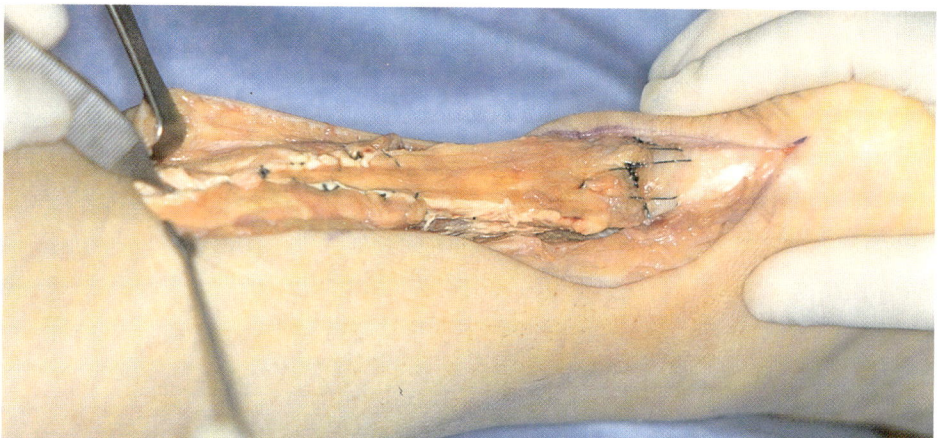

F

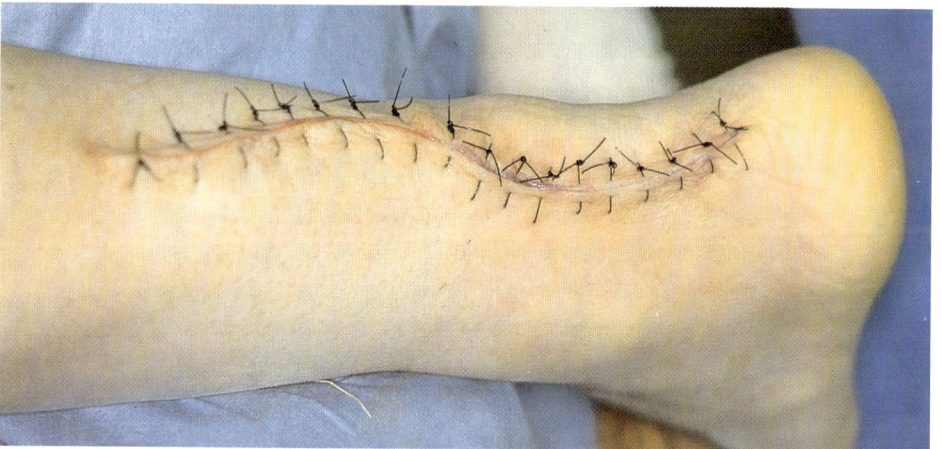

G

Figure 8. A: The hourglass-narrowed Achilles tendon has resulted from a complete tear that filled in with scar tissue between the true tendon tear ends. **B:** The tendon is cut where the normal tendon enters into the scarred area. **C:** A 7-cm gap was present after resection of the scar tissue. **D:** A proximal V in the gastrocsoleus aponeurosis was made. **E:** A zigzag (Bunnell) suture was placed in each end of the cut Achilles tendon. **F:** The advanced tendon ends are tied to close the gap of resected fibrous tissue. The proximal limb of the Y is closed. **G:** Careful wound closure with interrupted nylon mattress sutures.

RECOMMENDED READING

1. Abraham, E., and Pankovich, A. M.: Neglected rupture of the Achilles tendon: treatment by V-Y tendinous flap. *J. Bone Joint Surg.*, 57A: 253–255, 1975.
2. Hattrup, S. J., and Johnson, K. A.: A review of ruptures of the Achilles tendon. *Foot Ankle*, 6(1): 34–38, 1985.
3. Inglis, A. E., Scott, W. N., Sculco, T. P., and Patterson, A. H.: Ruptures of the tendon Achilles. *J. Bone Joint Surg.*, 58A(7): 990–993, 1976.
4. Justis, E. J., Jr.: Traumatic disorders. In: *Campbell's Operative Orthopaedics*, 7th ed., Vol. 3, edited by A. H. Crenshaw, C. V. Mosby, St. Louis, pp. 2226–2233, 1987.
5. Sarrafian, S. K.: *Anatomy of the Foot and Ankle. Descriptive, Topographic, Functional*. J. B. Lippincott, Philadelphia, pp. 313–316, 1983.

25
Plantar Fascia Release

W. Grant Braly

INDICATIONS/CONTRAINDICATIONS

The etiology of heel pain is controversial and treatment often frustrating for the patient and practitioner alike. More often than not, it follows a self-limiting course, but conservative treatment may be quite helpful in alleviating symptoms.

Typically, the patient is middle-aged, often overweight, and usually not able to recall any precipitating traumatic event. However, there may be a history of overuse or sudden change in activity level temporally related to the onset of symptoms.

It is generally accepted that the cause of heel pain, or "heel pain syndrome," is proximal plantar fasciitis. More precisely, this probably represents a degenerative attritional or fatigue interstitial tear of the plantar fascia in the proximity of its calcaneal insertion with associated chronic inflammation and eventual fibrosis. However, other possible causes of heel pain may be nerve entrapment, inflammatory arthritis with enthesitis, and stress fractures, among others. The significance of the "heel spur" is controversial, and may in fact be a normal variant, unrelated to the heel pain itself.

Conservative treatment modalities are numerous and varied. They include restriction of activities, especially repetitive impact loading sports, weight loss in the obese patient, heel cord/plantar fascia stretching exercises, heel pads or cups, arch supports, nonsteroidal antiinflammatory medications, steroid injections, physical therapy, and immobilization, among others. In the vast majority of patients, these measures are successful to varying degrees, but may require literally months of such treatment and a generous dose of "tincture of time" and patient reassurance. Surgical treatment is only considered after a diligent effort of conservative management for at least 6 to 12 months in the patient with intractable heel pain.

W. G. Braly, M.D.: Section of Foot and Ankle Surgery, Department of Orthopaedic Surgery, Baylor College of Medicine, Houston, Texas 77030; and *private practice*, Scurlock Tower, Suite 2100, Houston, TX 77030-2727.

Again, surgery is generally reserved for the patient who has failed various conservative treatment measures. Also the heel pain must be chronic and of such severity that it has significantly altered one's life-style and/or limited one's ability to participate in desired conditioning activities or sports.

Contraindications generally include such conditions for which surgical treatment (plantar fascia release) may not be effective. This may seem obvious, but a certain level of diagnostic finesse is necessary to exclude patients who may have an occult autoimmune disease, calcaneal stress fracture, structural hindfoot abnormality, senile heel pad atrophy, hindfoot tendon disorders, subtalar joint arthritis, tarsal tunnel syndrome, lumbar disk disease, and peripheral vascular disease with ischemia, among others.

The astute diagnostician must also be keenly aware of the patient with bilateral heel pain, particularly the younger male with no other predisposing factors. Such a patient profile may herald the onset of Reiter's syndrome. A thorough history investigating other signs and symptoms of this syndrome and screening laboratory serum tests will often suggest this diagnosis.

Morbid obesity may also be another contraindication for obvious reasons. Conversely, for these patients, weight loss should be encouraged as a conservative treatment measure.

Absolute contraindications include patients with ischemic peripheral vascular disease, especially those with diabetes, or localized heel pad infections or dermatological diseases that would compromise wound healing.

PREOPERATIVE PLANNING

As alluded to previously, the patient with heel pain often cannot recall any precipitating traumatic event, but an overuse pattern may be elicited historically. The pain usually begins gradually and may wax and wane in its intensity. Not uncommonly, it may resolve for an extended period of time only to return just as inexplicably as it perhaps began. Typically, the pain is worse upon rising in the morning or after significant periods of recumbency or sitting. The first few steps are often memorable, but gradually as the foot "warms up," the pain resolves or diminishes, only to return or intensify later in the day, especially with prolonged periods of standing or walking. Such a history is almost pathognomonic for heel pain secondary to plantar fasciitis.

The patient often presents with an antalgic gait and localizes the usually achy type pain in the central or anteromedial heel pad region. Occasionally, the discomfort radiates distally into the arch along the course of the plantar fascia. Symptoms are consistently reproduced by deep palpation at the point of maximal subjective tenderness and occasionally by passively hyperdorsiflexing the toes, which stretches the inflamed plantar fascia. Swelling is rarely encountered. Tight or even contracted heel cords are a common finding. For this reason, and also by unloading the heel, many patients, especially females, find relief by donning higher heel shoes.

The radiographic workup for heel pain is relatively simple. A complete weight-bearing foot radiographic series (AP, lateral, and oblique), including an axial heel view, is recommended. If bony pathology is suspected and not readily evident on plain films, then a bone scan may be helpful. There may also be an indication for a computed tomography (CT) scan or magnetic resonance imaging (MRI) in selected cases in which the diagnosis is not readily apparent by other means.

SURGERY

The theoretical rationale for the plantar fascia release procedure is to decrease the tension on the often tight and fibrotic proximal plantar fascia. This may also serve to decompress anatomical structures deep to it, specifically the intrinsic muscles and various nerves in the plantar heel region. The release of the conjoined ligament of the forearm extensor muscles for chronic lateral epicondylitis or "tennis elbow" is perhaps an analogous procedure.

The vast majority of cases can be accomplished in an outpatient setting unless significant medical problems dictate otherwise. The patient is placed in the supine position and an anteromedial heel pad field block or ankle block with intravenous sedation is administered. The author prefers to utilize a 50% solution of 2% lidocaine and 0.5% Marcaine without epinephrine; 10 to 12 cc will usually suffice. General anesthesia is also an alternative, but is usually not recommended, especially for outpatient cases. A pneumatic proximal thigh tourniquet is preferred for general anesthesia and a supramalleolar ankle tourniquet for local anesthesia (Fig. 1).

The foot and ankle is then prepped and draped. To exsanguinate the foot, the extremity may simply be elevated for several minutes. However, an elastic bandage (sterile Ace wrap or Esmarch) may also be utilized, especially in local anesthetic cases where an ankle tourniquet is employed. The pneumatic tourniquet is then inflated (250–300 mm Hg for ankle and 300–350 mm Hg for thigh tourniquets) after administration of an intravenous antibiotic (the author prefers Cephazolin).

The foot is left suspended over a padded wedge or bolster. An assistant is essential to keep the foot in a dorsiflexed or at least neutral position to enhance exposure and keep the plantar fascia taut during the procedure (Fig. 2).

Technique. Preferably under loupe magnification, an oblique incision 3 to 4 cm in length is made just distal and medial to the heel pad near the junction of the thicker plantar heel pad skin and the thinner skin of the proximal medial arch (Fig. 3A). The oblique incision is important so as to avoid transection of the medial calcaneal nerve branches, which can result in postoperative neuroma foundation with pain (Fig. 3B). Dissection proceeds through the subcutaneous tissue, coagulating bleeders as they are encountered. A self-retaining and/or small hand-held

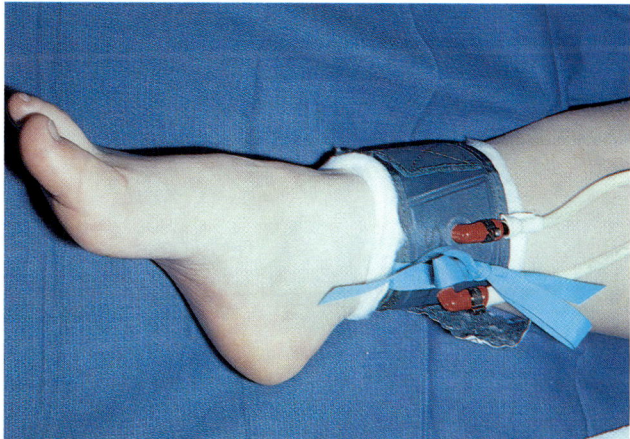

Figure 1. The patient is placed in the supine position with a supramalleolar pneumatic ankle tourniquet applied for local anesthesia with intravenous sedation. The author prefers injection of the local anesthetic prior to prepping and draping.

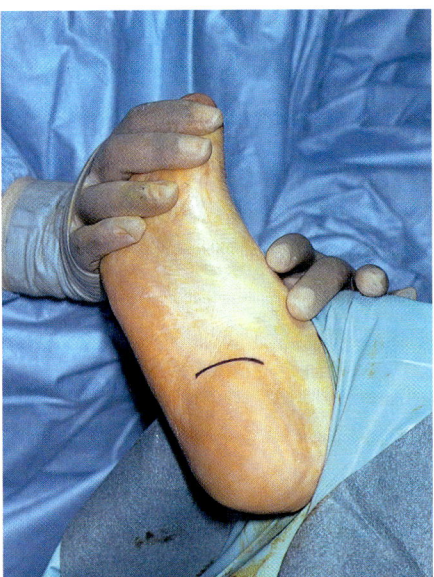

Figure 2. After prepping, draping, and inflation of the tourniquet, the foot is left suspended over a padded wedge. An assistant keeps the foot in a neutral or dorsiflexed position to enhance exposure and keep the plantar fascia taut.

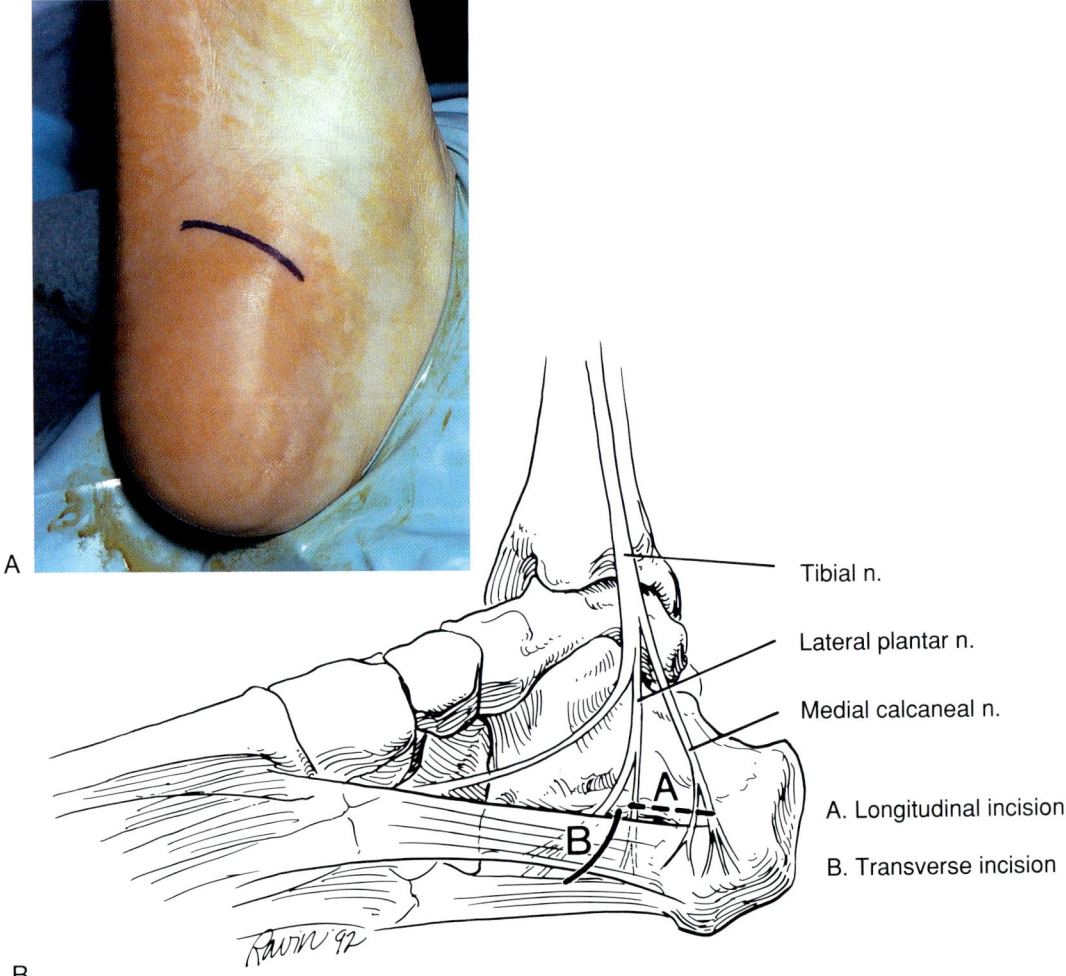

Figure 3. A: A 3- to 4-cm oblique incision is made just distal and medial to the heel pad in the proximal arch region. **B:** Incision location along alignment of medial nerve structures.

retractor for the billowing subcutaneous and heel pad tissue is recommended (Fig. 4). The medial and lateral borders of the proximal plantar fascia are then identified 1 to 2 cm distal to its origin from the calcaneus (Figs. 5A and 6A). The medial two-thirds of the plantar fascia is then cut sharply in this area, taking care not to violate the intimately underlying intrinsic musculature (Figs. 5B and 6B). Preserving the lateral one-third of the plantar fascia is recommended as releasing the entire structure may result in a soft tissue flatfoot deformity. Another reason release of the lateral plantar fascia is ill-advised and perhaps unnecessary is that the medial calcaneal insertion is usually thicker, more fibrotic, and thus tighter in the diseased plantar fascia. This corresponds clinically to the area of maximal tenderness in the majority of patients.

If a heel spur is to be removed, dissection proceeds from the cut edge of the plantar fascia posteriorly to the calcaneus between the fascia and intrinsic muscles. The spur is then removed piecemeal with a rongeur under direct visualization. All rough edges are smoothed with a manual rasp, power rasp, or burr instrument.

Surgical removal of a heel spur is controversial and may be of psychological importance to the patient. As alluded to previously, the presence of one correlates inconsistently with the presence of heel pain due to plantar fasciitis. However, to the patient, the heel spur is a tangible, easily recognized radiographic structure versus the nebulous concept of a degenerative "torn ligament." Therefore, he or she is often focused on the necessity of its removal. Perhaps the only absolute indication for excision is in the patient with an extremely large heel spur combined with chronic plantar fasciitis, heel pad atrophy, and a localized plantar callus directly over the spur. With perhaps this one exception, I discourage excision of the smaller heel spur since to do so requires deeper surgical dissection, thus significantly increasing the morbidity of the procedure and prolonging postoperative recovery.

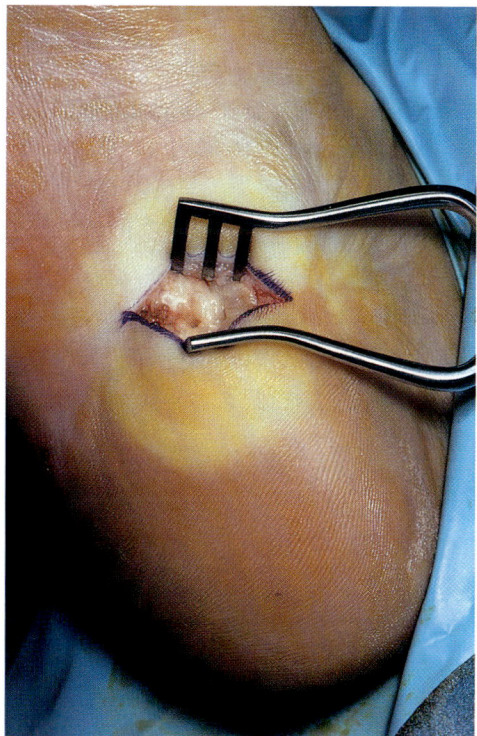

Figure 4. A self-retaining and/or small hand-held retractor displaces the billowing subcutaneous and heel pad tissue.

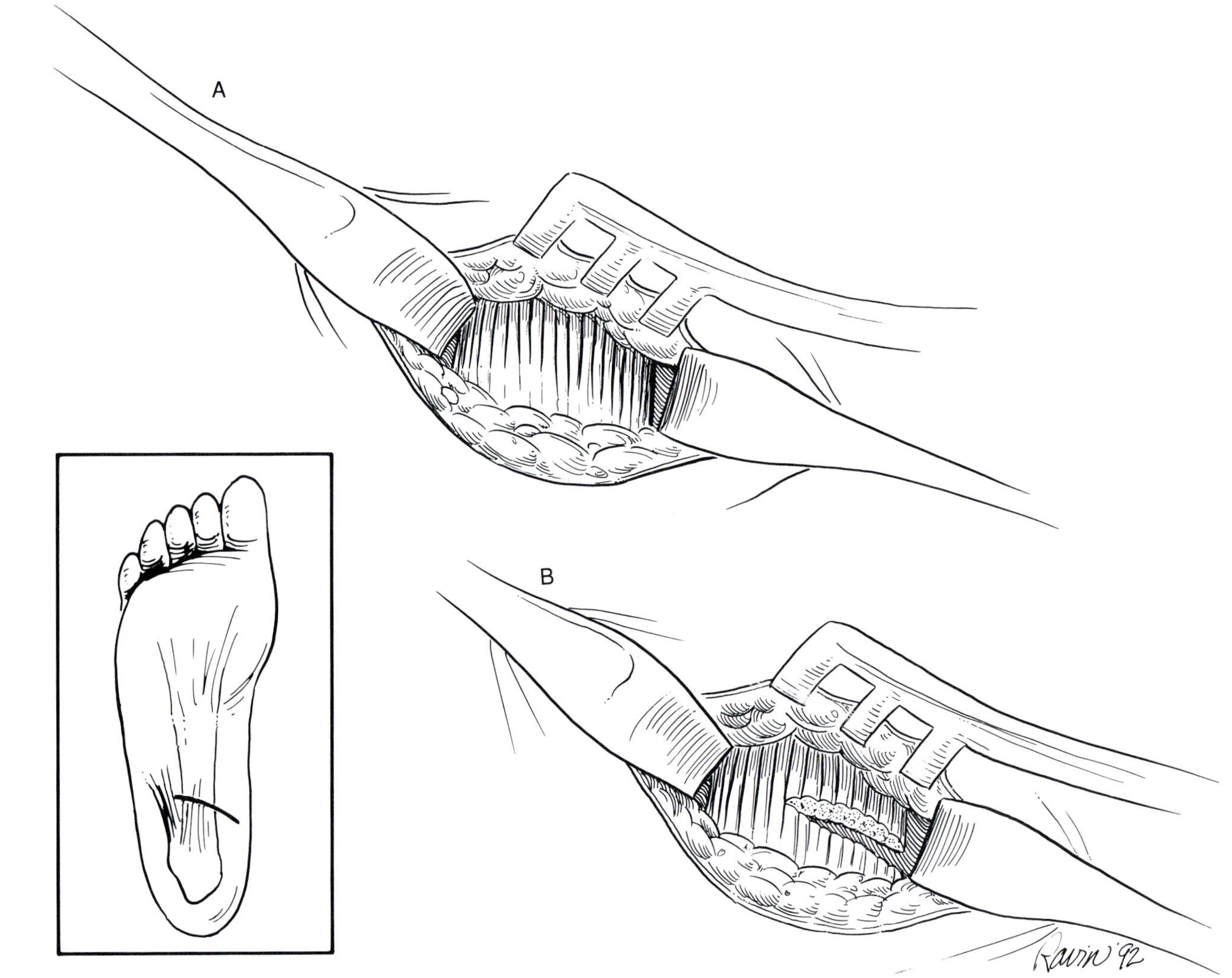

Figure 5. A: The medial and lateral borders of the proximal plantar fascia are identified 1 to 2 cm distal to its origin from the calcaneus. **B:** The extent of plantar fascia release is shown.

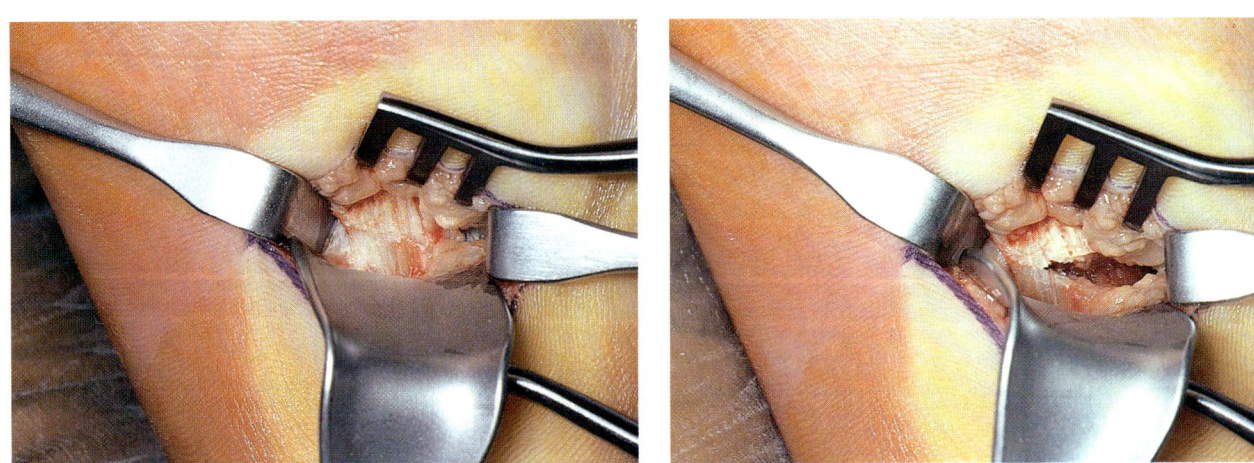

Figure 6. A: This intraoperative view shows the surgical exposure of the plantar fascia. **B:** The medial two-thirds of the plantar fascia is cut sharply, taking care not to violate the underlying intrinsic muscles. The lateral one-third of the plantar fascia is preserved.

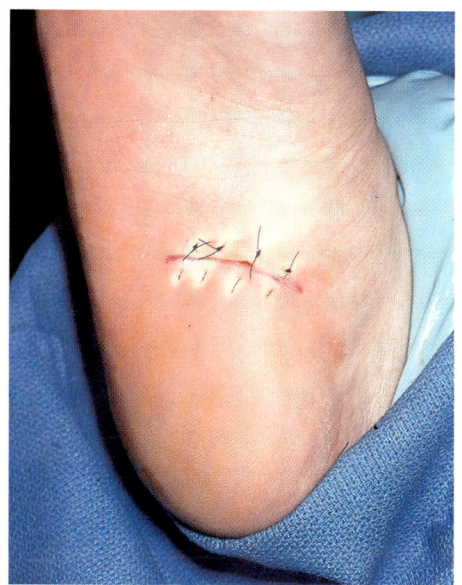

Figure 7. Hemostasis is achieved after release of the tourniquet and the skin closed with nonabsorbable monofilament type interrupted vertical mattress sutures.

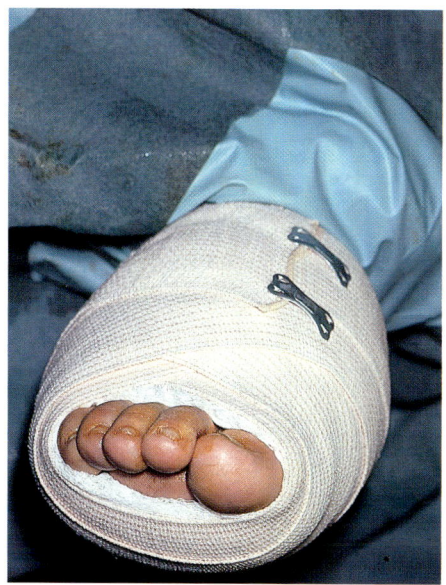

Figure 8. A bulky compression dressing is applied.

The wound is then thoroughly irrigated, the tourniquet released, hemostasis achieved, and the skin closed with nonabsorbable monofilament type (3-0 Prolene) interrupted vertical mattress sutures (Fig. 7). A bulky compression dressing is then applied comprised of Xeroform, 4″ × 4″ gauze pads, ABD pad, Kerlix, 3″ Kling, and a 3″ Ace wrap, in that order (Fig. 8).

POSTOPERATIVE MANAGEMENT

After leaving the recovery room, the patient is crutch or walker trained, non–weight bearing on the operated heel (Table 1). Some balance or touch-down weight bearing with a postop shoe is permitted on the forefoot. Oral antibiotics are prescribed for 3 days after surgery.

The dressing is usually changed in 3 to 5 days. The patient is then given instructions on local wound care with daily hydrogen peroxide cleansing of the wound and Kerlix, or similar dressing, application to protect the wound. Exposure to bath or shower water is forbidden until suture removal.

At approximately 1 week postop, progressive heel weight bearing as tolerated in the postop shoe is allowed. The patient is encouraged to wean from their crutches or walker and begin a normal gait pattern at this time. Sutures are removed 10 to 14 days postop.

Supportive soft-sole shoe-wear (e.g., athletic shoes) is encouraged at the point when sutures are out and heel weight bearing is consistently tolerated (generally 2 weeks postop).

No repetitive impact loading conditioning activities or sports are allowed until at least 6 weeks postop. Alternative non–impact loading forms of exercise before this time for the patient so inclined may include cycling or swimming.

Generally, most patients have "recovered" to their respective preoperative level of activity between 6 and 12 weeks postop. However, this greatly depends, perhaps obviously, on each patient's preoperative expectation. It is therefore criti-

TABLE 1. *Postoperative care for plantar fascia release*

Time postoperative	Care
Day of surgery	Soft bulky dressing
	Crutch or walker training, non–weight bearing on operated heel with postop shoe
3–5 days	Dressing changed
	Local wound care begins
7–10 days	Heel weight bearing permitted
	Wean from crutches or walker
10–14 days	Sutures removed
	Supportive, soft-sole shoe-wear encouraged
	Home program of physical therapy
2–4 weeks	Repetitive impact loading sports and activities proscribed (swimming or cycling permitted)
6–12 weeks	Formalized physical therapy, if necessary
	Resumption of all activities as tolerated
	Possible dismissal
12 weeks–12 months	Gradual resolution of postoperative swelling
	Probable dismissal

cal that the preoperative plantar fascia release patient be thoroughly counseled as to the anticipated recovery time. A significant minority of patients require a much longer period to recover, and the surgeon is well advised to allow a generous latitude of time. It is also recommended to emphasize the longer end point so as to lessen the patient's potential disappointment. Specifically, I allow 6 months to 1 year for complete recovery, especially in regard to the resolution of postoperative swelling. Unfortunately, chronic postoperative swelling is common in most significant foot surgery, and a plantar fascia release is no exception.

REHABILITATION

Beyond crutch or walker training, formalized physical therapy is not usually prescribed. At the time of suture removal with a well-healed wound (10 to 14 days postop), all patients are given instructions for at least twice daily warm soaks, gentle massage, and foot and ankle range of motion exercises.

However, for the patient who has persistent peri-incisional weight-bearing pain at 6 weeks postop, formalized physical therapy may be indicated. Special emphasis is given to whirlpool, massage, and ultrasound modalities. Such treatment is generally recommended for the patient who has an increased level of swelling and incisional fibrosis.

COMPLICATIONS

Although by no means an exhaustive or complete list, the following are some complications encountered in my experience with this procedure.

1. *Infection*. This is an exceedingly rare problem. Fortunately, if it does occur, it is usually superficial and responds readily to local wound care and oral antibiotics. I have never seen a deep infection requiring inpatient care, surgical debridement, or parenteral antibiotics. Meticulous aseptic technique and thorough hemostasis is essential and perioperative antibiotics are recommended to avoid this complication.

2. *Flatfoot.* By avoiding complete release of the plantar fascia and perhaps limiting early postoperative heel weight bearing, this complication may theoretically be avoided. When it occurs, the soft tissue support of the arch is lost to varying degrees. This may ultimately lead to changes of the bony arch, although this has not been proven in my experience. In my later experience with this procedure in which complete release of the plantar fascia was avoided, this complication has decreased.

   In addition to a sometimes subtle change in the arch height, the patient may also complain of dorsal and lateral midfoot pain. This is loosely referred to as a "settling phenomena", and is probably the result of chronic strain of the intertarsal and tarsometatarsal joint capsules that are subjected to greater weight-bearing forces due to loss of the support formerly provided by the intact plantar fascia. The symptoms associated with this complication eventually resolve, but may require up to a year to do so. The patient is encouraged to wear supportive shoes with stock or prescribed arch supports in the recovery period associated with this complication.

3. *Nerve damage.* Beyond necessarily sacrificing local cutaneous nerves associated with a primarily transverse incision, nerve damage is rare in this procedure. One of the primary reasons for development of the plantar surgical approach was to avoid the medial calcaneal nerve that was often damaged with the still popular longitudinal medial heel pad incision. Theoretically, the lateral plantar is the deep nerve most vulnerable to surgical damage.

   To avoid deep nerve damage, familiarity with the anatomy is essential and loupe magnification is recommended with meticulous hemostasis and surgical dissection under direct visualization.

4. *Plantar intrinsic muscle damage.* With time, this may resemble a mild intrinsic minus foot and is thought to be due to insertional detachment or severance of the plantar intrinsic muscles, usually associated with an amateurish heel spur excision.

   Therefore, with few exceptions, I discourage heel spur excision, associated with a plantar fascia release, not only to avoid this complication, but also for reasons explained previously. However, if it is elected to remove the heel spur, I again emphasize meticulous dissection under magnification, thereby avoiding or at least minimizing damage to the intrinsic muscles.

ILLUSTRATIVE CASE FOR TECHNIQUE

This patient is a 60-year-old man who had right heel pain approximately 1 year prior to surgical treatment. As is typical, he could not recall any traumatic event, was middle-aged and mildly overweight, and presented with pathognomonic signs and symptoms described previously. Preoperative radiographs revealed a small heel spur, but were otherwise unremarkable (Fig. 9A). The patient had undergone a period of conservative treatment, including activity restrictions, heel pads, custom-made arch supports, nonsteroidal antiinflammatory drugs, physical therapy (emphasizing heel cord/plantar fascia stretching exercises), and two steroid injections. Admittedly, he enjoyed some temporary success with several of these measures, but continued to have significant chronic heel pain to the degree that he could not play golf. For him, this was a disturbing restriction of his favorite recreational activity.

Therefore, a plantar fascia release and heel spur excision was performed as an outpatient procedure under ankle block anesthesia with intravenous sedation. Postoperative radiographs demonstrated resection of the heel spur (Fig. 9B). (This case was early in the author's experience with this procedure when heel spurs were more routinely removed.)

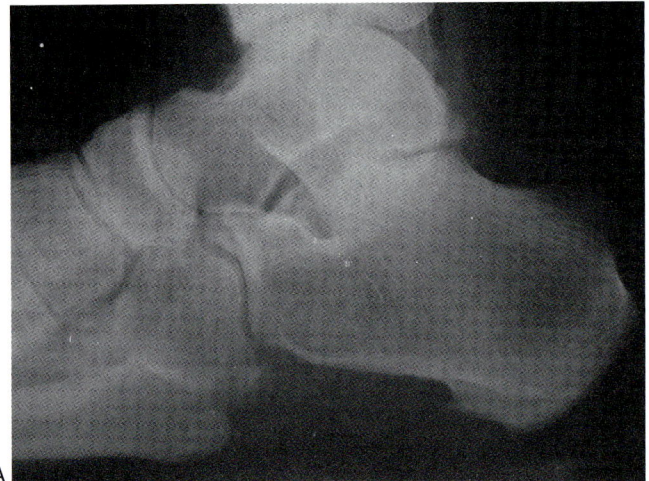 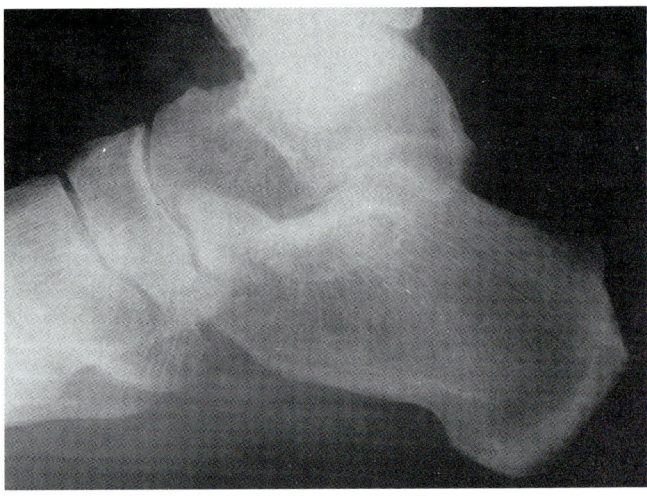

Figure 9. A: Preoperative lateral foot radiograph of illustrative case revealing heel spur. **B:** Postoperative film documenting resection of heel spur.

The postoperative course was uneventful, and he returned to all activities, including golf, approximately 6 weeks postop. Almost 1 year later, he had the same procedure on the left foot performed with similar success. Follow-up of approximately 4 years on the right and 3 years on the left foot confirmed the procedure's relatively long-term success for this patient.

RECOMMENDED READING

1. Anderson, R. B., and Foster, M. D.: Operative treatment of subcalcaneal pain. *Foot Ankle*, 9: 317–323, 1989.
2. Baxter, D. E., and Thigpen, C. M.: Heel pain-operative results. *Foot Ankle*, 5: 16–25, 1984.
3. Bordelon, R. L.: Subcalcaneal pain: a method of evaluation and plan for treatment. *Clin. Orthop.*, 177: 49–53, 1983.
4. Furey, J. G.: Plantar fasciitis: the painful heel syndrome. *J. Bone Joint Surg.*, 57A: 672–673, 1975.
5. Kahn, C., Bishop, J. O., and Tullos, H. S.: Plantar fascia release and heel spur excision via plantar route. *Orthop. Rev.*, 14:222–225, 1985.
6. Leach, R. E., Seavey, M. S., and Salter, D. K.: Results of surgery in athletes with plantar fasciitis. *Foot Ankle*, 7: 156–161, 1986.
7. Lester, D. K., and Buchanan, J. R.: Surgical treatment of plantar fasciitis. *Clin. Orthop.*, 186: 202–204, 1984.
8. Michetti, M. L., and Jacobs, S. A.: Calcaneal heel spurs: etiology, treatment, and a new surgical approach. *J. Foot Surg.*, 22: 234–239, 1984.
9. Snider, M. P., Clancy, W. G., and McBeath, A. A.: Plantar fascia release for chronic plantar fasciitis in runners. *Am. J. Sports Med.*, 11: 215–219, 1983.
10. Sundberg, S. B., and Johnson, K. A.: Painful conditions of the heel. In: *Disorders of the Foot and Ankle: Medical and Surgical Management*, edited by M. H. Jahss. Philadelphia: W. B. Saunders, 1991.
11. Ward, W. G., and Clippinger, F. W.: Proximal medial longitudinal arch incision for plantar fascia release. *Foot Ankle*, 8: 152–155, 1987.

26
Release of the Nerve to the Abductor Digiti Quinti

Donald E. Baxter

INDICATIONS/CONTRAINDICATIONS

The indication for release of the nerve to the abductor digiti quinti or the first branch of the lateral plantar nerve is chronic neuritic pain that does not resolve with conservative care. This neuritic pain is localized to the medial aspect of the heel underneath the inferior aspect of the abductor hallucis muscle. The pain often radiates proximally up into the ankle and may migrate across the foot on the plantar surface. After all other causes of heel pain have been ruled out and pain persists for an extended period of time (preferably 1 year) nerve release may be indicated.

Contraindications to this procedure include other causes of heel pain such as plantar fasciitis, stress fracture of the calcaneus, tarsal tunnel syndrome, sciatica, and various arthropathies.

PREOPERATIVE PLANNING

The diagnosis of entrapment of the first branch of the lateral plantar nerve or the nerve to the abductor digiti quinti is made on a clinical basis. The clinical expertise of the examiner is the main determinant of a painful heel that would benefit from operative decompression of the first branch of the lateral plantar nerve. It is important for the examiner to differentiate first branch entrapment from the other common causes of heel pain including heel pain syndrome, plantar fasciitis, and fat pad disorders.

D. E. Baxter, M.D.: Department of Orthopaedic Surgery, Baylor College of Medicine, Houston, TX 77074.

The pathognomonic sign of entrapment of the first branch of the lateral plantar nerve is maximal tenderness in the area where the nerve is compressed between the taut deep fascia of the abductor hallucis muscle and the medial caudal margin of the quadratus plantae muscle. Chronic inflammation of the plantar fascia may predispose to entrapment of the first branch of the lateral plantar nerve. Therefore, the patient may have some tenderness over the proximal plantar fascia and the medial calcaneal tuberosity. However, without maximal tenderness over the course of the nerve of the plantar medial aspect of the foot, the diagnosis of entrapment should not be made. Some patients may have paresthesias elicited with pressure over the nerve entrapment site.

Electromyographic (EMG) and nerve conduction studies are not always helpful. We have recently been doing nerve studies and have found that there are occasionally changes with chronic compression. The preoperative evaluation of the patient should include an EMG nerve test, not only to try to determine the point of entrapment, but to rule out more proximal disorders such as radiculopathy from the back or higher tarsal tunnel syndrome. Radiographs should be made to look for stress fractures of the heel or bone tumors. A bone scan may be helpful to determine whether a stress fracture exists. Lab work including a rheumatological workup should be considered in any patient who has any symptoms suggestive of an arthropathy.

SURGERY

The patient is placed in the supine position on the operating table. The hip and knee are flexed at 90° and externally rotated. An ankle block is used most frequently. No tourniquet is required, although an ankle tourniquet may be used. A 4-cm oblique incision is made (Fig. 1) on the medial heel over the proximal abductor hallucis muscle. The incision is centered over the course of the first branch of the lateral plantar nerve (Figs. 2 and 3). The sensory branches of the medial calcaneal nerve are not encountered as they course posterior to the incision. Care is taken, however, to preserve any aberrant branches.

The interval between the fascia overlying the abductor hallucis and the medial border of the plantar fascia is identified (Fig. 4). A small portion of the medial plantar fascia may be removed to facilitate exposure and clearly define the plane between the deep abductor fascia and the plantar fascia (Fig. 5). The superficial fascia of the abductor hallucis muscle is divided with a #15 blade and the muscle is retracted superiorly (Fig. 6). A section of the deep fascia of the inferior abductor hallucis is removed directly over the area where the nerve is compressed between the taut fascia and the medial border of the quadratus plantae muscle (Figs. 7 and 8). The deep fascia of the abductor hallucis is then divided from the inferior to superior to sufficiently free the nerve from the entrapment (Fig. 9). A heel spur, if present, is removed taking care to protect the freer nerve that runs superiorly (Fig. 10). The abductor hallucis muscle and most of its superficial fascia are left intact. The posterior tibial nerve more proximally in the tarsal tunnel is not explored.

If the plantar fascia is chronically inflamed and thickened, more of the proximal plantar fascia can be released or preferably resected. It may be necessary to release the entire fascia in addition to releasing the nerve. This is done should the preoperative evaluation and finding at surgery support a more extensive operation. The recovery is longer with complete release of the fascia. Even though the bone is not usually the cause of pain, care should be taken to remove any significant spur, which can easily be done at the time of nerve and or fascia release.

There are cases that I feel are primarily nerve compression cases. For these, I simply release the nerve. There are also cases that are primarily fascia and not nerve. I usually release fascia but also release the nerve to avoid a nerve compression that may occur as the fascia migrates distally.

At the end of the operation, a small hemostat is used to palpate along the course of the nerve to make sure that it is free from any adhesions proximally or distally. The wound is closed with 4-0 nylon interrupted horizontal mattress sutures (Fig. 11). A bulky compressive dressing is applied to the foot and ankle.

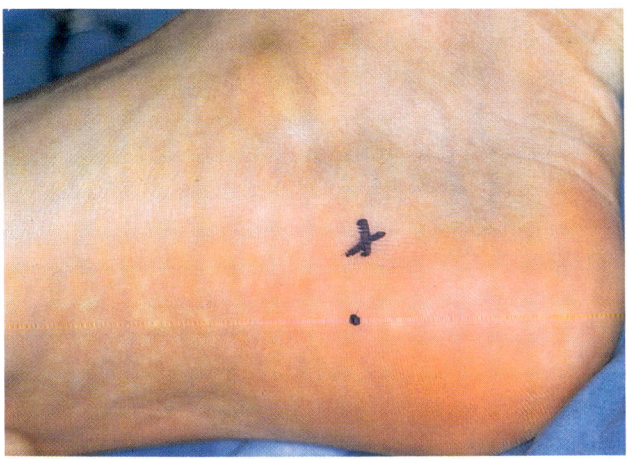

Figure 1. The location of the incision for release of the nerve to the abductor digiti quinti.

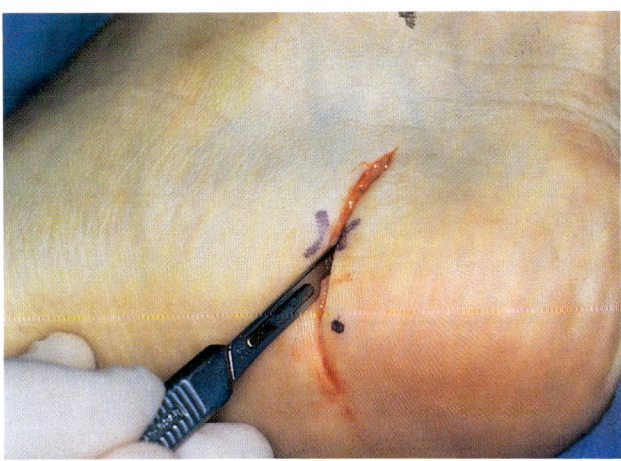

Figure 2. Line of incision over the nerve to the abductor digiti quinti. The X marks the point of maximum tenderness and the location of the nerve deep to this point.

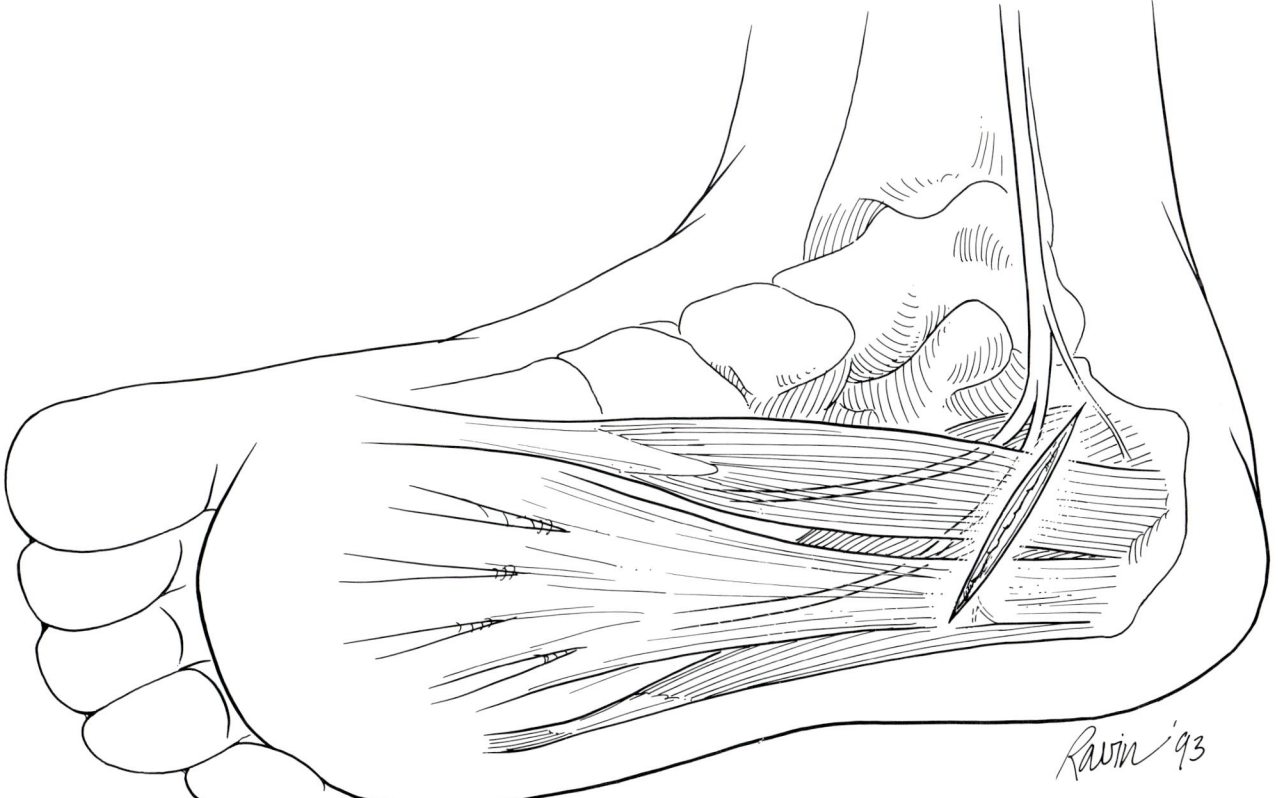

Figure 3. The relationship of the skin incision to the underlying bony structures.

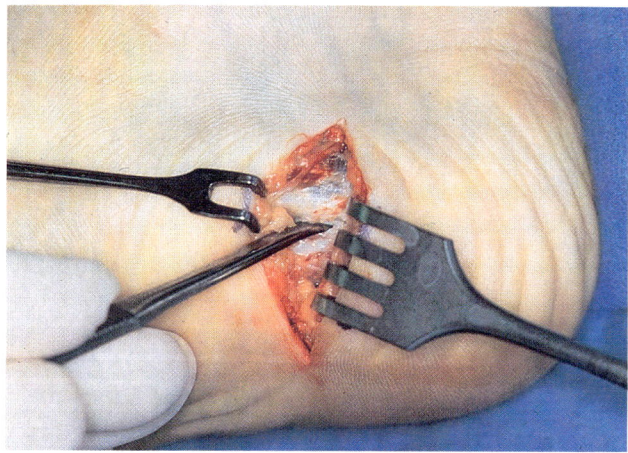

Figure 4. The interval between the plantar fascia and the investing fascia of the abductor hallucis muscle belly is developed.

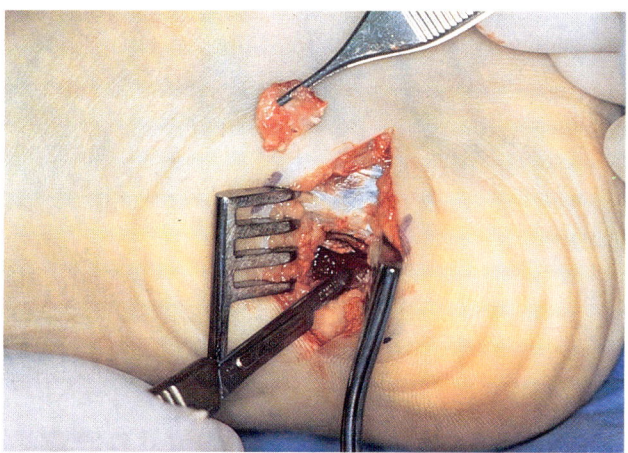

Figure 5. A portion of the plantar fascia is removed showing the quadratus plantae muscle deep to this structure.

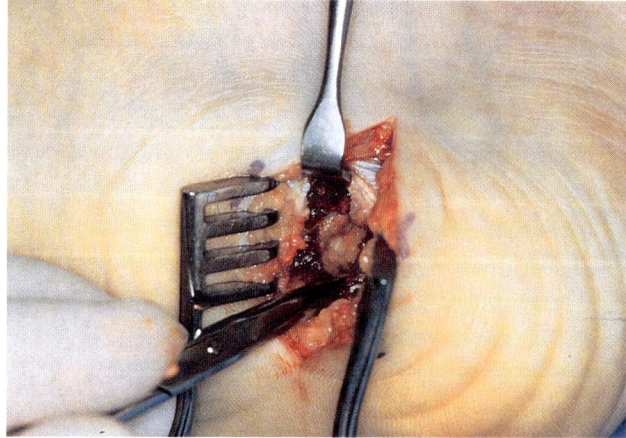

Figure 6. Retraction of the quadratus plantae to the lateral aspect of the foot and the abductor hallucis superiorly allows exposure to the nerve to the abductor digiti quinti.

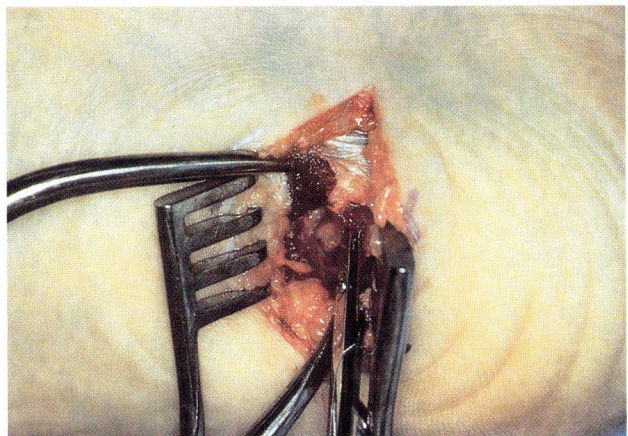

Figure 7. On the undersurface of the abductor hallucis fascia that tethers the nerve, the nerve to the abductor digiti quinti is released by taking out a section of the deep fascia.

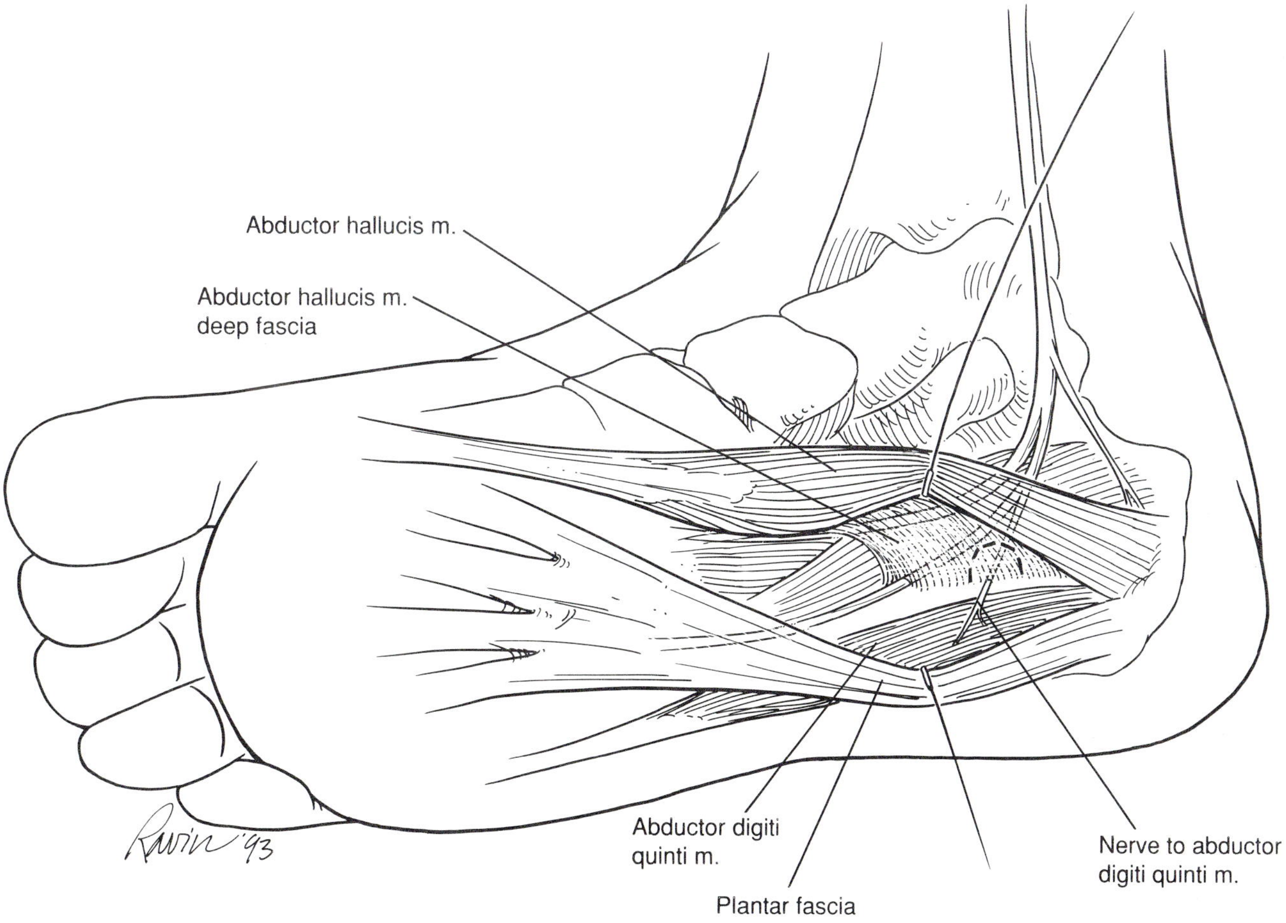

Figure 8. A diagrammatic representation of removing the tethering fascia over the nerve to the abductor digiti quinti.

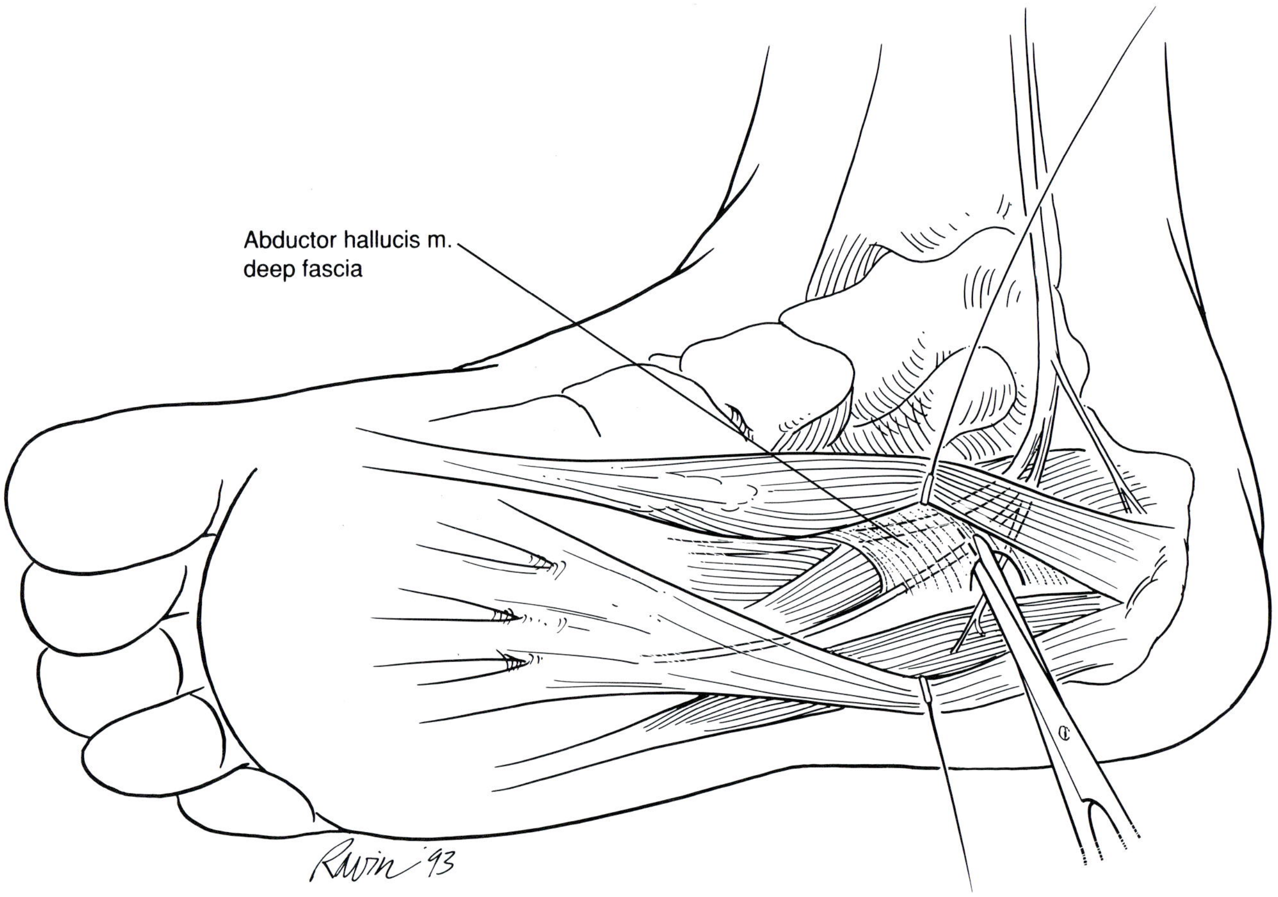

Figure 9. The investing fascia on the undersurface of the abductor hallucis is also released.

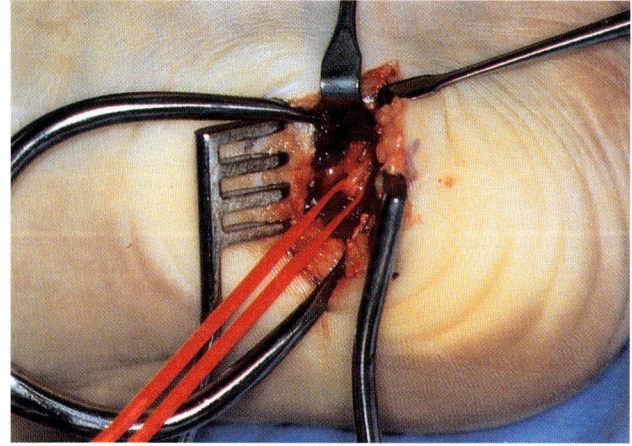

Figure 10. The nerve to the abductor digiti quinti is shown with the red retraction rubber. Care is taken to be certain this nerve is released at the end of the procedure.

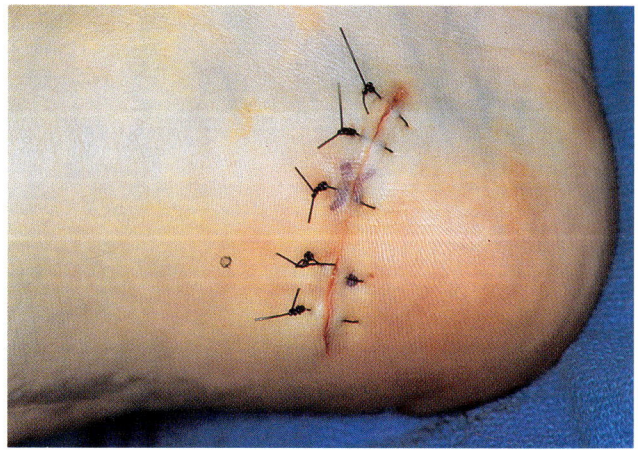

Figure 11. Careful skin closure coapting the skin edges is completed with nylon interrupted mattress sutures.

POSTOPERATIVE MANAGEMENT

Postoperatively, a bandage is maintained on the patient for 3 days. We ask the patient to elevate the foot for 2 days as much as possible, only getting up for short periods of time. Crutches are generally used for 4 to 5 days. A postoperative shoe is used over the bandage for 2 weeks.

When the bandage is changed at 3 days, a smaller bandage is applied to the foot and ankle. Compression is continued for 2 weeks until the stitches are removed. At that time, the patient gradually discontinues the use of the bandage and progresses to a jogging shoe with a soft heel pad. At 3 weeks stationary bicycling is allowed if there is no swelling. At 4 weeks, the patient is allowed to run or walk as tolerated. We have found that the average length of recovery is 3 months. The recovery can extend as long as 6 months or be as short as 1 month, but 3 months is the average.

The operative results of releasing the nerve to the abductor digiti quinti along with the associated aspects of this operation has been reported by Baxter and Thigpen (1). Of 34 operated heels, 32 had good results and 2 had poor results. The good results reported relief of the preoperative symptoms of pain. Those with poor results had continued difficulties with the pain problem. It should be noted that only 26 patients had this operative procedure done over a 6-year period in which the senior author had a very busy foot surgery practice.

COMPLICATIONS

The complications of operative treatment of heel pain by release of the abductor digiti quinti nerve are several. Inadvertent transection of the medial calcaneal nerve branch to the medial aspect of the heel will leave numbness along that medial and plantar aspect of the heel. This complication is avoided by making the incision parallel to the course of these medial calcaneal nerve branches and being aware of their location. Excessive dissection and bleeding in the wound may cause scarring about the nerve or in the skin. Meticulous hemostasis with or without the use of the tourniquet at the time of the operation is important. Also adequate postoperative compression dressing and limiting the early weight bearing can avoid this complication. It is possible that other branches from the lateral plantar nerve might be cut at the time of this surgical procedure. Again, being aware of the anatomy would obviate such a situation.

A potential complication would be to release too much of the plantar fascia and abductor muscle fascia and in this way create a flexible flatfoot. Theoretically the soft tissues tethering the branches of the tarsal tunnel would then compress the tibial nerve and create an iatrogenic tarsal tunnel syndrome. If this occurs, casting during the postoperative period in a short leg walking cast will hold the foot in the proper position while a stabilizing scar develops. Of course being careful to release only the proper amount of fascia about the abductor hallucis as well as the medial portion of the plantar fascia will avoid the possibility of such a complication.

ILLUSTRATIVE CASE FOR TECHNIQUE

In 1975 a world-class athlete was training for the Olympic 1500 meter run. He had participated in the 1972 Olympic 5000 meter run in Munich, Germany, and had been America's premier college miler for 3 years. In 1973 and 1974, there had been no resolution to a chronic heel condition. The pain was located in the inferior, medial, and plantar heel at the proximal medial plantar fascia in the proximal abductor muscle. The pain was described as local with occasional radiation into the lower medial leg and across the inferior heel. For over 1 year, conservative treatment was used. Orthoses, shoe modifications, therapies, medications, injections, acupuncture, and even hypnosis were tried. The heel pain was disabling.

After exhausting all forms of conservative treatment, surgery was considered. When planning an operation on this world-class runner, several problems were considered. Would cutting the plantar fascia lower the arch and affect the running speed? This runner had a small heel spur also. In the preoperative planning, we felt that he had some element of plantar fasciitis medially but the primary problem was chronic compression of the first branch of the lateral plantar nerve.

At surgery, the medial fascia was windowed at the junction of the abductor hallucis fascia and the plantar fascia. Two things were observed. The first was that the heel spur was dorsal to the fascial structure with the spur in the flexor brevis muscle. The second was that a nerve appeared to be compressed by the deep abductor fascia and the most medial plantar fascia. The spur was just plantar to the observed nerve and was thought to be contributing to nerve compression or irritation.

After release of the medial one-fourth of the plantar fascia and the deep inferior fascia of the abductor hallucis muscle, the nerve appeared to be "decompressed." A small spur that lay dorsal to the fascia was removed as the nerve displaced distally. The main structure of the fascia was left intact. The incision was closed.

The runner recovered. He was training again at 6 weeks. Even though he did not go back to the Olympics, he ran an under–4-minute mile 6 months later without pain in his heel.

RECOMMENDED READING

1. Baxter, D. E., and Thigpen, C. M.: Heel pain—operative results. *Foot Ankle*, 5: 16, 1984.
2. Bordelon, R. L.: Subcalcaneal pain: a method of evaluation and plan for treatment. *Clin. Orthop.*, 177: 49, 1983.
3. Graham C. E.: Painful heel syndrome: rationale of diagnosis and treatment. *Foot Ankle*, 3: 261, 1983.
4. Henricson, A. S., and Westlin, N. E.: Chronic calcaneal pain in athletes: Entrapment of the calcaneal nerve? *Am. J. Sports Med.*, 12: 152, 1984.
5. Lutter, L. D.: Surgical decisions in athletes subcalcaneal pain. *Am. J. Sports Med.*, 14: 481, 1986.
6. Mann, R. A.: Miscellaneous afflictions of the foot. In: *Surgery of the Foot*, 5th ed. St. Louis: C. V. Mosby, p. 247, 1986.
7. Rondhuis, J. M., and Huson, A.: The first branch of the lateral plantar nerve and heel pain. *Acta Morphol. Neerl. Scand.* 24: 269, 1986.

27

Calcaneal Prominence Resection

Carol Frey and Glenn B. Pfeffer

INDICATIONS/CONTRAINDICATIONS

Inflammation of the retrocalcaneal bursa can be the result of a prominent or sharply angled posterior superior margin of the calcaneus. In 1928, Patrick Haglund reported on the clinical condition of retrocalcaneal bursitis and described a calcaneus with a prominent posterior superior border that compressed the Achilles tendon and its surrounding bursa against the posterior shoe counter, causing irritation.

Initial treatment for "Haglund's syndrome" is nonoperative and includes anti-inflammatory medication, heel lifts, soft heel counters, and backless shoes. If the patient is a running athlete, mileage should be decreased and the runner is instructed to stop training on hills and hard surfaces. Since the shoe counter can irritate the posterior heel and aggravate the problem, external pressure should be decreased. This can be done by removing or softening the heel counter or by adding a small internal heel wedge to elevate the heel away from the shoe counter. Alternatively, a heel cup can be used to protect the area. Tight calf muscles, tight hamstrings, or a cavus foot may be associated with a symptomatic Haglund's deformity. Achilles tendon stretching is encouraged. If a biomechanical problem such as a cavus foot is noted on physical examination, proper orthotic devices can be used.

If the above measures are not successful, immobilization in a short leg walking cast often reduces acute symptoms. Steroid injections are discouraged as fluid will leak out of an inflamed bursa into the paratendinous structures of the Achilles tendon, even if placed into the bursae under image control.

C. Frey, M.D.: Department of Orthopaedic Surgery, University of Southern California, Los Angeles; and Orthopaedic Foot and Ankle Center, Los Angeles, CA 90007.

G. B. Pfeffer, M.D.: Department of Orthopaedics, University of California–San Francisco; and Orthopaedic Foot and Ankle Clinic, San Francisco, CA 94115.

Surgical treatment is indicated when adequate conservative or nonoperative treatment has failed to give relief. The surgical objective is to eliminate pain by relieving pressure from the underlying bony prominence. Although various angles and lines have been described for evaluating the posterior calcaneus, angles and graphics are difficult to measure due to the lack of consistent reference points on the calcaneus. Furthermore, the significance of such measurements has not been established.

Most patients will respond to nonoperative treatment within a 6-month period of time. It is only after this period of conservative treatment that surgery should be considered. One should avoid operating in an area where there is a blister, open wound, abrasion, or infection.

PREOPERATIVE PLANNING

With the patient in a prone position on the examining table and resting the foot in your hand, the index and thumb are used to palpate the medial and lateral aspects of the posterior superior tuberosity of the calcaneus. When inflammation

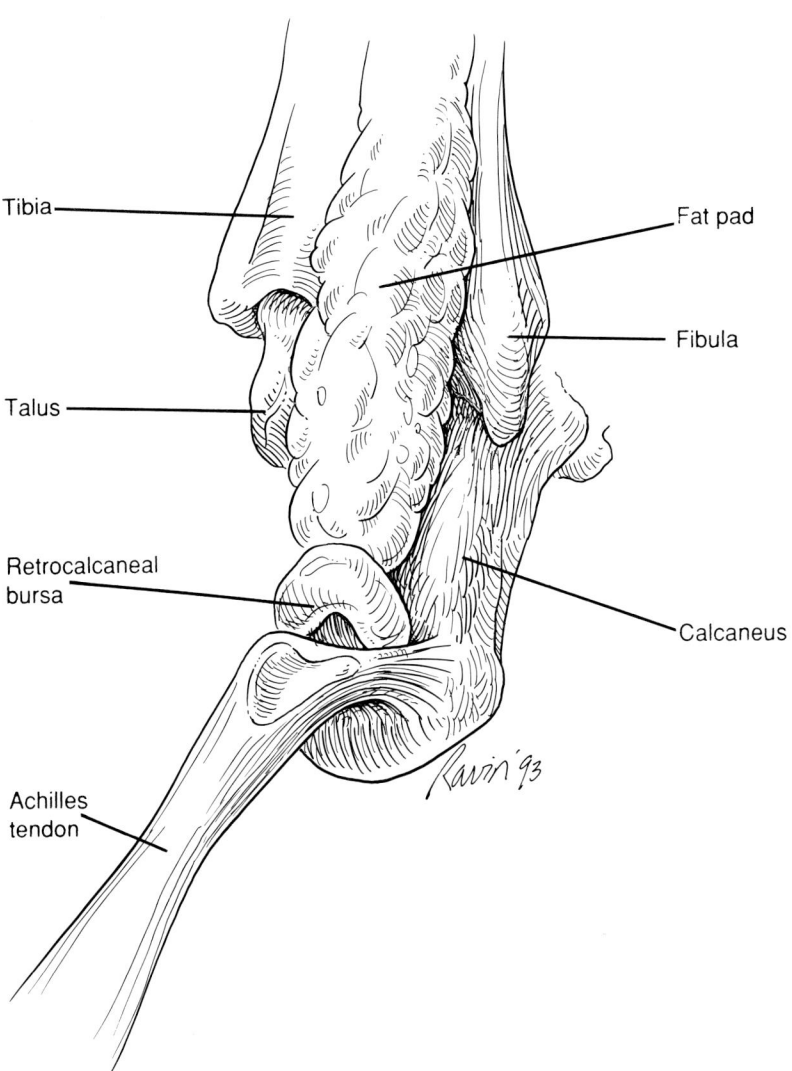

Figure 1. The Achilles tendon has been turned down and the horseshoe-shaped retrocalcaneal bursa as well as the fat pad anterior to the Achilles tendon is seen.

of the retrocalcaneal bursa is present, a soft fluctuant sensation will be felt and usually the patient will describe this test as eliciting the pain. On external inspection, loss of the skin lines due to distention of the retrocalcaneal bursa may also be evident. In severe cases, erythema and warmth may also be present.

With roentgenograms, between the tendon and bone on the standing lateral view of the heel, one can identify a thin strip of fat between the tendon and the bone proximal to the insertion of the Achilles tendon. Likewise, the anterior aspect of the Achilles tendon is sharply outlined throughout its extent by the pre-Achilles fat pad (PAFP). Retrocalcaneal bursitis is indicated when the sharp definition of the retrocalcaneal recess is lost and the lucency of the PAFP in this region is replaced by soft tissue density. The distended fluid-filled bursa often projects above the calcaneus and into the PAFP. In addition, erosion of the cortex of posterior superior aspect of the calcaneus may be evident with retrocalcaneal bursitis. Achilles tendinitis is noted by a thickening of the tendon and a loss of its sharp anterior interface with the PAFP.

The anatomy of the retrocalcaneal bursa (Fig. 1) can be demonstrated with bursography but magnetic resonance imaging (MRI) is more helpful in not only demonstrating anatomy but differentiating retrocalcaneal bursitis from Achilles tendinitis. Accurate recognition of these entities is necessary for proper management. On the MRI, the retrocalcaneal bursa is a potential space that is most clearly demarcated when inflamed. MRI is only recommended in those cases where making a diagnosis is difficult.

SURGERY

The preferred operative approach includes resection of the superior prominence of the calcaneus along with associated bursal tissue. A medial and lateral incision along the Achilles tendon can be used for resection of the superior prominence, although complete resection can usually be carried out using just a lateral incision. A single incision decreases the incidence of wound problems as well as the possibility of injury to the medial calcaneal sensory nerve.

Technique. The patient is placed in the prone position with a bolster under the distal leg (Fig. 2). An 8-cm longitudinal incision is made just anterior to the Achilles tendon on the lateral side of the heel (Fig. 3). The retrocalcaneal area and the superior aspect of the calcaneus (Fig. 4) are exposed by a combination of blunt and sharp dissection, being careful to avoid the sural nerve, which lies approximately 6 mm anterior to the lateral border of the Achilles tendon. The sural nerve should be protected by retracting it anteriorly with the subcutaneous tissues. The incision is carried down to the bone making sure that the insertion site is adequately exposed (Fig. 5). If there is extensive inflammation of the retrocalcaneal bursa, the bursal tissue should be removed. Removal of the bursal tissue is not as important as adequate decompression of the posterior calcaneal prominence. This decompression is carried out using an oblique osteotomy of the superior angle of the calcaneus starting approximately 1.5 cm anterior to the posterior border of the calcaneus and angling downward to the insertion of the Achilles tendon (approximately 2 cm distal to the superior margin of the calcaneus) (Fig. 5). The osteotomy is carried out with a power saw, keeping perpendicular to the longitudinal axis of the calcaneus (Fig. 6). A ridge of bone is always left at the insertion site of the Achilles tendon and must be carefully removed with a small curette and microreciprocating rasp.

To successfully decompress the retrocalcaneal space, adequate bone must be removed. Bone can be removed up to the insertion site of the Achilles tendon. Do not leave a ledge or spike of bone near the insertion site of the Achilles tendon. This is potentially painful and a source of irritation to the Achilles tendon.

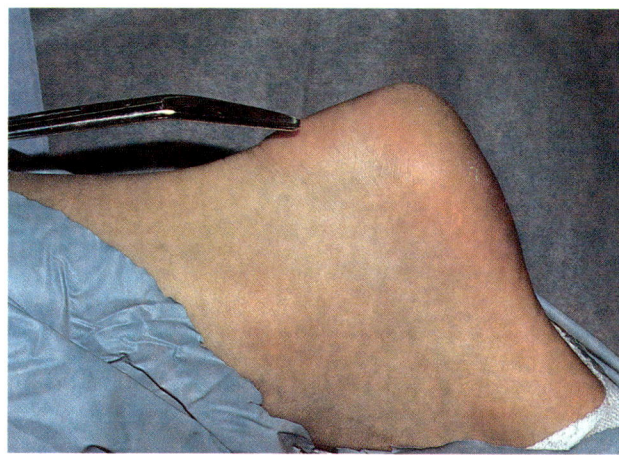

Figure 2. At the time of operation, with the patient in a prone position, the prominence of the posterior aspect of the calcaneus is at the end of the surgical instrument.

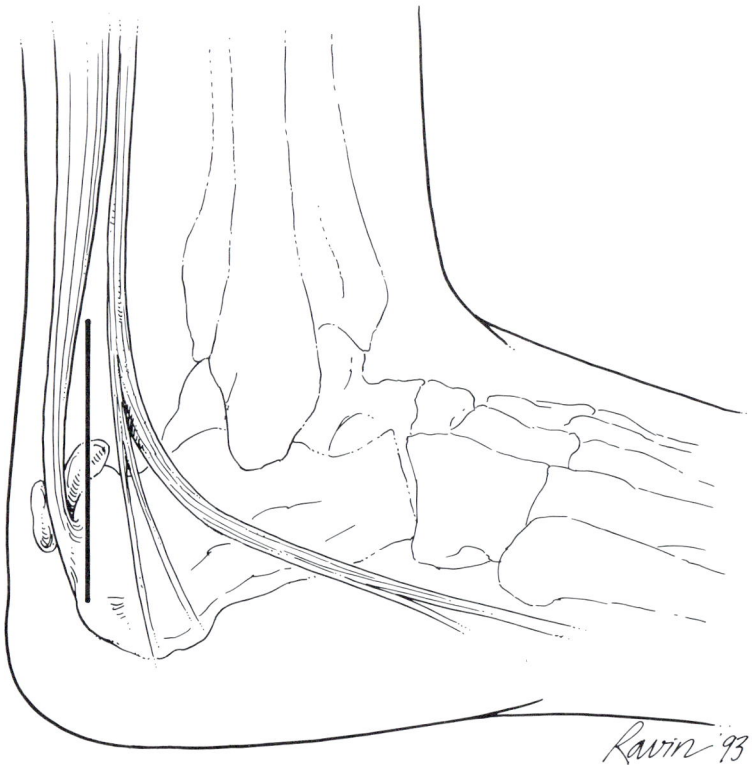

Figure 3. An incision is made along the lateral aspect of the heel centered over the posterior superior tuberosity of the calcaneus.

The microreciprocating rasp is also helpful in rounding off the margins of the calcaneus in all directions, especially on the medial side. If the medial ridge still cannot be reached adequately, a medial incision should be added. This is rarely necessary, however.

The area is palpated often through the overlying skin to make certain that all ridges and prominences are removed. The wedge of bone removed must be of adequate size to ensure thorough decompression of the retrocalcaneal area (Fig. 7). It should be kept in mind that the Achilles tendon does not insert at the superior

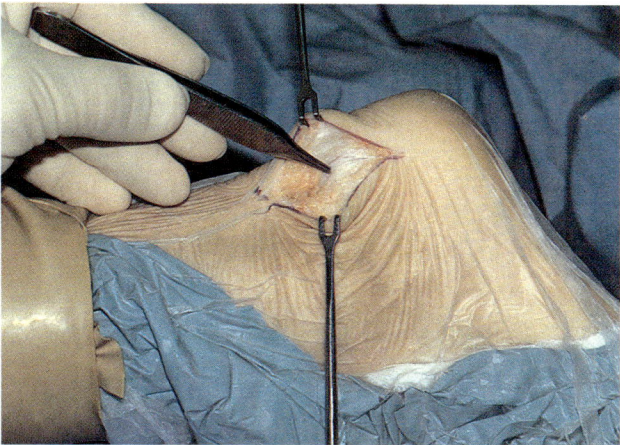

Figure 4. At the time of operation, the thumb forceps shows the prominent posterior lateral aspect of the superior calcaneus.

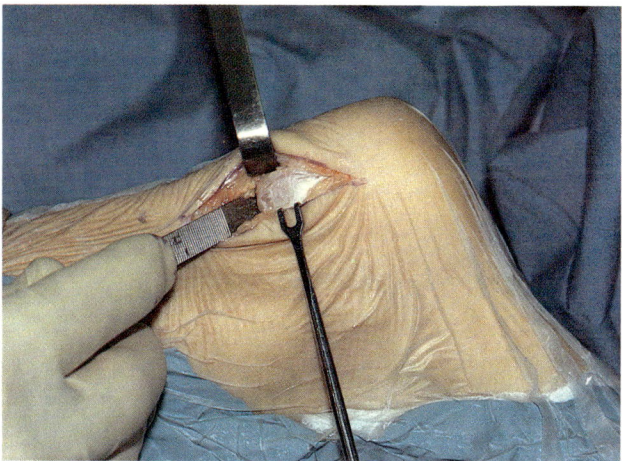

Figure 5. Subperiosteal dissection is done of the tuberosity of the calcaneus all the way to the medial side of the calcaneal tuberosity.

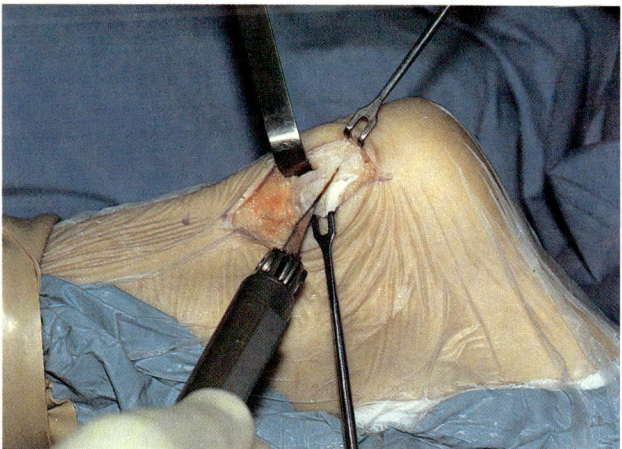

Figure 6. A saw is used to resect the posterior aspect of the calcaneus from the insertion of the Achilles tendon at a 45° oblique angle to the superior aspect of the posterior calcaneus.

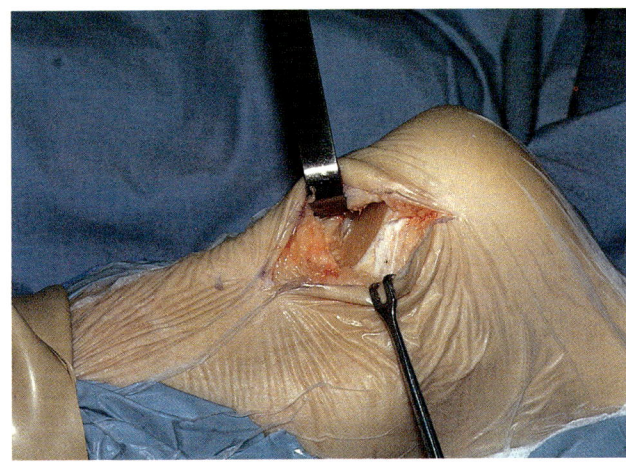

Figure 7. The amount of bone resected can be seen in the depths of the wound.

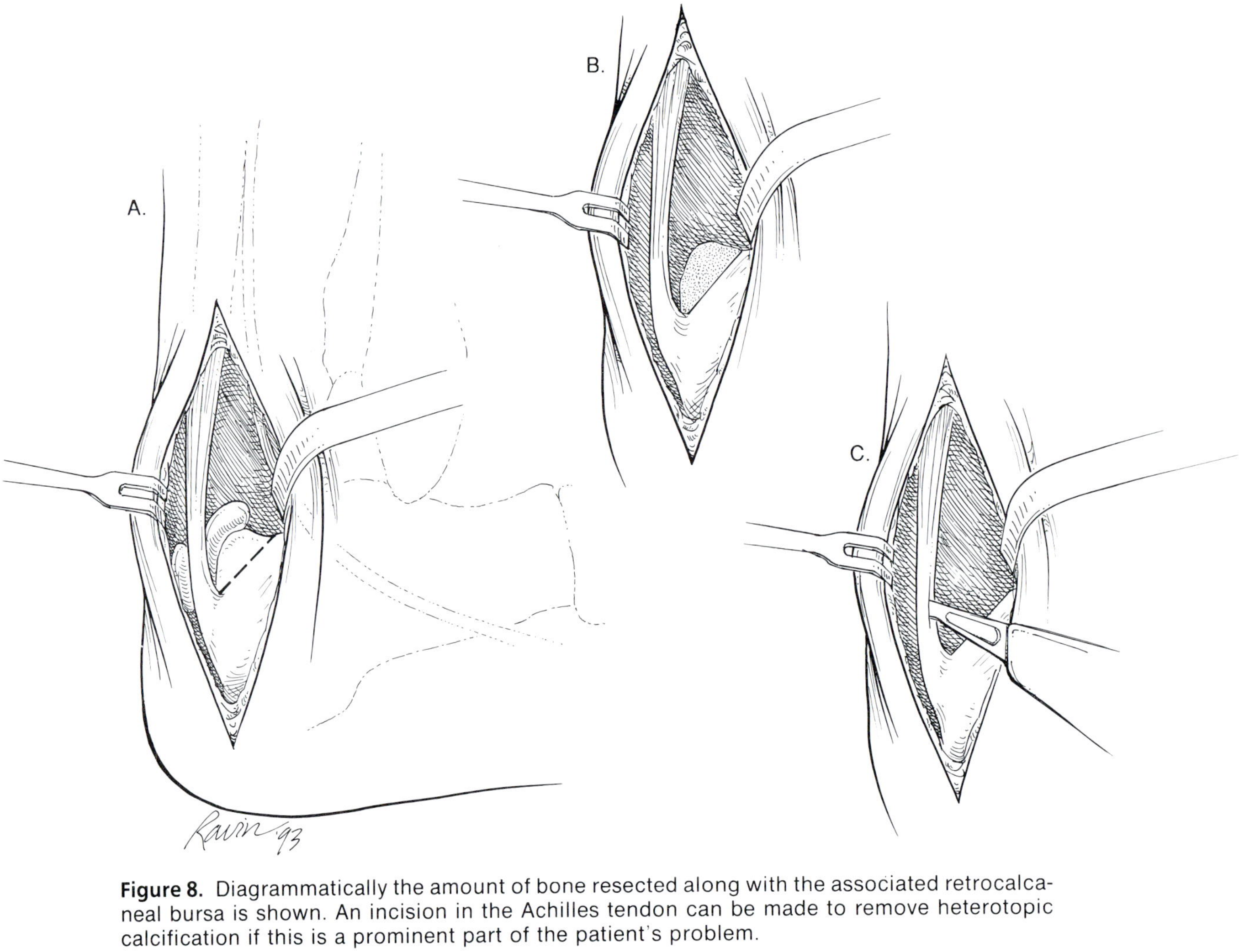

Figure 8. Diagrammatically the amount of bone resected along with the associated retrocalcaneal bursa is shown. An incision in the Achilles tendon can be made to remove heterotopic calcification if this is a prominent part of the patient's problem.

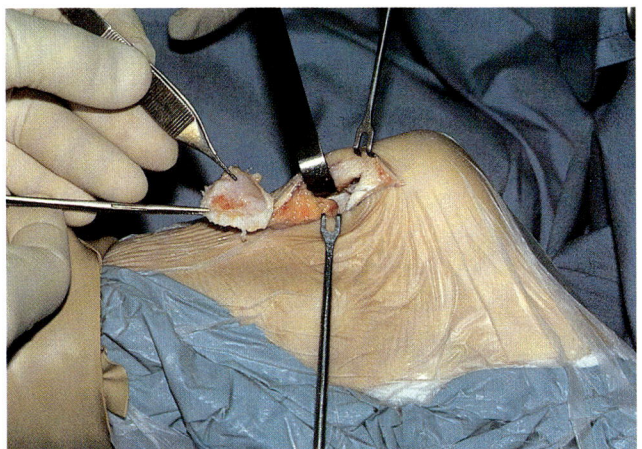

Figure 9. The excised tuberosity of the calcaneus is shown next to the surgical wound.

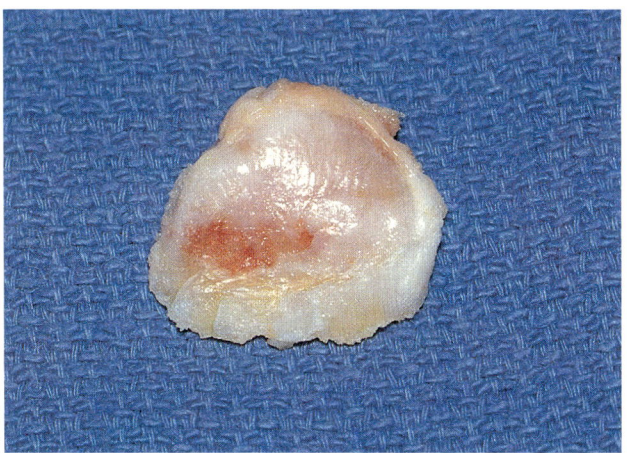

Figure 10. A close-up view of the excised tuberosity shows the result of chronic irritation of the calcaneus. Eburnation and hemorrhage of the bone is seen.

aspect of the calcaneus but significantly more inferior in the apophyseal portion of the calcaneus. The Achilles tendon sweeps backward and away from the tibia to meet the inclined calcaneus obliquely, the bone and the tendon forming an acute angle. By resecting bone down to the insertion site of the Achilles tendon, adequate decompression of the retrocalcaneal space can usually be obtained (Fig. 8).

It is possible to remove too much distal bone and cut into the insertion of the Achilles tendon. This could allow the tendon to avulse later. Careful exposure of the insertion site of the Achilles tendon at the time of surgery should help the surgeon avoid this pitfall.

The Achilles tendon should then be inspected for tendinosis. Longitudinal cuts with a scalpel in the anterior 50% of the tendon will often reveal necrotic areas of tendon that require debridement. After the tendon is debrided, it is repaired with buried 3-0 nonabsorbable suture such as Ethibond.

Inspection of the resected portion of the posterior superior process of the calcaneus (Figs. 9 and 10) will sometimes show the eburnation of the posterior superior aspect of the calcaneus by the Achilles tendon. This aspect of the calcaneal tuberosity almost has a cartilaginous appearance to it, particularly with prolonged inflammation.

The wound is closed routinely in layers over a small suction drain.

POSTOPERATIVE MANAGEMENT

The patient is placed into a short leg non–weight-bearing cast with the foot in mild plantar flexion for the first 4 weeks. He or she is then placed into the short leg walking cast with the foot gradually brought up to neutral position for the next 4 weeks. When the cast is removed the patient is placed into a shoe with a $7/16$-inch tapered internal heel lift that is gradually brought down to $3/16$ of an inch. This is worn for 3 months. General muscle conditioning is begun when the cast is removed.

The recovery period from this operative procedure can be quite prolonged, a period of 3 to 6 months. A possible reason for this is the dependent nature of the foot during the later postoperative period. The later result, however, is usually satisfactory for the majority of patients.

COMPLICATIONS

Problems that can be encountered include damage to the sural nerve or the medial neurovascular structures. This can be avoided by paying close attention to anatomy and using careful dissection technique. Wound problems are a source of worry around the Achilles tendon and great care should be taken when handling the soft tissues and posterior skin.

As mentioned previously, removing too much bone at the insertion of the Achilles tendon may result in avulsion of the Achilles tendon. Removing not enough bone from the posterior superior aspect of the calcaneus may result in inadequate decompression of the retrocalcaneal bursa. If the plane of resection of the posterior superior calcaneus is too oblique, the posterior facet of the subtalar joint may be inadvertently entered.

ILLUSTRATIVE CASE FOR TECHNIQUE

This 22-year-old woman described pain in the posterior lateral aspect of her heel. Although high-heeled shoes tended to be the most aggravating, she had pain even with low-heeled lace-up type shoes due to irritation of the posterior aspect of the lateral calcaneus (Fig. 11). This restricted her work as well as recreational activities and she sought permanent relief.

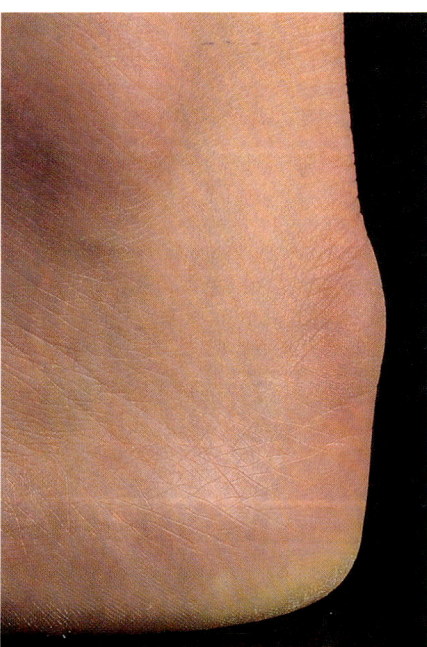

Figure 11. Profile view of the patient's posterior calcaneus showing the bony prominence posterior and lateral to the Achilles tendon.

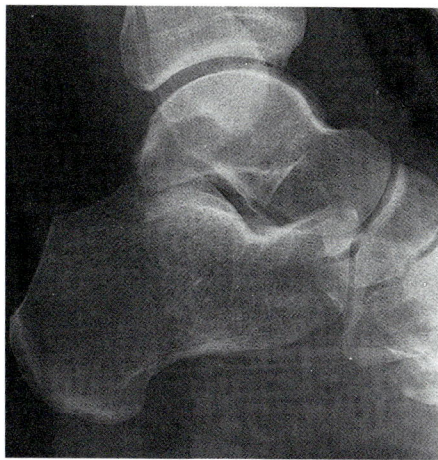

Figure 12. Appearance of the calcaneus following excision of the posterior superior aspect.

A resection of her posterior superior tuberosity of the calcaneus along with associated bursal inflammation was done (Fig. 12). Two years later she was asymptomatic on this side, but was starting to develop pain in the opposite heel region and thought she would have a similar procedure done on that side.

RECOMMENDED READING

1. Fiamengo, S., et al. Posterior heel pain associated with a calcaneal step and Achilles tendon calcification. *CORR*, 167: 203, 1982.
2. Fowler, A., and Philip, J. F. Abnormality of the calcaneus as a cause of painful heel. *Br. J. Surg.*, 32: 494, 1945.
3. Frey, C., Rosenberg, Z., Shereff, M. J., and Kim, H.: The retrocalcaneal bursa: anatomy and bursography. *Foot Ankle*, 13: 203–7, 1992.
4. Henneghan, M., and Pavlov, H. The Haglund painful heel syndrome. *CORR*, 187: 228, 1984.
5. Keck, S., and Kelley, P. Bursitis of the posterior part of the heel. *J. Bone Joint Surg.*, 47A: 267, 1965.
6. Pfeffer, G. B., and Baxter, D. E. In: *Surgery of the Adult Heel, Disorders of the Foot and Ankle*, edited by Jahss M. Philadelphia: W. B. Saunders, 1991.

28
Osteotomy of the Calcaneal Tuberosity

R. Luke Bordelon

INDICATIONS/CONTRAINDICATIONS

Abnormalities of position of the os calcis, whether congenital, developmental, or acquired, are important in determining foot function. The position of the tuberosity of the calcaneus influences the motion in the subtalar joint, and the position and function of the subtalar joint and associated transverse tarsal joints will determine whether the foot is supple or rigid.

With an osteotomy through the body of the os calcis going dorsal to plantar just posterior to the peroneal tendons, one can change the position of the os calcis to provide proper alignment of the subtalar joint. This osteotomy may be used to correct a deformity of the os calcis and to place the os calcis in a better functional position. This calcaneal osteotomy is used when there is an intrinsic deformity of the os calcis or a functional abnormality of the subtalar joint.

The calcaneal tuberosity can be moved to the desired position, which will allow the foot to function in an optimum manner (Fig. 1). For a flatfoot deformity with excessive eversion of the heel the tuberosity would be moved medially and inverted. For a cavus type of foot with an inversion of the heel, the tuberosity would be moved laterally and everted. For a cavus foot with increased inclination of the calcaneus but without an inversion or eversion deformity, sliding the tuberosity upward on the body of the calcaneus will decrease the cavus. Conversely, if one had a decreased angle of inclination of the os calcis, displacing the tuberosity plantarward would increase the arch of the foot.

With complex deformities such as inversion of the heel plus increased calcaneal inclination, a biplane type of repositioning of the tuberosity can be accomplished.

R. L. Bordelon, M.D.: Department of Orthopaedics, Louisiana State University School of Medicine, Opelousas, LA 70570.

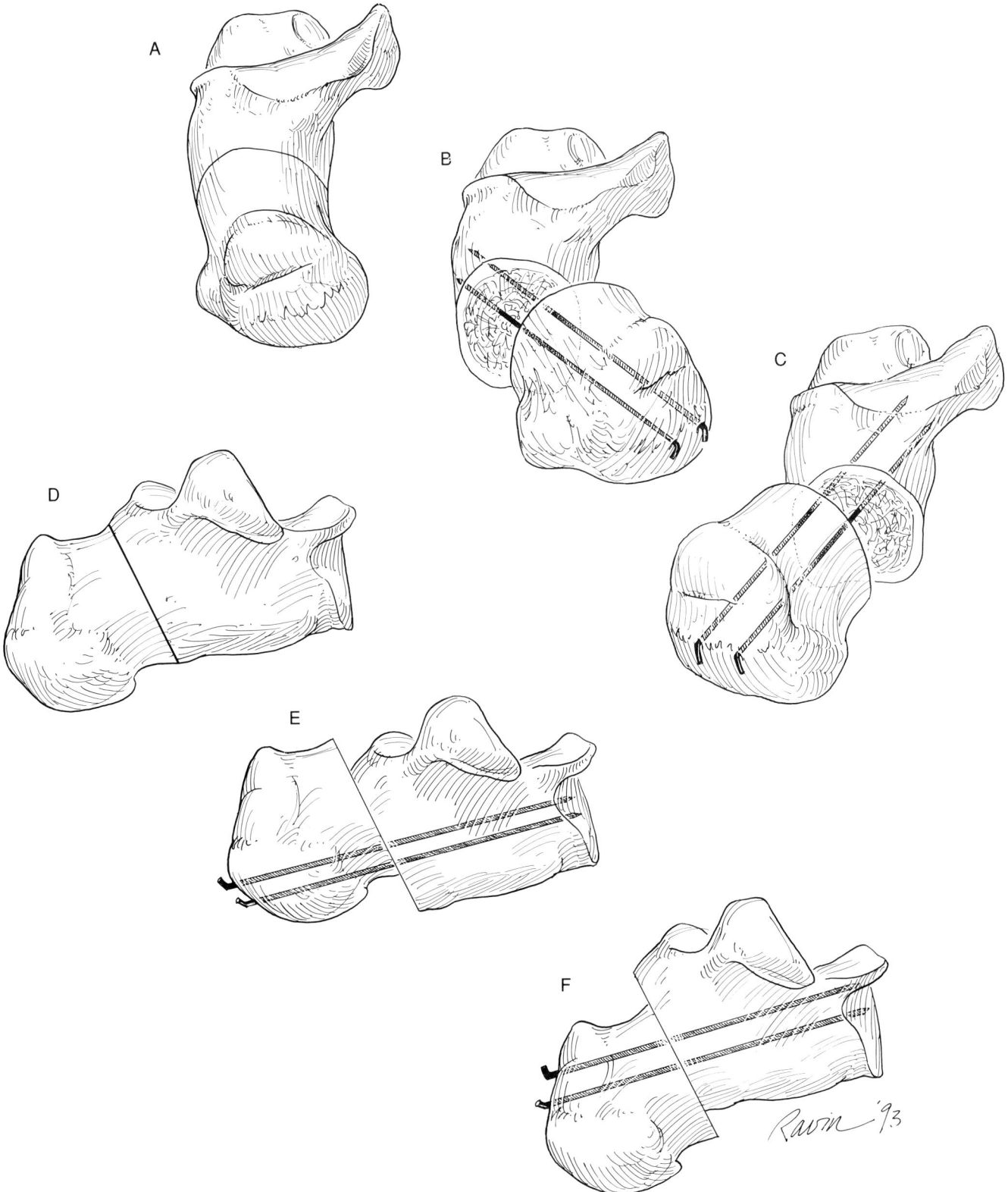

Figure 1. A: View from the posterosuperior aspect of the calcaneus shows the position of the osteotomy through the tuberosity of the calcaneus. **B:** The translocation of the tuberosity medially and then an inversion tilting of the calcaneal tuberosity. **C:** A lateral displacement of the calcaneal tuberosity and an eversion of the posterior tuberosity fragment. **D:** Lateral view of the calcaneus shows the position of the osteotomy in relationship to the tuberosity and body of the calcaneus. **E:** A dorsal displacement of the tuberosity of the calcaneus. It should produce a flatter foot. **F:** The tuberosity of the calcaneus has been slid plantarward to produce a more cavus foot.

The calcaneal tuberosity can be translocated dorsally or plantarly and shifted medially with an inversion angulation, or laterally with an eversion angulation.

Generally, shifting position of the os calcis is adequate and provides adequate stability and bony contact. Small appropriate wedges may be used, but it has been found that changing the position of the bone by cutting through and releasing the soft tissue provides better control and ability to place the heel in the position one desires than a closing wedge type of osteotomy.

PREOPERATIVE PLANNING

In order to properly plan for the positioning of the os calcis, the mobility of the joints of the foot and ankle, the position of the foot relative to the leg, and the position and motion of the leg and hip are determined. The mobility of the subtalar joint and ankle joints are particularly important. In a foot with a mobile subtalar joint, when the talonavicular joint is in a congruent alignment (neutral position), the surgical goal is to position the calcaneal tuberosity in about 0° to 5° of hindfoot valgus.

The osteotomy of the os calcis through the tuberosity is used to correct structural deformities of the foot around the subtalar joint complex. Using it in this manner can help to convert a rigid cavus foot to a more normal flexible foot and to convert an excessive flatfoot to a more normally supportive foot.

Weight-bearing radiographs of the feet are made. Also, posterior calcaneal views with the foot weight bearing will help evaluate the calcaneal tuberosity position.

SURGERY

General anesthesia with the patient supine is preferred. The entire lower leg and knee are draped out (Fig. 2). A sandbag is placed under the ipsilateral hip to allow better access to the lateral side of the foot.

Technique. The surgical approach for osteotomy of the calcaneal tuberosity is through an oblique incision dorsal to plantar posterior to the line of the peroneal tendons (Fig. 3). Care is taken to avoid injury to the sural nerve. The incision is carried down to the lateral aspect of the calcaneus (Fig. 4). Two hemostats are used, one dorsally and one plantarly, to identify the line of the calcaneal osteotomy (Fig. 5). The periosteum is incised and stripped from the lateral cortex of the

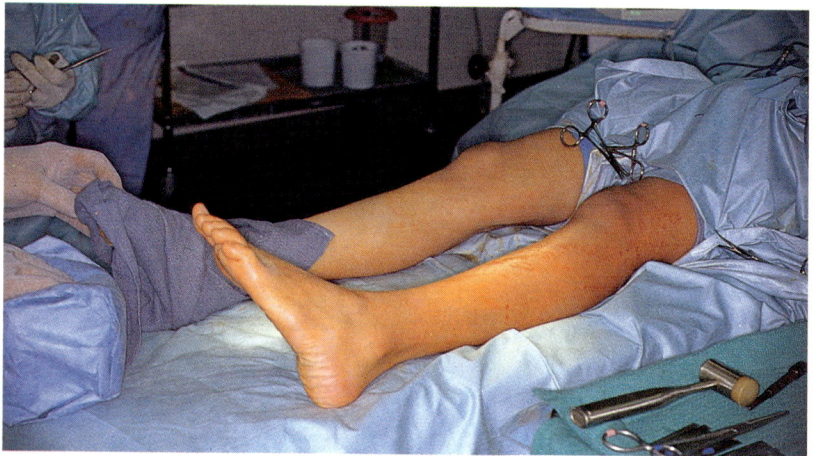

Figure 2. The entire lower extremity from above the knee down to the foot is draped free at the time of surgery.

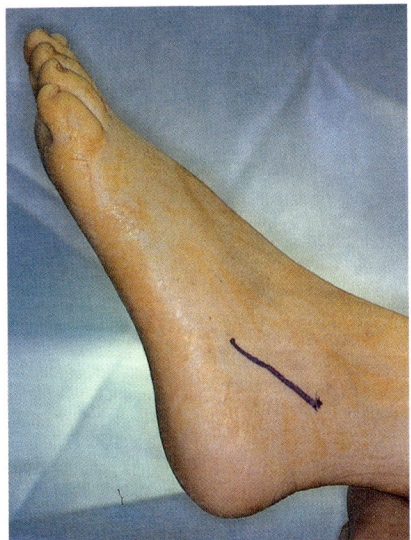

Figure 3. The skin incision just posterior to the peroneal tendons is marked.

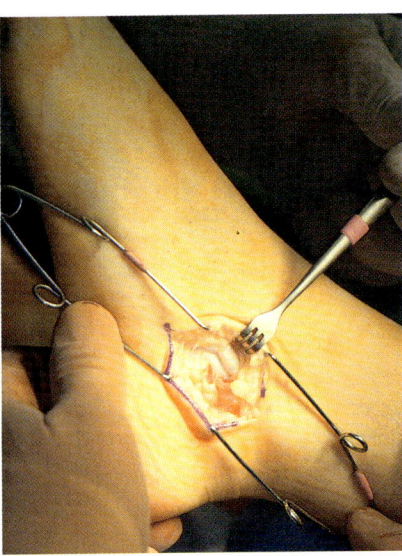

Figure 4. The skin and subcutaneous tissues are divided with care being taken to protect the sural nerve.

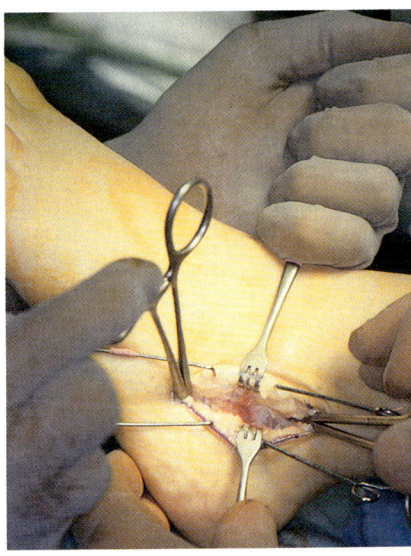

Figure 5. The superior and inferior aspects of the calcaneal tuberosity are identified and hemostats placed to orient for elevation the periosteum and subsequent osteotomy.

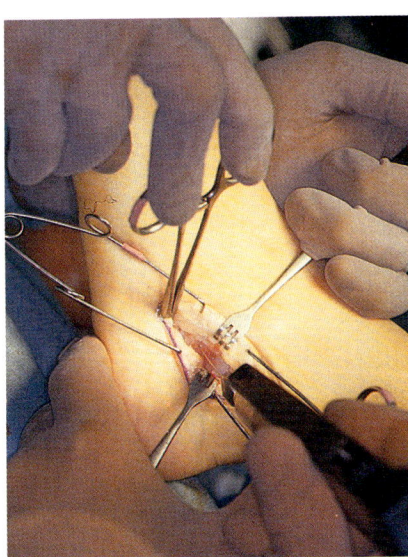

Figure 6. An overall view showing the reciprocating saw entering the tuberosity of the os calcis in a transverse direction.

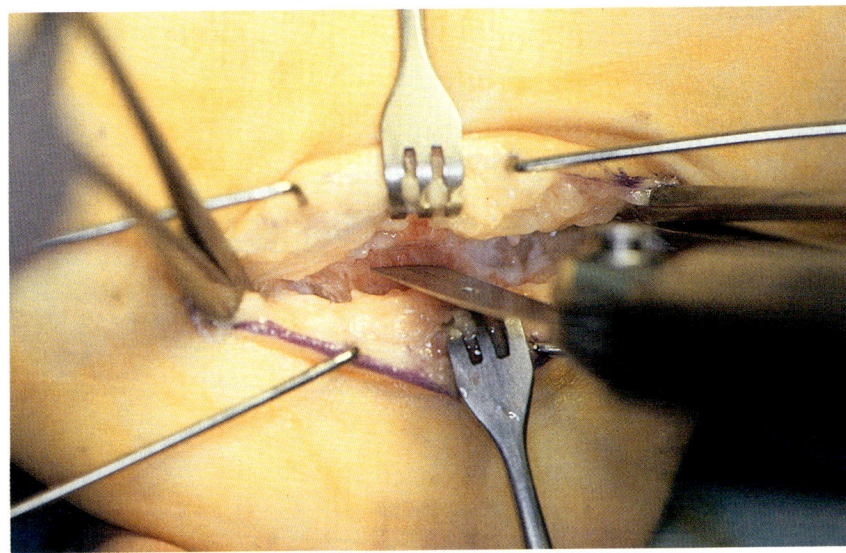

Figure 7. A close-up view showing the saw in the lateral aspect of the os calcis.

calcaneus. An osteotomy is then made through the tuberosity of the os calcis (Fig. 6). This osteotomy is made in line with the peroneal tendons and is perpendicular to the bone and may be made with either a saw or an osteotome (Fig. 7). Care is taken when cutting through the medial cortex not to go into the soft tissue as this might injure the tendons or the neurovascular structures of the tibial nerve and artery.

Once the cut is made through the medial wall, a periosteal elevator is used to strip the soft tissue from the medial side of the os calcis, prying the os calcis open. Thus one has the distal portion of the os calcis, which is now free and can be displaced into an improved position. The displacement will depend upon the hindfoot mobility and deformity that was present. Generally, the os calcis is moved over one-half the width and then tilted to the appropriate degree. Dorsal displacement and plantar displacement of the distal portion of the os calcis may be performed to increase or decrease the angle of calcaneal inclination.

Fixation is by two Steinmann pins (7/64th or 3/32nd), going from the posterior portion of the os calcis through the osteotomy into the body of the os calcis. The pins are bent and buried beneath the skin. These two pins are only in the os calcis and do not cross a joint. Once the os calcis is in its new position, a clinical examination will demonstrate how the talocalcaneal joint will function with the os calcis in its new position.

The wound is then irrigated and closed, taking care to avoid damage to the sural nerve.

Although there have been described different types of osteotomies of the os calcis with curves and positions, these are difficult. I find it easier to cut the os calcis in a single straight line and then position the os calcis exactly where I deem best. The most common surgical problem that I have encountered has been that of making the cut through the body of the os calcis too far distally, thus not having an adequate amount of bone in the distal portion of the os calcis to provide control and to adequately correct the deformity. Stripping of the soft tissue medially is extremely important in providing mobility of the distal fragment. This allows placement of the os calcis in the appropriate position to correct the deformity. Placing the two smooth Steinmann pins from posterior into the anterior part of the os calcis requires some dexterity. These pins provide secure fixation and do not interfere with any motion of the foot. This allows the examiner to determine the motion of the talocalcaneal joint as well as the position of the os calcis. I have not had any displacement using this method, and bone grafting has not been necessary.

POSTOPERATIVE MANAGEMENT

The patient's foot is placed in a well-padded posterior plaster splint. Elevation and pain control as needed are utilized. Active range of motion exercises as possible while in the splint are started within 48 hours and continued through the postoperative course to maintain mobility of the joints of the foot. At 2 weeks, the sutures are removed and the patient is placed in a well-padded short leg non–weight-bearing cast. Range of motion exercises, again as possible, are continued. The extent of activity that the patient may be up to depends upon the amount of swelling. If there is not much swelling, activity can be increased. If there is a great deal of swelling and pain, then the dependency is decreased. At 4 to 6 weeks, depending upon the age of the patient, stability of the fixation, and cooperation of the patient, weight bearing in a short leg cast is allowed. The pins are removed at about 8 weeks, generally under local anesthesia in the office. A short leg weight-bearing cast is usually used for 2 more weeks. Thus, the usual recuperation immobilization time is 4 weeks in a non–weight-bearing cast and 4 weeks in a weight-bearing cast with the pins in place, and then 2 weeks in a weight-bearing cast after the pins have been removed. Physical therapy is not used unless there are other factors and other conditions that necessitate its use. A period of 6 to 12 months is required to determine what the functional result will be following this procedure.

When the procedure is done for a structural condition where the other joints are normally mobile, satisfactory correction can usually be obtained. If the procedure is performed to try to provide a better functional foot but without complete mobility of the adjacent joints and especially with fibrotic and arthritic changes of the adjacent joints, then complete resolution of the problem might not be obtained. The patient has to know this prior to surgery.

COMPLICATIONS

If there is excessive correction, then the reverse deformity of the foot can be produced. If inadequate correction is performed, then the patient will have the same difficulty as before. It is important to determine by clinical examination how much correction to obtain.

With a medial displacement osteotomy, skin necrosis may be a problem because of pressure on the skin due to displacement. This problem if it occurs will heal by secondary intention.

Pin tract infection may occur. If there is increasing pain and tenderness, then the site of the pins must be inspected. In order to try to prevent pin tract infection, the pins are bent and buried beneath the skin and the cast well padded. Sometimes they will protrude through the skin in spite of this. If there is evidence of infection, then antibiotics are utilized, the area is cleaned, and if necessary the pins are removed.

ILLUSTRATIVE CASE FOR TECHNIQUE

A 16-year-old male football player had a history of recurrent sprains of the left ankle (Fig. 8). There was an inversion deformity of the os calcis that was structural. There was decreased eversion of the os calcis. Forefoot position was normal. When the patient ambulated, because of the inversion of the heel and inability to evert the heel, the foot and ankle collapsed inward, producing abnormal stresses on the ankle joint. Stress radiographs of the ankle revealed some instability of the tibiotalar joint (Fig. 9).

A Chrisman-Snook repair was performed of the ligaments of the ankle to provide ligamentous stability of the ankle.

To provide a hindfoot that functioned properly and would not produce additional stress on the ankle joint, an osteotomy of the calcaneal tuberosity was done dis-

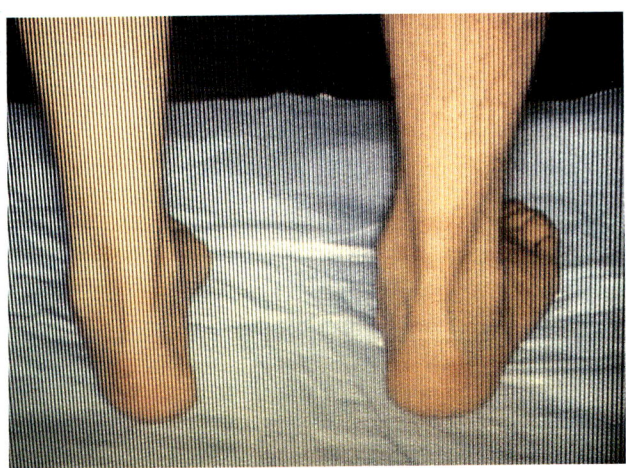

Figure 8. The structural inversion of the patient's left calcaneal tuberosity.

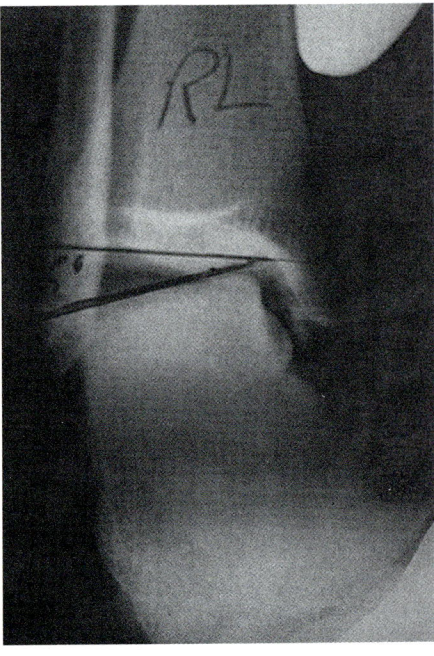

Figure 9. Inversion and stress testing of the left ankle was 15° more than that of the unaffected right.

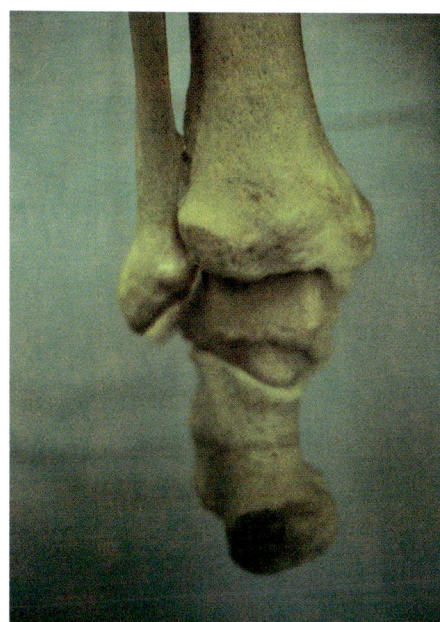 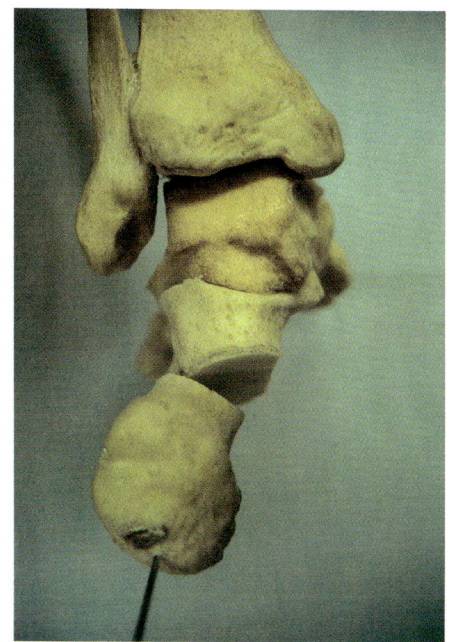

Figure 10. A: Skeletal model showing an inversion deformity of the tuberosity of the os calcis such as was present in this patient. **B:** A calcaneal osteotomy has been done in this model and the new corrected position of the tuberosity of the os calcis is seen.

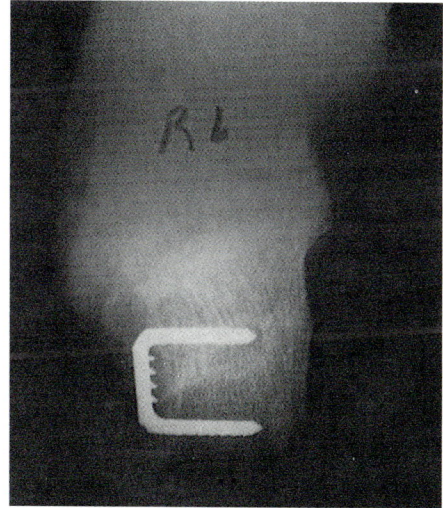

Figure 11. Radiograph after healing of the calcaneal osteotomy. In this instance a staple was used for fixation instead of the two Steinmann pin technique.

placing the tuberosity laterally and in eversion (Fig. 10). This corrected the abnormal structural position of the calcaneal tuberosity and provided the patient with a functional foot (Fig. 11). The heel functioned in eversion during the early part of stance phase and allowed normal motion of the midfoot. The result was avoidance of excessive strain on the hindfoot and the repaired lateral ligaments.

RECOMMENDED READING

1. Bordelon, R. L.: Hypermobile flatfoot in children: Comprehension, evaluation and treatment. *Clin. Orthop.*, 181: 7–14, 1983.
2. Bordelon, R. L.: Hypermobile flatfoot in children: present status of diagnosis and treatment. *Semin. Orthop.*, 5(1): 13–22, 1990.
3. Bordelon, R. L.: *Surgical and Conservative Foot Care*. Slack, Thorofare, NJ, 1988.
4. Dwyer, F. C.: The treatment of relapsed club foot by the insertion of a wedge into the calcaneum. *J. Bone Joint Surg.*, 45B: 67, 1963.
5. Elftman, H.: The transverse tarsal joint and its control. *Clin. Orthop.*, 16: 41, 1960.
6. Koutsogiannis, E.: Treatment of mobile flat foot by displacement osteotomy of the calcaneus. *J. Bone Joint Surg.*, 53B: 96, 1971.
7. Lord, J. P.: Correction of extreme flatfoot: value of osteotomy of os calcis and inward displacement of posterior fragment (Gleich operation). *JAMA*, 81: 1502, 1923.
8. Mann, R. A.: *DuVries Surgery of the Foot*, 5th ed. C. V. Mosby, St. Louis, 1986.
9. Mann, R. A., and Coughlin, M. J.: *Surgery of the Foot and Ankle*, 6th ed. Mosby, St. Louis, 1993.
10. Silver, C. M., Simon, S. D., Spindell, E., Litchman, H. M., and Scala, M.: Calcaneal osteotomy for valgus and varus deformities of the foot in cerebral palsy: a preliminary report on twenty-seven operations. *J. Bone Joint Surg.*, 49A: 232, 1967.

29

Talocalcaneal (Subtalar) Arthrodesis

Michael J. Shereff

INDICATIONS/CONTRAINDICATIONS

Arthrodesis of the talocalcaneal joint serves to stabilize the deformed or arthritic hindfoot. The operation described enables the clinician to correct varus or valgus deformities of the subtalar joint. Subtalar fusion also eliminates the painful crepitant motion of the incongruous articular surfaces during weight-bearing activities. The surgical technique recommends a moldable bone graft first described by K. A. Johnson. It has proved itself to be an effective method of obtaining arthrodesis of this articulation. The moldable subtalar arthrodesis minimizes shortening of the height of the hindfoot. A pin or screw is utilized to provide adequate fixation. The moldable bone graft provides rapid healing and a high incidence of union.

The limitations of the technique include the fact that it can be utilized to correct only varus or valgus deformities. Pathologic disorders involving the talonavicular and calcaneocuboid joint require incorporation of these articulations in the fusion in the form of a triple arthrodesis.

Isolated subtalar arthrodesis is utilized for correction of posttraumatic arthritis of the subtalar joint as is typically seen following fractures of the talus or the calcaneus. Isolated degenerative arthritis would also provide a reasonable indication for this surgical procedure. Rheumatoid arthritis and other inflammatory disorders with subtalar involvement might also be addressed by this technique. Other potential indications include infectious arthritis or metabolic disorders of the talocalcaneal joint.

Localized arthritis secondary to malalignment of the subtalar joint, as well as talocalcaneal coalition with secondary subtalar arthritis, may be treated with this

---

M. J. Shereff, M.D.: Division of Foot and Ankle Surgery, Department of Orthopaedic Surgery, Medical College of Wisconsin, Milwaukee, WI 53226.

technique. This surgical procedure may also be used to correct varus or valgus deformity of the hindfoot secondary to congenital abnormalities, neurologic disorders, or other acquired disorders.

Contraindications to subtalar arthrodesis include advanced age, vascular insufficiency, neuropathic disorders, as well as active local or systemic infections. The presence of pathologic disorders or deformities involving the ankle, Chopart's joint, or the midfoot are not amenable to correction by fusion of the subtalar joint alone.

PREOPERATIVE PLANNING

Planning for the isolated subtalar arthrodesis requires meticulous evaluation of the patient. Patients typically describe pain and swelling quite localized to the region of the subtalar joint. Physical examination enables identification of localized tenderness in the region of the sinus tarsi. Motion of the subtalar joint most often reproduces the patient's pain. The normal range of motion is often restricted and attempted passive motion may be associated with palpable crepitus.

Anteroposterior (AP), lateral, and oblique radiographs are helpful in identifying changes associated with articular destruction and incongruity at the subtalar joint. Narrowing of the joint space with loss of articular cartilage and cystic erosions in subchondral bone may often be identified. Periarticular osteophytes may be seen. Lateral tomographs of the hindfoot, as well as computed tomography (CT) scans in the coronal plane, enhance evaluation of this region.

To assess the contribution of the subtalar joint to the patient's symptomatology, diagnostic injections of that joint can be performed. An injection of local anesthetic under image intensification may increase diagnostic accuracy. An oblique approach at the dorsolateral aspect of the hindfoot by means of the sinus tarsi is most often utilized. Preoperative injection will provide both the orthopaedic surgeon and the patient with some insight as to the role of the subtalar joints in the patient's problem.

Physical examination also requires evaluation of the neurovascular status of the foot since vascular or neurologic dysfunction may be contraindications to extensive hindfoot reconstruction.

SURGERY

Hindfoot arthrodesis can be performed under a spinal or general anesthesia. This operation is usually done in an inpatient setting since postoperative care requires neurovascular observation, significant postoperative analgesic medications and ambulation training and physical therapy.

The patient is placed supine on the operating table. The use of a pneumatic thigh tourniquet is utilized to obtain hemostasis. It is helpful to place several folded sheets under the buttocks to increase the prominence of the iliac crest from which the bone graft will be obtained. The leg and iliac graft site are prepped in the usual manner and the leg is draped free.

Technique. An oblique skin incision is made that is centered over the sinus tarsi (Fig. 1). The incision begins 1 cm distal to the tip of the lateral malleolus and is then extended anteriorly and distally. Subcutaneous tissue is incised along the line of the skin incision.

The extensor retinaculum is incised longitudinally and the extensor tendons are retracted superiorly (Fig. 2).

The origin of the extensor digitorum brevis muscle is incised and reflected distally to allow exposure and excision of fatty tissue from the sinus tarsi (Fig. 3).

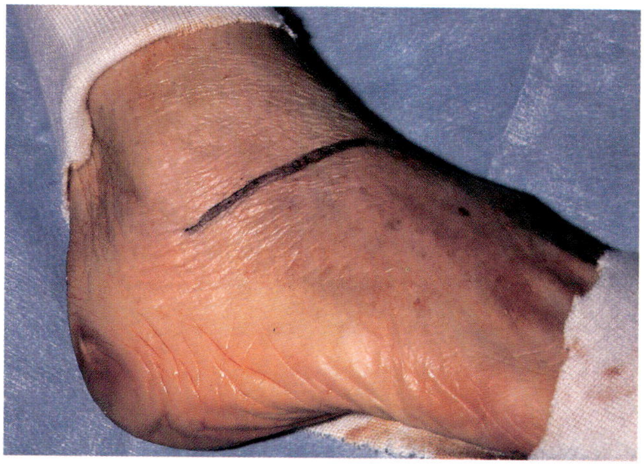

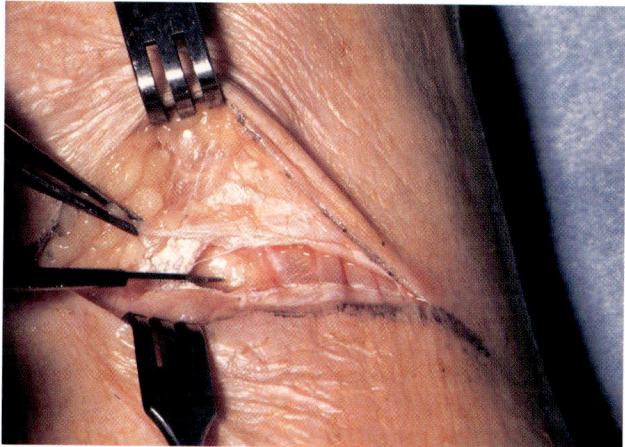

Figure 1. The oblique skin incision is shown.

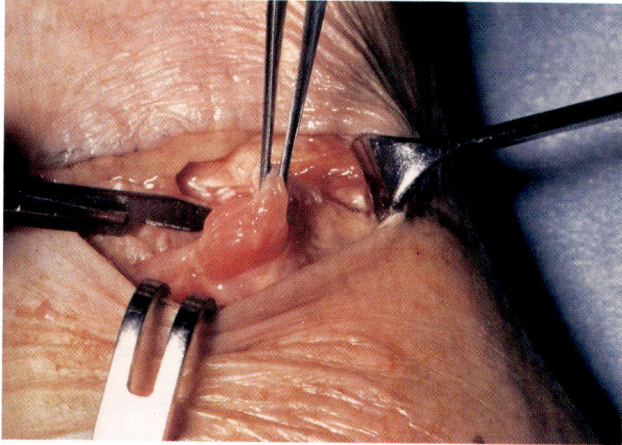

Figure 2. The incision extends from the extensor digitorum longus tendon anteriorly to the peroneal tendon posteriorly.

Figure 3. The extensor digitorum brevis muscle is reflected distally to expose the sinus tarsi.

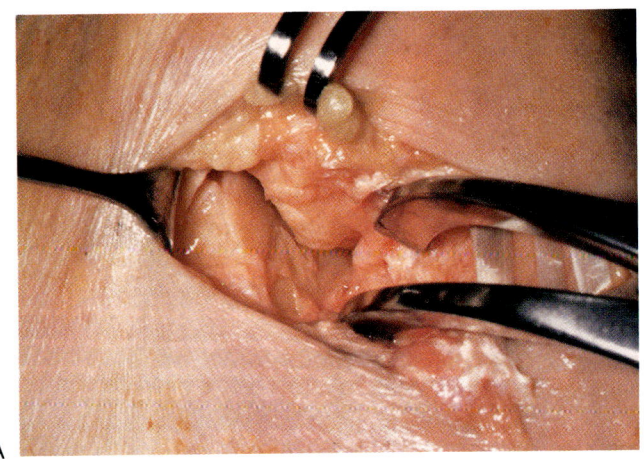

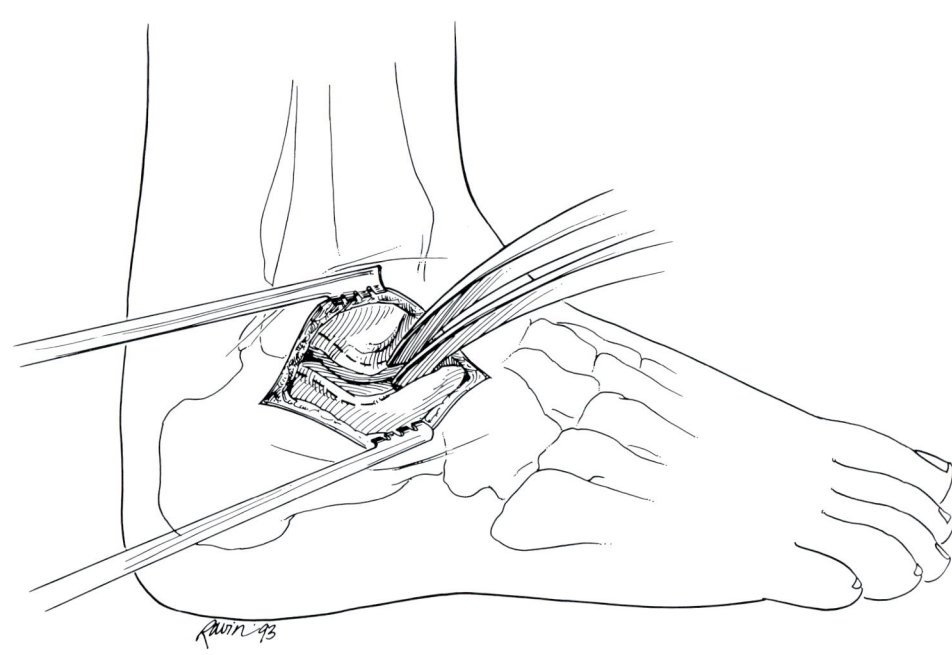

Figure 4. A: A laminar spreader is inserted in the sinus tarsi. **B:** The positioning of the laminar spreader and the planned line of joint removal.

Retraction of the peroneal tendons posteriorly allows excellent exposure of the posterior subtalar joint.

The joint capsule of the talocalcaneal joint is incised and a lamina spreader is inserted into the sinus tarsi to expose the entire articulation of the subtalar region (Fig. 4).

With an osteotome articular cartilage and subchondral bone of the subtalar joint is excised (Fig. 5). Care should be taken to insure excision of articular cartilage from the anterior, middle, and posterior facets. The location and relative position of these facets are easily identified through this exposure (Fig. 6).

All nonarticular surfaces of the sinus tarsi are also decorticated with an osteotome.

While holding the ankle in neutral dorsiflexion/plantar flexion and the calcaneus in neutral varus-valgus, a smooth Steinmann pin is inserted for varus-valgus fixation (Fig. 7). The pin is inserted medial to the anterior tibial tendon from the neck of the talus into the calcaneus. It is important that the Steinmann pin be inserted through the neck of the talus while the ankle is in dorsiflexion. If the fixation pin

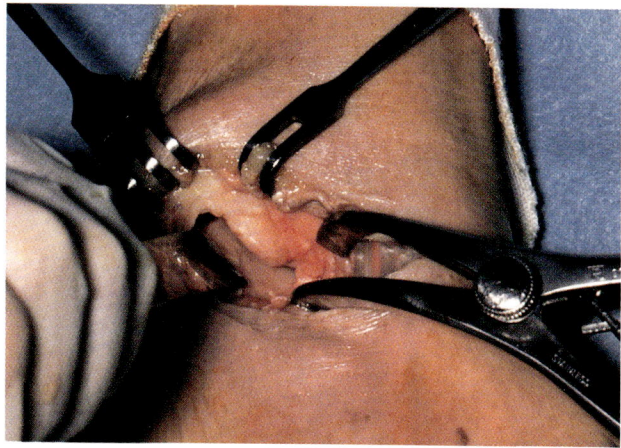

Figure 5. Articular cartilage and subchondral bone is excised from the subtalar region with an osteotome.

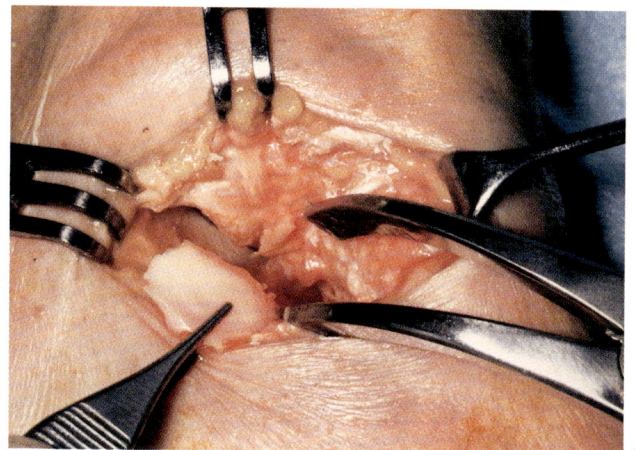

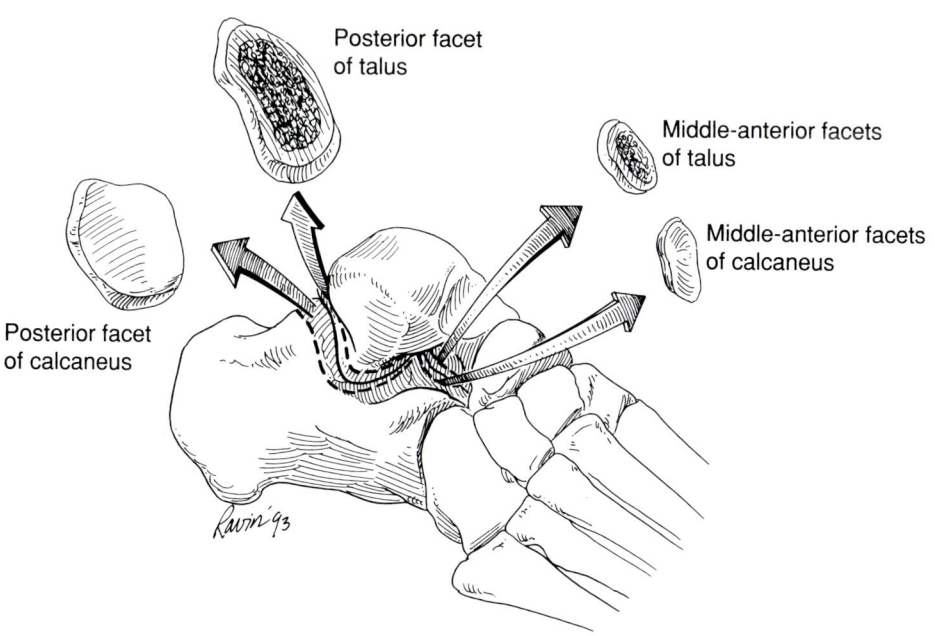

Figure 6. A: Excision of a portion of the articular surface of the posterior facet. **B:** Schematic diagram of the relative size of the facets that are removed from the subtalar region, posterior, middle, and anterior.

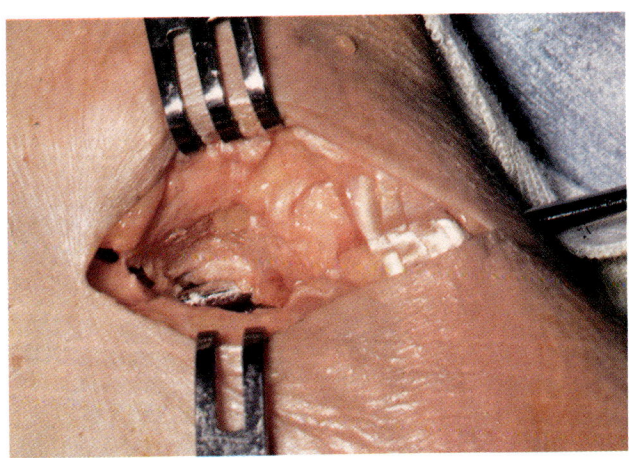

Figure 7. Fixation is obtained by use of a smooth Steinmann pin inserted from the neck of the talus into the calcaneus through the interval between the tibialis anterior and extensor hallucis longus.

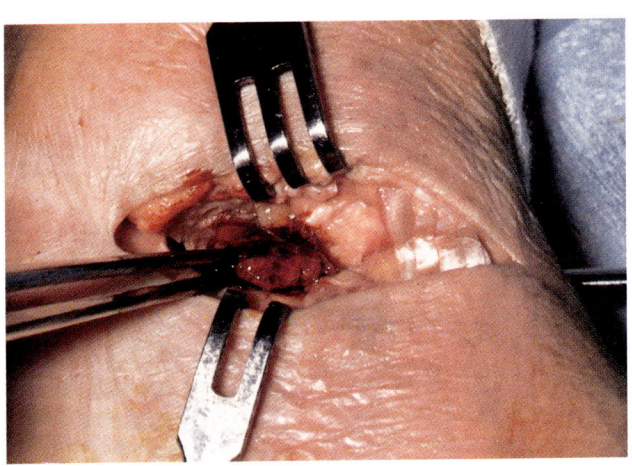

Figure 8. The arthrodesis sites are packed with the autogenous iliac crest bone graft.

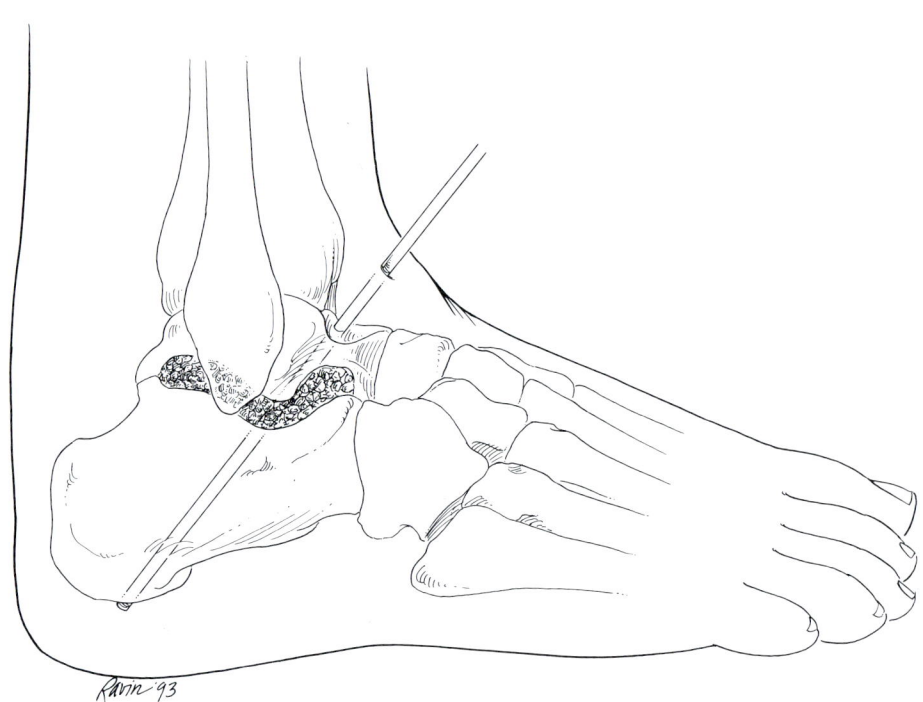

Figure 9. The position of the bone graft in the resected subtalar joint is seen. A ridge of bone in the posterior medial aspect of the joint will prevent extrusion of the bone graft in the medial aspect of the foot in an undesired location about the neurovascular structures.

is inserted with the ankle in plantar flexion and is located too close to the anterior margin of the tibia, it will have the effect of blocking dorsiflexion. This can lead to a later plantar flexion deformity of the ankle and prolonged period of recuperation. The Steinmann pin is inserted through the neck of the talus and then is visualized as it goes through the sinus tarsi region into the calcaneus. The bulge of the pin under the skin of the heel region is then felt and the pin is retracted back about 2 cm. This makes the use of an intraoperative radiography unnecessary. When cutting the pin off beneath the skin, again the ankle should be placed in dorsiflexion. If the ankle is in plantar flexion and the pin is cut off it will make removal of the pin at a later time difficult since it will be quite far below the level of the skin.

Curvilinear incision is made over the anterior iliac crest. This is done on the same side as the foot being treated with subtalar arthrodesis. The patient will then have only one operative side, which will be less limiting for postoperative ambulation. Bone graft is removed from the outer aspect of the ilium only. The soft tissues are meticulously removed since any residual fibrous tissue in the arthrodesis site can inhibit healing. This bone graft is then run through a bone mill, breaking the bone into pieces from 2 to 5 mm in diameter. Cancellous graft is harvested for transfer to the recipient area of the subtalar joint. The iliac crest wound is closed over a suction drain after Gelfoam impregnated with thrombin is inserted into wound. The arthrodesis site is packed with the autogenous bone graft (Fig. 8).

The flap of the extensor digitorum brevis muscle is reapproximated with interrupted figure-of-eight 2-0 Vicryl sutures. Subcutaneous tissue is reapproximated with interrupted simple 3-0 Vicryl sutures. Skin is closed with interrupted vertical mattress 3-0 nylon sutures. The relative position of the Steinmann pin and bone graft is shown (Fig. 9).

POSTOPERATIVE MANAGEMENT

A soft compression dressing is applied for the first 48 hours after surgery. At that point the dressing is removed, the wound examined, and a well-padded, short leg cast is applied. The cast is changed and the sutures are removed at 3 weeks after the surgery.

During the first 6 weeks postoperatively, patients are kept on crutches non–weight bearing. At 6 weeks the pin is removed under local anesthetic and a short leg walking cast is applied. The patient is allowed to bear weight in the cast as tolerated for the second 6-week period. At 12 weeks after surgery the short leg walking cast is removed.

A slow gradual return to weight-bearing activities is permitted. Generally, patients begin with crutches partial weight bearing and then progress to crutches full weight bearing. Once the patient is comfortable, a cane may be utilized in the opposite hand. Generally, patients require a soft rubber-sole wedgie shoe with a soft flexible arch support to decrease the impact loading on the foot during the stance phase of gait. Gentle progressive range of motion exercises are included in the postoperative regimen.

Using this technique Russotti et al. (2) reported 90% of the patients were satisfied with their relief of pain symptoms. Only one of 45 arthrodeses went on to nonunion, and that was in a patient with severe rheumatoid arthritis and bone loss. This surgical technique provides consistent arthrodesis and associated relief of pain symptoms.

COMPLICATIONS

Complications of a subtalar arthrodesis can occur. If excessive bone is removed from the both the medial and lateral aspects of the subtalar joint, collapse of the hindfoot and shortening may occur. This is prevented by being careful not to remove the cortical struts from the medial aspect of the subtalar joint, and by bone grafting sufficiently to maintain the hindfoot height.

Improper positioning of the subtalar joint can lead to later difficulties in ambulation. If a hindfoot valgus position is obtained, the patient may complain of pain in the arch region. The opposite deformity of a hindfoot varus can lead to significant lateral margin foot pain. Resecting enough bone in the subtalar joint to provide some medial hindfoot varus-valgus mobility, followed by fixation of the hindfoot in the desired position of about 7° to 10° of valgus, will prevent the complication of improper positioning.

As with any arthrodesis procedure, nonunion can occur. With this particular technique, however, nonunion is very unusual. The surface area of exposed bleeding bone in the subtalar joint is quite large. Utilizing the patient's own iliac crest bone for grafting enhances the success of the union. A period of adequate immobilization is also necessary to allow the arthrodesis to progress satisfactorily.

If excessive bone is placed into the subtalar joint region it may extrude out beneath the subfibular area and give later pain. Such a complication is avoided by placing the graft carefully so that it does not protrude beyond the lateral margin of the subtalar joints.

ILLUSTRATED CASE FOR TECHNIQUE

This patient is a 27-year-old man who presented with a history of problems related to the left hindfoot after injury. He was driving a truck when it turned over. His foot was caught in the forepart of the cab and then twisted. The patient developed pain and swelling at the lateral aspect of the hindfoot and was seen in the emergency room. A diagnosis of sprain was made and the patient was treated with external immobilization and non–weight bearing.

Unfortunately the patient noted persistent pain at the dorsolateral aspect of the hindfoot that increased with weight bearing and ambulation. Pain was associated with swelling and a limp.

Physical examination revealed tenderness in the sinus tarsi and pain and crepitus with subtalar motion.

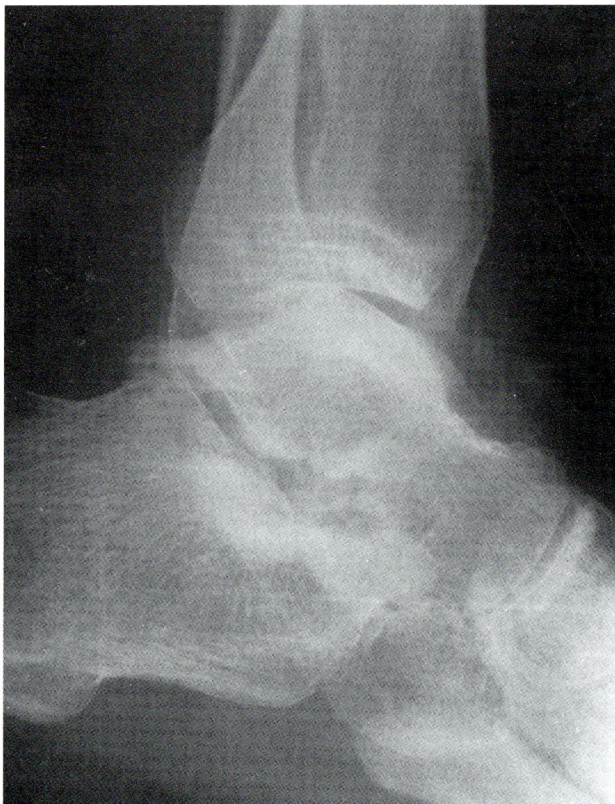

Figure 10. Preoperative lateral radiograph showing the arthritis of the subtalar joint.

Radiographs revealed arthrosis of the subtalar joint (Fig. 10). CT scans in the coronal plane showed articular incongruity that was most pronounced in the region of the middle facet (Fig. 11). A diagnosis of traumatic arthritis in the subtalar joint was made. Initial treatment included the use of a UCBL hindfoot orthosis to eliminate motion in the subtalar joint. This provided partial relief.

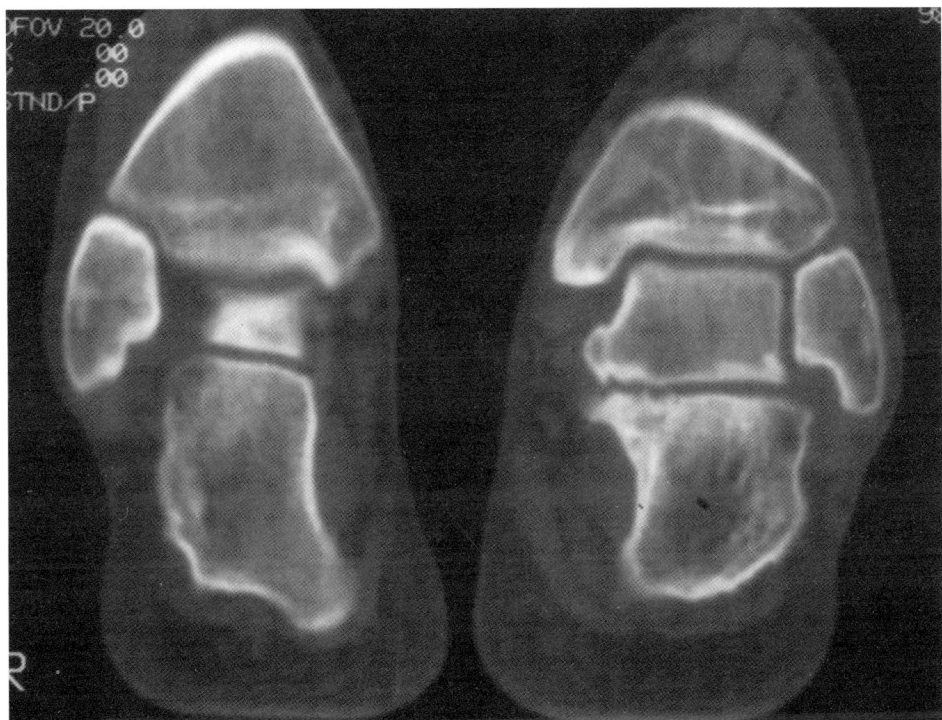

Figure 11. Preoperative CT scan shows the degeneration located primarily in the region of the middle facet.

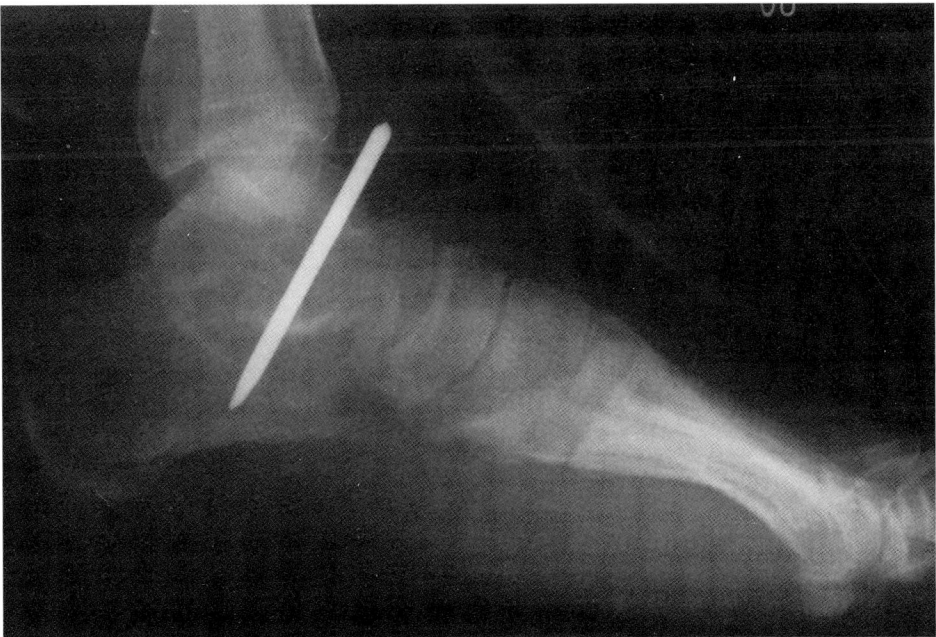

Figure 12. This postoperative radiograph shows the Steinmann pin, which stabilizes the subtalar joint in varus-valgus position. A more oblique insertion of the pin inserting down into the tuberosity of the calcaneus would have been more appropriate.

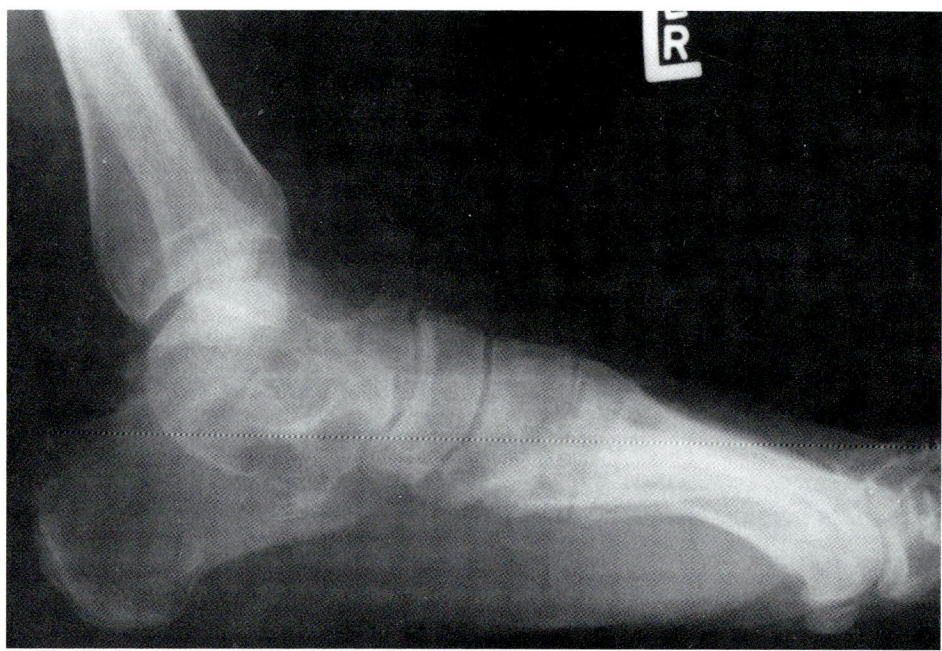

Figure 13. Lateral radiograph shows a solid arthrodesis extending throughout the subtalar region.

After failure of conservative modalities surgical intervention was performed. Subtalar arthrodesis was utilized by means of the technique described in this chapter. Note the use of a smooth Steinmann pin for fixation (Fig. 12). Radiographs at 6 months after surgery reveal solid arthrodesis of the subtalar joint (Fig. 13).

RECOMMENDED READING

1. Russotti, G. M., Johnson, K. A., and Cass, J. R.: Tibiocalcaneal arthrodesis, a salvage procedure. *J. Bone Joint Surg.*, 69A(9): 1304–1307, 1988.
2. Russotti, G. M., Johnson, K. A., and Cass, J. R.: Isolated talocalcaneal arthrodesis, a moldable bone graft technique. *J. Bone Joint Surg.*, 70A(10): 1472–1478, 1988.
3. Shereff, M. J.: Isolated subtalar arthrodesis. In: *Atlas of Foot and Ankle Surgery*. Philadelphia: W. B. Saunders, in press.

30

Talus-Calcaneus-Cuboid (Triple) Arthrodesis

James A. Amis

INDICATIONS/CONTRAINDICATIONS

A triple arthrodesis is the fusion of the subtalar, calcaneocuboid, and talonavicular joints. In general, this demanding procedure is only indicated when conservative measures have failed.

The majority of indications for a triple arthrodesis fall into the following three broad categories: (a) correction of a fixed hindfoot deformity, such as that resulting from a posterior tibialis tendon rupture and an acquired flat foot; (b) arthritis, most commonly rheumatoid arthritis or osteoarthritis; and (c) control of progressive hindfoot deformities such as Charcot-Marie-Tooth or the imbalances following a cerebrovascular accident. Additionally, more specific indications for triple arthrodesis include posttraumatic osteoarthritis subsequent to a calcaneus or talus fracture, painful flexible flatfoot, and tarsal coalition.

Contraindications for a triple arthrodesis include the cases when a more appropriate procedure would suffice. Examples include a tendon transfer for correction of a hindfoot deforming process or a single joint arthrodesis such as a subtalar arthrodesis when a transverse tarsal joint need not be included for correction of a particular problem. Another contraindication is vascular disease, especially in elderly patients and diabetics. When vascular insufficiency is suspected, an adequate workup with noninvasive vascular studies is requisite.

PREOPERATIVE PLANNING

It is important that the surgeon determine and discuss with the patient the goals of the triple arthrodesis that may be considered as a solution of the problem.

J. A. Amis, M.D.: Department of Orthopaedics, University of Cincinnati Medical College, Cincinnati, OH 45220.

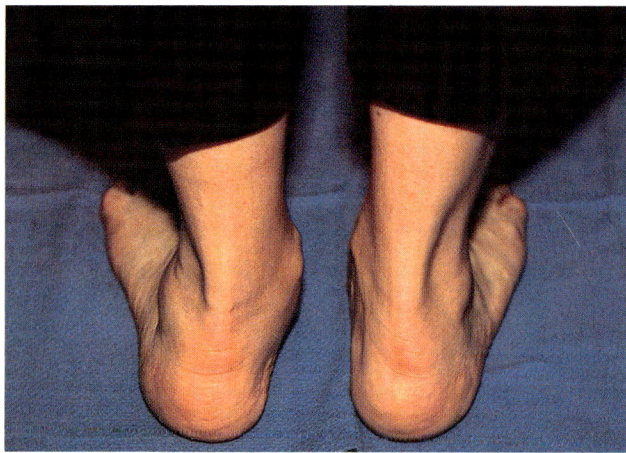

Figure 1. Severe hindfoot valgus is noted on the left foot. Also note the abduction of the forefoot producing "too many toes" sign.

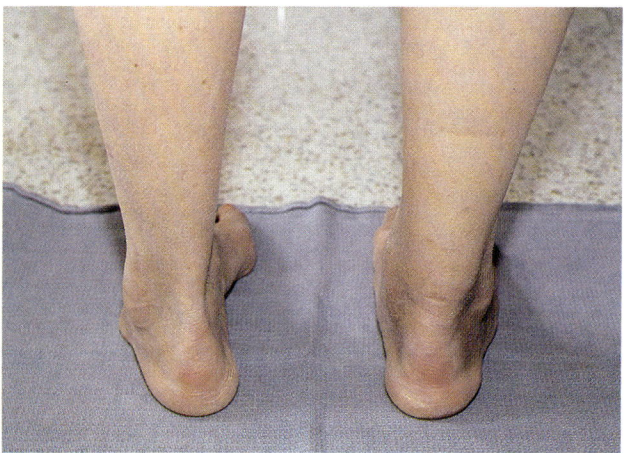

Figure 2. Hindfoot varus as a component of a cavus type deformity, left foot.

These goals might include correcting a deformity, stabilizing a deforming force, reducing pain, or a combination therein depending on the patient's problem. It is critical that the surgeon discuss the severity of this surgery, the lengthy recovery, and the potential complications that can occur as a result. I make it clear to my patients that even when all goes well and no complications have occurred, the recovery can be very difficult and lengthy. The patient's expectations must be realistic and tempered for the long recovery or they may be unsatisfied even if, in the surgeon's eye, a satisfactory result has been obtained.

The history obtained should be specific for the diagnosis for which a triple arthrodesis is being considered. On proceeding to physical examination it is important to observe the patient in a standing position both anteriorly and posteriorly. Look for any deformity, such as hindfoot varus or valgus (Figs. 1 and 2). A varus hindfoot will usually have a compensatory forefoot valgus with a plantar flexed first ray. Hammertoes may also be present. This cavus type of foot would be consistent with a Charcot-Marie-Tooth disorder.

A valgus hindfoot will usually be associated with a varus forefoot deformity to compensate (Fig. 3), along with an abducted forefoot via the hindfoot joints. Quite often there is an Achilles tendon contracture with this pronated deformity of the foot. Presence of an Achilles contracture can best be tested by placing the hindfoot into the maximal varus position, locking the subtalar joint, and then attempting dorsiflexion. This maneuver may be difficult if the hindfoot deformity is fixed in a pronated position, thereby preventing placement of the hindfoot in varus.

Observing the patient's gait may reveal such problems as the substitution of the long extensors of the toes with dynamic hammertoe formation in the cavus type of foot. In the acquired flatfoot there may be an accentuation of midfoot collapse at midstance just prior to heel raise.

Once the deformity is identified, the flexibility of the hindfoot is tested. If the foot can be reduced to a satisfactory position then an in situ type of arthrodesis may be considered. If the hindfoot deformity is fixed and cannot be brought back to a satisfactory position, a corrective type of triple arthrodesis will be necessary.

As a routine, I use standing anteroposterior (AP) radiographs of both ankles including a major portion of the distal tibias. This is done with a relaxed stance and with the patient evenly weight bearing on both sides. These views can help

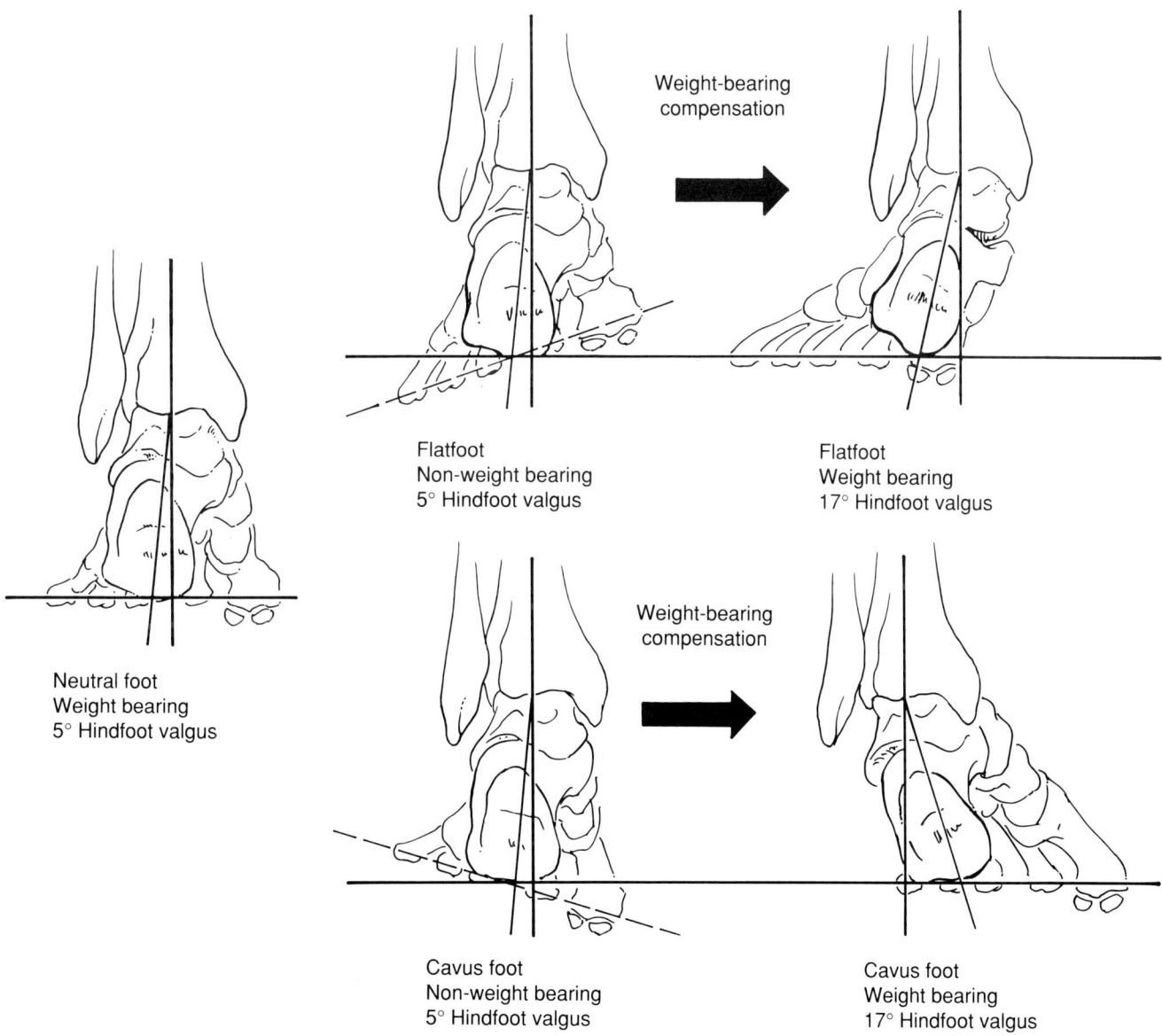

Figure 3. Generally the hindfoot and forefoot are linked and one will compensate for the other. For example, the "flatfoot" with its hindfoot valgus attains a plantar grade position by a compensatory forefoot varus.

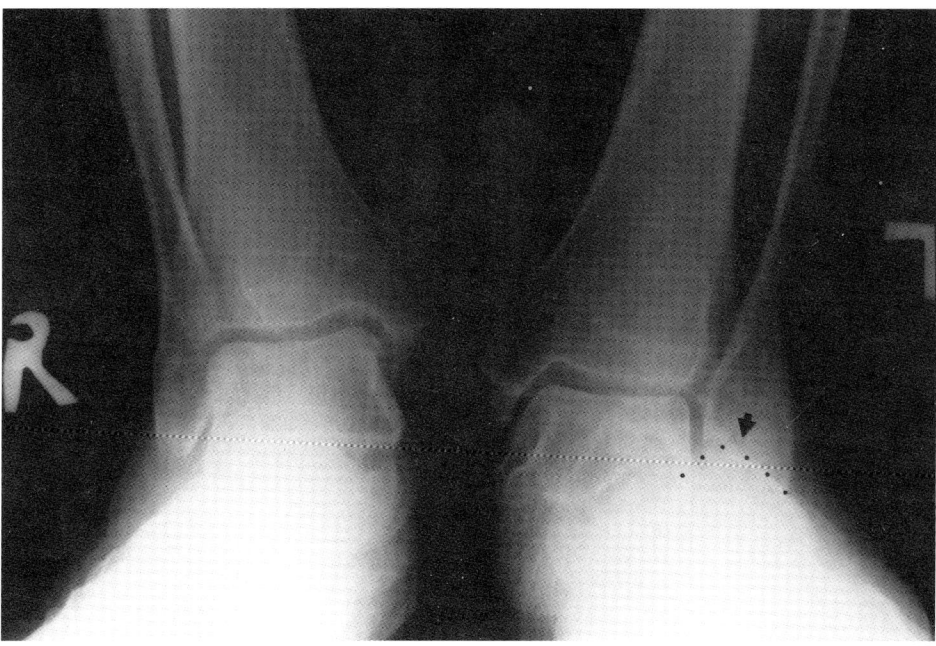

Figure 4. Standing bilateral ankle anteroposterior (AP) radiographs are an essential part of the workup. The left hindfoot demonstrates calcaneofibular impingement *(black arrow)* compared to the normal right. The *black dots* demonstrate the outline of the calcaneal tuberosity.

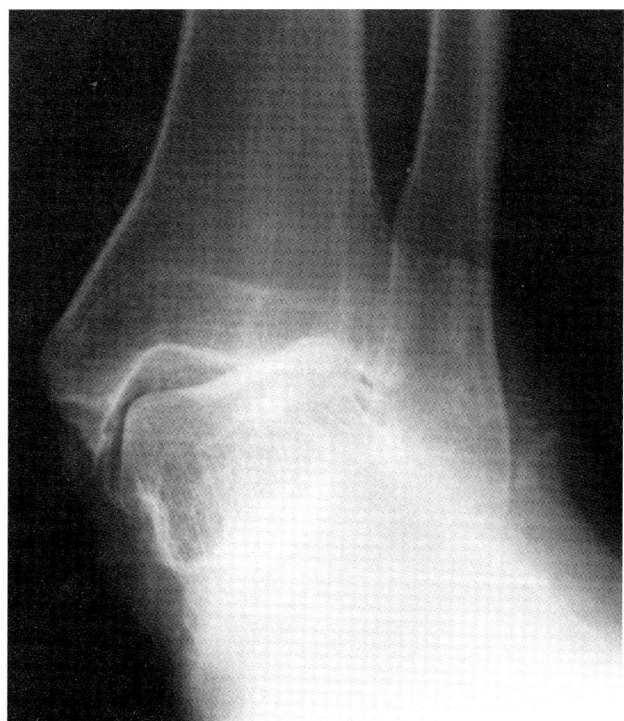

Figure 5. Ankle valgus as shown may produce all or part of the "flatfoot" deformity noted clinically. Standing AP ankle radiographs again should be part of the routine workup.

detect certain amounts of calcaneofibular impingement in the acquired flatfoot (Fig. 4) as well as any varus or valgus deformities at the ankle joint (Fig. 5). These findings do occur from time to time either secondary to the prolonged hindfoot deformity or as a primary ankle deformity with a compensatory hindfoot deformity.

Most importantly this view shows the axis of the tibia as it relates to the ground or what I call the "tibial mechanical axis." This tibial mechanical axis will make a major impact on how much forefoot correction is needed. For example, if a patient has physiologic genu varum with a tibia that has a varus tibial mechanical axis, then an appropriate or compensatory increase in forefoot valgus must be obtained at the time of surgery (Fig. 6). This tibial alignment to the ground is not to be confused with the mechanical axis that has been popularized in total knee surgical procedures.

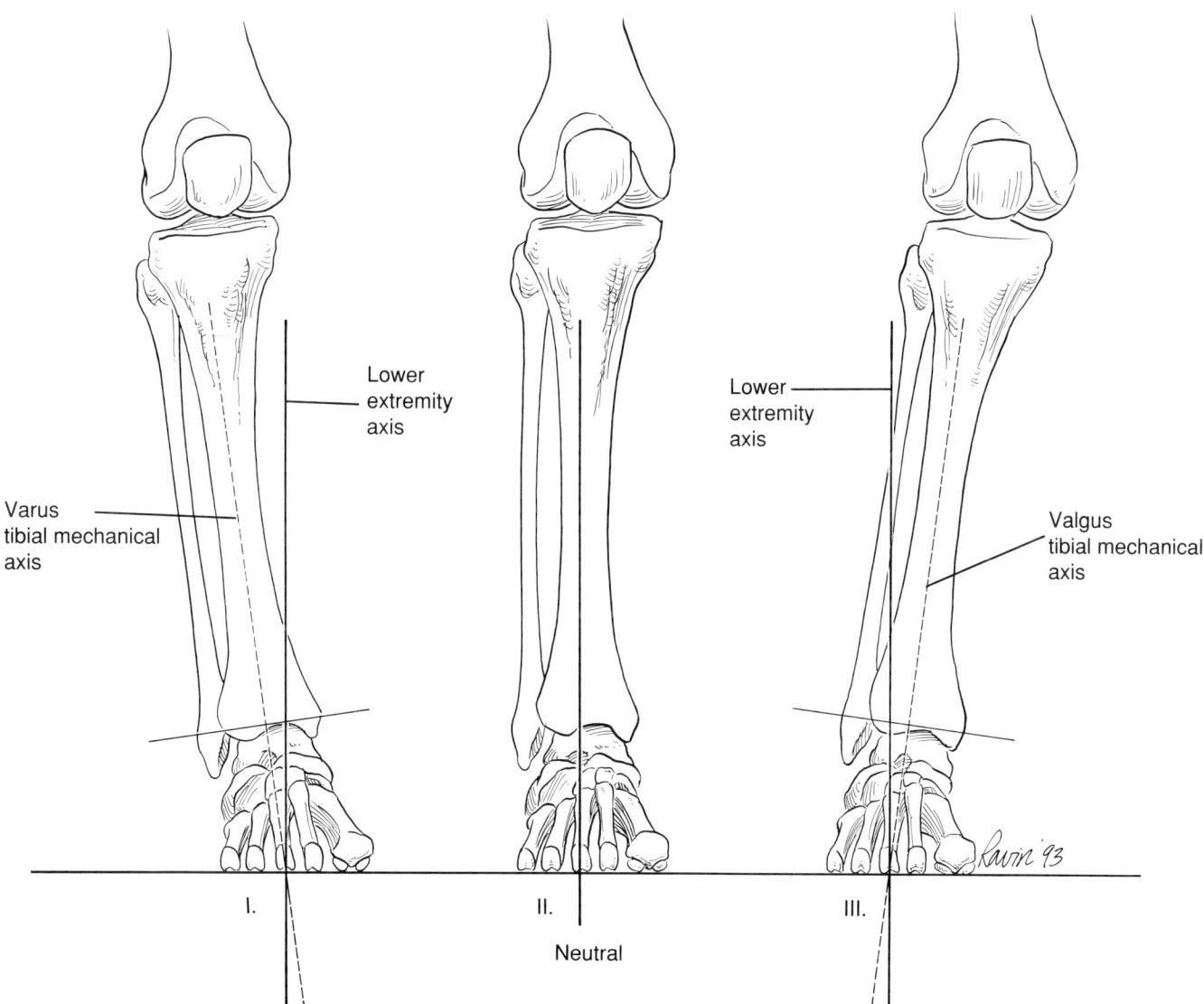

Figure 6. The tibial mechanical axis is demonstrated in its three basic forms: I. Varus tibial mechanical axis; II. Neutral tibial mechanical axis; III, valgus tibial mechanical axis. The position of the forefoot at the time of a triple arthrodesis must take into consideration the angle of the tibial mechanical axis and its relationship with the forefoot axis.

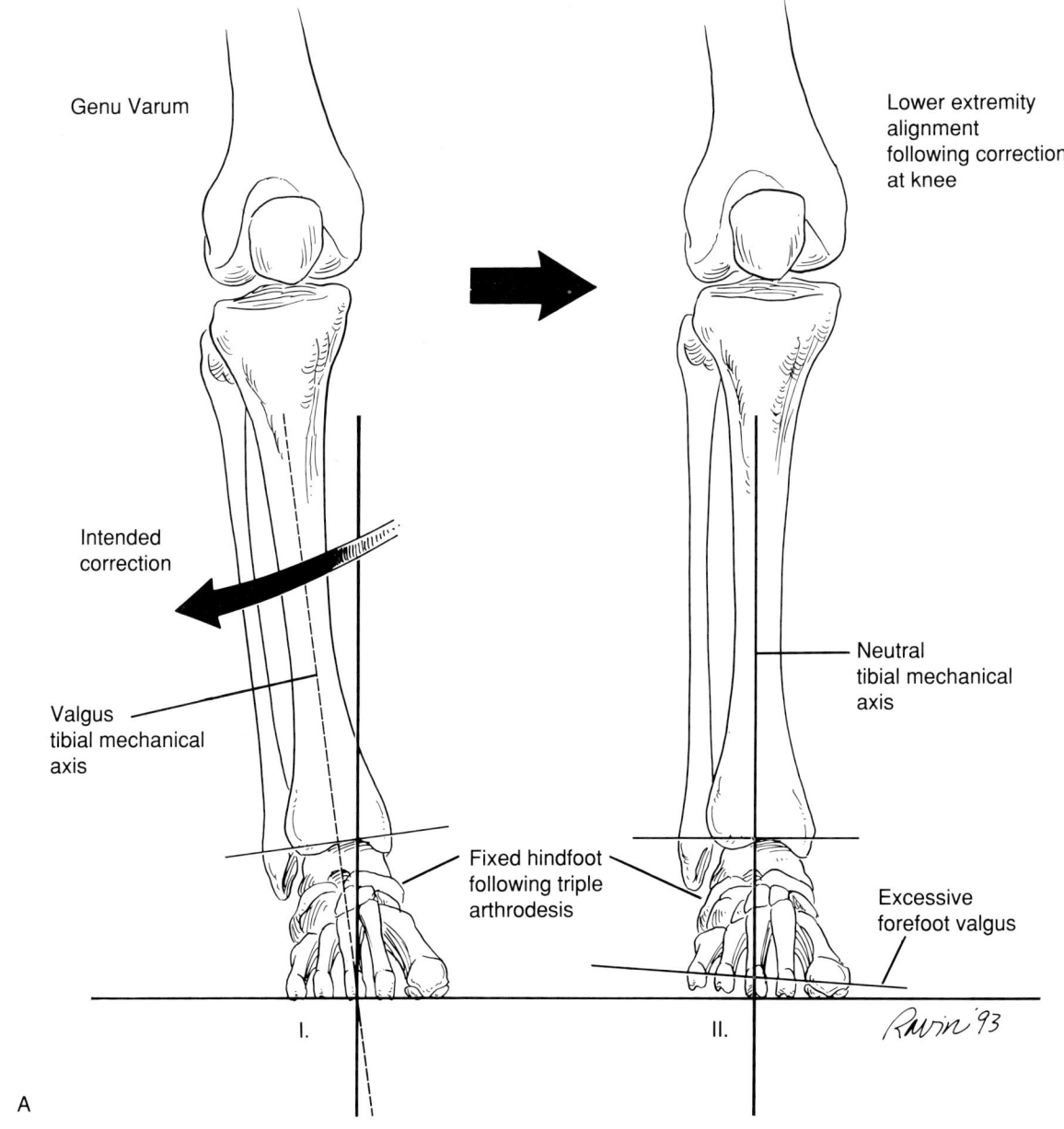

Figure 7. A and **B:** These two diagrams demonstrate the need for knee correction prior to a triple arthrodesis, when both the knee and foot present with concomitant problems that may result in angular correction. A fixed hindfoot will move with correction of the knee, thereby placing the forefoot in a malalignment following knee correction.

It is essential that the patient be viewed either in a gown or shorts during the course of the examination so that the general alignment of the lower extremities can be observed. If any major deformities, especially unilateral deformities of the alignment particularly at the knee are observed, radiographs of the knee may be needed. Preexisting knee deformities of problems that may ultimately require a corrective surgical procedure [e.g., total knee replacement (TKR), high tibial osteotomy], thereby changing the tibial mechanical axis, must be recognized. Any corrective procedure that changes the angle at which the tibia approaches the ground will have a profound change on a foot that has had a triple arthrodesis and therefore a fixed *noncompensatory hindfoot* (Fig. 7A).

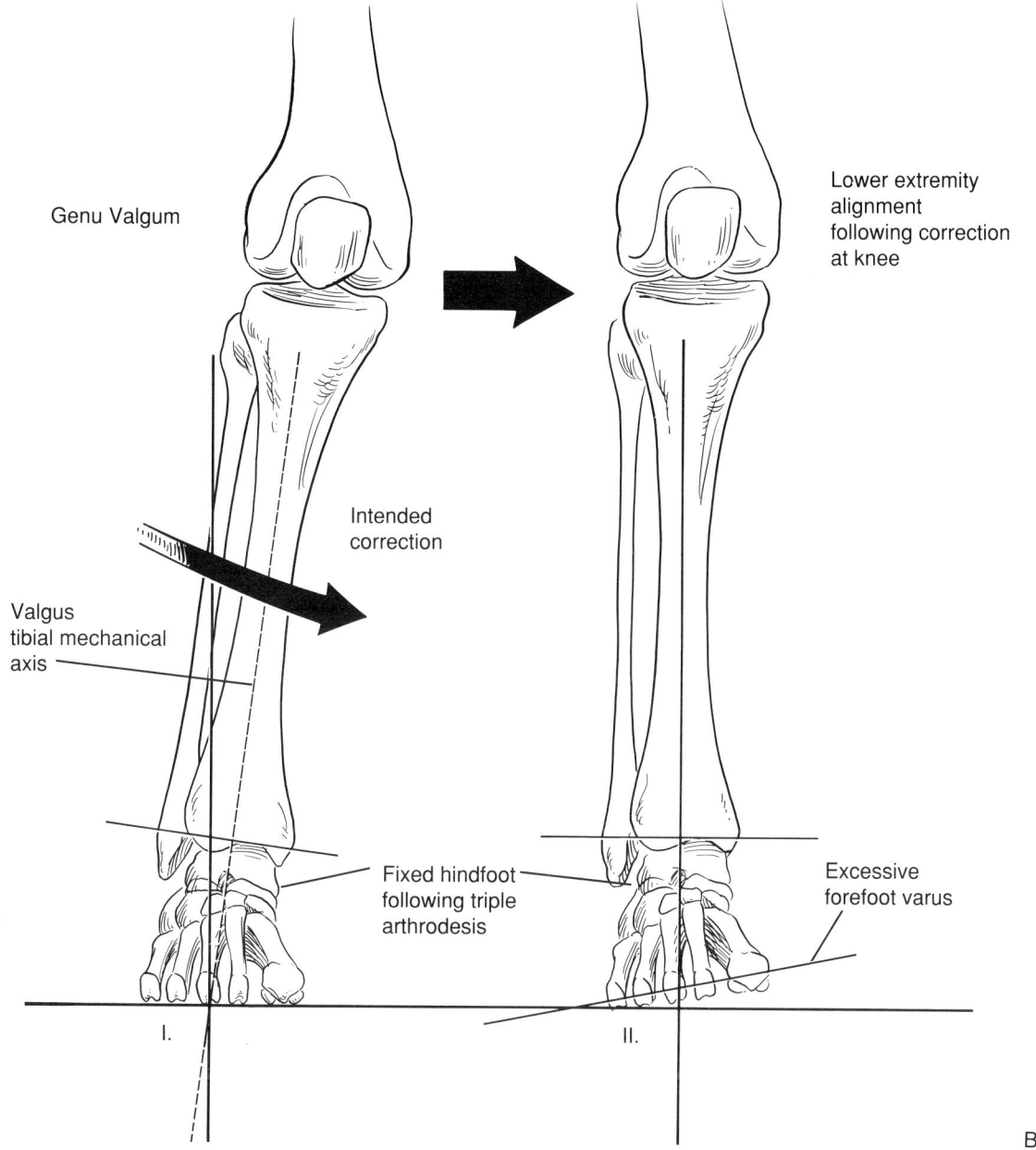

Figure 7. *Continued.*

It is generally recommended that if a knee replacement or corrective surgery at the knee is contemplated, it should be done prior to any major hindfoot corrective surgery so that this critical combined knee and foot alignment can be matched. For example, if a patient has a genu varum with a tibia approaching the ground in a few degrees of varus, this patient must be placed in more forefoot valgus at the time of a triple arthrodesis. Suppose now the patient with the same genu varum and a post–triple arthrodesis plantar grade foot has either a high tibial osteotomy or a knee replacement that corrects this genu varum deformity and brings the tibia into a more direct perpendicular alignment and will contact the ground on the medial column or first metatarsal on the forefoot excessively. The reverse of this situation holds true as well (Fig. 7B).

Standing foot radiographs must be obtained. In the pronated or acquired flatfoot, the AP (Fig. 8) and lateral talocalcaneal angles (Fig. 9) will be noted to diverge, while in the more cavus foot these angles tend to be parallel or converge.

A computed tomography (CT) scan, a bone scan, and magnetic resonance imaging (MRI) may be necessary as well. A bone scan may be particularly helpful when determining exactly what joints are involved. We use a standardized process, displaying eight views of the foot at 1.5× magnification thereby obtaining high detail of the foot and ankle.

Selective injections are very useful diagnostically and may be necessary to determine the exact joints involved and their role in the patient's pain process. A long-acting local anesthetic should be used such as mepivacaine (Carbocaine) or; bupivacaine (Marcaine).

Quite often other procedures are necessary in conjunction with a triple arthrodesis for adequate results and these must be identified and discussed with the patient preoperatively. The two most common procedures that are performed concomitantly include an iliac crest bone graft harvesting and an Achilles tendon lengthening, especially in patients with acquired flat foot deformities. I cannot emphasize enough that iliac crest bone graft is a useful and often necessary adjunct to the triple arthrodesis and should be employed without hestitation.

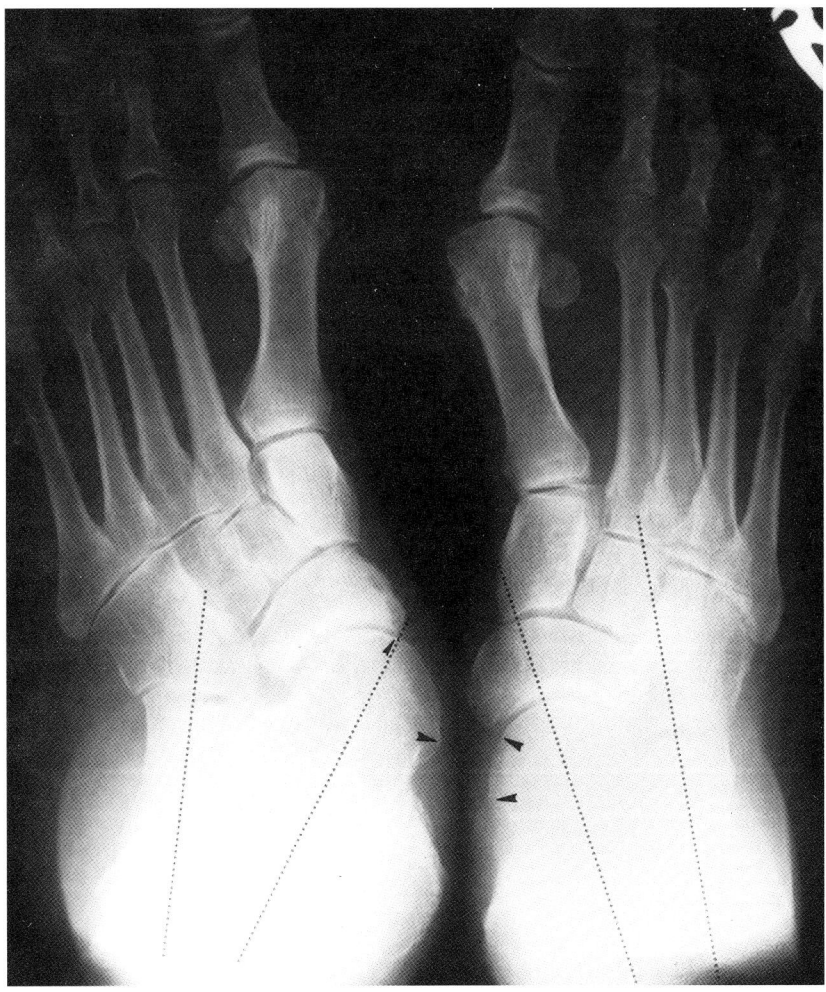

Figure 8. Standing foot radiographs may reveal talocalcaneal divergence *(dotted lines)* as shown on the left foot. Also note the talar head "uncovering" *(arrows)*.

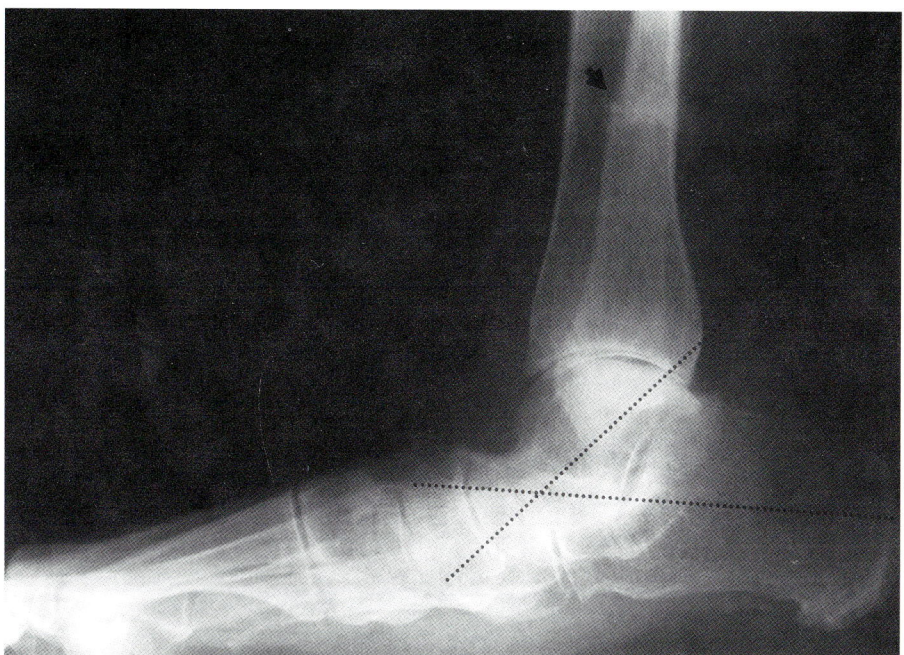

Figure 9. Standing lateral foot radiographs show divergence of the lateral talocalcaneal angle *(dotted lines)*. Note the "sag" of the foot at the talonavicular joint. There is also a stress fracture of the fibula *(arrow)* as a result of prolonged lateral impingement.

The long duration and difficulty of recovery from a triple arthrodesis must be actively stressed to each and every patient. The patient should be counseled on preparing his or her family and home for the postoperative period so that transition from the hospital will be as smooth as possible. One final note is that patients will quite often try to compare a triple arthrodesis with other standard procedures such as a spine procedure or a total joint replacement. I make it very clear to them that those procedures are typically quicker in recovery and much easier to tolerate. A satisfactory result will only arise out of realistic expectations.

SURGERY

The surgeon must first determine whether an in situ or corrective triple arthrodesis is to be performed. Any additional procedures required, such as iliac crest bone graft or Achilles tendon lengthening must be determined. In principle, an in situ and a corrective triple arthrodesis are the same with the exception of the preparation of the joints and the degree of correction desired.

An in situ triple arthrodesis implies that the foot can be placed in the proper position preoperatively and no aggressive correction is necessary. Preparation of the joint requires that the peripheral aspect of it be maintained while the central portion of the joint is debrided in order to allow for the fusion process (Fig. 10). The depth of debridement must be through the subchondral plate into healthy cancellous bone (Fig. 11). This is usually done with a 4 mm round bone cutting bur on a high-speed drill. During the burring process the operative field is completely submerged in a constant flow of cooled normal saline to prevent burning from the heat generated by the bur tip. Once the joints are definitively fixed, iliac crest bone graft is firmly tamped within the debrided area of the joint, thereby providing an expansive force to further increase stability as well as to facilitate the fusion process. The more involved corrective triple arthrodesis is described in the Technique section.

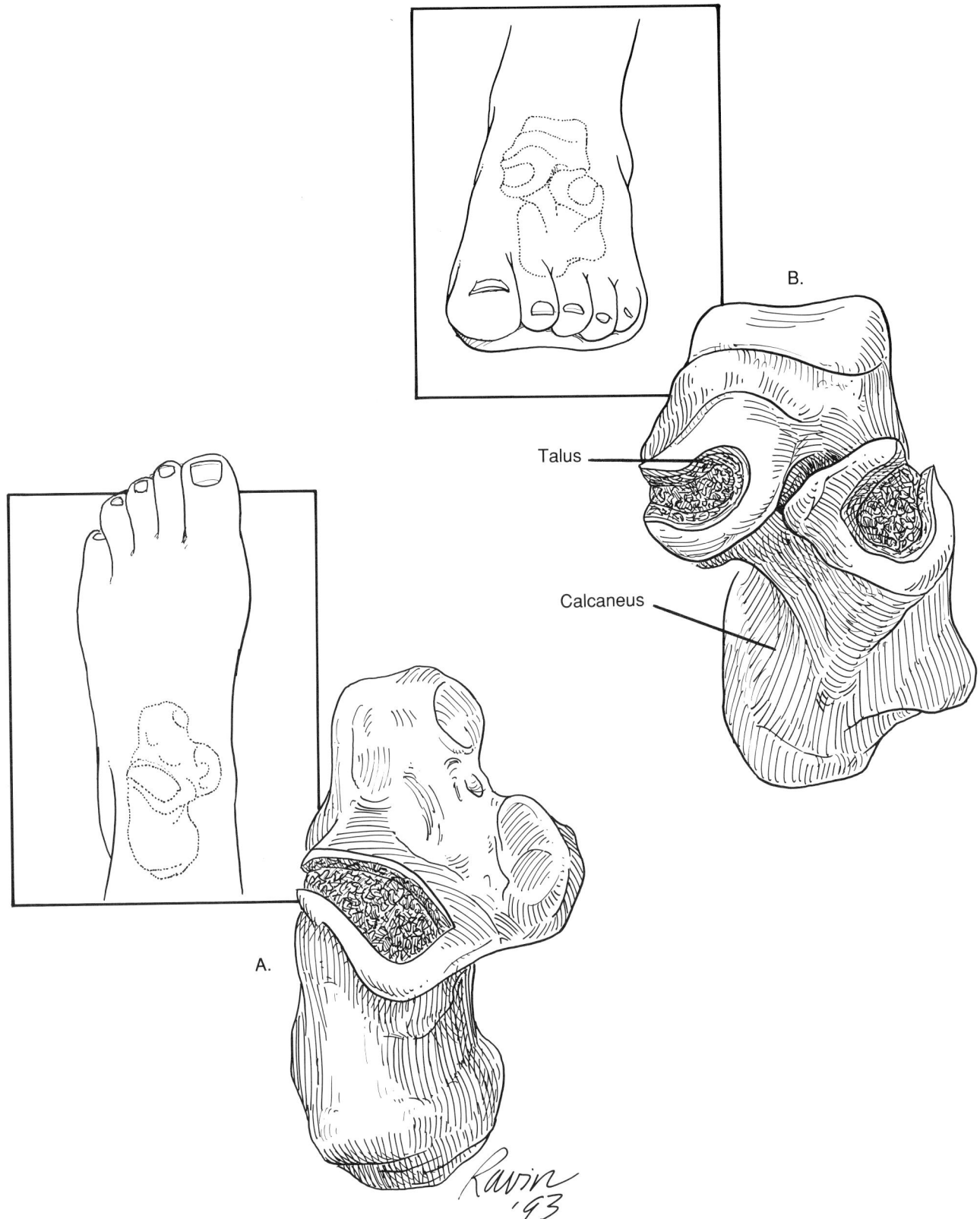

Figure 10. Surface areas of central joint debridement in situ of the calcaneus (dorsal view) **(A)** and the talonavicular, calcaneocuboid, and subtalar joints (frontal view). **(B)**. Note the central area of debridement and retained peripheral joint cartilage.

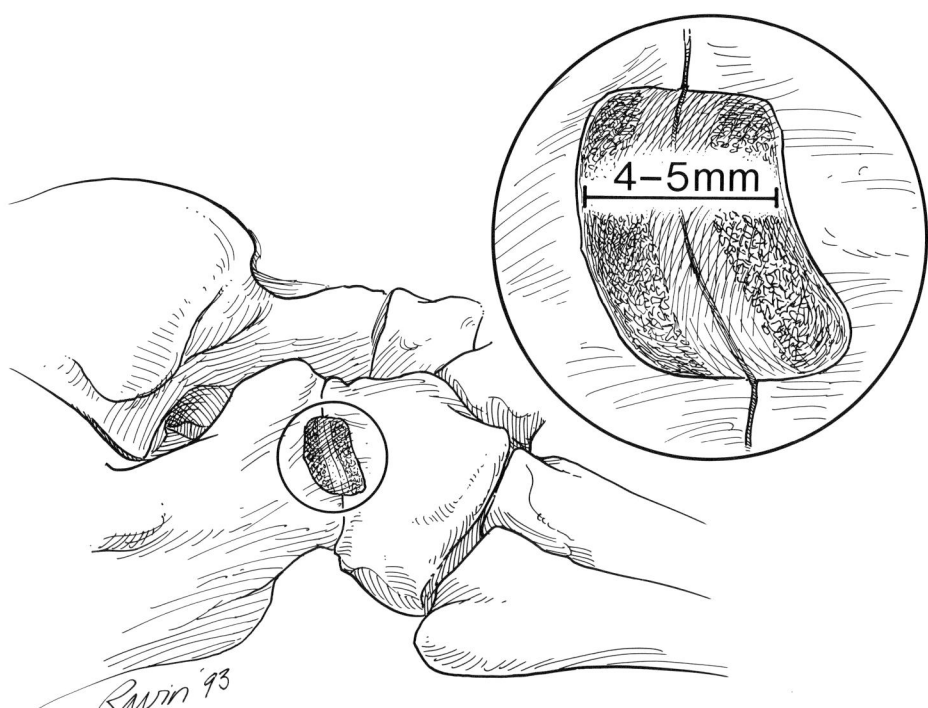

Figure 11. This central joint debridement must pass through the cartilage and dense subchondral bone to deeper vascular cancellous bone.

Several unique tools are used in conjunction to facilitate a smooth uncomplicated operative procedure:

1. 0.062″ smooth double ended K-wires for provisional fixation.
2. Power wire driver (Hall) (not a drill with a chuck, as this method of placing K-wires is too cumbersome while the correction is temporarily held).
3. Hall micro 100 power set or equivalent.
4. Synthes large fragment 6.5 mm cancellous or equivalent cannulated screws.
5. Staplizer 3M or equivalent barbed bone fixation staples.
6. A 4 to 5 mm round bone cutting bur.
7. High-speed bur (Hall, micro 100 drill or Surg-Airetome Two) or an Ansbach or Midas Rex power.
8. Beanbag positioner.
9. A 6½″ baby Inge lamina spreader.

After the general or spinal anesthetic is administered, the patient is situated on the beanbag positioner in a semilateral debucitus position. The toes must point straight to the ceiling to 20° of internal rotation (Fig. 12). If any external rotation of the foot is allowed on the table, an assistant will be needed to hold the foot in internal rotation for the more demanding lateral exposure of the foot. This positioning also facilitates access to the ipsilateral anterior iliac crest for bone graft harvesting. The external rotation necessary for adequate exposure of the talonavicular joint is easily achieved.

A tourniquet is placed proximally on the thigh, followed by a routine sterile prep and drape to the tourniquet. The leg is exsanguinated using a Martin bandage to the tourniquet, followed by inflation of the tourniquet. The surgeon should be positioned facing lateral to medial. Positioning will be slightly different depending on whether the right or left foot is being done.

Technique. Corrective Triple Arthrodesis. The lateral incision (Fig. 13) is longitudinal and placed on a line drawn connecting the points between the tip of the

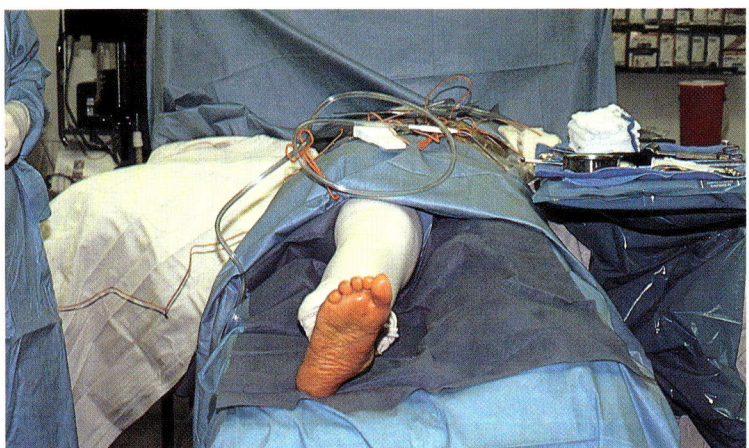

Figure 12. The optimal position of the patient on the beanbag positioner places the foot in internal rotation facilitating the lateral exposure. This also positions the patient for ipsilateral iliac crest harvesting.

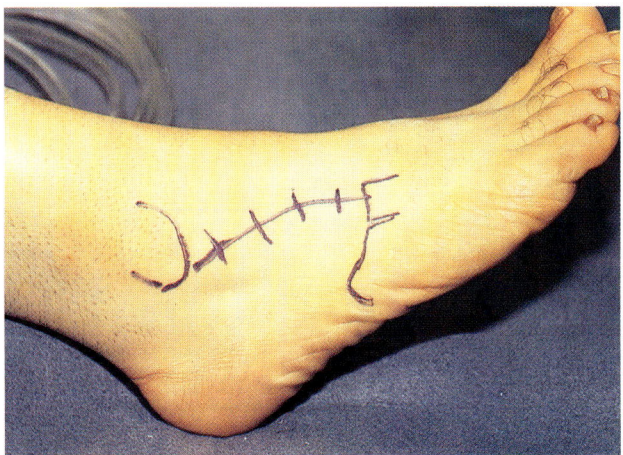

Figure 13. Lateral skin incision.

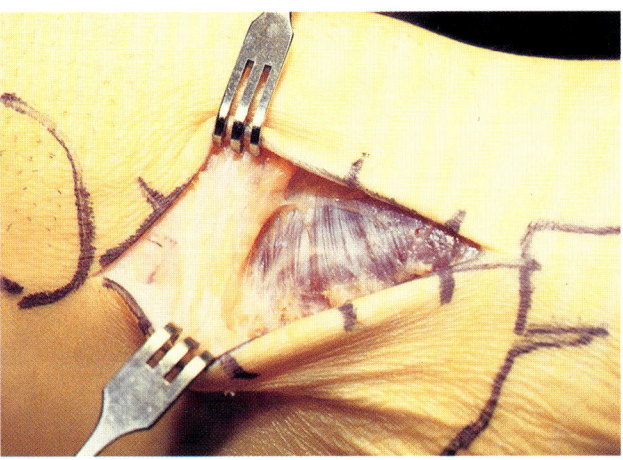

Figure 14. Superficial lateral exposure demonstrates the proximal fat pad over the sinus tarsi and the extensor digitorum brevis and its fascia.

lateral malleolus to the base of the fourth metatarsal. The base of the fourth metatarsal is easily located about 1 inch dorsal and ½ inch distal to the tip of the fifth metatarsal tuberosity. Curving the incision slightly between these two lines, making it convex toward the dorsomedial aspect of the foot, can make the exposure more extensile. This longitudinal approach is favored owing to wider exposure over the more aesthetically pleasing transverse exposure, described by Ollier. Of further disadvantage, the Ollier approach has a much higher risk of damage to the sural and superficial peroneal nerves.

This dorsolateral incision is extended deeply using sharp dissection, except in its most distal portion. In the distal 1 to 2 cm of the incision, a small anterior branch of the sural nerve may course from lateral to medial and must be freed and retracted safely. The fat overlying the sinus tarsi is identified as well as the fascia overlying the extensor digitorum brevis (EDB) muscle belly, which should be preserved (Fig. 14). The dissection is continued over the muscle belly to its plantar lateral and dorsomedial extents. The lateral extent of the EDB is achieved upon identification of the peroneal tendon sheath. The dissection is thus well deep to the sural nerve. The proximal extent of the EDB is noted as it disappears into the sinus tarsi, beneath the fat pad and the inferior extensor retinaculum (Fig. 14). The medial extent of the EDB is followed until the peroneus tertius tendon is identified (Fig. 15). At this point, a knife or cautery is used to cut the sinus tarsi

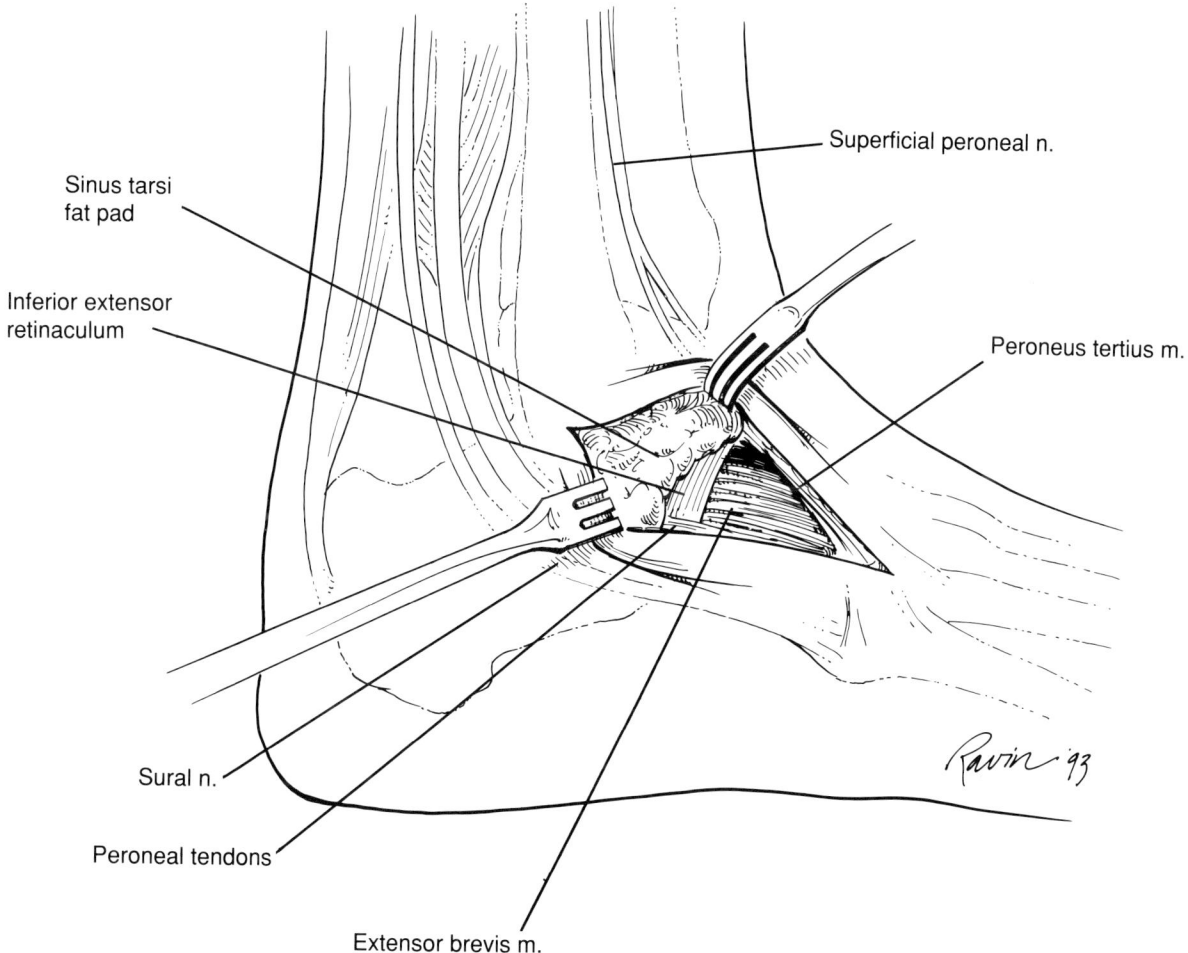

Figure 15. Superficial lateral exposure is bordered by (a) plantar: peroneal tendons; sural nerve, especially distal; (b) dorsal: peroneus tertius tendon; superficial peroneal nerve, lateral branch; (c) proximal: sinus tarsi fat pad; lateral limb of inferior extensor retinaculum; (d) base: extensor brevis fascia and muscle.

fat pad up to the tip of the lateral malleolus in the same line as the skin incision was made (Fig. 16). The surgeon must be careful around the lateral malleolus not to incise too far anterior toward the ankle joint in order to avoid transection of the anterior talofibular ligament. These two corners of the fat pad must be preserved as they will later be used to suture the proximal portion of the extensor digitorum brevis muscle belly for closure. I do not favor removing the so-called oyster or sinus tarsi contents. This fat pad provides excellent vascularized coverage for the sinus tarsi, while closing the dead space.

By this point, the posterior facet of the subtalar joint should have been entered and identified (Fig. 17). The outline of the extensor digitorum brevis muscle is now completed by encircling it at its extents as noted above and raising it up from proximal to distal forming a distally based flap (Fig. 18A). I take the dissection along the plantar border of the EDB while retracting the peroneal tendons out of their tendon sheath plantarly and laterally using them as my lateral guide. The dissection is now taken to the cuboid and distal calcaneus bones through the deep portion of the peroneus sheath. Care must be taken distally, as there is a venous plexus in that region which may necessitate heavy cauterization. I prefer to bring the deeper contents of the sinus tarsi out, keeping them connected to the extensor

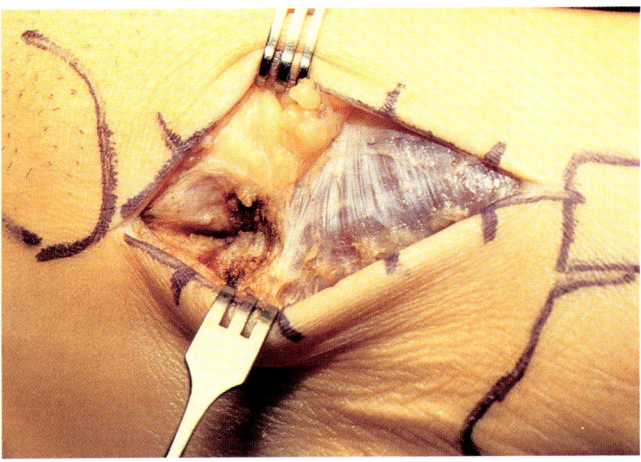

Figure 16. The sinus tarsi fat pad is divided in same line as skin incision up to tip of lateral malleolus. This facilitates both exposure and closure.

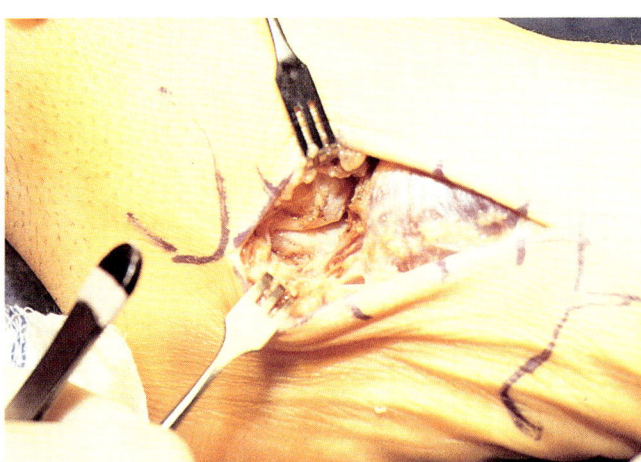

Figure 17. Reflection of the fat pad clearly identifies posterior facet of the subtalar joint.

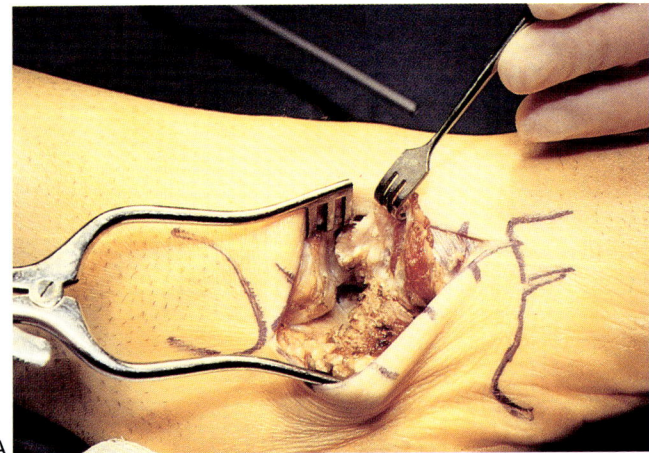
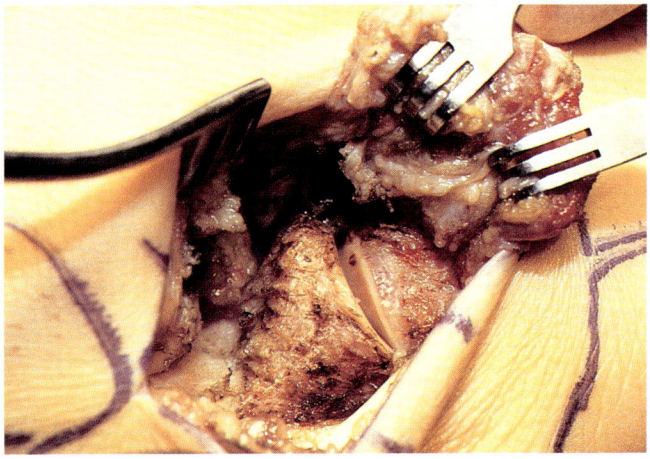

Figure 18. **A** and **B:** Proximal to distal subperiosteal reflection of the extensor digitorum brevis (EDB) creates a distally based flap and exposes the lateral talonavicular and calcaneocuboid joints.

digitorum muscle belly for later closure (Fig. 18A). As the extensor digitorum muscle belly is brought out of the sinus tarsi by subperiosteal dissection using cautery or a sharp knife, it is dissected over the anterior process of the calcaneus as well as the lateral wall of the calcaneus uncovering the calcaneocuboid joint (Fig. 18B). Medially, the dissection is continued in a deeper fashion uncovering the talonavicular joint and its lateral border as well as the dorsum of the calcaneocuboid joint. This dissection, which raises the EDB muscle belly, is taken to the midportion of the cuboid bone in order to facilitate debridement of the calcaneocuboid joint and fixation. In the more medial and dorsal dissection of the extensor digitorum muscle, care must be taken to remain in the subperiosteal space as the neurovascular supply of this muscle enters here, approximately 1.5 cm medial and distal to the anterior process of the calcaneus. Additional exposure of the posterior facet may be obtained by dissection posteriorly, and can be taken along the lateral border of the calcaneus underneath the peroneal tendon sheath, thereby uncovering the lateral portion of the posterior facet.

A sharp osteotome is used to remove the dorsal 7 or 8 mm of the anterior process of the calcaneus (Fig. 19) to facilitate visualization medially as well as the placement of staple fixation later (unless screw fixation of the calcaneocuboid joint is used). The joint capsule that is attached to the lateral neck of the talus must be dissected in a plantar to dorsal direction subperiosteally, moving distally to the corresponding area of the navicular. This is all done from the lateral side. Care must be taken not to go too far dorsally so as to avoid any damage to the blood supply entering through the talar neck. At this point, Homan retractors are inserted from the lateral side at the talonavicular joint to improve lateral visualization (Fig. 20). With the retractors in place and the lateral portion of the talonavicular joint identified, the process of debridement of the laterally exposed joints can be undertaken (Fig. 21).

Some fine points of joint debridement must be made. It is my feeling that the primary failure of fusion of any joint is due to inadequate debridement of the subchondral bone. Osteoarthritic bone has a less vascular, thicker, and harder subchondral base and needs to be debrided more deeply to obtain a healthy cancellous substrate for fusion. Certainly, a softer bone, such as that found in a patient with rheumatoid arthritis, may need relatively less debridement; however, healthy cancellous bone well beyond the subchondral plate is still necessary. The debridement must include all of the joint surfaces on both sides of the joint. Failure to completely debride the joint by leaving peripheral rims of cartilage may result in

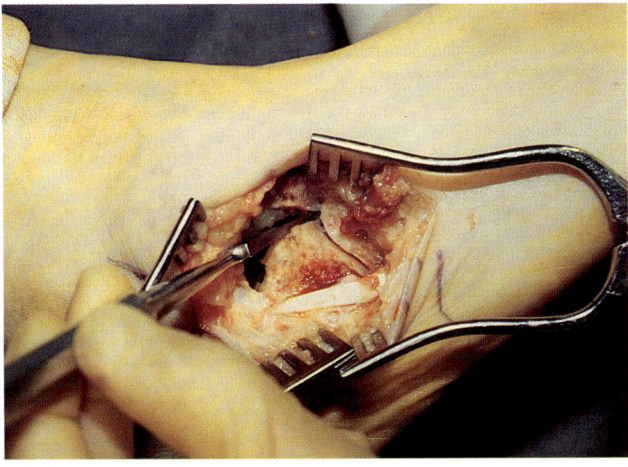

Figure 19. Removal of the dorsal tip of the anterior process is essential for deeper exposure, especially the plantar portion of the talonavicular joint laterally.

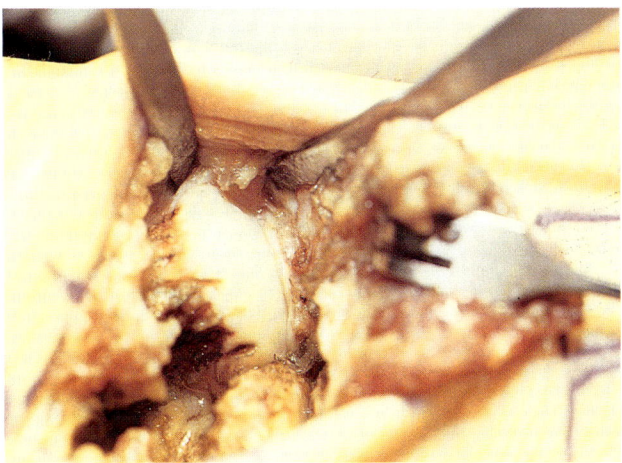

Figure 20. Placement of Homan retractors dorsal over the navicular and talar head.

poor contact of the bone and poor correction. The goal is to obtain anatomically correct surfaces that have been debrided with the same amount of kerf throughout.

The lateral portion of the talonavicular joint is then debrided using a 5-mm round bone cutting bur while cooling with a copious flow of cool normal saline. Because use of saline obscures direct visualization of the operative field, the depth of this blind burring is checked often and necessary adjustments are made. The lateral half of the talonavicular joint is debrided in this manner, which can be facilitated by placing a baby Inge lamina spreader laterally in the talonavicular joint for distraction (Fig. 22). Whenever the lamina spreader is used care must be taken to avoid crushing the bone by excessive distraction. This is especially true in the softer bone such as in a rheumatoid patient. In the talonavicular joint is it important for the surgeon to be aware that the talar head is made of softer bone than the navicular, which creates a path of lesser resistance for the bur. Thus, drifting of the bur into the softer talar bone should be actively avoided, and the navicular side of this joint debrided a bit more aggressively.

Once the lateral portion of the talonavicular joint is debrided, the retractors are removed and the calcaneocuboid joint is debrided in a similar fashion. The lamina spreader can be inserted after the joint is entered dorsolaterally to help facilitate debridement of the deeper portions of the joint (Fig. 23). The calcaneus bone of

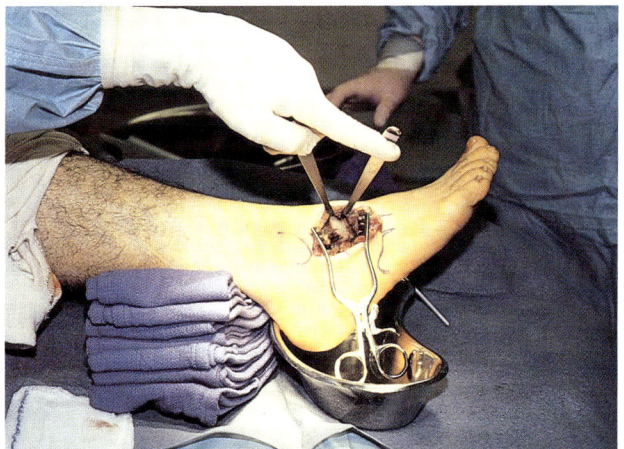

Figure 21. The setup for joint debridement laterally using towel bolster, and emesis basin for heavy flow of normal saline during burring process.

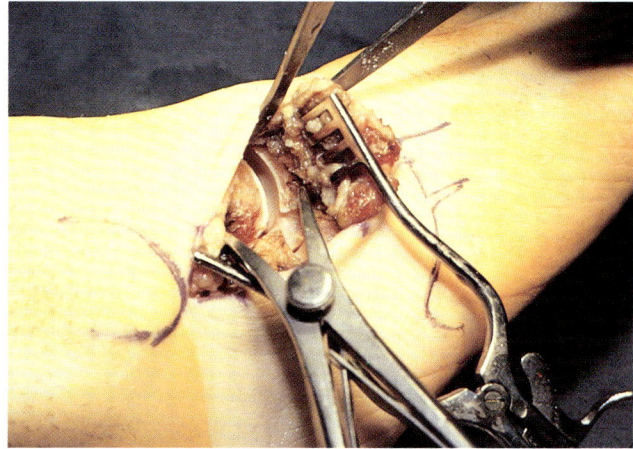

Figure 22. Deeper talonavicular joint resection can only be accomplished by placement of a lamina spreader.

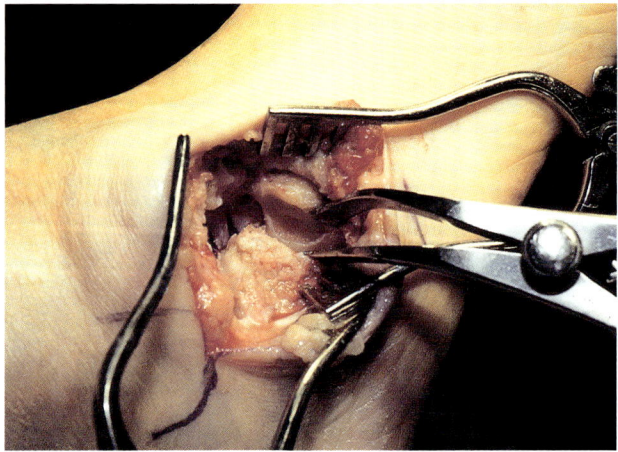

Figure 23. Calcaneocuboid joint resection follows completion of lateral talonavicular resection. Note the use of the lamina spreader.

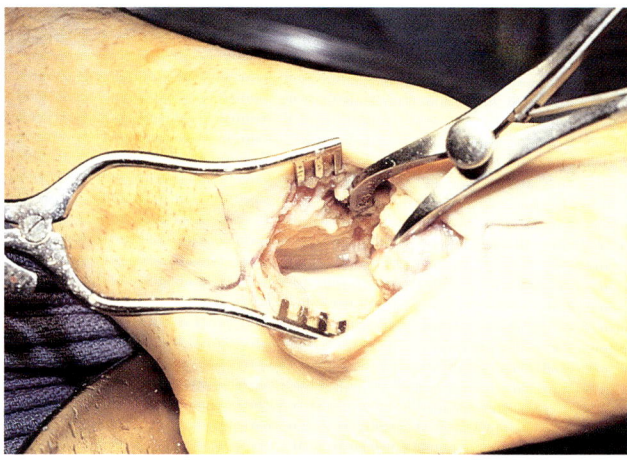

Figure 24. Exposure of the anterior, middle, and posterior facets of the subtalar joints require use of a lamina spreader. Full view of the posterior facet is shown.

this joint is usually the hardest bone, thus particular attention must be paid to the debridement in this area. Both the talonavicular and calcaneocuboid joints have thick rich plantar capsular ligaments and the tendency to plow into the depths of the foot with the bur should be resisted by these ligaments.

Next, the subtalar joint should be debrided. This debridement will include the anterior and medial facets of the subtalar joint, which lie anterior to the interosseous ligament under the talar head, followed by the posterior facet, which lies posterior to the interosseous ligament. It is best to raise the table another 12 to 18 inches, as the surgeon is now positioned near the foot of the table and is facing cephalad. The burring process at this point must be carefully performed to avoid damage therein. Lying very close to the middle facet is the neurovascular bundle. Anterior to the interosseous ligament the softer subchondral bone is on the side of the talar head, while both calcaneal and talar sides of the posterior facet are dense. The posterior facet should be debrided laterally first by placing a Homan retractor around the lateral side of the calcaneus. This retraction will facilitate visualization of the lateral and posterolateral aspect of the posterior facet. Both sides of the joint are debrided while a lamina spreader is placed under the neck of the talus (Fig. 24). The entire posterior facet should be debrided.

Once the lateral and posterolateral centimeter or so of the posterior facet is adequately debrided, the Homan retractors can be removed and the lamina spreader is moved over to the lateral side of the joint. This allows maximal exposure at the posterior aspect of the posterior facet. The rest of the joint is subsequently debrided paying close attention to the posteromedial corner of the joint. When debriding in this area, I use a curette or debride without the flow of water in order to avoid impaling the capsular wall and damaging the neurovascular bundle. Manipulation of the great toe, resulting in movement of the flexor hallicus longus tendon or capsule is helpful in localizing the exact location of the tibial artery and nerve, since they reside slightly anteromedial to the course of the flexor hallucis longus tendon at the level of the subtalar joint.

When necessary, either prior to or at this point, an Achilles tendon lengthening is performed in the manner of choice. For example, in the situation of an acquired or flexible flatfoot deformity, placing the hindfoot out of its extreme valgus position into a neutral position can only be acceptably achieved by an Achilles tendon lengthening. If not performed, the hindfoot reduction will be incomplete, dictating that the only remaining way to gain plantar grade position is by dorsiflexing the forefoot at the transverse tarsal joint, thus producing a rocker bottom deformity. I prefer a step cut percutaneous tenotomy as described by Hoke for Achilles tendon lengthening.

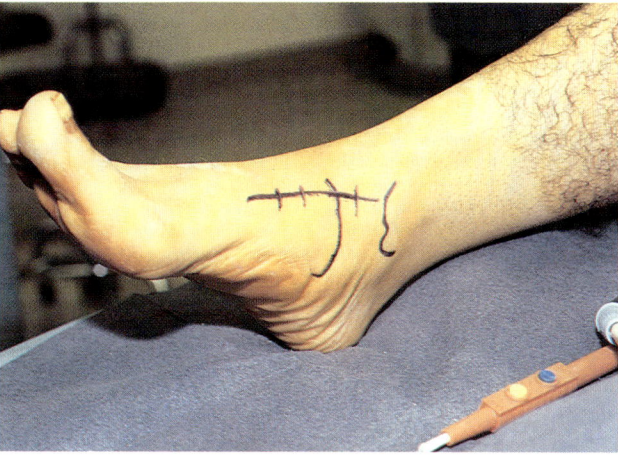

Figure 25. Dorsomedial skin incision.

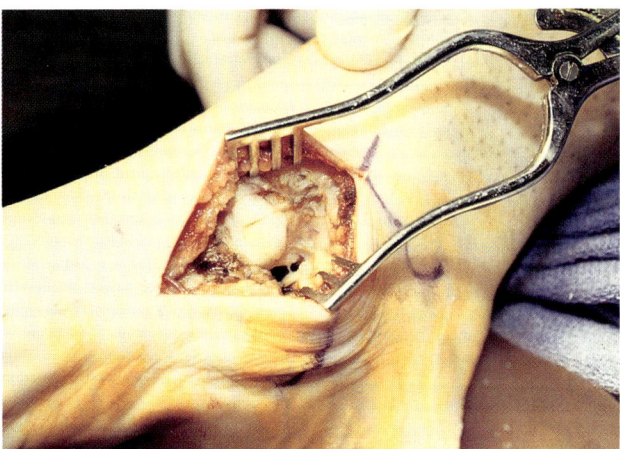

Figure 26. Deeper exposure dorsomedially shows the navicular distally and the medial talar head proximally.

The surgeon next positions himself on the opposite side of the operating table and a 4-inch bump is placed under the distal portion of the calf to raise the foot in order to facilitate exposure. The incision is made dorsomedially, beginning at the tip of the medial malleolus and in line with the medial border of the foot, extending 6 to 7 cm toward the great toe longitudinally, and ending between the insertions of the posterior and anterior tibialis tendons (Fig. 25). The saphenous vein typically courses close to the incision and should be identified during the subcuticular dissection and retracted safely, usually dorsally. Then the dissection can be continued deeply to the bone and through the joint capsule in the same line as the skin incision. At this point careful attention should be directed toward identification of the talonavicular joint and confirmation of location. Subperiosteal dissection is carried out both plantarly and dorsally from the navicular (Fig. 26). Here, too, the dorsal dissection is limited in order to avoid damage to the vascular supply of the dorsal neck of the talus. Even so, the dissection must be taken at least 1.0 to 1.5 cm over the talar head and neck in order to facilitate exposure of the dorsomedial aspect of the talonavicular joint and to localize the area in which a screw will be placed that will eventually be utilized in fixing the subtalar joint. If there are osteophytes around the peripheral medial rim of the navicular, they may be removed with an osteotome or a rongeur, thus facilitating exposure into this joint.

The cavus foot is particularly troublesome in this area given the fact that the navicular is usually well medial "over hanging" the talar head and so obscures the surgeon's view into the joint. A wider navicular soft tissue dissection is most often necessary. Once the talonavicular joint is in good view, Homan retractors are placed in the joint dorsally and plantarly. The joint debridement technique as described previously is utilized including use of the lamina spreaders to debride the medial half of the talonavicular joint. Another helpful maneuver is just to have an assistant pull on the foot since the lamina spreader is sometimes difficult to insert into the medial talonavicular joint. Do not forget that the navicular subchondral bone is significantly more dense than the talar head subchondral bone. Therefore, the surgeon should carefully monitor the bony debridement in order to avoid drifting toward the path of least resistance, into the talar head. It is essential that adequate subchondral bone be obtained on the navicular side of this joint due to its density. It is my opinion that one reason for a high rate of talonavicular nonunions is secondary to the inadequate debridement of the navicular. All of the joints are irrigated copiously with normal saline prior to reduction.

The reduction is first approximated by placing the foot in the general position desired. At this point, if an Achilles tendon lengthening has not been performed, the decision to do so can still be made if the reduction is found to be difficult. It is absolutely mandatory that the reduction be done in two stages and not attempted as a single-stage reduction. The easiest method is to reduce and fix the subtalar joint first, followed by reduction of the transverse tarsal joint. When done in this manner the reduction is actually quite simple and reliable.

When reducing the subtalar joint two factors must be addressed. First, the hindfoot position should be about 5° of valgus. With more severe deformities, however, more valgus can be accepted while still obtaining a good result. When reducing the subtalar joint as in the case of a planovalgus foot, it is not simply a varus-ward correction but also an internal rotation of the calcaneus underneath the talus. Second, the width between the talar head and the distal portion of the calcaneus (or the AP talocalcaneal width) should match the transverse tarsal width (Fig. 27). This is estimated by placing the thumb in the lateral wound and index finger in the medial wound or the reverse depending on which foot is involved and comparing the width between the medial head of the talus and the lateral border of the more distal calcaneus to the width of the corresponding navicular and cuboid. These should match fairly closely or the reduction of the transverse tarsal joint will be difficult and the fit may be poor.

Once the reduction of the subtalar joint is complete, it is provisionally fixed in the manner of choice. I use two percutaneous 0.062" K-wires extending from the plantar lateral calcaneus to the dorsal medial talus (Fig. 28). One pin starts more distally and is directed proximally, while the second pin starts more proximally

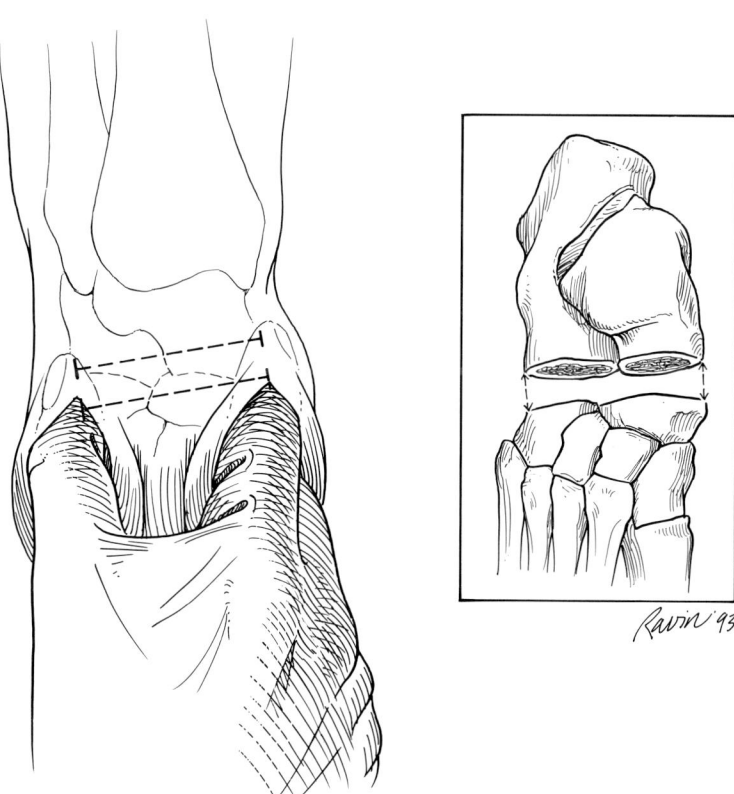

Figure 27. Before permanent fixation the surgeon must check the talocalcaneal width and make sure it approximates the soon to match up navicular-cuboid width. This can be done as shown.

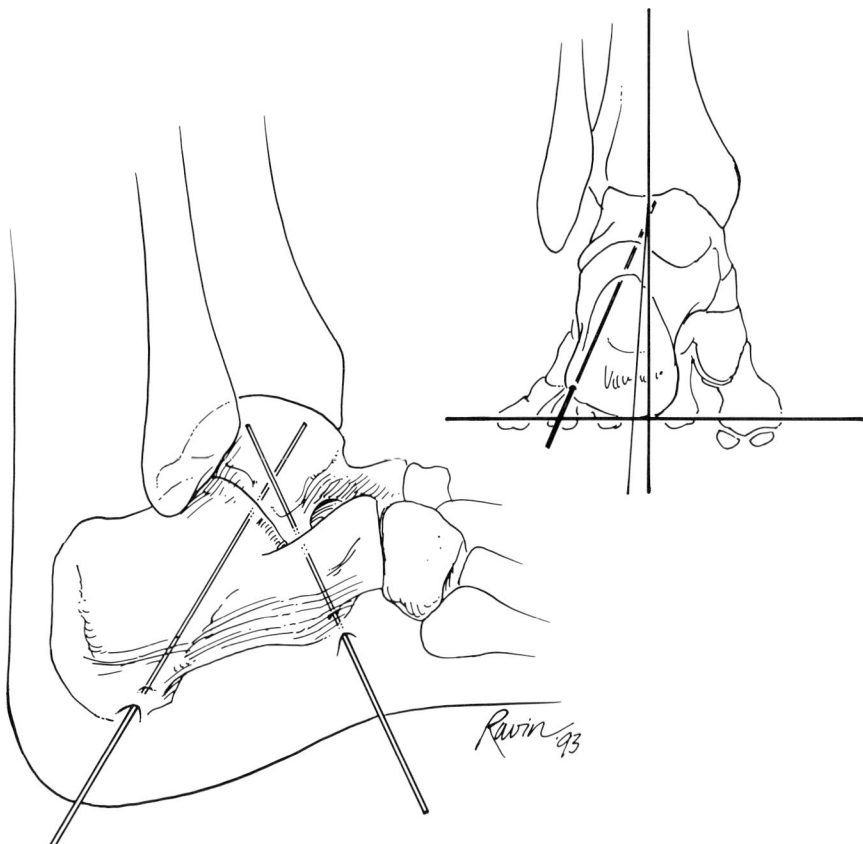

Figure 28. Hindfoot valgus of approximately 5° is desirable. Provisional subtalar joint fixation can be accomplished by two 0.062" smooth Kirschner wires as shown.

on the heel and is directed distally, resulting in a cross-pin configuration. Care must be taken to ensure that they do not penetrate the ankle joint. This fixation is more than adequate for provisional purposes and while the position of the hindfoot is being checked.

The hindfoot position is checked by raising the leg high in the air to approximately 45° to 60° from horizontal. The surgeon remains seated and backs away from the table while observing the hindfoot position as the assistant holds the ankle in a neutral position (Fig. 29). Lines can be drawn on the heel to further confirm the positioning of the calcaneal tuberosity relative to the line of the calf or tibial shank. At this point, if the reduction is not acceptable any necessary repositioning can be achieved by repeating the process outlined above. It is fairly obvious that if the ankle joint is provisionally fixed in a varus or valgus tilt, the entire correction during the triple arthrodesis will be in error to the corresponding degree of the talar tilt.

Definitive fixation of the talonavicular joint can be performed using many methods. The method that I prefer utilizes an A-O 6.5 cancellous screw (32 mm threads), and a 3.2 mm drill bit. The surgeon may also choose to use cannulated screws. The placement of this screw is actually quite easy. Anatomically, the position of the screw should be about 5 mm distal to the point where the medial talar dome corner meets the talar neck (Fig. 30). Once the starting point is identified, the drill bit is inserted about 2 mm so that the surgeon is able to focus on the trajectory of the drill. The trajectory of the drill should be toward the posterolateral corner of the heel. I have noticed that visually it appears as though the screw is

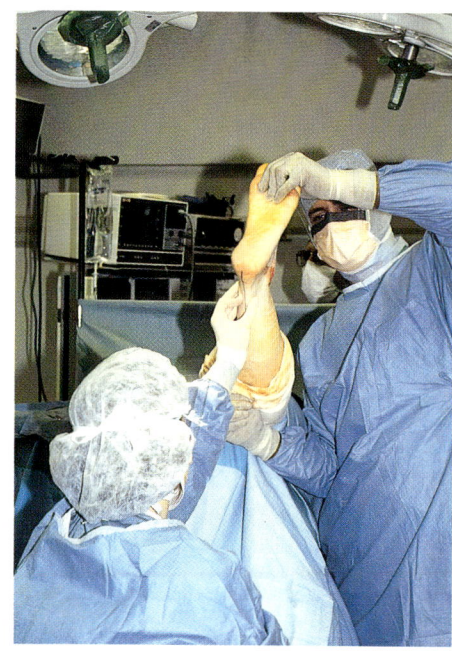

Figure 29. The assistant places the ankle in neutral and raises the leg high while the seated surgeon confirms hindfoot position visually.

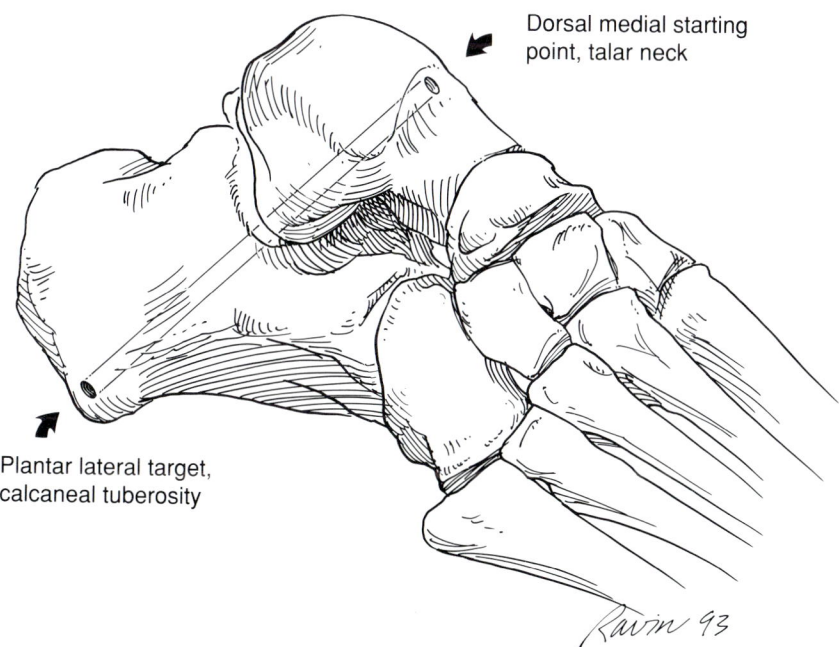

Figure 30. Starting point and trajectory of the subtalar fixation screw. Find the starting point and aim toward your finger tip at the plantar, posterior, and lateral heal.

heading too laterally and my instinct tells me to place the screw more medially. However, if one must err one way or the other, the screw should be placed more laterally than medially, as the offset of the calcaneus is lateral and the neurovascular bundle is medial. The length of the screw should be measured and is usually 60 ± 5 mm for females and 65 ± 5 mm for males (Fig. 31).

The starting hole through the neck of the talus is tapped with the large 6.5 mm A-O tap to avoid any expansile damage or cracking of the neck. The screw is now inserted, resulting in the outstanding amount of compression and stability of this fixation in nearly all cases. The provisional fixation pins or K-wires can then be removed and the screw tightened one additional time. The hindfoot position is

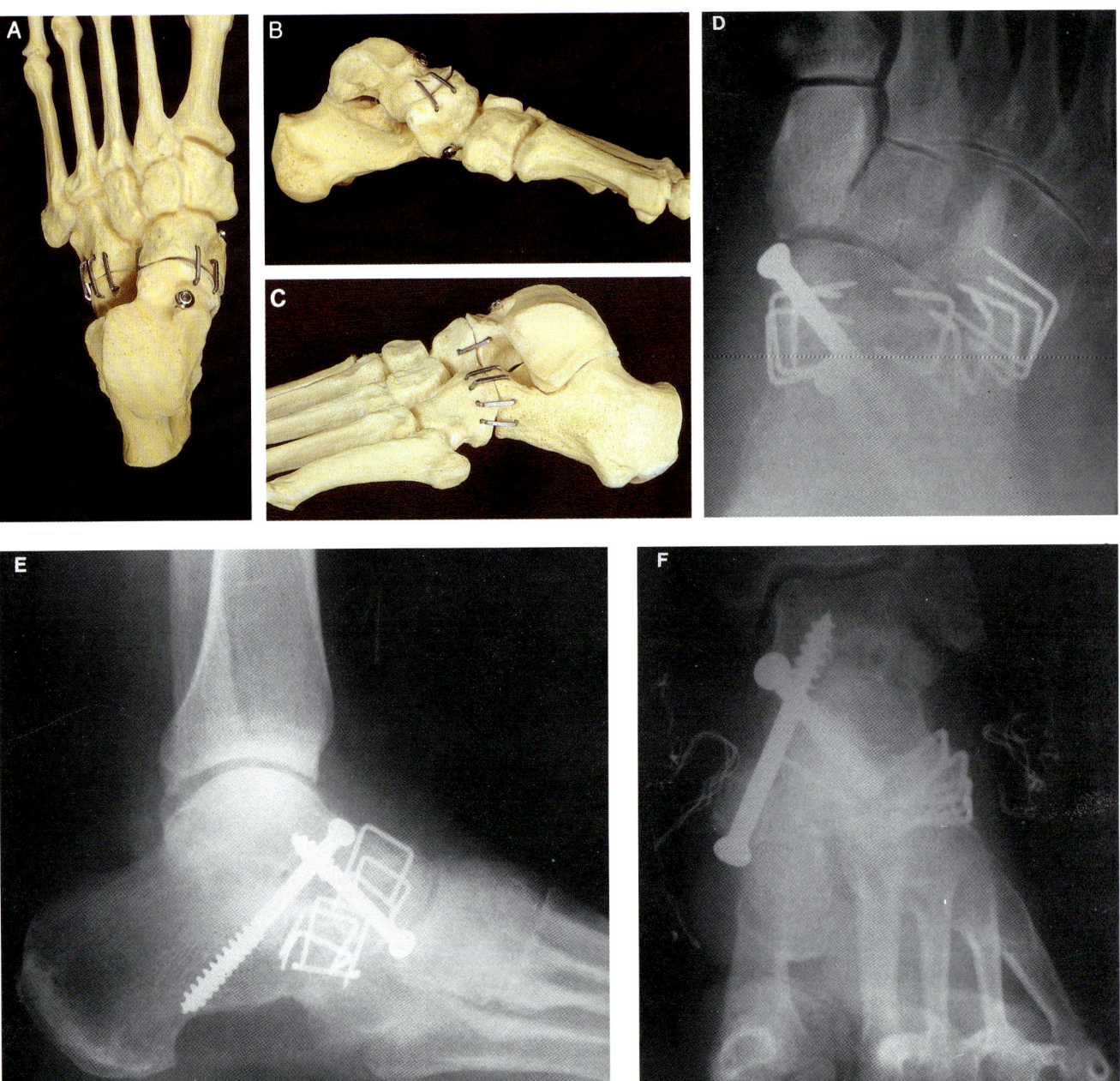

Figure 31. Standard fixation of the triple arthrodesis is shown. **A:** AP view of prepared model. **B:** Medial view of prepared model. **C:** Lateral view of prepared model. **D:** AP foot radiograph with fixation. **E:** Lateral foot radiograph with fixation. **F:** AP ankle radiograph with fixation. Slight overpenetration shows foot fixation.

rechecked because the placement of screws or other fixation can alter the positioning once obtained (Fig. 32). For this reason, the position of the foot must be checked repeatedly from here on out.

The transverse tarsal joint is now reduced. I usually reduce the calcaneocuboid joint anatomically, which if the other joints have been resurfaced properly, should fit accurately. At times, the bony area between the calcaneocuboid and the talonavicular joints can be "high" and cause the transverse tarsal joint to rocker between them (Fig. 33). In this case, the central portion of these two joints should be debrided down using a bur or osteotome. The calcaneocuboid joint is provisionally

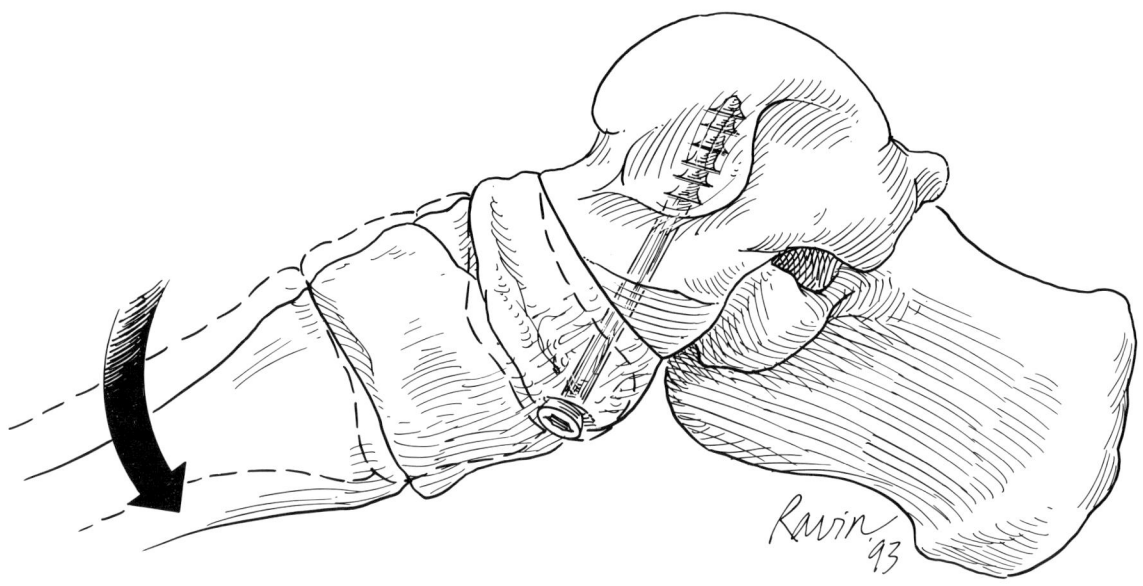

Figure 32. A plantarward correction of the navicular on the talar head (after calcaneocuboid prefixation) is essential to achieve medial column depression and therefore valgus forefoot positioning.

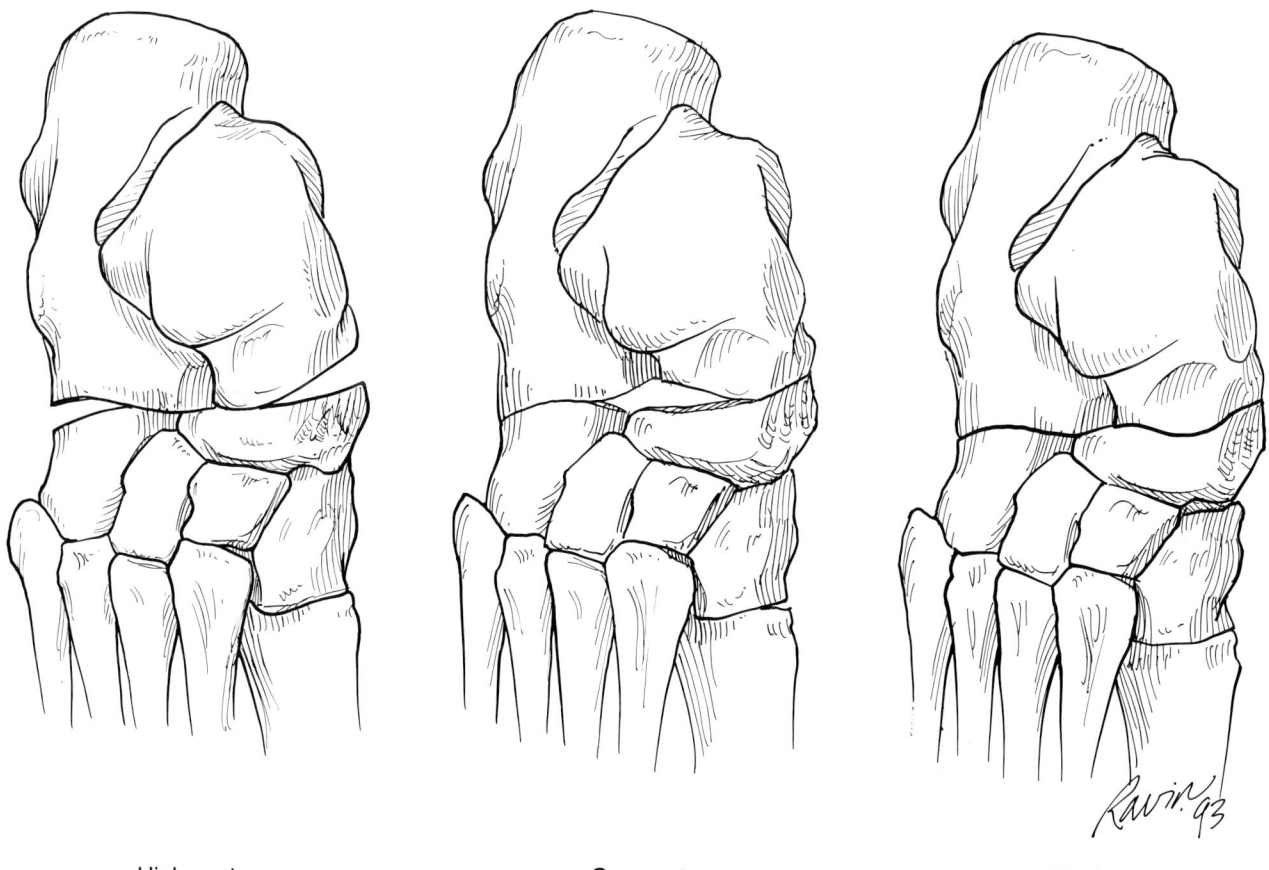

High center   Gap center   Ideal

Figure 33. A center contact area that is proud can reduce bone contact and stability of the ultimate fixation.

fixed using crossed percutaneous 0.062" K-wires. The exact trajectory of this provisional fixation is not standard. I usually place the first pin through the fifth metatarsal tuberosity toward the joint and the second pin starting at the lateral portion of the anterior process heading distally to cross-fix the calcaneocuboid joint. If a stable fixation is achieved, the surgeon's attention can be turned to the critical talonavicular or medial side. This joint is placed as close as possible to an anatomic position, attempting what amounts to near overcorrection of the medial forefoot downward (Fig. 34). To do this properly the heel must be stabilized in one hand while the navicular is manipulated in the other hand. If there is a tendency to err in one plane, err to place the medial forefoot more plantarly than the lateral forefoot or place the forefoot in a slight degree of valgus. When I'm finished, I prefer to see the forefoot in about 3° to 5° of valgus when the ankle is in a neutral position (Fig. 34). This valgus forefoot positioning is much more easily overcome by the patient than a varus forefoot positioning, which is the most common complication of this procedure. The talonavicular joint can now be provisionally fixed using two additional 0.062" K-wires, which are usually inserted from separate skin areas and which cross the joint.

At this point, the surgeon should stabilize the transverse tarsal joint in one of two ways. One utilizes staples alone, the other consists of screws with or without staples (Fig. 31). I prefer the latter. Screw fixation of the talonavicular joint is performed first by making a separate 1 to 1.5 cm incision on the prominent tuberosity of the navicular plantarly and medially, and slightly more distally than you think it needs to be. Dissection is continued deeply without fear of any neurovascular structure as long as the incision has been made medially enough and not straight plantarly. An area is cleared on the navicular tuberosity remaining distal to make sure an adequate area of navicular tuberosity is traversed by the screw. At this

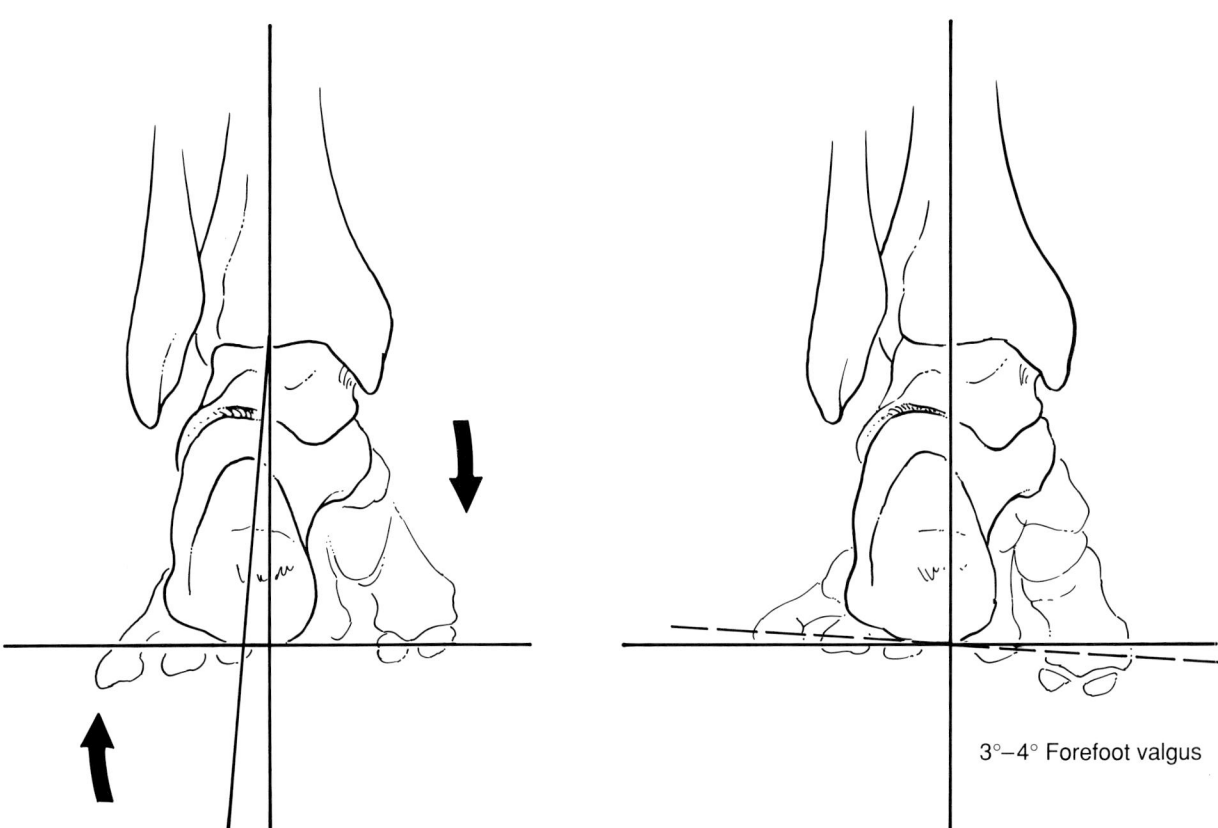

Figure 34. Mild forefoot valgus must be achieved. The plane of the forefoot is determined through the transverse tarsal correction.

point, a 3.2-mm drill bit is used with an angular trajectory aiming from the tuberosity to the center of the talar dome. If the subtalar joint screw is directly in the way (and it usually is), place a screwdriver in that screw to serve as the trajectory to avoid. Insertion of the drill bit can now be directed either medial or lateral to the subtalar joint screw. Once the drill hole is made, the hole is measured (usually requires a 50 ± 5 mm screw). I use a 16-mm threaded 6.5 A-O cancellous screw. In the same manner as described for the talar head, the drill hole in the navicular is tapped to avoid splitting this bone. If the area of the drill hole is made too far proximally, the purchase will be poor and this bone may split. I have found that if the screw starting point is made very close to the medial cuneiform navicular joint, the purchase is excellent and the bone will not split. One additional function that this screw serves when tightened is plantar flexion of the medial column of the foot a few extra degrees (Fig. 32), which helps in attaining the lowering of the medial column and therefore valgus positioning of the forefoot, which is highly desirable (Fig. 34). At this time I prefer to insert one to two 16×20 mm 3M titanium staples in the dorsomedial aspect of the talonavicular joint. The calcaneocuboid joint is fixed in a similar fashion using three to five of the same type of staples. Alternately, the calcaneocuboid joint can be fixed in a similar fashion using a 6.5 mm A-O screw going through the anterior process of the calcaneus plantarly, into the cuboid. The provisional fixation pins are removed at this time.

All of the joints are now checked for their fit and for positioning of the foot. I highly recommend that radiographs not be used to determine positioning of the foot but that the positioning be evaluated based on visual reference by the surgeon at the table. Depending on the fit of the joint surfaces, the decision is made whether or not to proceed with a bone graft.

Iliac crest bone graft is placed in the small areas of poor fit that will be present quite often. Bone graft is tamped into these areas of the joints as well as into the deeper portion of the sinus tarsi. In the more osteoporotic patients such as those with rheumatoid arthritis, the need for iliac crest bone graft can be reduced while with the more dense bone of osteoarthritis I tend to use bone graft more readily.

Next, the foot is prepared for closure and deflation of the tourniquet. The wound margins are injected with 0.5% Marcaine with or without epinephrine, using between 15 and 20 cc. This will aid in postoperative pain relief. We prefer to spray the wound with topical thrombin as well. The only closure done prior to tourniquet deflation is that of the two tabs of the sinus tarsi fat pad to the proximal portion of the extensor digitorum brevis muscle belly in a purse string fashion using 2-0 Vicryl (Fig. 35). Additional sutures can be placed plantarly and dorsally along corresponding borders of the extensor fascia. Care must be taken not to take bites that are too large in either direction and to keep them deep in order to avoid damaging the superficial peroneal nerve dorsally and the sural nerve plantarly. Provisional dressings are packed in the wounds and a lightly compressive ace bandage is placed on the foot. The tourniquet is now released and the reactive hyperemia time is allowed to pass over about 10 minutes. During this time, radiographs are obtained and checked for positioning of the fixation as well as for the fit of the joints. Standard radiographs that I obtain intraoperatively are an AP and lateral of the foot and an AP of the ankle to verify the position of the talonavicular screw angled toward the dome of the talus.

The wound is now closed over two medium suction drains, one placed medial and one placed lateral through separate skin stab incisions. I use 3-0 undyed Vicryl for subcutaneous closure followed by 4-0 nylon in a horizontal mattress fashion. After closure, the foot is placed in a sterile slightly bulky dressing with a Seabrook cooling blanket close to the skin layer but not directly on it. Then the type of immobilization is chosen based on the age of the patient and the reliability of the fixation. If the patient is younger and the fixation is felt to be optimal, an off of the shelf orthosis such as a 3-D Brace can be used. If the fixation is not felt to be as satisfactory or the patient is older, a posterior plaster splint may be used.

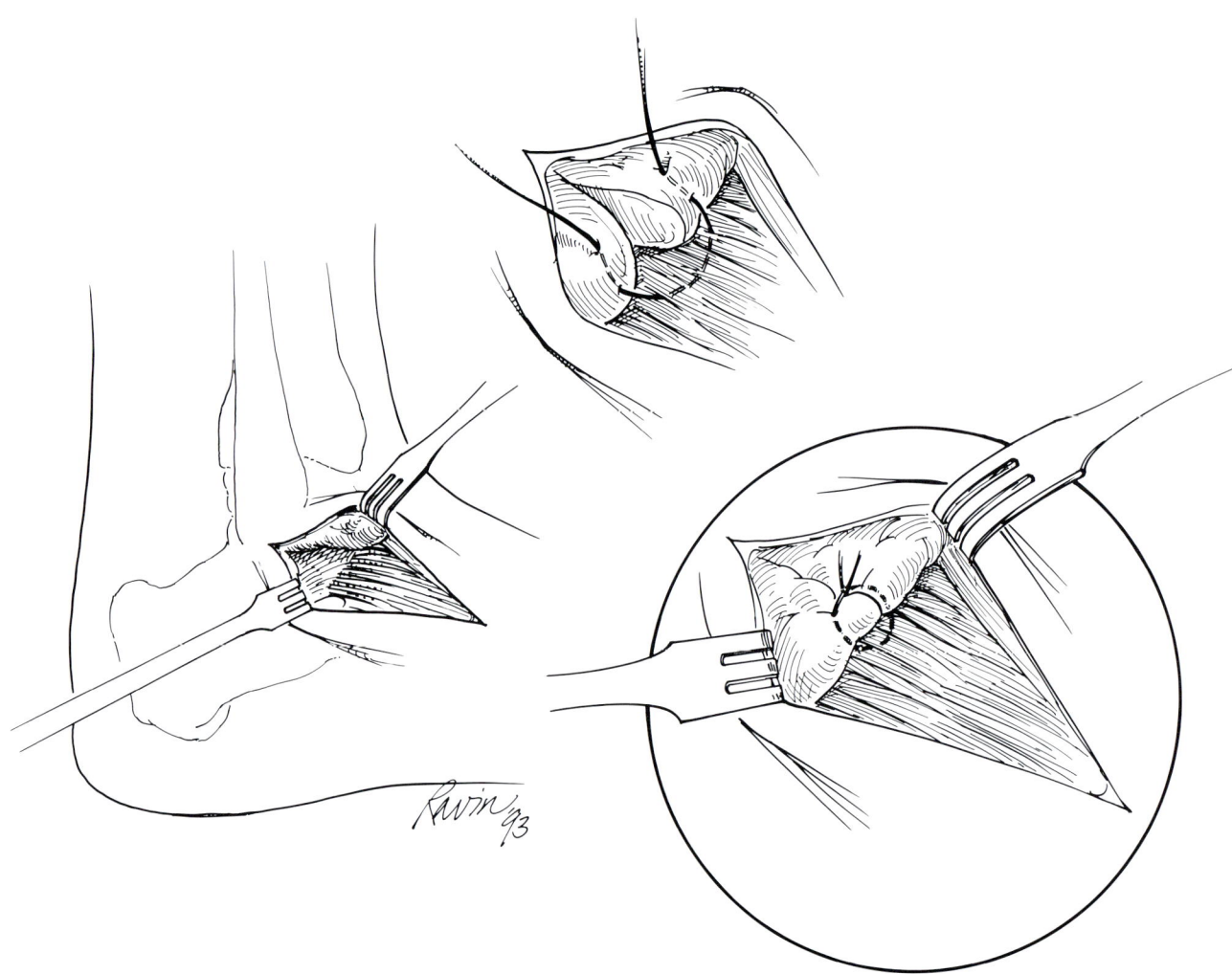

Figure 35. A purse string type suture is used for the deep closure of the lateral wound.

If a percutaneous Achilles tendon lengthening is done at the same time, it is important that the ankle be placed in a precisely neutral position to allow the proper length for Achilles tendon healing.

POSTOPERATIVE MANAGEMENT

The patient is maintained on patient controlled anesthesia (PCA) postoperative analgesia for no more than 18 hours, as I have found that this device makes the patient groggy and unable to do physical therapy the day after surgery. Physical therapy is started the first postoperative day for gait training. Preoperative gait instruction is highly desirable. The patient is instructed in a foot flat gait, bearing only the weight of the leg on his or her foot. Deep venous thrombosis prophylaxis should be maintained in the manner of choice postoperatively.

The patient continues a foot flat gait for 6 weeks with the sutures having been removed upon return 2 weeks postoperatively. In the steroid or methotrexate-dependent rheumatoid patient, suture removal should be delayed to 3 to 4 weeks. Radiographs are used as an objective measure of recovery thereafter. If they show bridging union at 6 weeks, the patient is allowed to bear weight while in immobilization (such as a cast or an off the shelf orthosis) for an additional 6 weeks. If the radiographs are not satisfactory at 6 weeks, a delay of 2 to 4 weeks can be determined by the surgeon at that time before weight bearing is allowed while in immobilization. At the 3 month check, if the radiographs are satisfactory, the patient is allowed to wean out of the brace at will. If the operation is done properly, no special shoe wear is required; however, tennis shoes will be the most comfortable for the patient for many months to come owing to residual swelling and thickness of the foot.

It is extremely important, not only preoperatively but during each visit, that the patients be counseled on the slow recovery that they will make. The first year after a triple arthrodesis can be very frustrating to a patient even when all is going well from the surgeon's standpoint. The patient must understand that he or she will never be "normal" again. The patient must be asked to look back and determine whether there has been improvement relative to both the preoperative and postoperative states. It is amazing that a patient easily forgets his or her earlier problems and feels as though there has been no improvement until looking back in an objective manner.

In general, I tell patients that 50% of their recovery will occur at 3 months, 75% at 6 months, with their maximal medical improvement plateauing somewhere around 2 years. However, even with the apparent plateau, it is important to inform patients that recovery will in some minor ways continue indefinitely. Only patience and time passage will reveal to what extent.

REHABILITATION

Long-term rehabilitation for maximal recovery is not necessary. Physical therapy is used after this procedure only for gait training. Calf strength and bulk will return somewhere between 12 and 24 months naturally, although exercise such as heel raises to enhance both can be done.

COMPLICATIONS

Complications that are specific to triple arthrodesis can be maddening not only to the patient but to the surgeon. Luckily, most of these are technique dependent and as the surgeon gains experience, these complications can be reduced.

1. *Malpositioning.* If absolute and meticulous attention is not paid to detail of positioning after surgery, the forefoot can be left in a varus position causing contacting on the base of the fifth metatarsal and at times on the fifth metatarsal head. Unfortunately, this is an all too common complication; however, it can be alleviated by making an osteotomy through the transverse tarsal fusion in order to rotate the foot in a valgus or neutral position. Other methods of correction of the varus positioning, if slight, include plantar flexion osteotomy of the first metatarsal and plantar flexion first metatarsal cuneiform arthrodesis.
2. *Nonunion.* Nonunion rates have been reported to be as high as 15% to 20%. By using the described method of anatomic joint resection with the addition of iliac crest bone graft, the nonunion rate drops to well below 5%. In many years of performing the triple arthrodesis, which seems to be a frequent foot and ankle surgical procedure, I have noted two common denominators contributing to nonunion. The depth of joint debridement is most notable. If the healthy vascular cancellous bone, which is well below the layer of the subchondral bone, is not obtained over a large area through adequate depth of debridement, it does not matter how much iliac crest graft is placed in the joint, bony fusion is not likely to occur. The second common denominator is failure to utilize iliac crest bone graft. One should never let the patient's per-

ception of performing a second operative procedure such as an iliac crest bone graft alter the surgeon's ability, when using proper technique, to achieve the best result possible for the patient. The method of correcting a nonunion is to simply perform the fusion again taking advantage of iliac crest graft to aid bony fusion.

3. *Marginal skin slough along the incisions.* Skin sloughing occurs in nearly all patients to at least minor degrees and must be discussed preoperatively. The treatment almost always includes patience, and normal saline wet to dry dressing changes or wound management of choice. Given time these skin sloughs will always heal by secondary intention.
4. *Sensory nerve damage.* Damage to the sural and superficial peroneal nerves can occur intraoperatively in the lateral aspect of the wound. Measures to avoid damage to these nerves have been discussed previously.
5. *Late osteoarthritis of adjacent joints.* Osteoarthritis of adjacent joints such as the tarsometatarsal joints or the ankle may occur late and are usually the result of increased demand for flexibility and use of these joints. This is an unavoidable problem and should be discussed with the patient prior to surgery. If the patient does develop arthritis in an adjacent joint, this should be dealt with when it occurs on an individual basis.

ILLUSTRATIVE CASE FOR TECHNIQUE

This patient is a 61-year-old woman who is referred by a local rheumatologist. She presents with a 2-year history of pain and progressive deformity in her left foot. During the previous 2 years, she has tried a variety of custom-molded inlays as well lace-up type ankle braces.

Physical examination upon presentation revealed marked hindfoot valgus on the left and tenderness under the lateral malleolus. On heel raise testing her left hindfoot did not invert when done bilaterally. This attempted single stance heel raising on the left was not possible due to pain and weakness. This was easily done on the contralateral right side. There was tenderness in the area just distal to the lateral malleolus corresponding to the area of calcaneofibular impingement seen on radiographs. The Achilles tendon was found to be contracted. There was also a fixed hindfoot contracture noting the patient's hindfoot could be everted greater than the right side but inversion fell well short of neutral, whereas the contralateral right side could be inverted 15°.

Standing radiographs of the foot and ankle reveal a talonavicular sag, an increased lateral talocalcaneal angle, and a calcaneofibular impingement (Figs. 36 and 37). Moderate to advanced hindfoot degenerative arthritis was noted in the radiographs. During the course of several follow-up visits and further conservative management with an additional solid ankle-foot orthrosis (AFO), the patient expressed her dissatisfaction with her rapidly declining life-style. The AFO was no longer effective. Her function and quality of life was now unacceptable. At this point, as we had discussed on the first visit, a triple arthrodesis along with iliac crest bone graft harvesting and a percutaneous Achilles tendon lengthening was the surgical treatment of choice. The patient returned two additional times with family members present to discuss this surgery.

The patient ultimately underwent the triple arthrodesis obtaining a successful correction using ipsilateral iliac crest bone graft. The percutaneous Hoke tenotomy was performed as well. The immediate perioperative and postoperative periods were uneventful, with removal of the suction drains in the foot and hip on the first postoperative day. The patient was immobilized in a posterior plaster splint for 2 weeks. Upon return at 2 weeks the sutures were removed and she was given further advice to continue to be foot flat (touchdown) weight bearing only. She returned at 6 weeks postoperatively when we obtained the first non–weight bearing

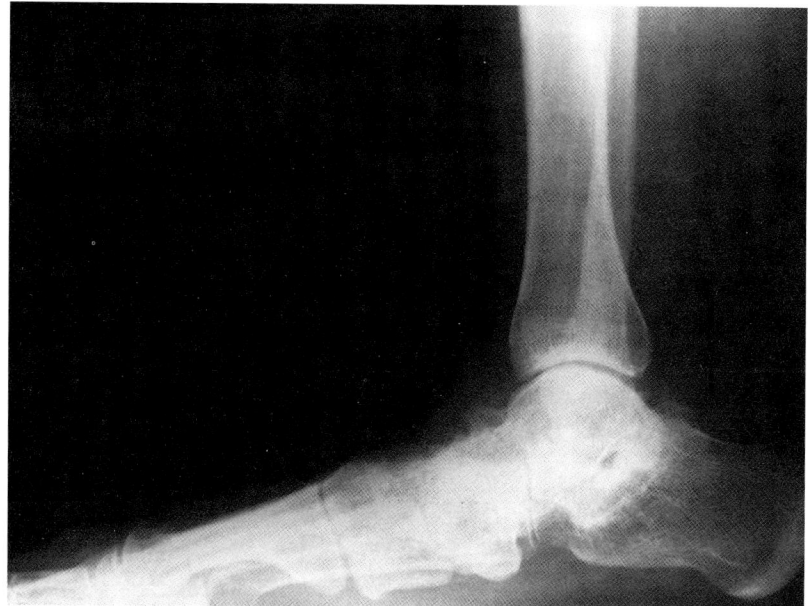

Figure 36. Illustrative case: preoperative lateral left foot radiograph, standing.

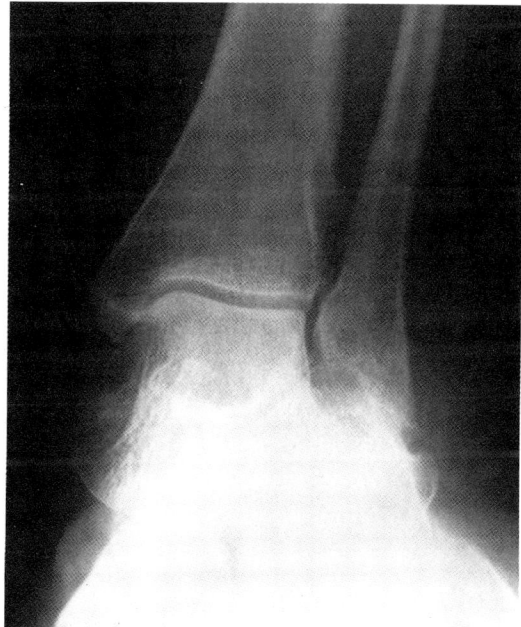

Figure 37. Illustrative case: preoperative AP radiograph left ankle.

radiographs of the foot and ankle (Figs. 38–40). It was noted that all three areas of fusion were solid radiographically. The patient had a powerful plantar flexion of the ankle indicating an intact Achilles tendon. In addition, the correction was noted to be satisfactory to the patient. At this point, she was instructed to weight bear as tolerated in an off the shelf orthosis for 6 weeks, weight bearing about 25% for the first week moving to 100% weight bearing thereafter. She returned at 12 weeks postoperatively and repeat radiographs revealed solid fusion just as was noted from the 6 week postoperative radiographs.

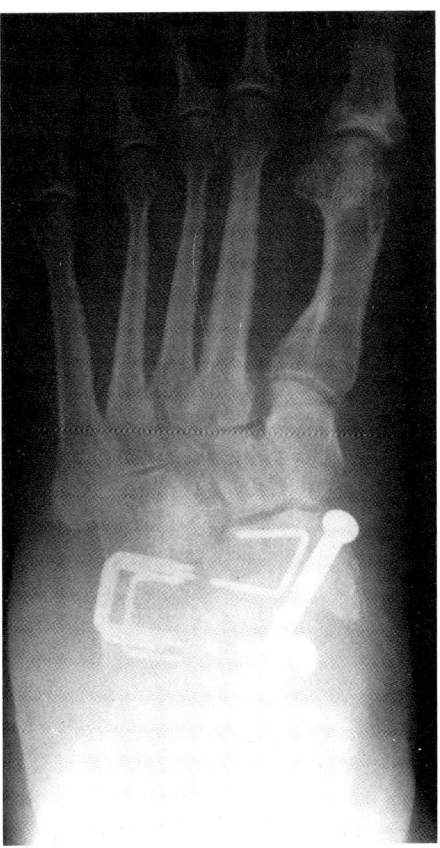

Figure 38. Illustrative case: 6 weeks postoperative non—weight bearing AP foot radiograph.

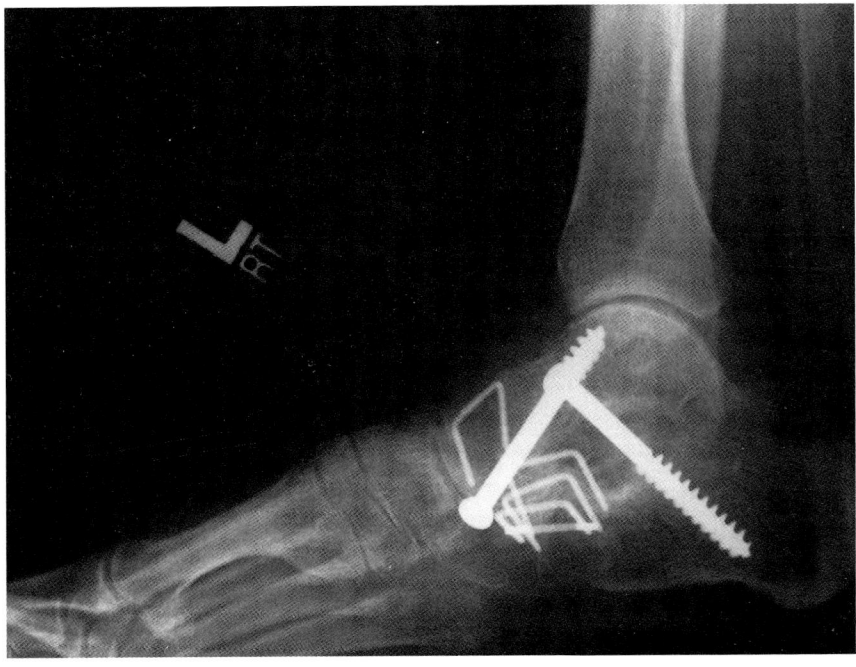

Figure 39. Illustrative case: 6 weeks postoperative non—weight bearing lateral foot radiograph.

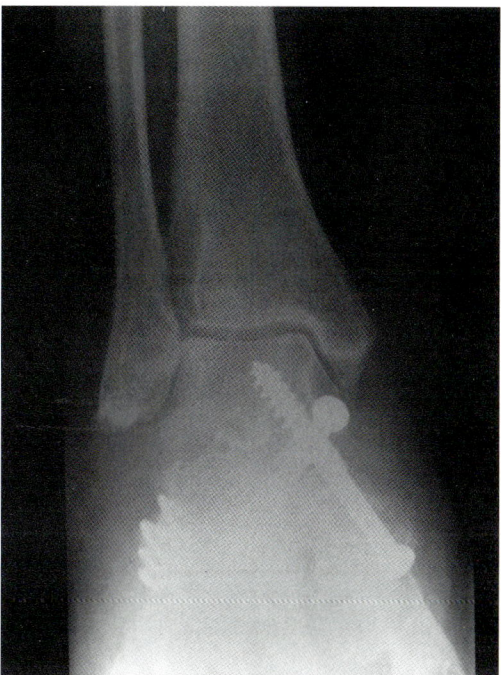

Figure 40. Illustrative case: 6 weeks postoperative non–weight bearing AP radiograph of ankle.

This patient was instructed at 3 months after surgery to perform normal activities as her foot would tolerate but to progress slowly and allow the foot to accommodate to its new activities. She was also instructed to use the brace if needed to allow her activities to rise rapidly.

The patient is now approximately 18 months postsurgery and has no complaints whatsoever, having resolved her calcaneofibular impingement and having achieved a plantar grade foot. Moreover, she has been playing golf at approximately 1 year and feels quite satisfied by the whole process.

The success for this patient clearly stemmed from adequate preoperative preparation and counseling so that there were no surprises for her. Even though the foot treated with the triple arthrodesis is clearly not normal, it is a considerable improvement over what she presented with, and so has returned to the life-style she desired.

RECOMMENDED READING

1. Adam, W., and Ranawat, C.: Arthrodesis of the hindfoot in rheumatoid arthritis. *Orthop. Clin. North Am.*, 7(4): 827–840, 1976.
2. Johnson, K. A.: *Surgery of the Foot and Ankle*. New York: Raven Press, 1989.
3. Mann, R. A.: *Surgery of the Foot*. St. Louis: C.V. Mosby, 1986.
4. Sammarco, G. J.: Technique of triple arthrodesis in treatment of symptomatic pes planus. *Orthopedics*, 11(11): 1607–10, 1988.
5. Wetmore, R. S., et al.: Long-term results of triple arthrodesis in Charcot-Marie-Tooth disease. *J. Bone Joint Surg.*, 71A(3): 417–422, 1989.

31

Calcaneal Fracture Open Reduction and Fixation

Michael M. Romash

INDICATIONS/CONTRAINDICATIONS

The indication for open reduction and internal fixation of a calcaneal fracture is controversial. As the fracture patterns and displacements of the fragments have been clarified by sophisticated imaging, newer classification patterns have developed. These classifications in general are based upon the amount of comminution of the posterior facet of the subtalar joint (6). The result of open reduction and internal fixation has been correlated with each of these various classifications. In general, the more severe the injury as defined by the amount of fragmentation of the posterior facet, the less satisfactory is the surgical result.

The pain that may result from malunited calcaneal fracture cannot completely be explained as a posttraumatic arthritis of the posterior facet (4,17). Other factors responsible for pain and disability may include the loss of height of the calcaneus, which causes abnormal spatial relationships at the hindfoot joints, and dorsiflexion of the talus with tibiotalar impingement and loss of ankle motion. Also with a malunited calcaneal fracture displacement of the calcaneal tuberosity fragment will shorten the heel lever arm, whereas widening of the heel can cause lateral impingement on the distal fibula and peroneal tendons and make the use of shoes difficult.

Operative reduction of a calcaneal fracture can reconstruct in general the architecture of the calcaneus and restore appropriate spatial relationships. Even if a later salvage is necessary, having the calcaneus in a somewhat normal arrangement will be helpful. For these reasons, primary surgical treatment of a calcaneal fracture becomes reasonable. It is necessary that fracture fragments be large enough to allow fixation.

M. M. Romash, M.D.: Department of Surgery, Uniform Services University of Health Sciences, Bethesda, Maryland; and Suite D, North Battlefield Boulevard, Chesapeake, VA 23320.

Contraindications to surgical treatment of the calcaneal fractures include the presence of fracture blisters, decreased vascularity of the limb, and bony fragments of insufficient size to accept fixation.

PREOPERATIVE PLANNING

The plan for surgical treatment is based on understanding the fracture pattern and fragment displacement. This is truly an exercise in three-dimensional anatomy (3,7,15,16).

The concave medial wall of the body of the calcaneus places the center of the tuberosity slightly lateral to the center of the calcaneus. When a vertical compressive injuring force is applied injuring the calcaneus, a shearing stress occurs through the body resulting in a primary fracture line that in a coronal plane runs from superior-lateral to inferior-medial. With this primary fracture the sustentaculum and medial portion of the posterior facets stay anatomically related to the talus, and the tuberosity fragment moves proximal, lateral, anterior, and rotates into varus. A secondary fracture line then occurs in the posterior calcaneal facet

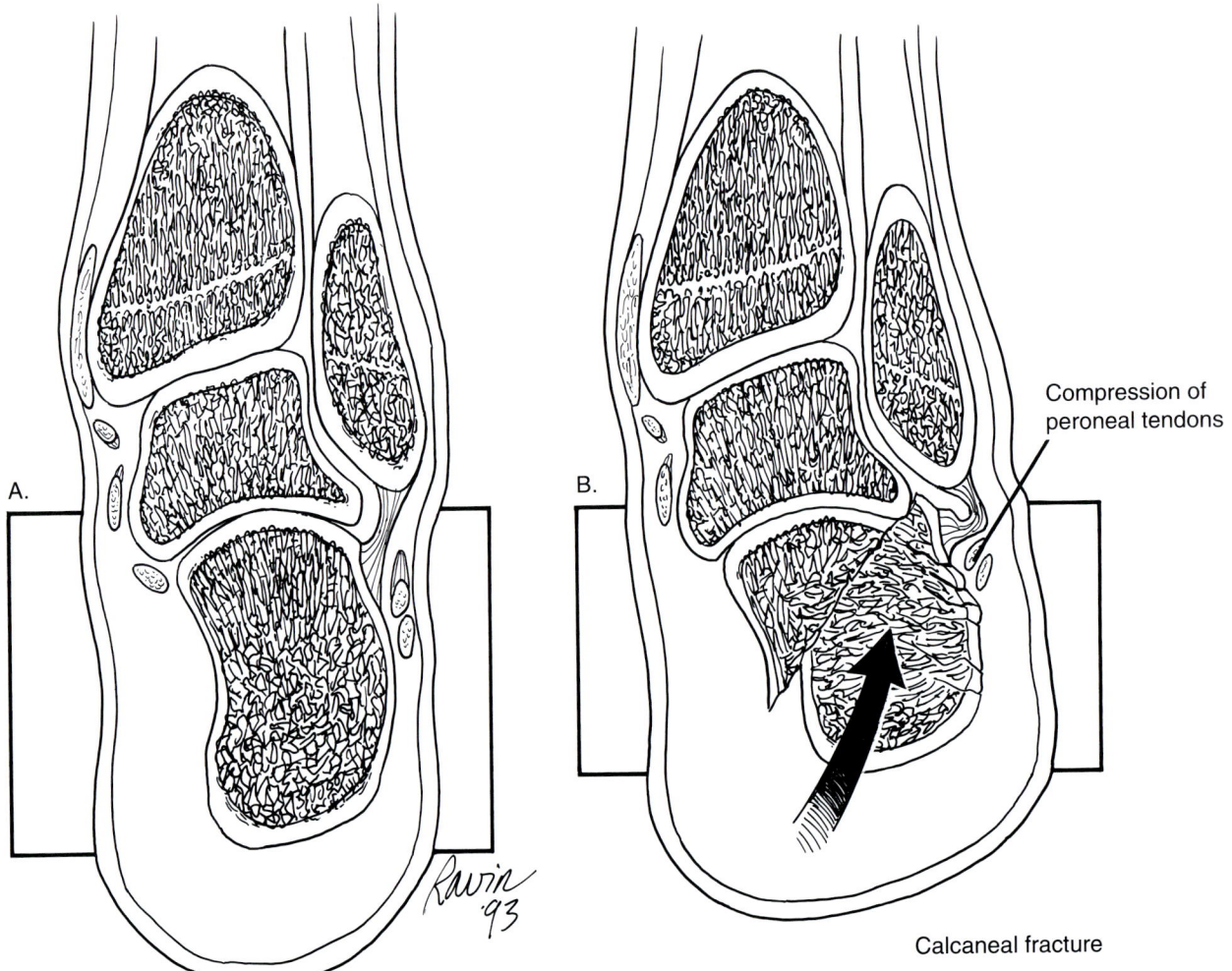

Figure 1. A: Normal calcaneal prefracture demonstrating relationships—axial view. **B:** Fractured calcaneus, axial view, demonstrating the shift of the tuberosity, articular disruption, secondary fracture lines, and peroneal impingement. Note that the sustentacular or medial side remains in anatomic position.

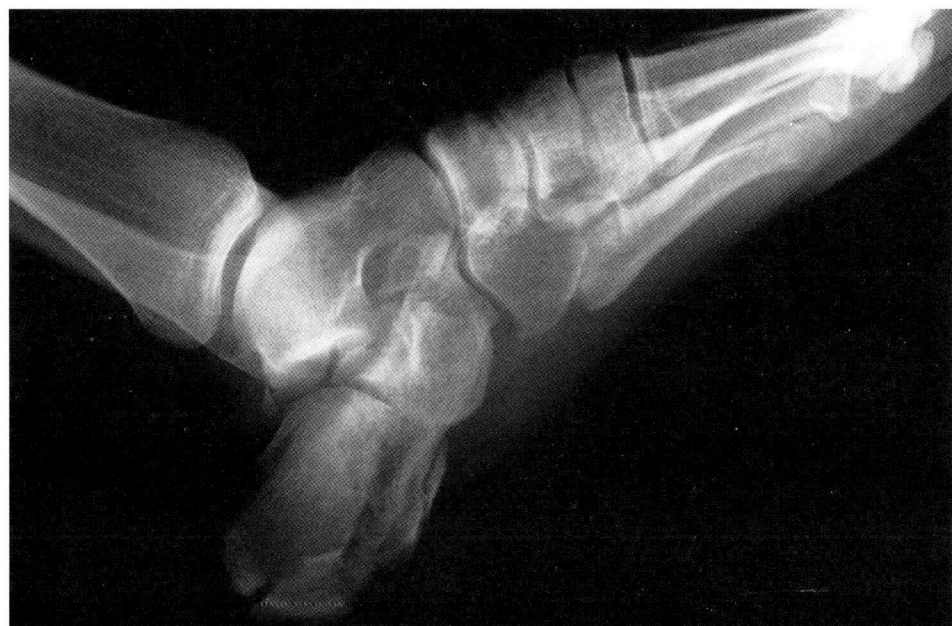

Figure 2. Lateral radiograph of displaced calcaneal fracture demonstrating dorsiflexed talus and talonavicular subluxation; the navicular is plantarly displaced.

causing it to be depressed down and often rotated severely. The lateral wall of the calcaneus can also be comminuted and bulge outward. The displacement of the tuberosity fragment up against the fibula causes the calcaneus-to-fibula impingement as well as displacing the peroneal tendons (Fig. 1). The loss of the posterior height of the heel dorsiflexes the talus, which can lead to limited ankle motion as the neck of the talus impinges on the anterior tibia. Also, talar dorsiflexion causes talonavicular joint subluxation with the navicular moving inferiorly in relation to the head of the talus (Fig. 2). The secondary fracture can also extend anteriorly with comminution at the calcaneocuboid joint.

Operative reduction is aimed at reestablishing the normal height and width of the heel by bringing the tuberosity fragment back to its normal position in relation

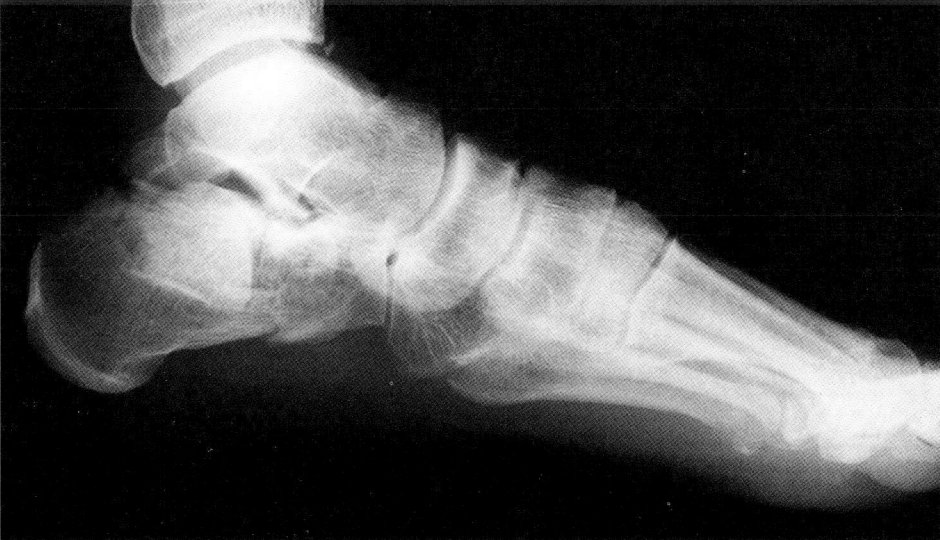

Figure 3. Lateral radiograph demonstrating loss of Böhler's angle and secondary fracture line depressing and rotating the lateral portion of the posterior facet.

to the undisplaced sustentacular fragment. Also, at surgery, the articular surface of the subtalar joint and the length of the calcaneus is reestablished. The method for this reduction and the means of fixation can be planned after appropriate radiographic images are obtained.

Routine radiography of the fractured calcaneus has been well described (1,3). The lateral view demonstrates the loss of height of the heel, which may be measured by Böhler's angle and compared to the contralateral foot. An idea of the displacement of the secondary fractures can be obtained from this film looking for the joint depression or tongue-type secondary fracture pattern (Fig. 3). The axial view of the heel often demonstrates the shearing fracture line, lateral and proximal displacement of the tuberosity fragment, and may demonstrate the articu-

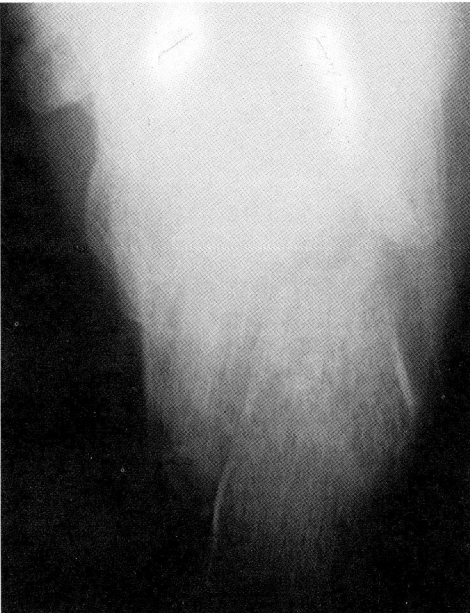

Figure 4. Axial view of the calcaneus radiograph demonstrating primary shearing fracture.

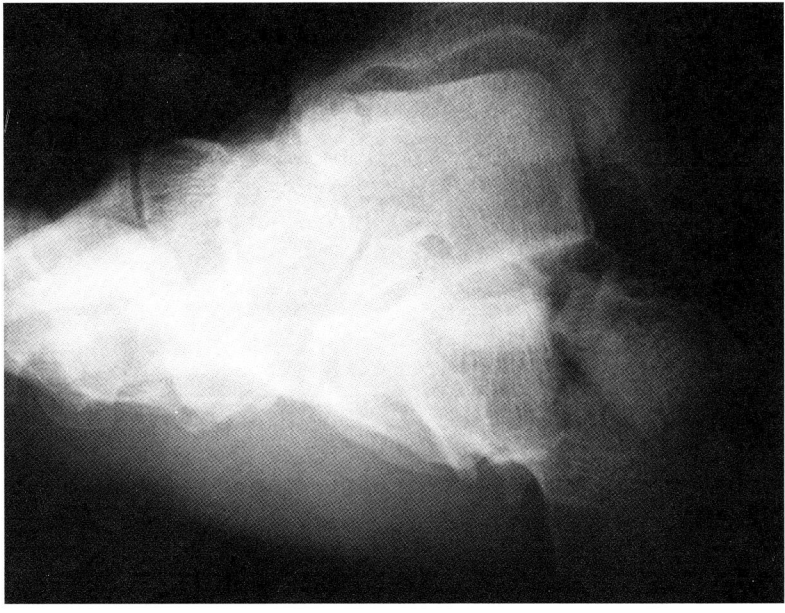

Figure 5. Broden's view of the calcaneus demonstrating the split of the posterior facet.

lar surface of the posterior facet (Fig. 4). The anteroposterior view of the foot may show comminution into the calcaneocuboid joint. The oblique or Broden's view of the foot will give information as to the disruption or splitting of the posterior facet of the calcaneus (Fig. 5).

Computed tomography (CT) of the foot is very helpful in axial, coronal, and sagittal planes (2,4,9,16). This allows three-dimensional object reconstruction (4) to be made. The axial and coronal views will demonstrate the shift of the tuberosity laterally, the rotation of the posterior facet fragments, and the lateral calcaneal wall displacement. The sagittal cuts will show the rotational displacement of the posterior facet fragment (Fig. 6). The three-dimensional reconstruction will dem-

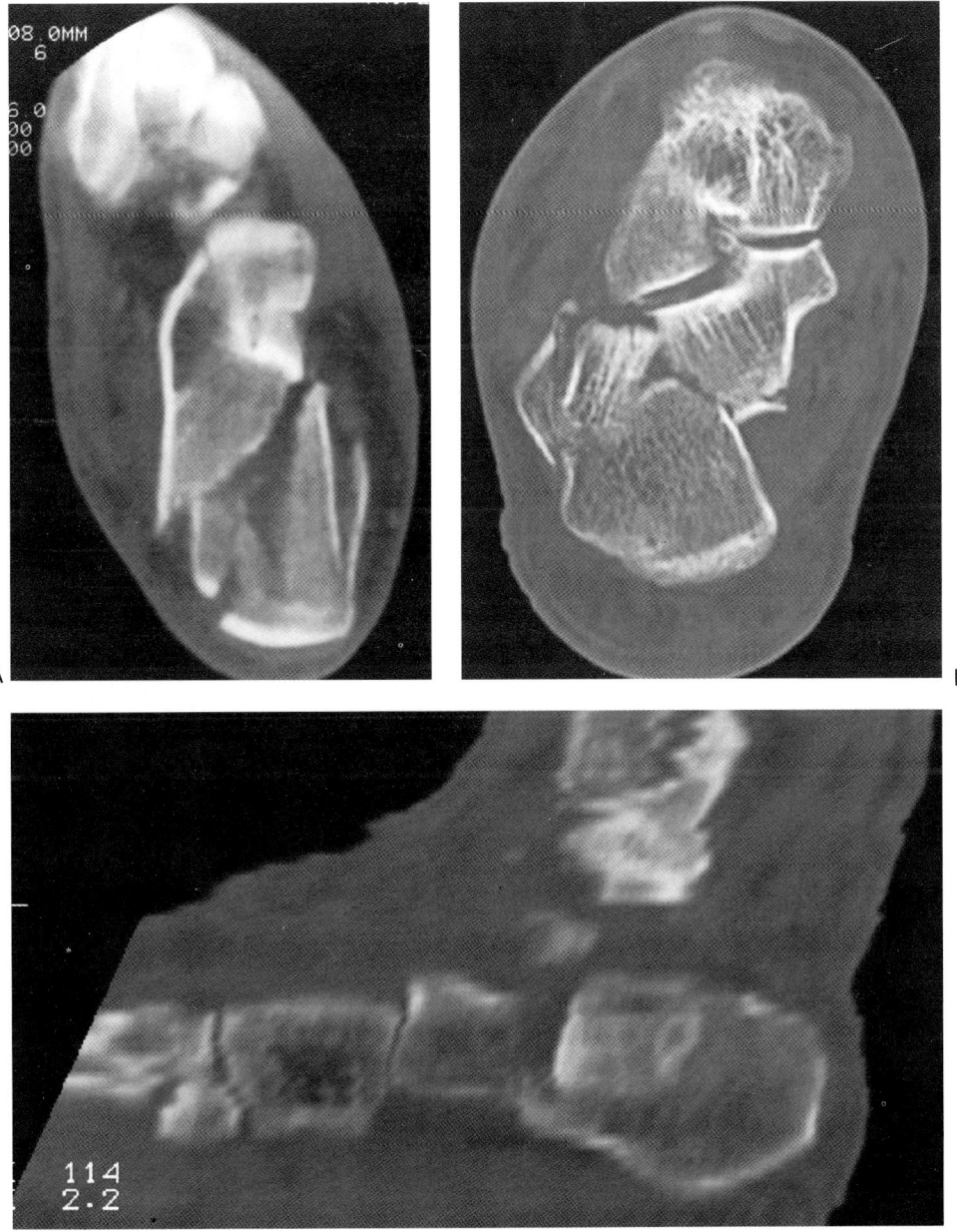

Figure 6. A: Axial cut CT scan demonstrating oblique shear fracture and shift of the fragments, overhang or "shingling" of medial wall. **B:** Coronal cut CT demonstrating shift of fragments rotation of posterior facet, and extension of fracture anteriorly to calcaneocuboid joint. **C:** Sagittal reconstruction demonstrating depression and rotation of posterior facet fragment.

onstrate the external architecture of the heel and the bony plates or surfaces that will accept fixation devices (Fig. 7).

During examination of the patient, the physician should be aware that a calcaneal fracture has a concomitant significant soft tissue injury as well as possible spinal compression fracture. The possibility of a plantar compartment syndrome associated with this fracture as described by Manoli and Weber (12) or significant tenting of the skin by fracture fragments may make early surgery necessary.

It is not uncommon to delay surgery 1 to 2 days while the appropriate CT scans and radiographs are performed. During this time, fracture blisters may occur. A bulky, circumferential compressive dressing rewrapped twice daily has been helpful in decreasing the development of fracture blisters. The technique of placing the padded, injured foot inside a cryocuff, which provides controlled compression with iced water, seems to have some promise in diminishing fracture blister formation (Fig. 8). If fracture blisters develop about the operative site, I prefer to delay surgery until the blisters have been resolved by unroofing of the blisters and sterile dressings. Delay of up to 3 weeks in reducing these fractures does not seem to compromise the result of surgery.

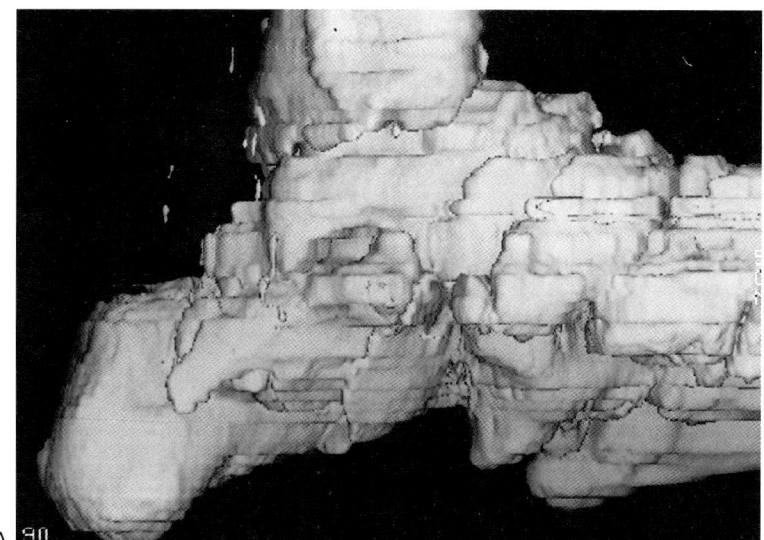

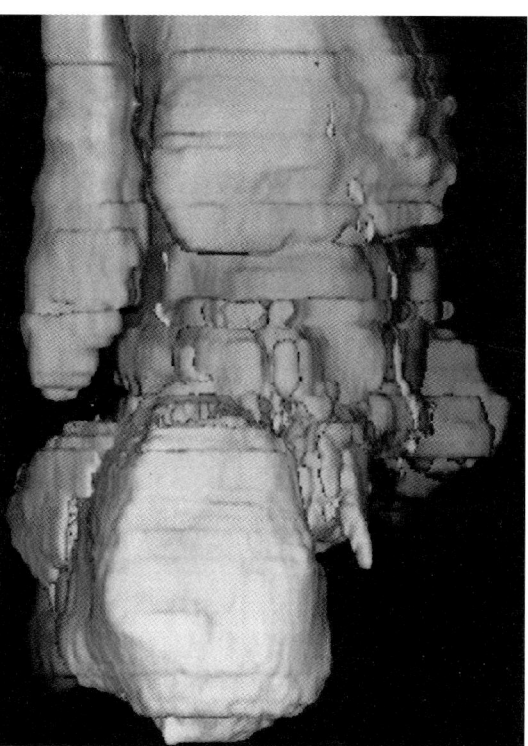

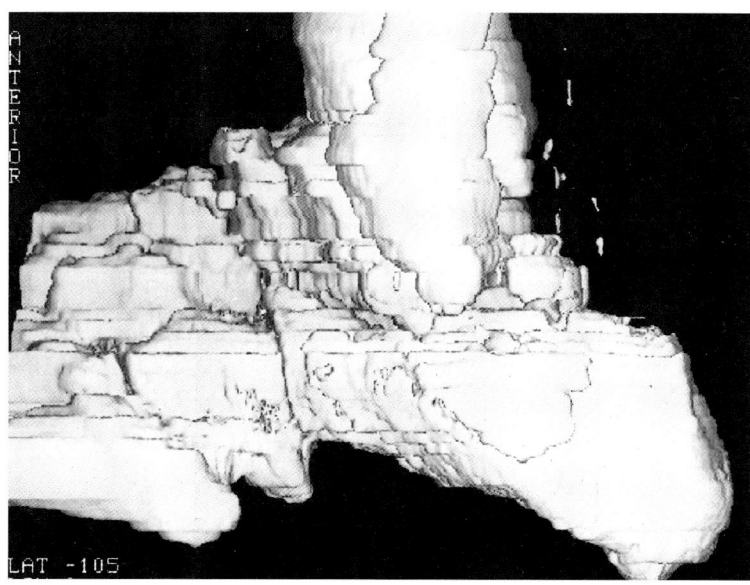

Figure 7. A: Three-dimensional object reconstruction, medial view demonstrating external bony plates, displacements of the fractures, "shingling," and impingement. **B:** Three-dimensional object reconstruction, axial view demonstrating external bony plates, displacements of the fractures, "shingling," and impingement. **C:** Three-dimensional object reconstruction, lateral view demonstrating external bony plates, displacements of the fractures, "shingling," and impingement.

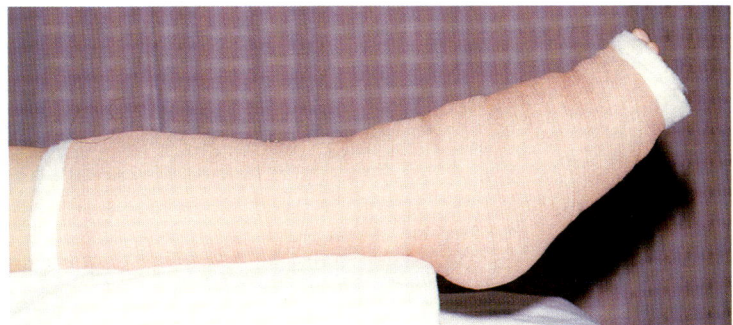 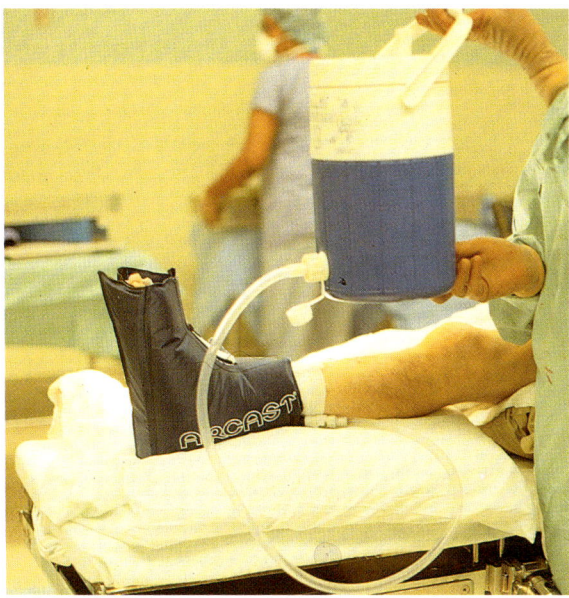

Figure 8. A: Bulky "Jones" type dressing. **B:** Cryocuff ice water compression dressing.

SURGERY

The important surgical concept to understand is that the sustentacular fragment that remains with the talus is the fragment that is in a normal anatomic position, and that the other fragments must be reduced to it (8,10,11,13,14,16,18–20). The tuberosity fragment must be reduced to its proper position relative to the sustentacular fragment and the fragments of the posterior facet articular surface are repositioned. It is important that before the tuberosity fragment can be reduced, disimpaction of the fragments must occur. In fact, the articular surface fragments that have rotated inferiorly must be elevated to prevent them from blocking the movement and reduction of the tuberosity fragment. As the calcaneus is brought out to normal height and length, the walls of the calcaneus, either medial or lateral, also move into appropriate alignment.

The calcaneus may be surgically approached either medially (3,9), laterally anterior to the peroneal tendons, or in a combination medial and lateral approach. Another surgical approach is by Sangeorzan's modification of the Letournel's lateral extensible approach (10). Each approach has its advantages and disadvantages.

My personal preference for the more common calcaneal fracture open reduction and internal fixation is through the medial approach combined usually with a lateral approach anterior to the peroneal tendons.

It is my practice to approach foot surgery as though it is hand surgery and use appropriate small surgical instruments. Number 15 scalpel blades, small tenotomy scissors, Freer elevators, small Key elevators, and Joker elevators are necessary. Joseph skin hooks (10 mm wide), ragnel retractors, somewhat larger 90° (right-angle) retractors, such as Mason's or Army-Navy's, and a baby Inge lamina spreader are used. Also available should be a small drill, such as a 3M type mini-driver, Kirschner wires, Steinmann pins, and standard fracture wire staples. A small fragment screw set is also used.

Under general or spinal anesthesia, the patient is placed supine on the operating table with a small lift underneath the buttock of the affected side. During the procedure on the medial side, the patient's injured limb is flexed at the knee and externally with the fractured foot placed across the opposite uninjured extremity and rested on the padded leg. During the lateral approach, the patient's injured extremity is placed on a towel booster with internal rotation at the hip.

Technique. It is helpful to mark the anatomic structures preoperatively so as to maintain orientation after draping (Fig. 9). Anatomical landmarks easily palpable are the medial aspect of the navicular and the medial malleolus. The line of the posterior tibial tendon can be represented, going from the area of the overlapping posterior aspect of the medial malleolus directly to the navicular tuberosity. Just posterior to this line is the flexor digitorum longus and then the neurovascular bundle. The medial incision is made two to three fingers' breadth below the medial malleolus parallel to the plantar surface of the foot. The neurovascular bundle often crosses in the anterior one-third of this incision. The incision should be below the level of the sustentaculum tali.

The first structure encountered is fascia overlying the abductor hallucis, as well as the short flexors of the foot (Fig. 10). This fascia is split and the underlying muscle belly is split along the line of its fibers using blunt dissection. This uncovers the neurovascular bundle in the anterior portion of the wound (Fig. 11). The calcaneal branch of the posterior tibial nerve is located in the posterior aspect of the wound, and should be preserved. Neurovascular structures are retracted with a rubber vessel loop and mobilized proximally and distally. Once the neurovascular structures are identified and mobilized, a small Key elevator can be used to expose the fracture fragments along the medial wall of the calcaneus (Fig. 12).

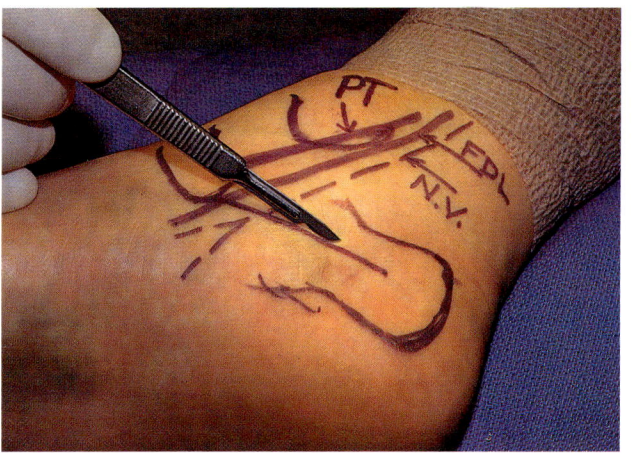

Figure 9. Preoperative marking of the medial side of the foot for McReynolds medial approach.

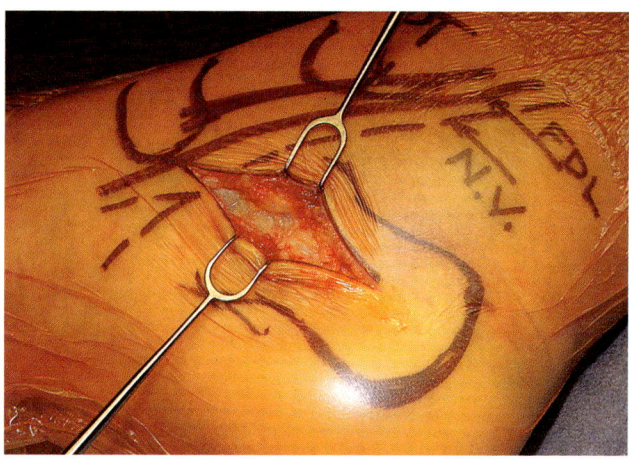

Figure 10. Fascia of the abductor hallucis is exposed.

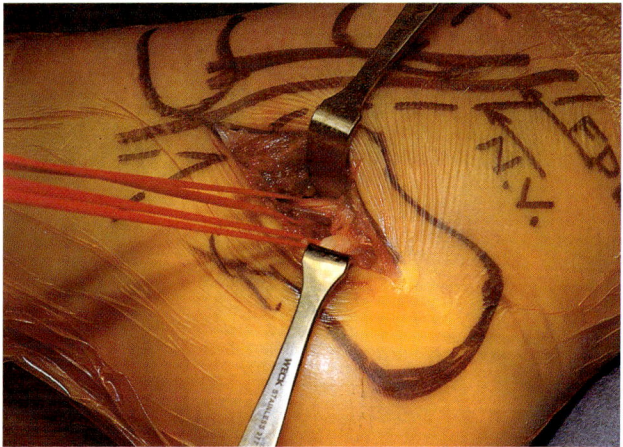

Figure 11. Posterior tibial neurovascular bundle is exposed and marked/protected.

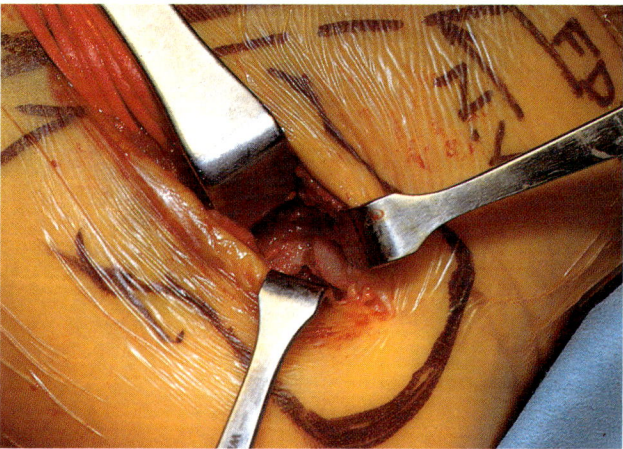

Figure 12. Medial wall fracture fragments—initial exposure.

It is at this point that a good three-dimensional orientation of the fracture must be present in the surgeon's mind, as only a small portion of the bone will be exposed. The key point is that the sustentacular tali fragment is the fragment that is in an anatomic position and the remainder of the fragments must be reduced to this sustentacular tali fragment. As the fracture is exposed from the medial side, the most medial fragment will be the sustentacular fragment and its medial wall. This will be overlying the medial wall of the calcaneal tuberosity, just like shingles on a roof. The tuberosity has shifted laterally, anteriorly, and proximally and into varus rotation. Hence, dissection of the medial calcaneal wall proceeds in a plantar direction, initially exposing the edge of the overlying sustentacular fragment until the medial wall of the tuberosity fragment can be palpated and then visualized. There is often depression of the tuberosity fragment of 5 mm or more from the sustentaculum tali fragment (Fig. 13). The fracture of this medial wall is not always a single fracture line.

Once the fracture line and calcaneal fragments have been identified, it is necessary to disimpact the fracture to allow reduction of the tuberosity fragment to the sustentacular fragment. If the lateral portion of the posterior facet has been markedly rotated down into the body of the calcaneus, this will block reduction of the tuberosity fragment because of the interposition. This disimpaction is accomplished by inserting a Freer or Joker elevator into the fracture line across the calcaneus and passing it posterior and inferior to the lateral portion of the posterior facet. The posterior facet fragments are then disimpacted and pushed upward

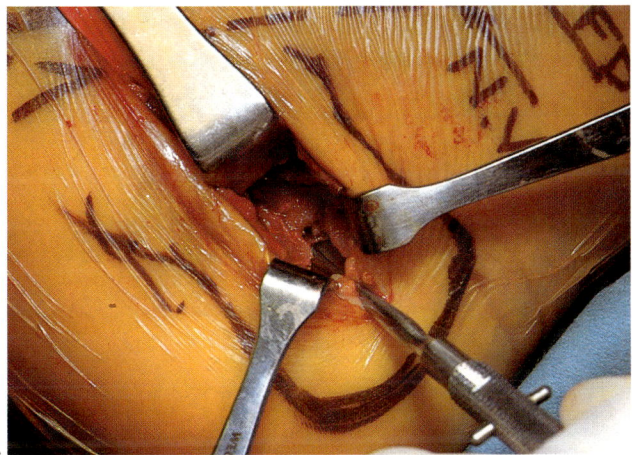
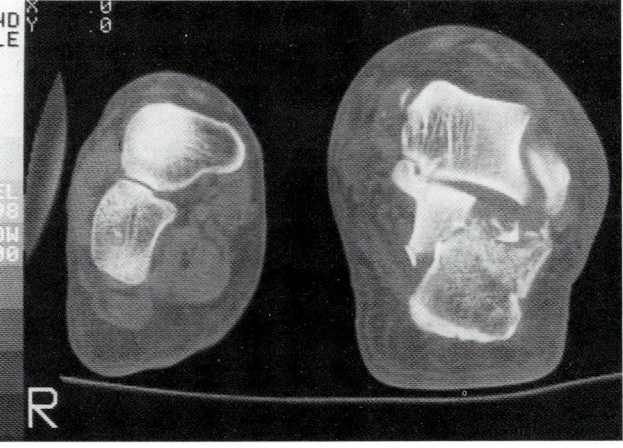
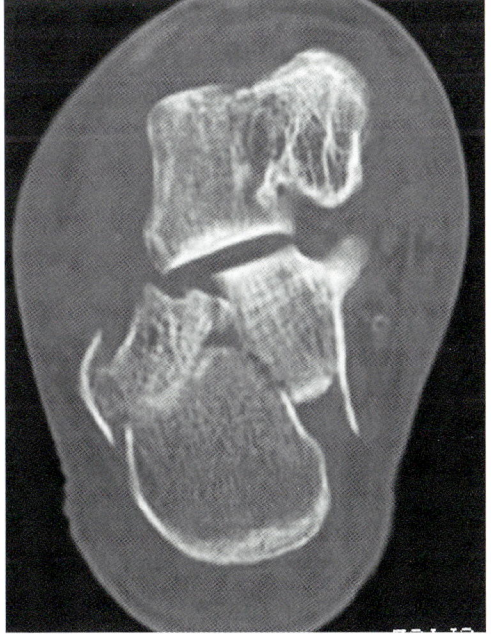

Figure 13. A: Medical wall "shingling" actual bone with Freer under "shingle of sustentaculum." **B** and **C:** CT scans of coronal view demonstrating "shingle" at exposed bone.

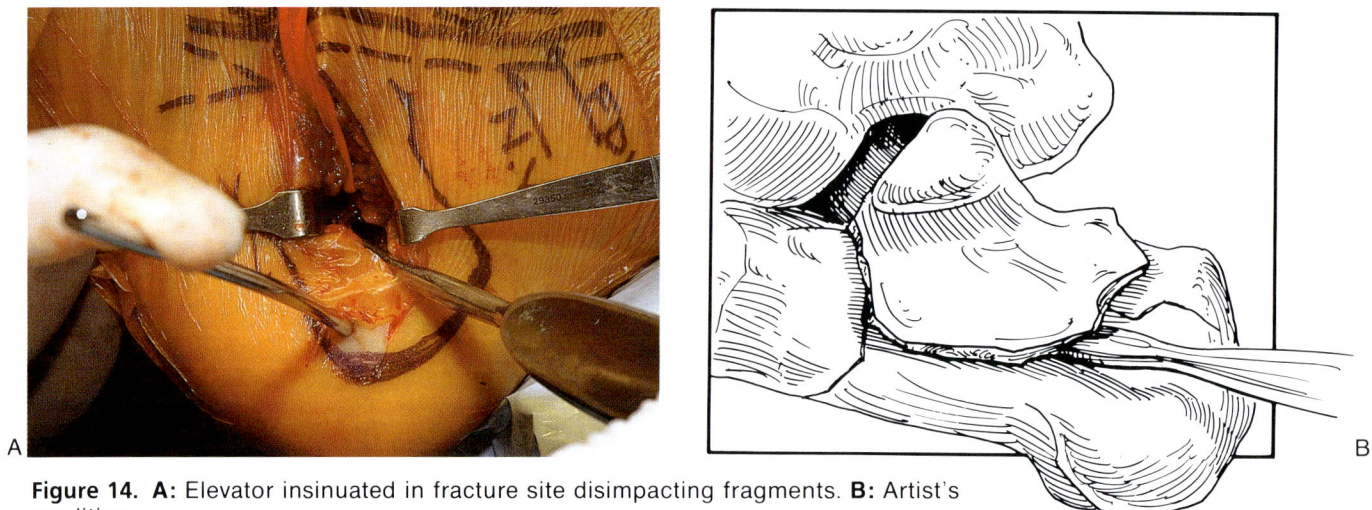

Figure 14. A: Elevator insinuated in fracture site disimpacting fragments. **B:** Artist's rendition.

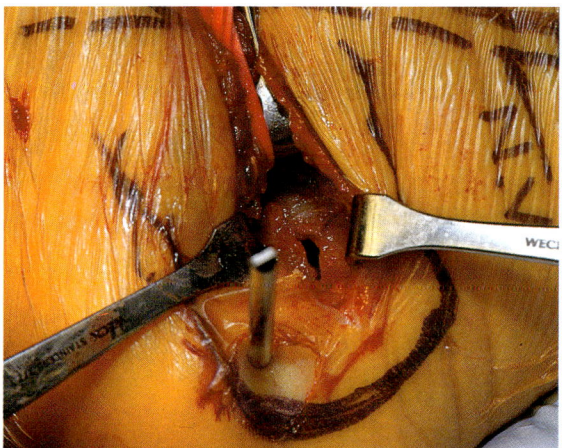

Figure 15. Reconstitution of the medial wall. Steinmann's pin through the tuberosity fragment for control and traction is visible.

toward the talus. At the same time, the tuberosity fragment is disimpacted posteriorly and inferiorly and out of varus (Fig. 14).

It is frequently helpful to place a Steinmann pin transversely through the most posterior and inferior aspect of the tuberosity to allow control of the tuberosity fragment as it is manipulated. Through these maneuvers, the tuberosity can usually be shifted back medially until it is reduced to the sustentacular fragment. At this point, the medial wall has been reconstituted (Fig. 15). The normal concavity and smooth aligned surface of the medial wall should be visualized and palpated by the surgeon at this time. Small comminuted fragments that may have worked free during the reduction are useful as spacers, much like placing a jigsaw puzzle together on the medial side, ensuring appropriate relationships to the two large fragments.

Once the position of the tuberosity to the sustentaculum tali has been established, a staple is used, not for compression, but rather as a bridging or spacing device to hold the tuberosity out to appropriate length and appropriately aligned. It is necessary to predrill the cortical holes for the staple, as there is not enough inherent stability in the medial calcaneal wall to allow the staples to be directly driven into the bone. The predrilling may be done either with a drill point or

Steinmann pin with the drill point appropriately sized to the staple. It is important that the staple be only impacted partially at this time. If the staple is completely impacted, and it is long enough to effect or penetrate fracture fragments on the lateral half of the calcaneus that are still displaced, subsequently repositioning these displaced fragments through the lateral approach will be difficult (Fig. 16). Standard staple drivers and holders are often too large for the incision. The staple is held and controlled with a 7-inch needle holder that is used for impaction.

Once the staple is in place, radiographs are made in the operating room. The views made are a lateral view of the heel, an axial view of the heel, and Broden's views (Fig. 17). If one can be certain from the Broden's view that the posterior facet is in an anatomic position, the fracture reduction portion of this surgical procedure is complete and the staple is completely impacted. However, if there is incongruity of the posterior facet, the lateral exposure of the calcaneus is done.

On the lateral side of the foot, the reference points marked are the head of the talus, the anterior process of the calcaneus, the lateral malleolus, and the base of the fifth metatarsal. The peroneal tendons course from the posterior aspect of the lateral melleolus to the base of the fifth metatarsal. An incision is made in the skin lines centered over the sinus tarsi and the anterior process of the calcaneus (Fig. 18). Through this incision, the fat over the sinus tarsi and the origin of the extensor digitorum brevis are reflected distally. The posterior facet of the calcaneus is exposed by opening the subtalar joint. Placement of a baby Inge lamina spreader into the sinus tarsi to distract the calcaneus from the talus is helpful. The lateral aspect of ligamentous restraint of the subtalar joint is opened and aids the exposure. Structures in the sinus tarsi should be opened completely to the medial wall so that an adequate exposure of the posterior facet of the calcaneus is made. Now the lateral aspect of the posterior facet will be exposed. It is often depressed and rotated with the anterior aspect of the facet more depressed than the posterior aspect (Fig. 19). Through this exposure, a Freer elevator or Joker elevator can be placed underneath this lateral aspect of the posterior facet and the fragment elevated to an anatomic position. Once this has been accomplished, the lateral wall of this facet, which previously had been buried in the body of the calcaneus, will be apparent with peroneal tendon retraction (Fig. 20). When this has been accomplished and with the lamina spreader in place, a view of the posterior facet in toto from lateral to medial is possible and anatomic restoration of the articular surface can be done. When an anatomic position has been obtained, the

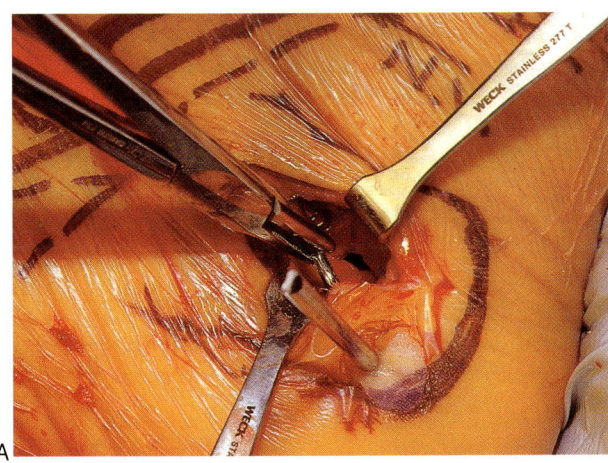
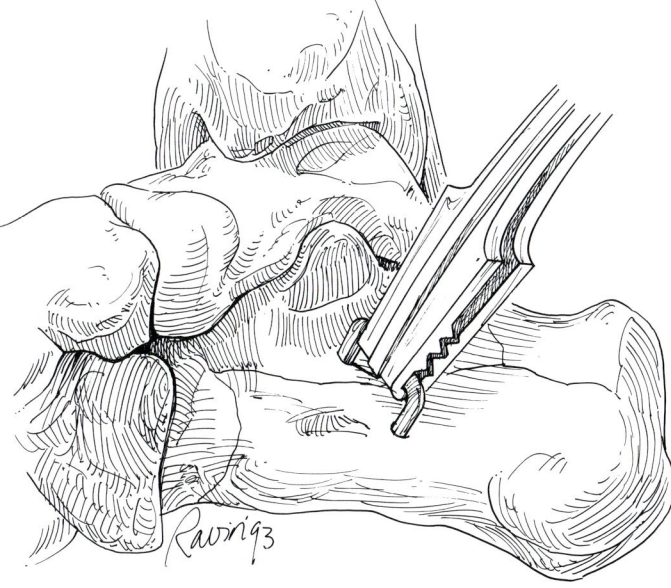

Figure 16. **A:** Staple placed initially. **B:** Artist's rendition and staple fixation.

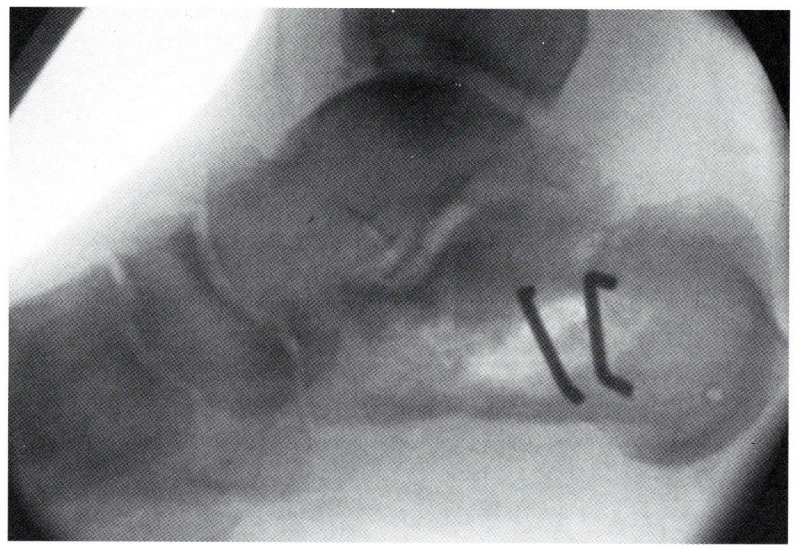

Figure 17. A: Intraoperative radiograph lateral-Böhler's angle reconstituted. **B:** Axial-medial wall reconstituted. **C:** Broden's view with the posterior facet split and unreduced.

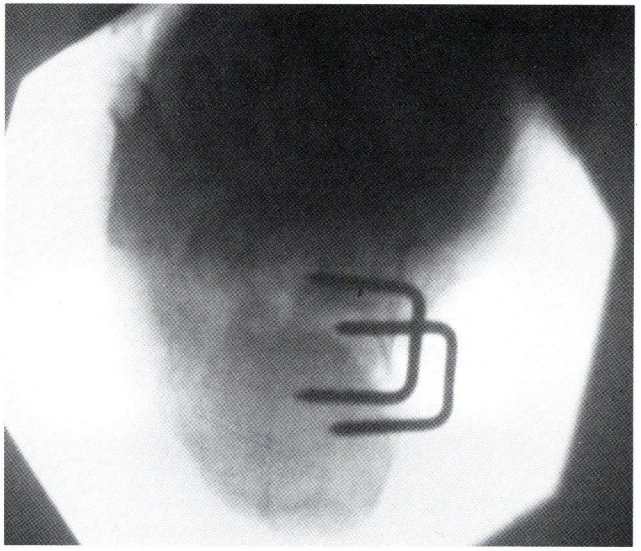
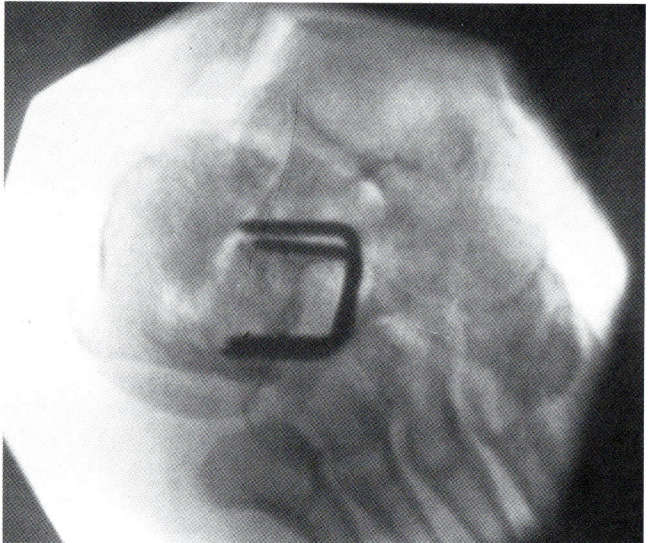

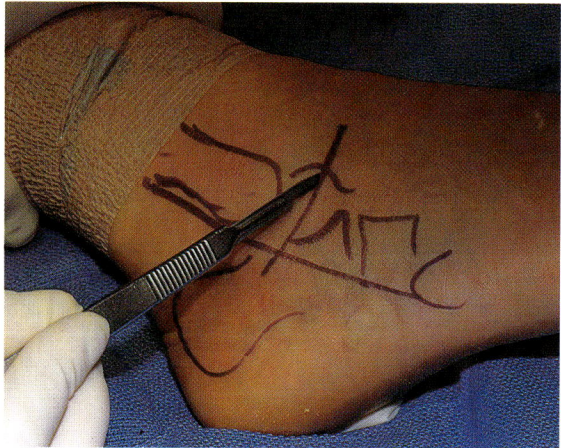

Figure 18. Lateral side of the foot marked for incision.

31 CALCANEAL FRACTURE

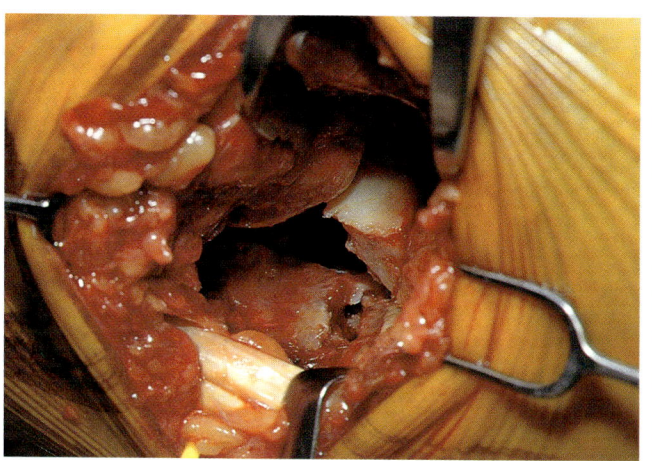
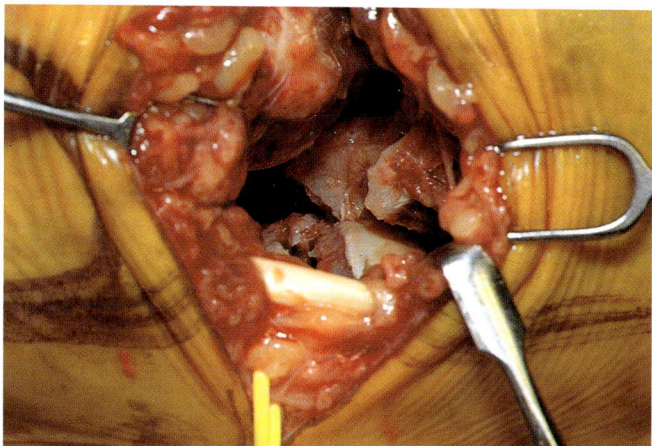

Figure 19. **A:** Lateral exposure. **B:** Lateral articular surface buried in body under anterior process.

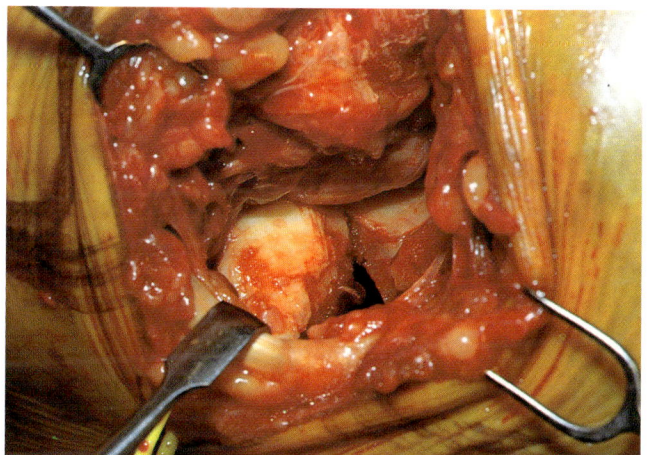
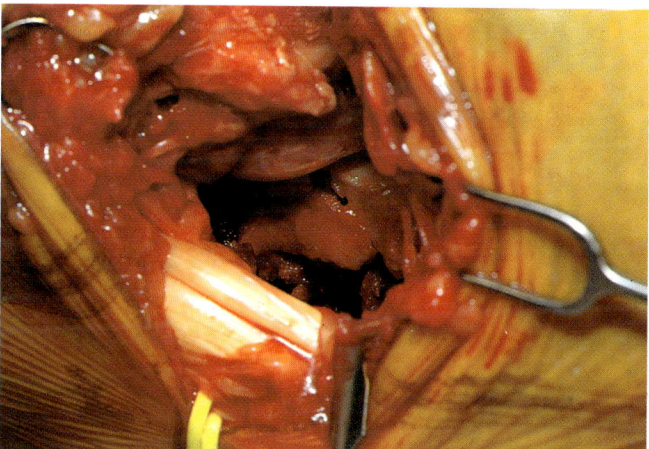

Figure 20. **A:** Lateral aspect of the posterior facet reduced visualized form lateral side partial reduction. **B:** Complete reduction.

pieces on the lateral wall should compress together and in fact the superior or dorsal cortical wall of the lateral side of the calcaneus has been reconstructed. Now the calcaneal tuberosity is in its proper position and the posterior facet is reduced.

Fixation is made from lateral to medial. Kirschner wires may be used to hold the fragments in place while radiographs are made. Final fixation is often obtained with transverse 4 mm diameter cancellous screws in the subchondral region of the posterior facet. Additional fixation can be secured from lateral to medial across the anterior aspect of the calcaneus into the area of the sustentaculum. An oblique wire may also be placed from anterolateral to posteromedial securing the anterior aspect of the calcaneus to the sustentacular fragment (Fig. 21). The medial wall is then reinspected, and the staples there are then completely impacted (Fig. 22). Radiographs now show the fracture reduction (Fig. 23). Once the radiographs are satisfactory, the Kirschner wires are cut off at a subcutaneous level, the tourniquet is released, and final hemostasis is obtained.

Anticipate a significant amount of bleeding from the bone, both medially and laterally. On the medial side, the fascia overlying the neurovascular bundle is closed loosely with three or four sutures of 3–0 Vicryl and the skin is closed in

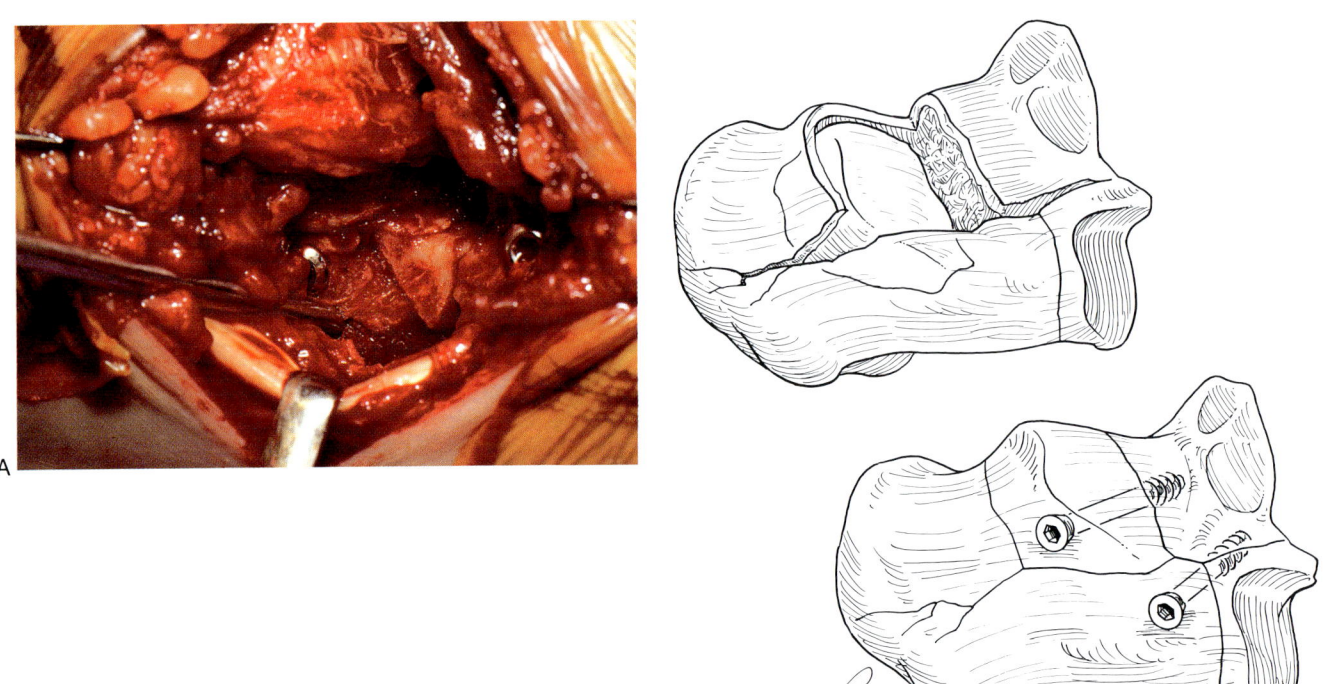

Figure 21. A: Lateral fixation viewed from lateral. **B:** Artist's rendition of lateral reduction and fixation.

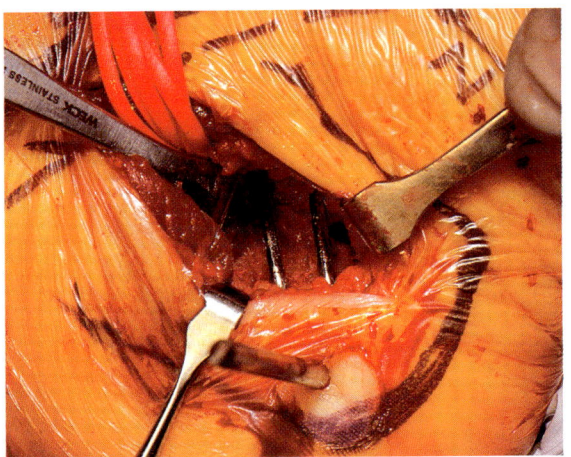

Figure 22. Medial staples impacted.

interrupted sutures so as not to impede the wound drainage that is anticipated. On the lateral side, the extensor brevis is tacked back to the point of origin on the peroneal sheath, and again the skin is closed with interrupted suture to allow wound drainage. The dressing applied in the operating room is a compressive dressing made up of multiple fluff-type sponges wrapped with sterile Webril. Over this, the foot and ankle cryocuff unit is placed, and the foot and ankle then splinted with plastic strips in a position of slight equinus. This is done so as not to place tension on the Achilles tendon and triceps surae, which would tend to disrupt the fracture reduction by pulling the tuberosity back into its displaced position and apply pressure on the posterior facet.

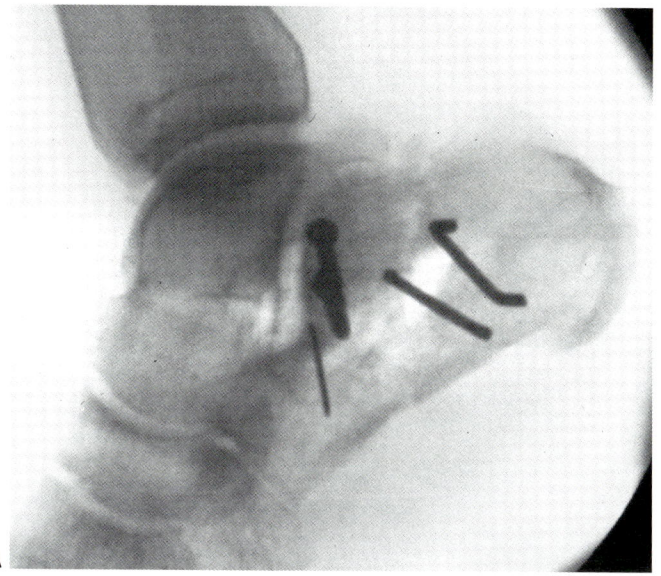
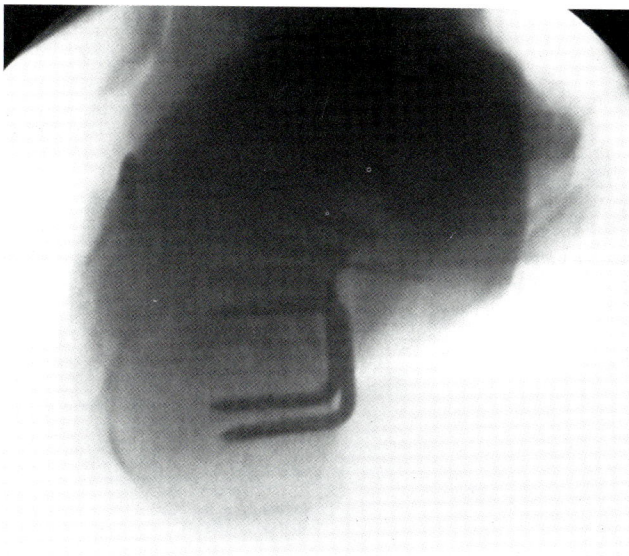
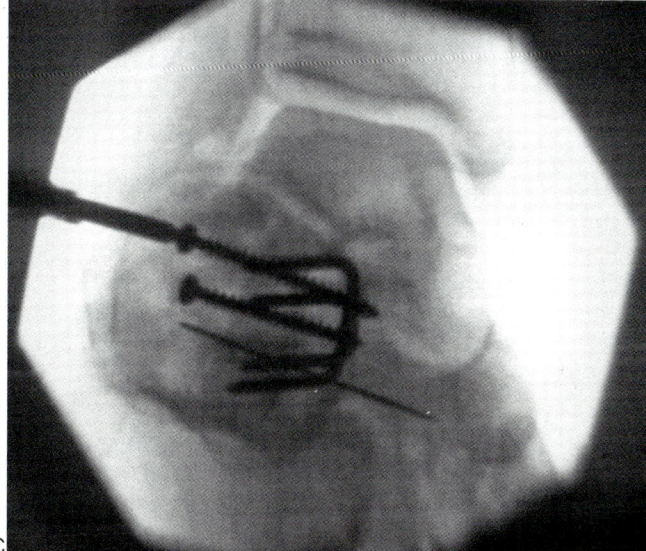

Figure 23. Radiographs after lateral and final medial fixation. **A:** Lateral view. **B:** Axial view. **C:** Broden's view.

POSTOPERATIVE MANAGEMENT

At 48 to 72 hours, the dressing is removed and the wound inspected. A short leg cast can then be applied with the foot in slight equinus. This cast is changed in about 10 days when the sutures are removed, and the foot is then again held in a position of slight equinus. At about 4 weeks postoperative the cast is removed and the foot brought up into a more neutral position as much as can be accomplished easily by the patient, and another cast is applied. At 6 weeks postoperatively, the patient is placed into the last short leg cast in a neutral position and partial weight bearing is allowed. At 8 weeks, casting is discontinued and the patient is usually full weight bearing at this time. Then a sneaker with a padded heel is used and the patient sent to physical therapy. At physical therapy, range of motion exercises of the ankle and subtalar joint is instituted along with gastrocoleus muscle strengthening.

The results expected to be obtained from open reduction and internal fixation of acute calcaneal fractures with a comminuted posterior facet do not vary according to the surgical approach used. Instead if the principles governing reduction are followed and a satisfactory fracture reduction obtained, the results of surgical care are similar. If the external architecture of the calcaneus is reconstructed, the patients can be expected to get back into standard shoes without the problems of peroneal impingement or impingement of the distal fibula on the calcaneus or on the shoe. If the height and proper talar inclination is regained, ankle motion will be unaffected. The patient can expect approximately 50% of the subtalar motion of the unaffected side to remain about a neutral position. This amount of motion is satisfactory for normal gait and foot function. In my experience, occurrence of symptomatic subtalar posttraumatic arthritis is low. However, no good studies exist at this time that compare injuries of equal magnitude treated with and without surgical care to determine the possible benefits of surgical calcaneal fracture treatment.

COMPLICATIONS

Infection is a possible postoperative complication of surgical treatment of the calcaneus fracture. Prevention of infection starts with preoperative prevention of fracture blister formation by application of a compressive dressing with elevation of the foot. Avoidance of surgery through early fracture blister formation is also felt to help avoid the complication of infection.

Wound necrosis is a possible complication that again is prevented by appropriate intraoperative and postoperative care. It is important to avoid creating successive layers of tissue, but to instead raise the skin flap in as thick and well vascularized a flap as possible. A postoperative dressing that prevents swelling in the wound along with adequate immobilization is also felt to be important.

The medial approach to the calcaneus does involve retraction of the tibial nerve. Transient hypesthesia in the sensory distribution of this nerve may occur during the postoperative period. The fracture reduction, however, will relieve pressure on the tarsal tunnel and in fact decrease the possible complication of the acute tarsal tunnel syndrome as a result of the calcaneal fracture.

With the lateral approach to the calcaneus, particular care is given to protect the sural nerve, which is located just inferior to the peroneal tendons. Awareness of this nerve position will decrease the likelihood of inadvertent transection of the nerve in the posterior aspect of the incision.

The decreased range of motion in the subtalar joint following surgical care is an expected result and really not a complication. It is important that the patient understand before surgery is undertaken that this is expected.

ILLUSTRATIVE CASE FOR TECHNIQUE

The patient is a 45-year-old man who fell 10 feet from a pole injuring his heel. He did not have any associated injury to his back or legs. The hindfoot was swollen and tender with medial and lateral ecchymosis. The dorsal pedis was palpable. There was no neurologic deficit. There were no signs of compartment syndrome. There were no fracture blisters.

The original plain films that accompanied the patient demonstrated the comminuted intraarticular joint depression type fracture. The lateral view (Fig. 24) demonstrates the loss of Böhler's angle. The axial view (Fig. 25) demonstrates the oblique shearing fracture, the lateral shift of the tuberosity, and suggests lateral impingement. Broden's view (Fig. 26) demonstrates the split of the posterior facet.

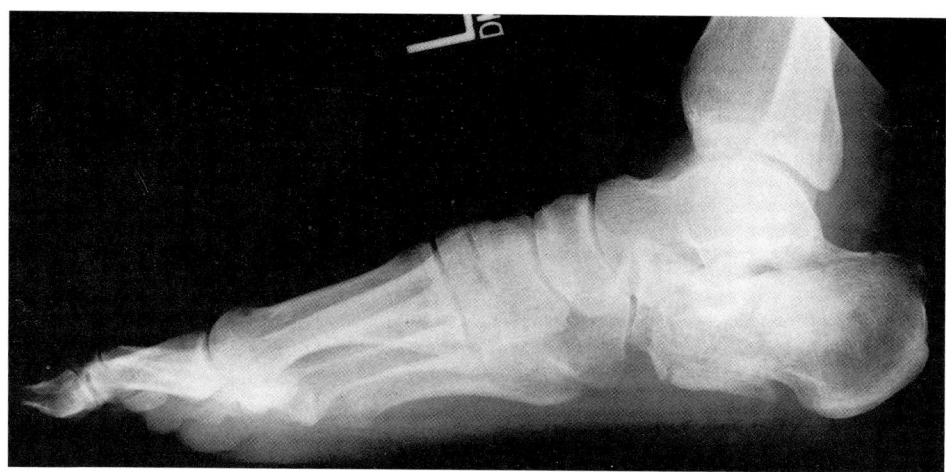

Figure 24. Radiograph of lateral view, acute fracture.

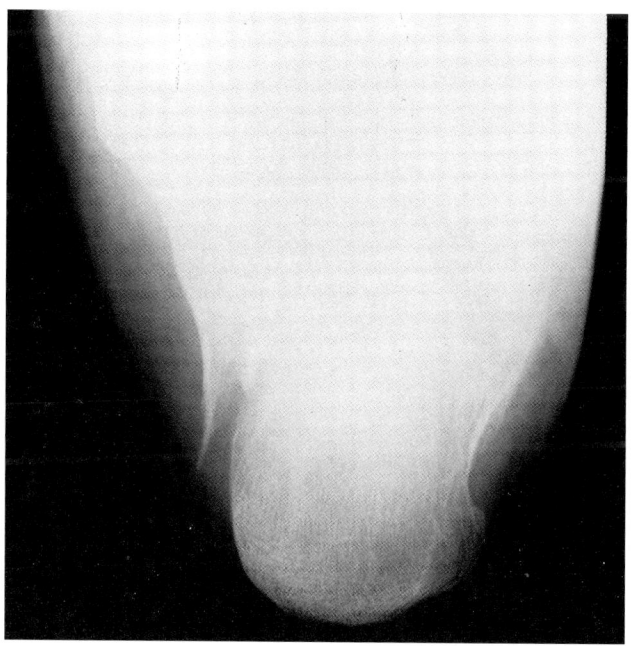

Figure 25. Radiograph of axial view, acute fracture.

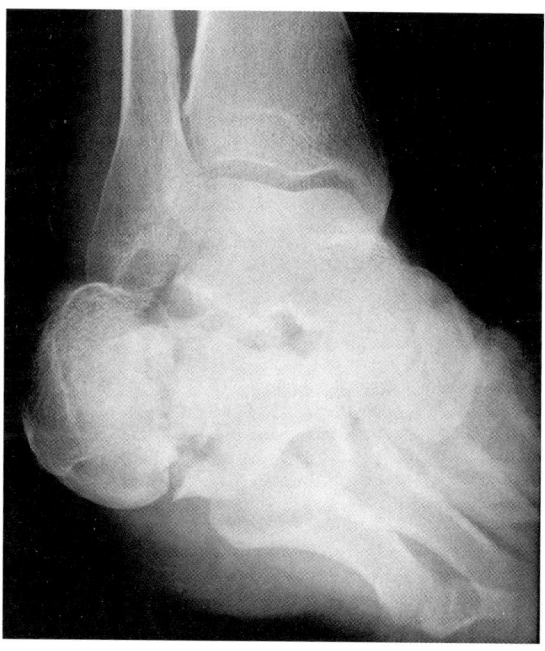

Figure 26. Radiograph of Broden's view, acute fracture.

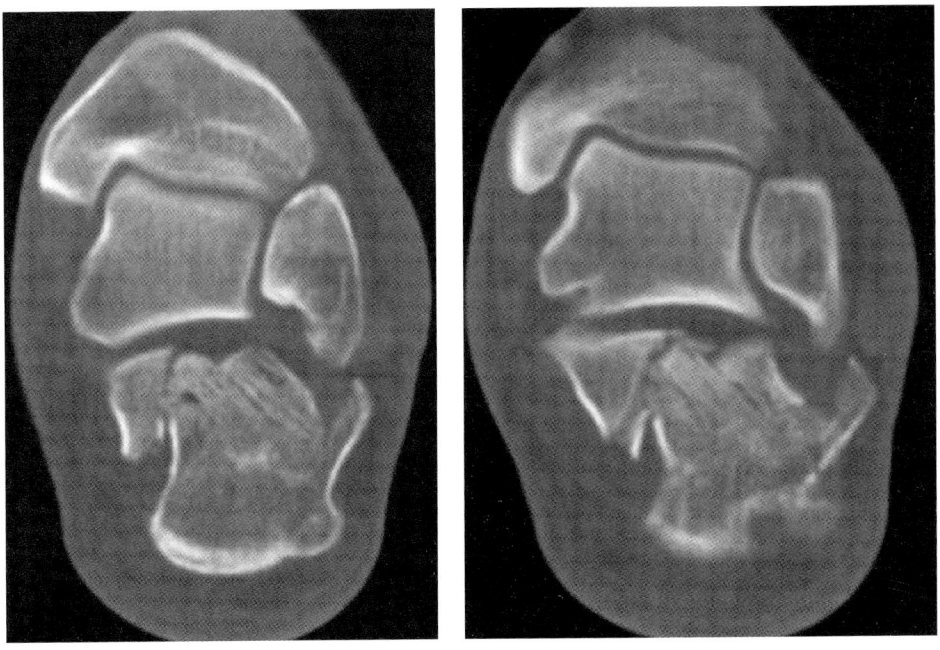

Figure 27. A and **B:** CT scan, acute fracture, coronal cut demonstrating lateral shift of tuberosity, anatomic position and sustentaculum, lateral impingement, comminution of posterior facet, and shingle effect medially.

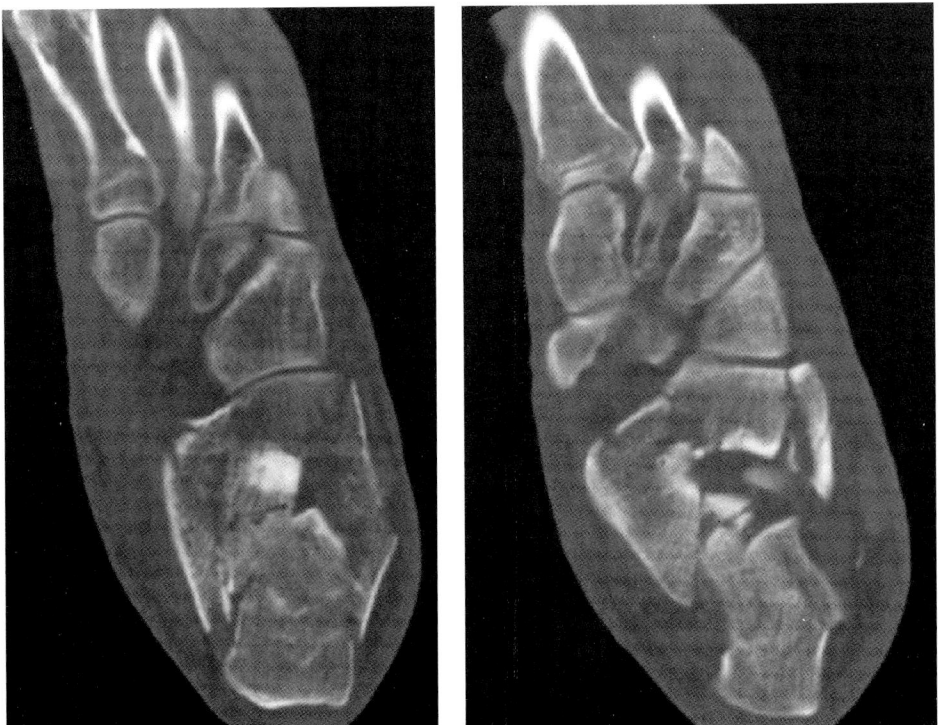

Figure 28. A and **B:** CT scan, acute fracture axial cuts demonstrating shortening of heel, medial shingle effect, and rotation of posterior facet.

More sophisticated imaging was performed using CT. Coronal and axial cuts were made. Sagittal and three-dimensional reconstructions were performed. Coronal cuts (Fig. 27) demonstrated the lateral shift of the tuberosity, anatomic position of the sustentaculum, lateral impingement, comminution of the posterior facet, and the "shingle" effect medially. Axial cuts (Fig. 28) demonstrated shortening of the heel, the medial shingle, and rotation of the lateral aspect of the posterior facet, which is seen on edge. The sagittal reconstruction (Fig. 29) demonstrated depression and rotation of the lateral aspect of the posterior facet. The three-dimensional reconstructions shed further light on the external architecture of the fracture. When viewed from the rear (Fig. 30) the magnitude of the medial shingle, lateral shift of the tuberosity, and lateral impingement are appreciated. When viewed medially (Fig. 31), the overlap of the sustentaculum (shingle) and the shift of the tuberosity are seen. When viewed laterally (Figs. 32 and 33), the shingle is seen from the oblique perspective, whereas the impaction of the posterior facet can be seen from the direct lateral view.

An open reduction and internal fixation using combined medial and lateral approaches was planned. While awaiting surgery, the limb was elevated, and cryotherapy and compression were applied using the cryocuff. Surgery was performed 10 days postinjury.

The medial approach was made first, and reduction of the tuberosity fragment to the sustentaculum was accomplished. This reestablished the height and length of the calcaneus (Fig. 34). Initial fixation was provided by a staple that was only partially impacted so as not to interfere with manipulation of the lateral fragments. The lateral approach and reduction was then performed. The lateral aspect of the posterior facet was disimpacted and derotated and the articular surface was

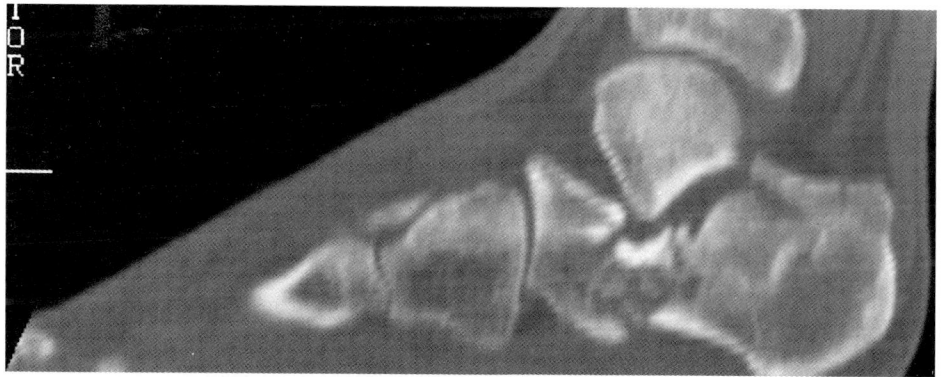

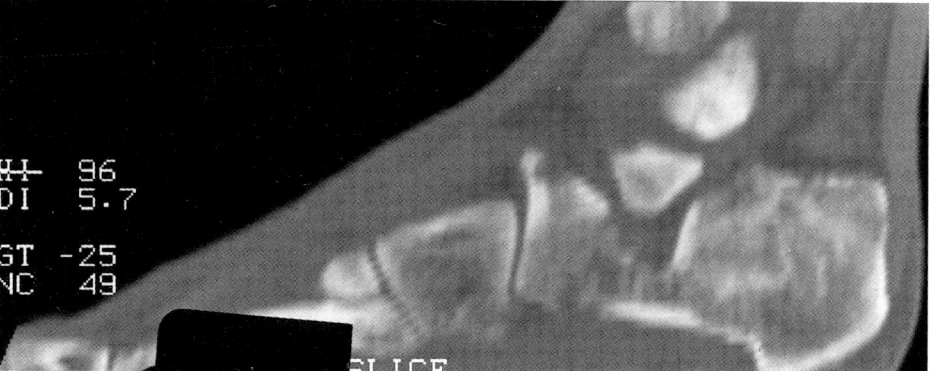

Figure 29. A and **B:** CT scan, acute fracture, sagittal reconstruction demonstrating depression and rotation of lateral aspect of posterior facet.

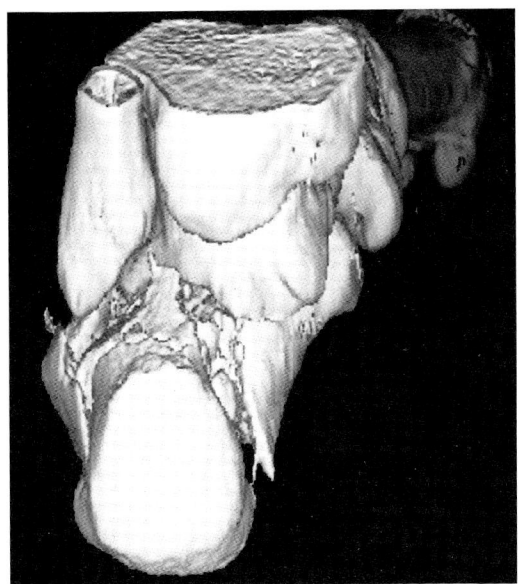

Figure 30. CT scan, three-dimensional reconstruction axial view showing medial shingle, lateral shift of tuberosity, and lateral impingement.

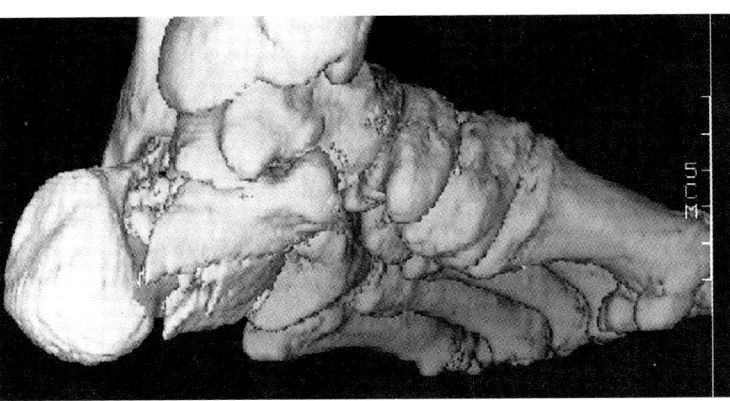

Figure 31. CT scan, three-dimensional reconstruction, medial view, demonstrating shingle effect and shift of tuberosity.

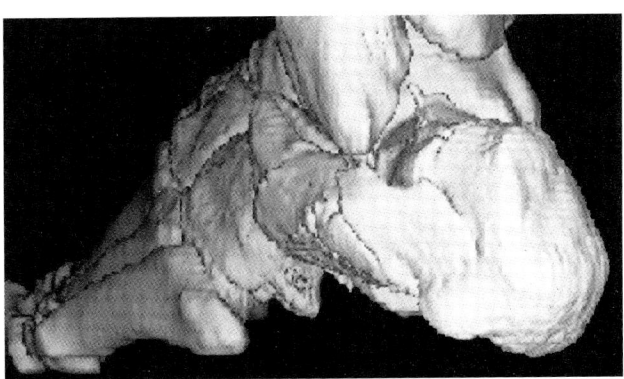

Figure 32. CT scan, three-dimensional reconstruction oblique lateral view, demonstrating shingle effect and shift of tuberosity.

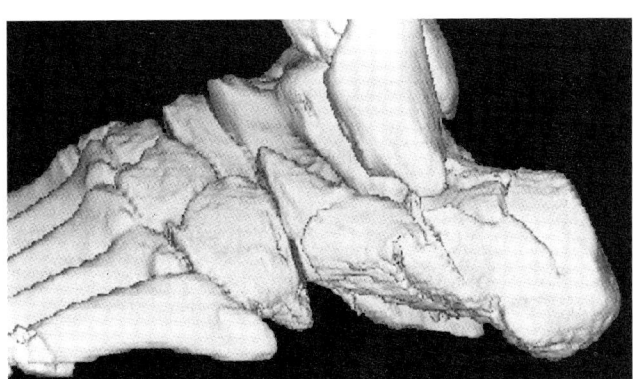

Figure 33. CT scan, three-dimensional reconstruction, lateral view demonstrating impaction of the posterior facet.

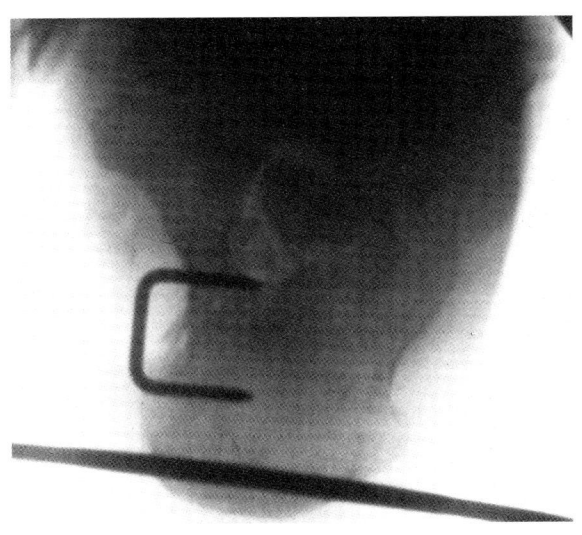

Figure 34. Intraoperative radiograph, axial view demonstrating horizontal Steinmann pin for traction and control, medial reduction and staple partially impacted.

reconstructed despite comminution. Temporary fixation was secured with K-wires (Fig. 35). Once this had been accomplished, final fixation was made with lag screws going from lateral to the sustentaculum medially and the staple was fully seated on the medial side. Two ancillary K-wires were used anteriorly (Fig. 36).

Postoperative management was immediate elevation using compressive cryotherapy (cryocuff) and splints. At 3 days postoperative, a short leg cast was applied with the ankle in mild plantar flexion to relieve tension on the tuberosity. Sutures were removed at postoperative day 10. The foot was held slightly plantar flexed for 4 weeks, at which time it was gradually brought to a neutral position by cast changes at 4 and 6 weeks. Touch weight bearing was permitted at 6 weeks and casting was discontinued at 8 weeks. At 8 weeks, physical therapy was instituted. Ankle and subtalar range of motion are aided by use of the BAPS board. Gastrocnemius and soleus strengthening are also performed.

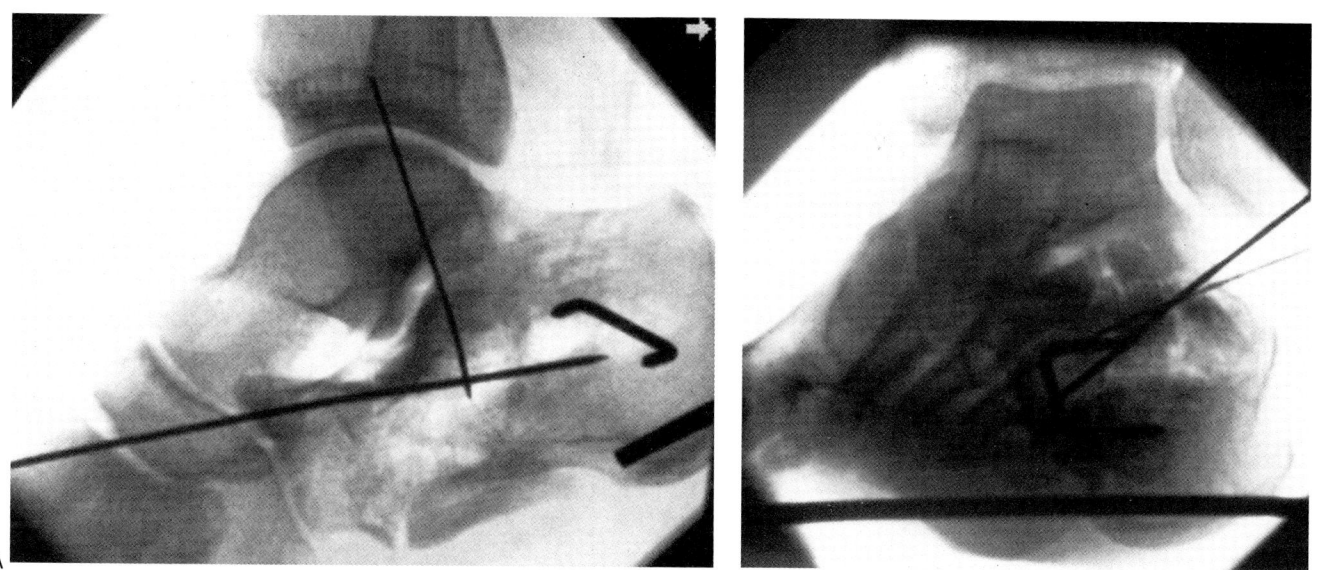

Figure 35. A and B: Intraoperative radiograph after lateral approach and reduction lateral view with temporary K-wire fixation. Broden's view demonstrating reduction of posterior facet.

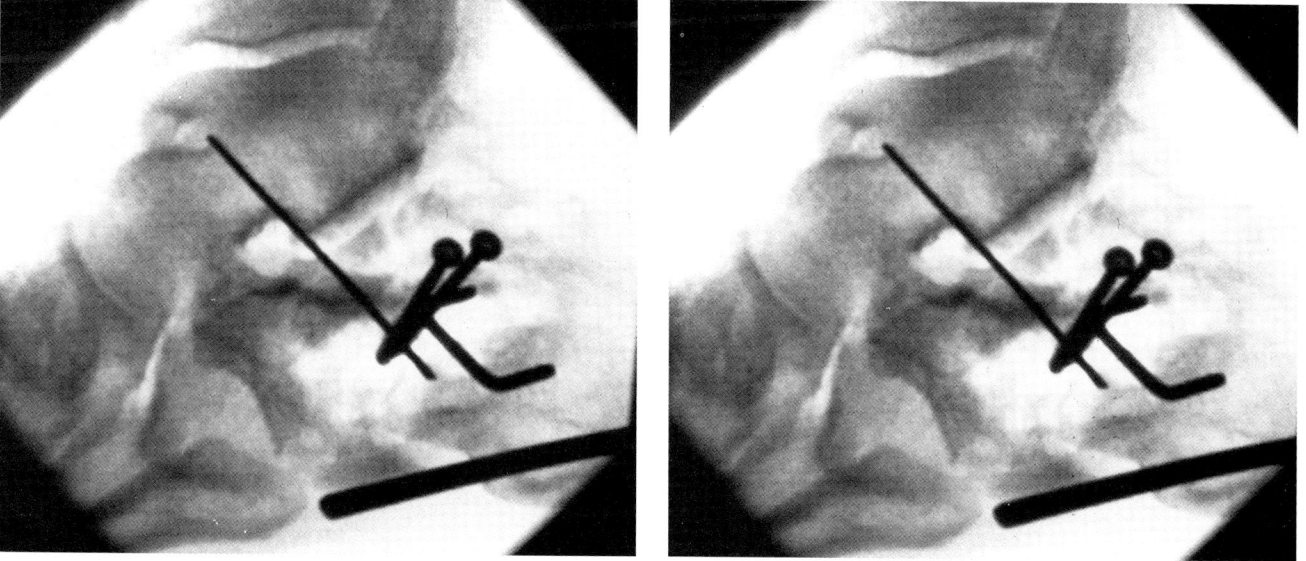

Figure 36. Intraoperative radiograph—final fixation. A: Lateral view. B: Broden's view.

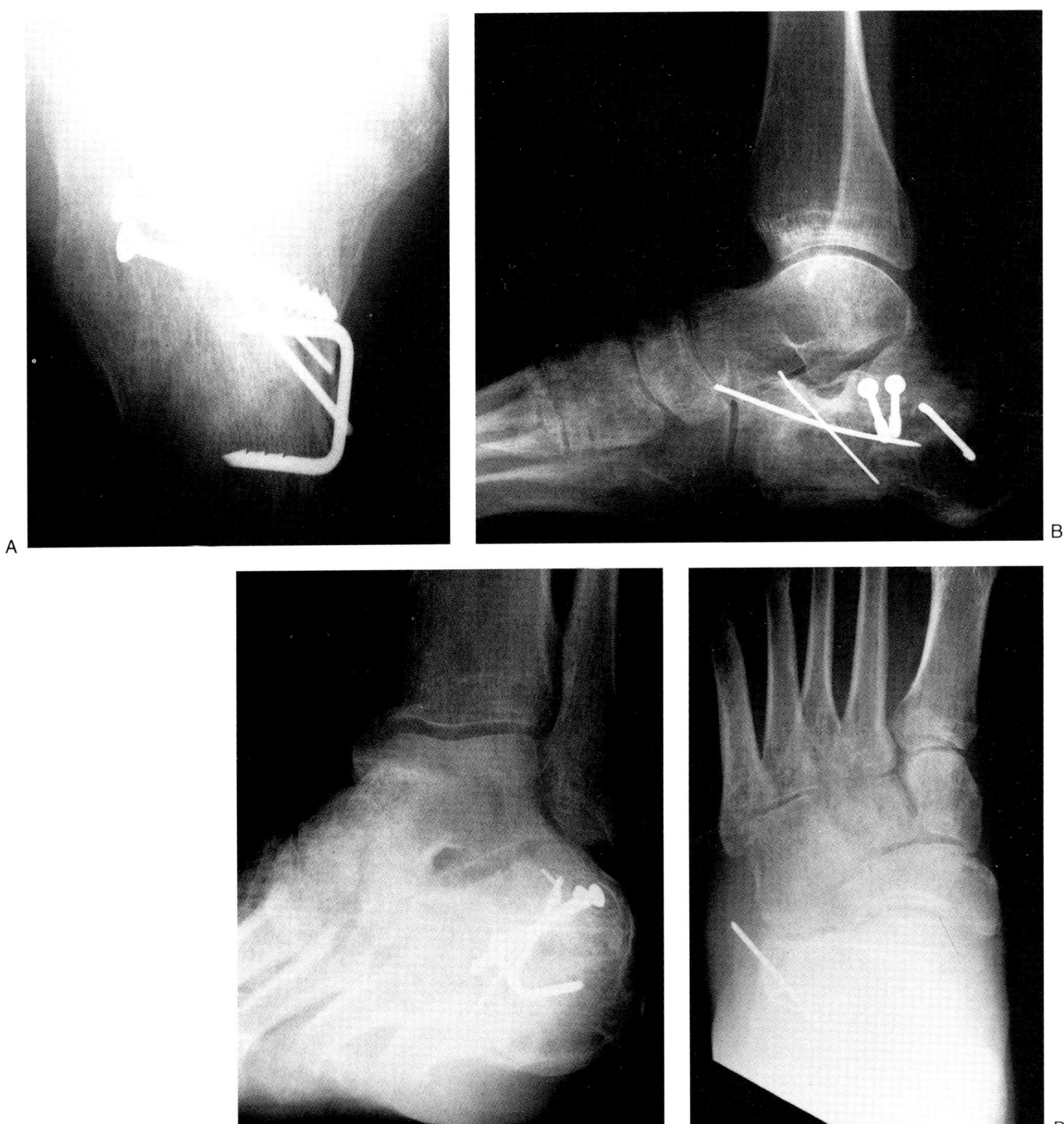

Figure 37. Final result radiographs demonstrating reestablishment of Böhler's angle, congruent posterior facet, normal width and length of heel, intact calcaneocuboid joint. **A:** Axial view. **B:** Lateral view. **C:** Broden's view. **D:** AP view.

The final radiographs demonstrate the maintenance of the reduction (Fig. 37). The patient has returned to his profession of surveyor. He wears normal shoes, and is able to raise his body weight on the toes of the injured foot. Ankle motion is normal. Subtalar motion is 50% of normal from a neutral position, and the patient tolerates uneven terrain. A K-wire became prominent subcutaneously as the swelling diminished and was removed. He is without significant pain.

RECOMMENDED READING

1. Bohler, M.: Diagnoses, pathology and treatment of fractures of the os calcis. *J. Bone Joint Surg.*, 13: 75–89, 1931.
2. Bradley, S. A., and Davies, A. M.: Computerized tomographic assessment of old calcaneal fractures. *Br. J. Radiol.*, 63: 926–933, 1990.
3. Burdeaux, B. D.: Reduction of calcaneal fractures by the McReynold medical approach technique and its experimental basis. *Clin. Orthop.*, 17: 87–103, 1983.
4. Carr, J. B., Hansen, S. T., and Benirshke, S. K.: Subtalar distraction bone block fusion for late complications of the os calcis fractures. *Foot Ankle*, 9: 81–86, 1988.
5. Carr, J., Nato, A., and Stevenson, S.: Volumetric three-dimensional computed tomography for acute calcaneus fractures: preliminary report. *J. Trauma*, 4: 346–348, 1990.
6. Crosby, L. A., and Fizbiggons, T.: Computerized tomography scanning of acute intra-articular fractures of the calcaneus: a new classification system. *J Bone Joint Surg.*, 72A: 852–859, 1990.
7. Essex-Lopresti P.: The mechanism, reduction technique, and results in fractures of the os calcis. *Br. J .Surg.*, 39: 395–419, 1952.
8. Gianchino, A. A., and Uhthoff, H. K.: Intra-articular fractures of the calcaneus. *J. Bone Joint Surg.*, 71A: 784–787, 1989.
9. Gilmer, P. W., Herzenberg, J., Frank, L., et al.: Computerized tomographic analysis of acute calcaneal fractures. *Foot Ankle*, 6: 184–193, 1986.
10. Letournel, E.: Open reduction and internal fixation of calcaneus fractures. In: *Techniques of Orthopaedics: Topics in Orthopaedic Trauma* edited by P. Spiegel, University Park Press, Baltimore, pp. 173–192, 1984.
11. Leung, K., Chan, W., Shen, W., et al.: Operative treatment of intraarticular fractures of the os calcis. The role of rigid internal fixation and primary bone grafting: preliminary results. *J. Trauma*, 3: 232–240, 1989.
12. Manoli, A., and Weber, T. G.: Fasciotomy of the foot: an anatomical study special reference to release of the calcaneal compartment. *Foot Ankle*, 10(5): 267–275, 1990.
13. Mast, J., Jakob, R., Ganz, R.: *Planning and reduction in fracture surgery.* Springer-Verlag, Berlin, pp. 185–192, 1989.
14. Miller, M.: Surgical management of calcaneus fractures: indication and techniques. In: *American Academy of Orthopaedic Surgeons Instructional Course Lectures*, XXXIX, 9th ed., edited by W. B. Gree, pp. 161–165. American Academy of Orthopaedic Surgeons, Park Ridge, IL, 1990.
15. Palmer, I.: The mechanism and treatment of fractures of the calcaneus. Open reduction with the use of cancellous grafts. *J. Bone Joint Surg.*, 8: 180–197, 1948.
16. Romash, M. M.: Calcaneal fractures: three dimensional treatment. *Foot Ankle*, 8: 180–197, 1988.
17. Romash, M. M.: Reconstructive osteotomy of the calcaneus with subtalar arthrodesis for malunited calcaneal fractures. *Clin. Orthop.*, 1993. [In Press.]
18. Stephenson, J. R.: Displaced fractures of the os calcis involving the subtalar joint: the key role of the superior medial fragment. *Foot Ankle*, 4: 91–101, 1983.
19. Stephenson, J. R.: Treatment of displaced intra articular fractures of the calcaneus using medial and lateral approaches, internal fixation, and early motion. *J. Bone Joint Surg.*, 69A: 115–130, 1987.
20. Whittaker, A. H.: Treatment of fractures of the os calcis by open reduction and internal fixation. *Am. J. Surg.*, 74: 687–696, 1947.

32
Calcaneal Osteotomy and Arthrodesis for Malunited Calcaneal Fracture

Michael M. Romash

INDICATIONS/CONTRAINDICATIONS

The problems caused by the malunited calcaneal fracture become clear once the pathomechanics of this fracture are understood. An axial load on the foot causes the shearing fracture across the calcaneus. This fracture line often runs from superior-lateral to inferior-medial from a lateral view and in an anterior-lateral to posterior-medial direction through the posterior facet from a dorsal view of the calcaneus. As explained in Chapter 31 by Romash, "Calcaneal Fracture Open Reduction and Fixation," the sustentaculum tali stays in anatomic relationship to the remainder of the foot and the talus. The tuberosity fragment of the calcaneus displaces laterally, upward, anteriorly, and into varus. As this tuberosity displacement occurs, the lateral half of the talus impacts the lateral aspect of the posterior facet causing secondary fracture lines in the calcaneus. The result is a depression and rotation of the posterior facet. Also, anterior fractures through the anterior aspect of the calcaneus occur. This resultant displacement and destruction of the posterior facet, if not reduced, interferes with the function of the calcaneus (Fig. 1).

The calcaneus is a primary point of support for the body's weight in initial heel contact and mid-stance during ambulation. It is a pedestal in that it supports the posterior aspect of the talus at an appropriate height relative to the mid- and

---

M. M. Romash, M.D.: Department of Surgery, Uniform Services University of Health Sciences, Bethesda, MD; Suite D, 700 North Battlefield Boulevard, Chesapeake, VA 23320.

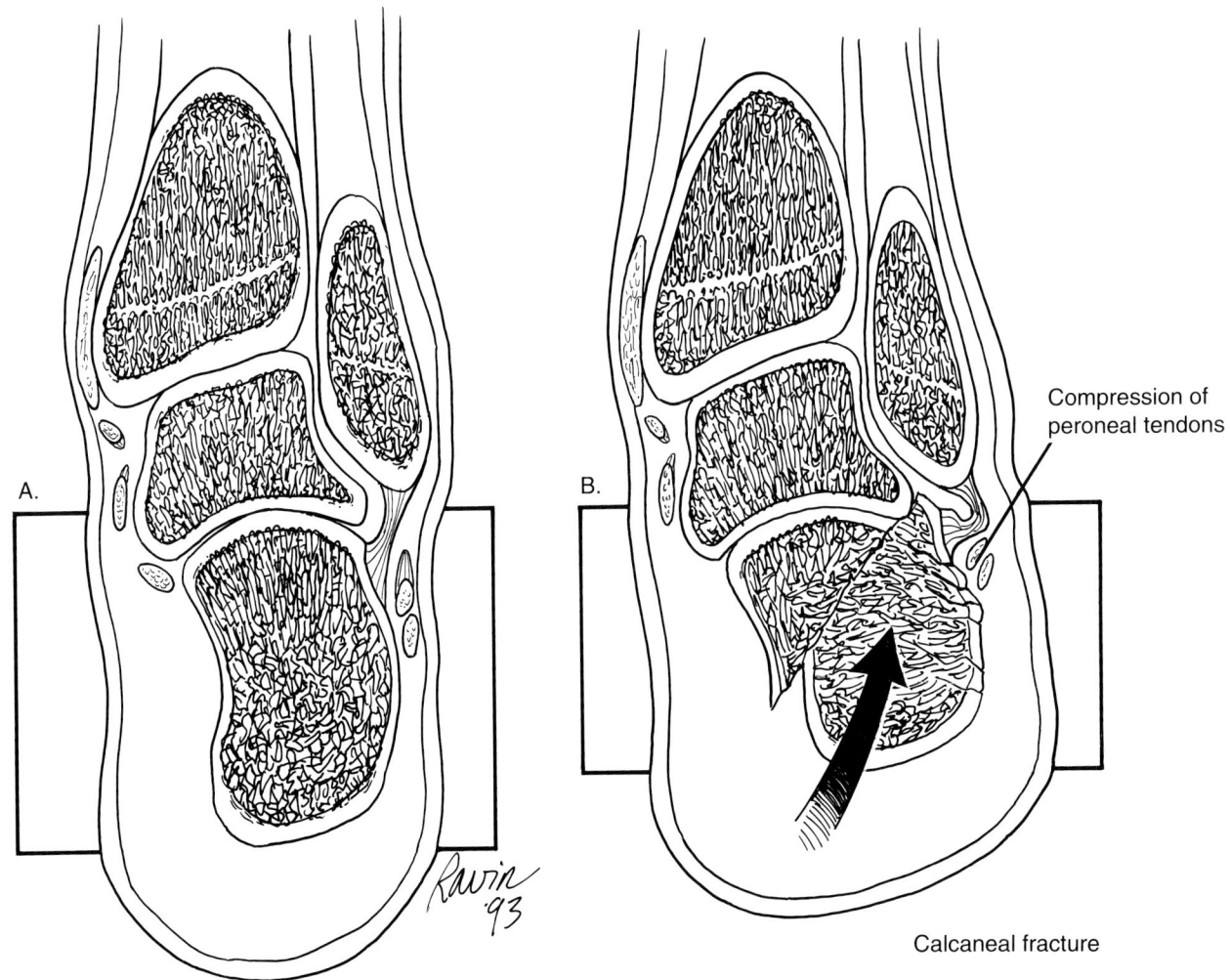

Figure 1. A: Normal shape of calcaneus—axial view. **B:** Displacement after fracture—axial view.

forefoot. This support of the talus by the calcaneus establishes the inclination of the talus relative to the floor and presents the appropriate portion of the articular surface of the talus to the tibia. Satisfactory ankle motion in plantar flexion and dorsiflexion is thus dependent to some degree on the proper height of the calcaneus. The calcaneus is also important as a center for hindfoot motion. Its joint surfaces articulate with the talus, cuboid, and the navicular tarsal articulations. These articulations must not only be smooth, but correctly arranged in their three-dimensional spatial array to ensure that the coordinated movement about these joints occurs with normal inversion and eversion of the foot. The shape of the calcaneus also permits unfettered passage of tendons about its medial and lateral sides and permits standard shoes to be worn. The relationship of the tuberosity to the foot provides the lever arm for the triceps surae and establishes appropriate length relationships for normal gait.

The malunited calcaneal fracture has multiple functional losses. Shortening of the foot diminishes the lever arm for the triceps surae, making it inefficient in plantar flexion of the foot. With the loss of support for the posterior aspect of the talus, the foot becomes flat as the pedestal function of the calcaneus is lost. The talus then undergoes relative dorsiflexion and changes its relationship in the ankle joint. As a result, there may be impingement anteriorly between the tibia and the neck of the talus and limited ankle dorsiflexion. The talonavicular joint is also adversely affected as the talus is dorsiflexed while the tarsal navicular remains in its normal position relative to the midfoot. This causes a subluxation at the talonavicular joint. The disruption of the posterior facet of the calcaneus results in a posttraumatic arthritis. The lateral, cephalad, and anterior displacement of the tuberosity fragment can cause direct impingement against the fibula and peroneal tendons (Fig. 2). Calcaneal tuberosity displacement also causes widening of the foot and loss of its height. This makes standard shoeing very difficult as the flat, short, and wide foot will impinge the malleoli on the normal counter of a shoe. The disruption of the three-dimensional spatial arrangement of the subtalur, calcaneocuboid, and talonavicular joints will disrupt coordinated multicentric motion through these joints.

Surgical treatment of the malunited calcaneal fracture must address all the above functional losses. It is necessary that operative correction will ablate the arthritis, and will reestablish the architectural relationships of the hindfoot to the midfoot. That is, it should reestablish both the height of the calcaneus and the normal inclination of the talus and its relationship to the navicular. Finally, it is important to relieve the fibular impingement and concomitantly narrow the heel.

It is my feeling that procedures such as arthrodesis in situ, whether they be subtalar or triple arthrodeses, are met with limited success. These procedures do not reestablish the height of the calcaneus and its relationship to the other tarsal bones. Also, I feel that a limited procedure to diminish the width of the heel by removing bone about the peroneal tendons and fibula would also meet with limited success, as the posttraumatic arthritis and architectural derangement of the foot are not corrected (Fig. 3).

The procedure described here corrects the malunited calcaneal fracture by recreating with an osteotomy the primary oblique shearing fracture. Then the tuberosity fragment is shifted medially, caudally, and posteriorly under the talus. In addition, a subtalar arthrodesis is also done (6). This procedure restores height and length to the heel, decompresses the lateral side by shifting the tuberosity away from the fibula, and ablates the posttraumatic arthritis by the arthrodesis.

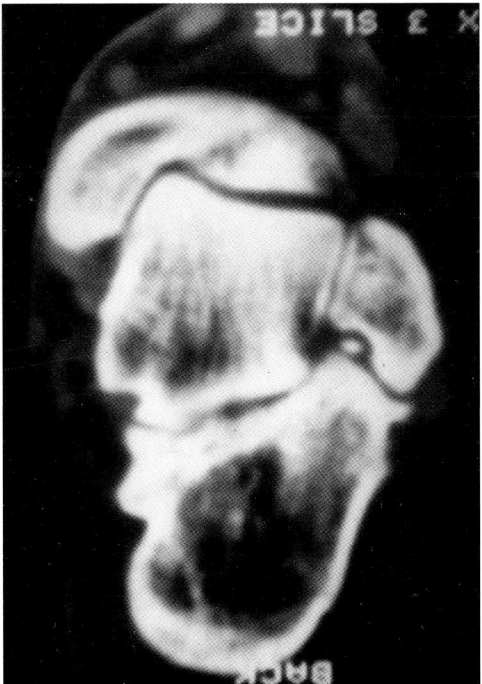

Figure 2. Coronal CT scan demonstrating displaced subtalar arthritis and fibular impingement.

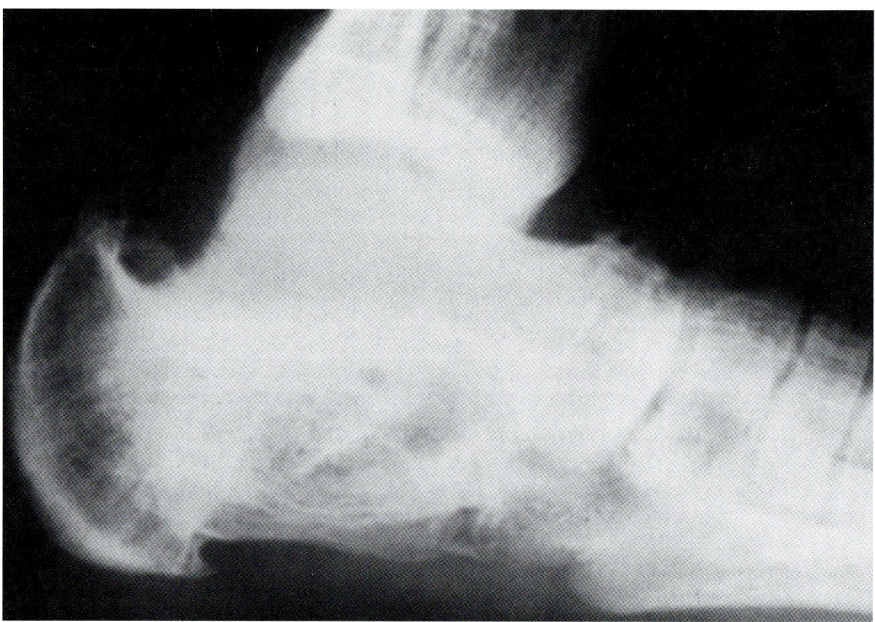

Figure 3. Triple arthrodesis done in situ with resultant abnormal architecture and talar inclination.

The ideal patient for this procedure would have a painful calcaneal fracture that had healed in a malposition. The primary displacement fracture line should be along the plane of the proposed osteotomy. A calcaneal fracture with many secondary fracture lines and comminution is not appropriate.

PREOPERATIVE PLANNING

Preoperative evaluation for this particular surgical procedure focuses on the patient's symptoms and radiographic evaluation.

The patient's pain should be of a degree to justify the procedure. In addition, problems such as difficulty with fit of shoes because of impingement on the malleoli or decreased ankle motion should be noted. Location of the patient's pain at the anterior ankle suggests anterior impingement; at the sinus tarsi suggests subtalar arthritis; at the subfibular region indicates possible impingement; and at the calcaneocuboid joint, direct fracture involvement and arthritis.

Radiographic evaluation is much the same as for the acute calcaneal fracture. Weight-bearing anteroposterior and lateral views of the foot along with the non–weight-bearing oblique and Broden's view are obtained. Also a computed tomography (CT) scan in the axial, coronal, and sagittal planes is necessary. A three-dimensional CT reconstruction is very helpful in planning the fracture's repositioning.

If the calcaneocuboid joint is involved with the fracture it may also need to be arthrodesed at the time of surgery. In an equivocal instance, a technetium bone scan may help determine whether or not the calcaneocuboid joint should be arthrodesed. If the calcaneocuboid joint does show activity on the technetium scan, it should probably also be arthrodesed.

SURGERY

It is my practice to use appropriate small surgical instruments. Number 15 scalpel blades, small tenotomy scissors, Freer elevators, small Kay elevators, and

Joker elevators are necessary. Joseph skin hooks (10 mm wide), ragnel retractors, somewhat larger 90° (right-angle) retractors, such as Mason's or Army-Navy's and a baby Inge lamina spreader are used. Also available should be a small drill, such as a 3M type minidriver, Kirschner wires, Steinmann pins, and standard fracture wire staples. A small fragment screw set is also used. Particularly helpful are small curved osteotomes and motorized burs to denude the subtalar cortical and articular surfaces. A cannulated cancellous 7-mm screw for tuberosity fixation and an external fixator distraction device facilitates tuberosity shift.

This procedure is done with the patient placed in a lateral debucitus position and the affected limb toward the surgeon on a bolster. This position allows easier passage of the final fixation screw through the tuberosity of the calcaneus into the talus. Both the extremity below the knee and the ipsilateral iliac crest are sterilely prepared and draped with a pneumatic tourniquet about the thigh.

Technique. After exsanguination and tourniquet inflation, a longitudinal incision is made centered over the sinus tarsi (Fig. 4). This allows access to the anterior process, body, and posterior facet of the calcaneus. The extensor digitorum brevis is reflected and the fat in the sinus tarsi is excised as necessary. Incision of the lateral ligament structures between the talus and calcaneus is done proceeding from anterior to posterior deep to the retracted peroneal tendons (Figs. 5 and 6). A baby Inge lamina spreader in the sinus tarsi between the talus and calcaneus provides distraction of the joint and exposure medially to the sustentaculum tali (Fig. 7).

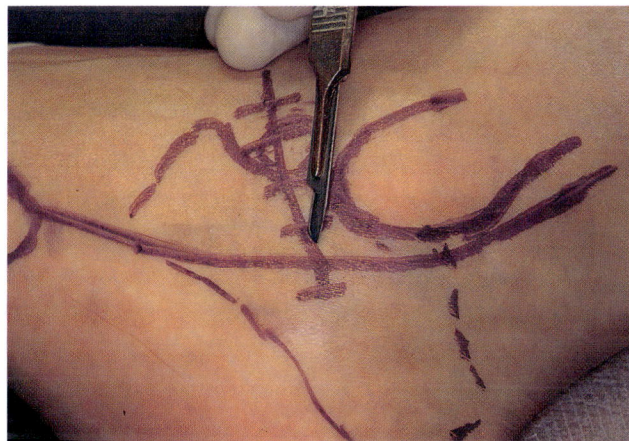

Figure 4. Diagram of skin incision.

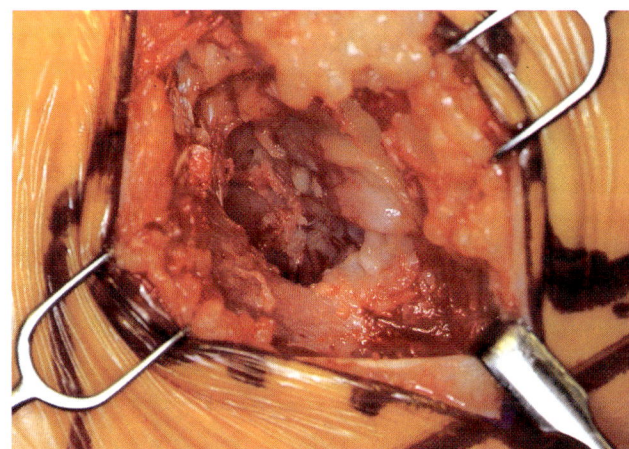

Figure 5. Sinus tarsi cleared, anterior lip of talus *(right)*.

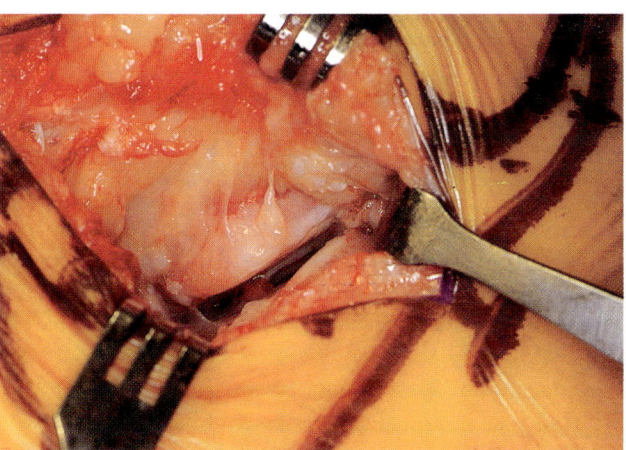

Figure 6. Lateral aspect of subtalar joint opened.

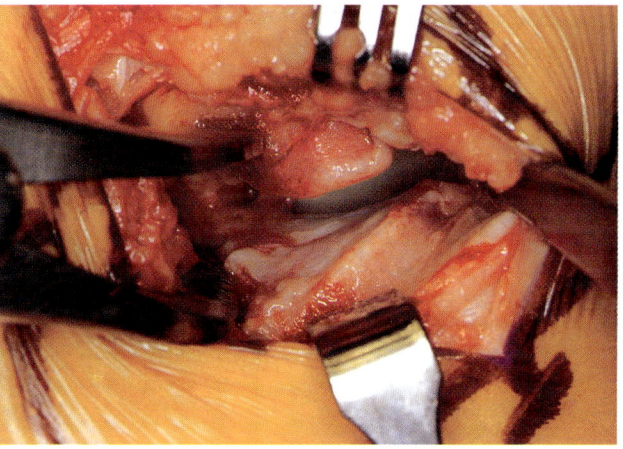

Figure 7. Subtalar joint spread with baby Inge lamina spreader.

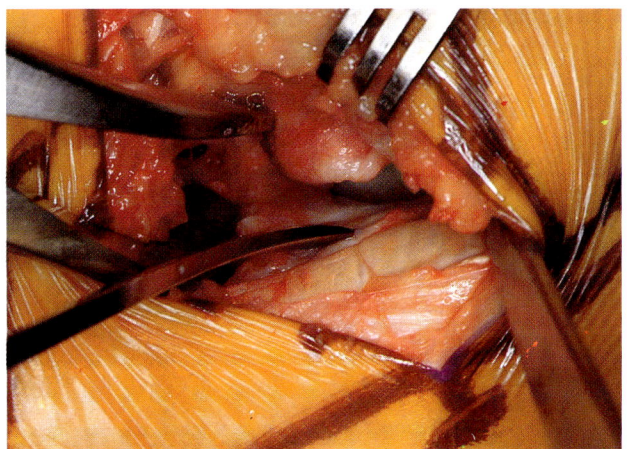

Figure 8. Curved Lambotte osteotome to decorticate calcaneus and talus.

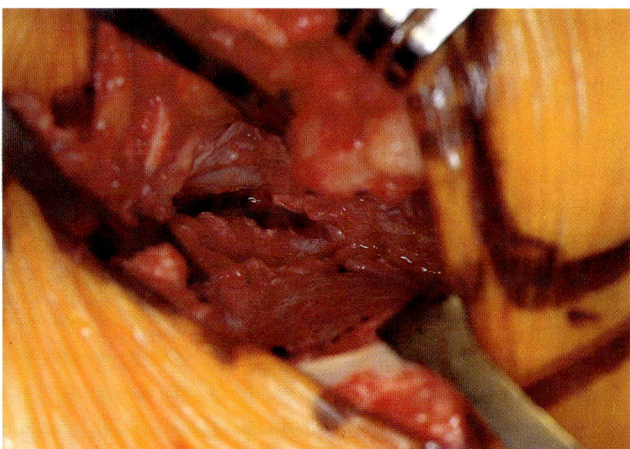

Figure 9. Surfaces decorticated.

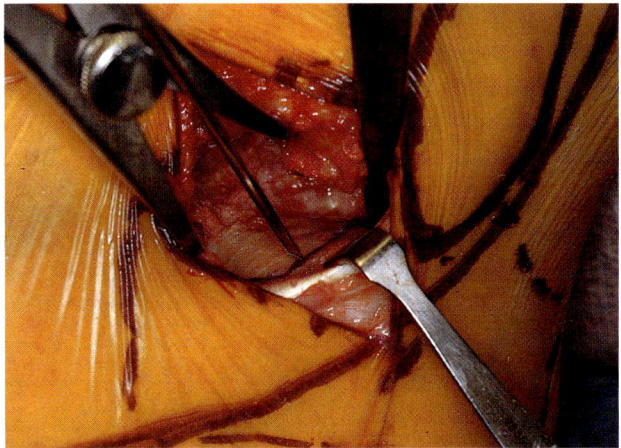

Figure 10 Fracture line marked with ink, Steinmann pin marking obliquity of the fracture.

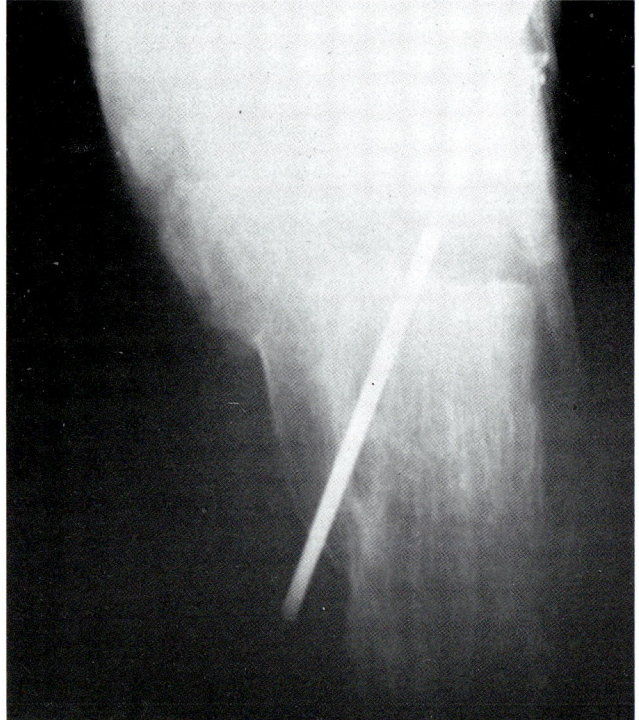

Figure 11. Intraoperative radiograph confirming placement.

At this point, the displaced articular surface of the posterior facet is exposed. The scarring within the joint is removed with a pituitary rongeur. Once the posterior facet surface has been uncovered, the site of the primary fracture line, which runs obliquely across the calcaneus from dorsolateral to plantar medial and anterolateral to posteromedial, can be identified.

Now remaining articular cartilage and cortical surfaces from the subtalar surface of the talus and calcaneus are removed. Special care is taken to go across to the sustentaculum tali of the calcaneus and to include the undersurface of the talar neck. Small curved osteotomes and a powered bur are particularly helpful in preparing the subtalar arthrodesis surfaces (Figs. 8 and 9).

A Steinmann pin is then placed across the calcaneus in the plane of the primary fracture line (Fig. 10). The position of this pin is confirmed by an axial radiograph in the operating room (Fig. 11). Once the pin position is satisfactory, an osteotomy of the calcaneus is then performed in the plane of the previous fracture. This frees the tuberosity from the sustentaculum (Fig. 12). The osteotomy exits the calcaneus anteriorly through the lateral wall. Posteriorly and inferiorly it exits through the medial wall of the calcaneus beneath the neurovascular bundle (Figs. 13 and 14). The tuberosity fragment is then released as necessary to permit its shift.

The most difficult portion of the operation is the shifting of the tuberosity fragment relative to the sustentacular fragment. It is helpful to obtain provisional

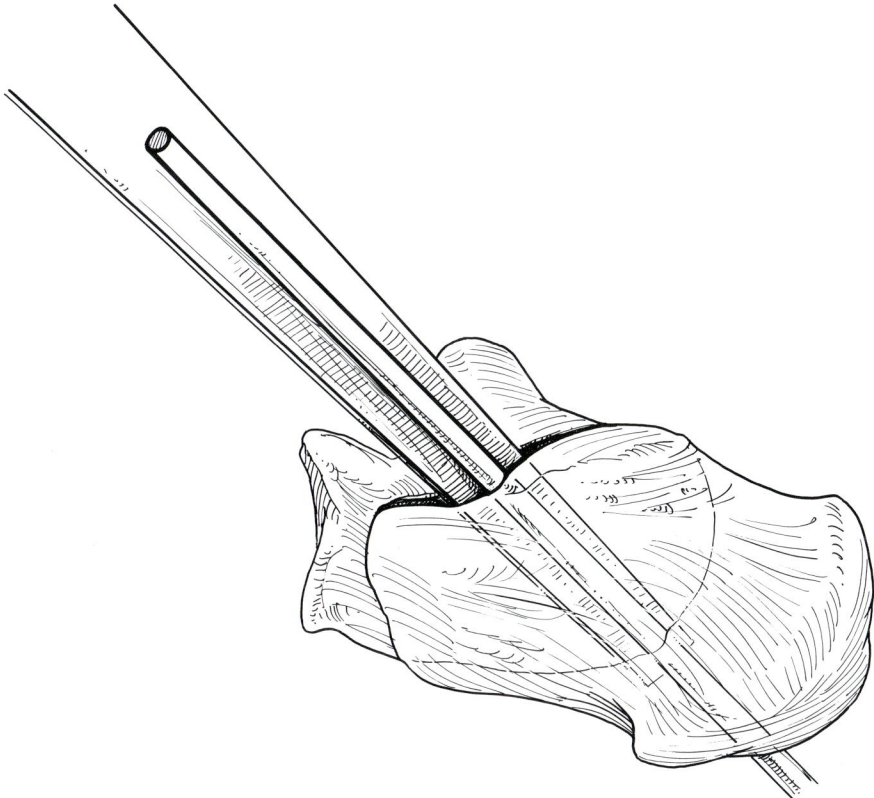

Figure 12. Osteotomy performed along Steinmann pin.

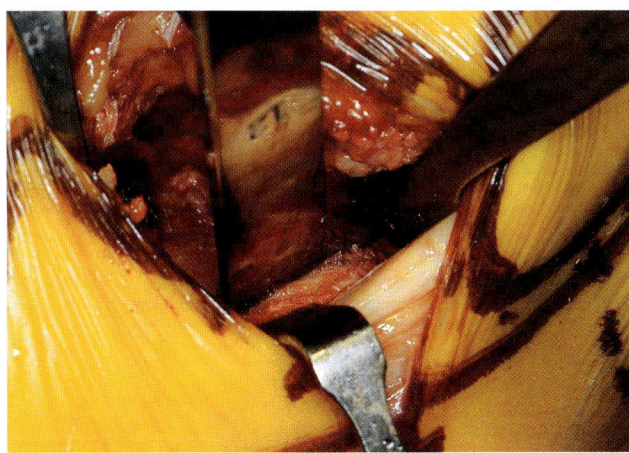

Figure 13. Osteotome in osteotomy Steinmann pin not visible.

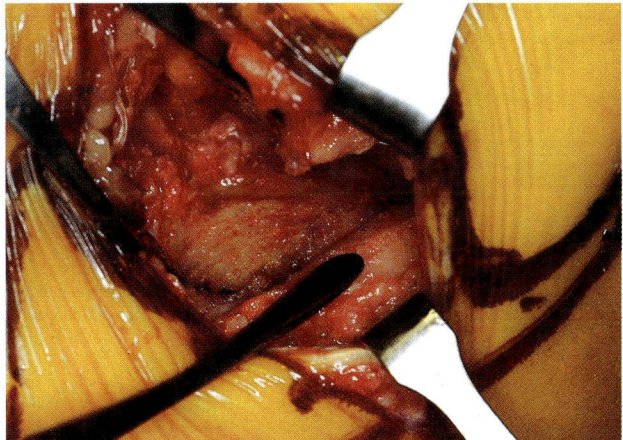

Figure 14. Osteotomy complete—no shift.

fixation of the sustentacular fragment to the talus. This can be done with screws, Steinmann pins, or Kirschner wires that are placed through the lateral body of the talus and into the sustentacular fragment. This will stabilize the sustentacular fragment and prevent its motion as the tuberosity is manipulated.

It is often helpful to use osteotomes as levers to distract the tuberosity from the sustentaculum. Also, a Steinmann pin is often placed through the tuberosity from anterolateral to posteromedial, parallel to the plane of the osteotomy, to give control of this fragment as the shift is done (Fig. 15). A baby Inge lamina spreader between the sustentaculum and the tuberosity fragment will help push the tuberosity into its new position. Even placing an Inge lamina spreader between the tip of the fibula and the sustentaculum posteriorly will help effect the shift (Fig. 16). If necessary an external fixation-type distractor can be applied between the tibia and the tuberosity fragment to help in moving the tuberosity fragment into its new position. Plantar flexion of the midfoot and talus helps effect the appropriate translation and rotation of the tuberosity fragment. Because of the obliquity of the osteotomy from dorsolateral to plantarmedial, the tuberosity fragment will move away from its impinging location on the peroneal tendons and the fibula as it is displaced. A space will be developed under the lateral aspect of the talus and the lateral aspect of the shifted tuberosity fragment (Fig. 17).

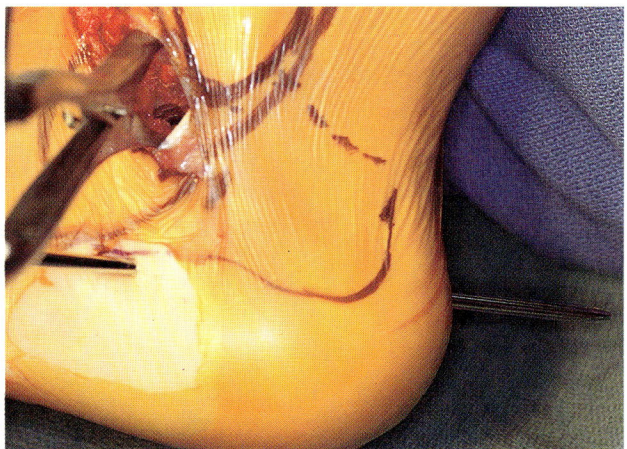

Figure 15. Steinmann pin through tuberosity for control.

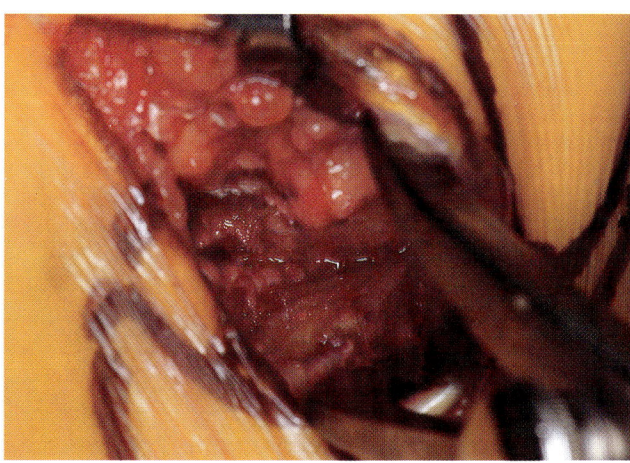

Figure 16. Osteotomy shifted—lamina spreader between tip of fibula and tuberosity fragment.

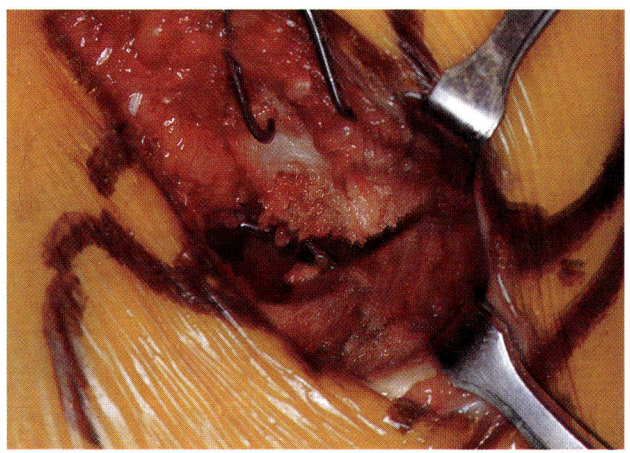

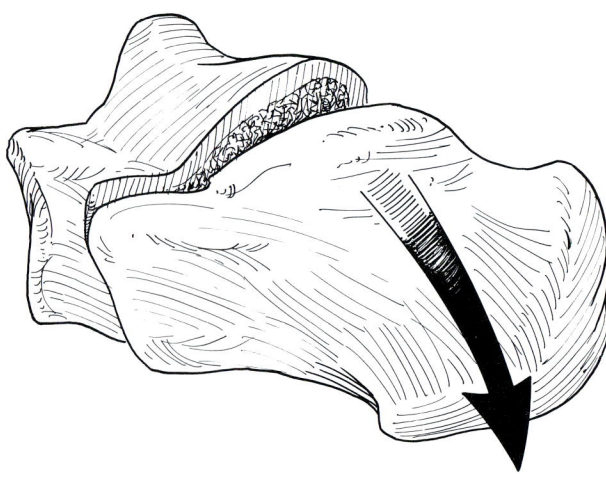

Figure 17. A: Shift of osteotomy held by K-wires. B: The tuberosity is shifted along the osteotomy plane—posterior, inferior, and medial.

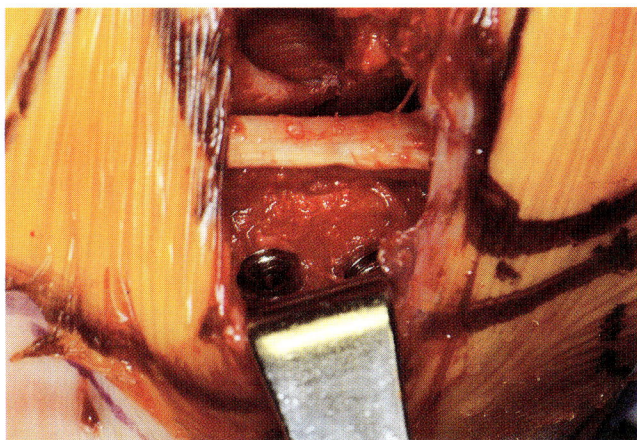

Figure 18. Osteotomy, fixation by two screws.

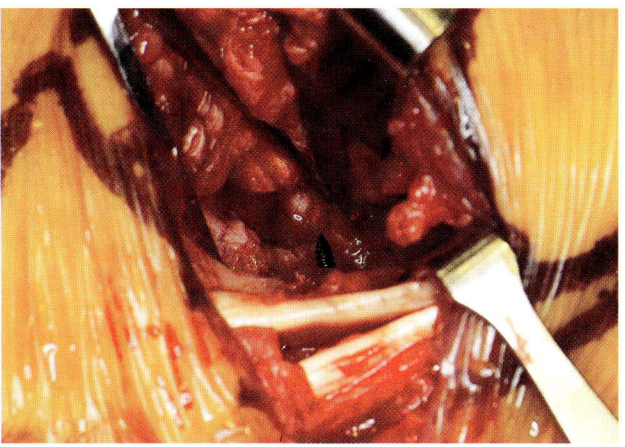

Figure 19. Tip of cannulated screw guide pin in sustentacular fragment.

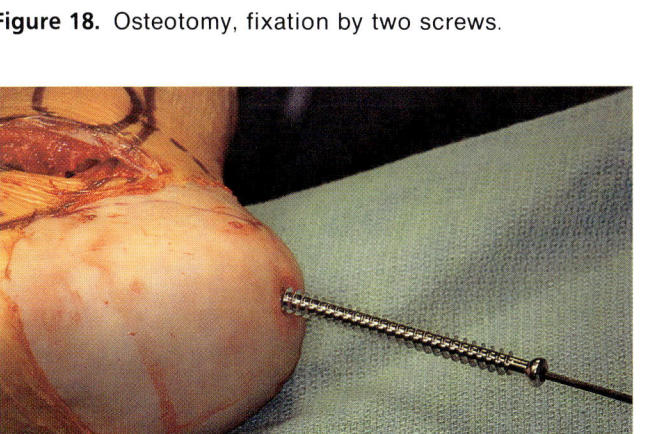

Figure 20. Screw into heel with guide pin.

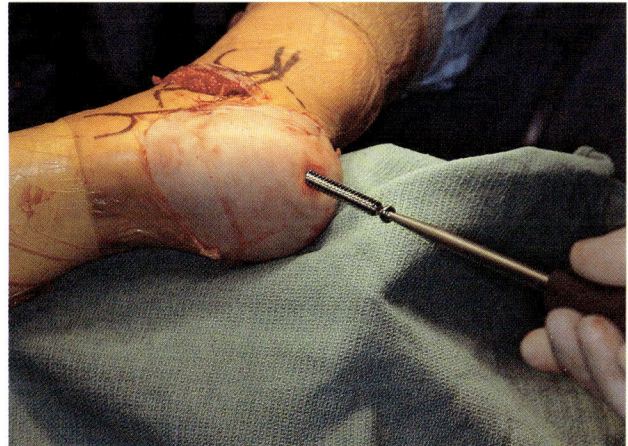

Figure 21. Screw being placed into heel, screwdriver.

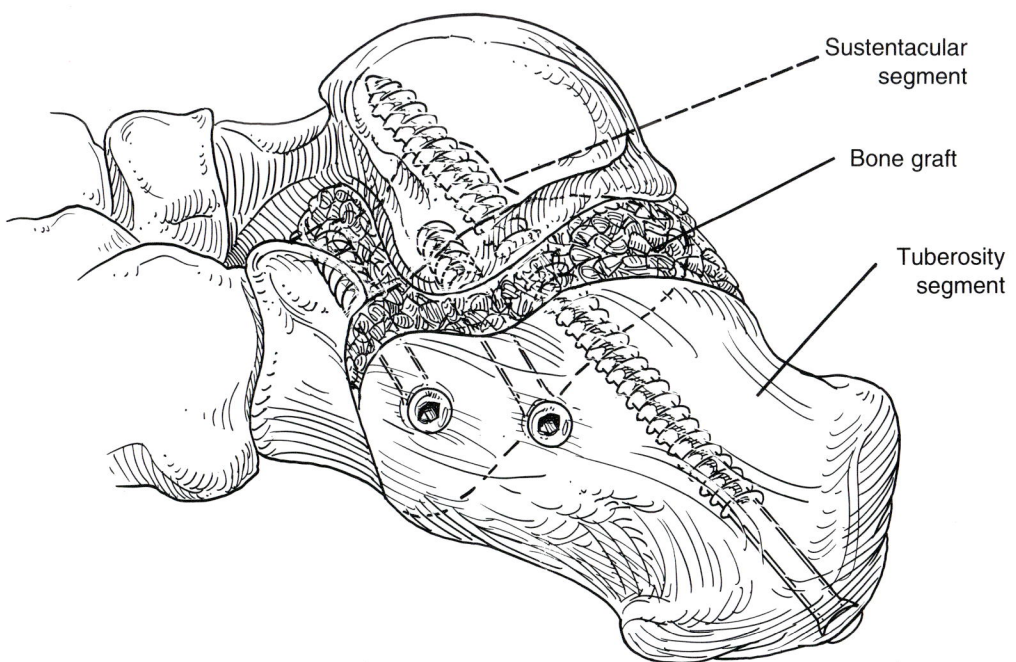

Figure 22. Axial transfixation screw—lateral view.

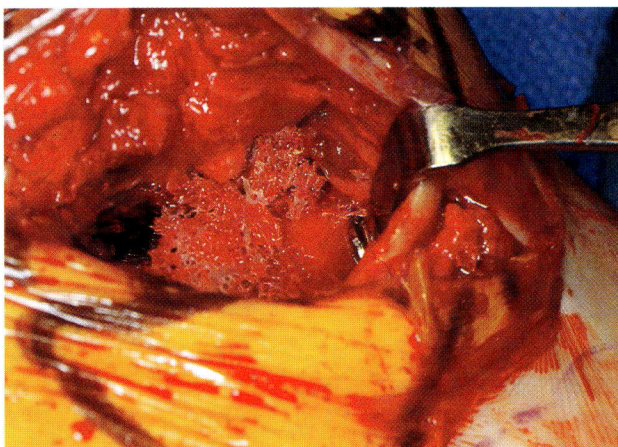

Figure 23. Cancellous bone graft in dead space.

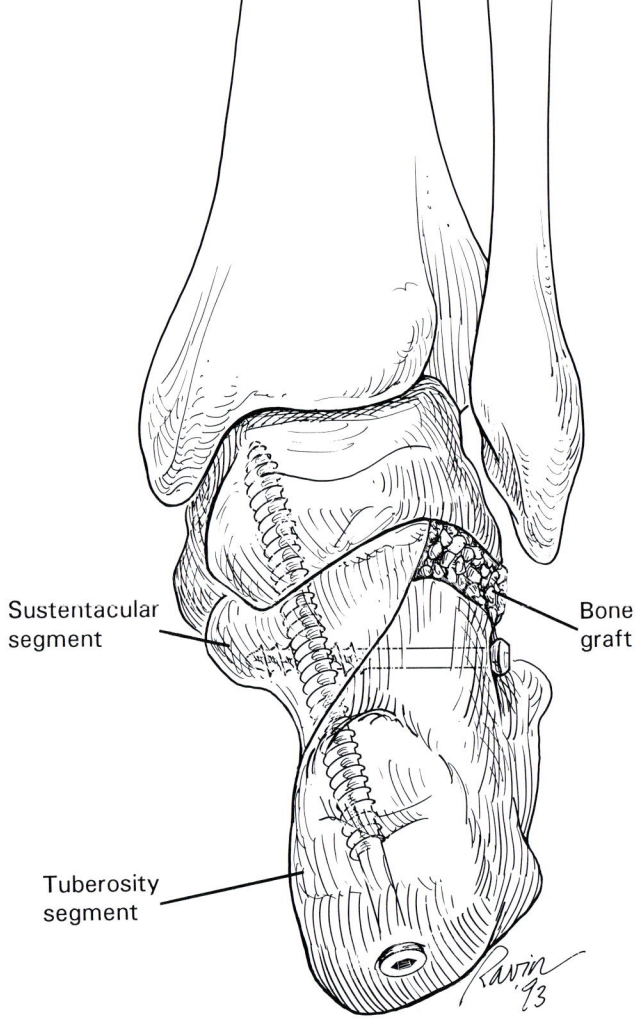

Figure 24. Final construct—axial view.

Once the shift has been obtained, transverse fixation is made through the lateral wall of the calcaneus into the sustentaculum tali with small fragment screws (Fig. 18). Next, a large cannulated 7-mm screw is placed through the tuberosity, the sustentacular fragment, and into the body of the talus. This screw placement can be done with direct visualization as well as with a radiographic control arm (Figs. 19–22). Once satisfactory position has been obtained, the decorticated subtalar joint and the dead space created laterally is packed with morcellated cancellous bone graft (Fig. 23). The bone graft is obtained from the ipsilateral iliac crest. The respositioned tuberosity is not structurally dependent upon the bone graft for maintenance of its position (Fig. 24). The wound is closed using absorbable suture in the subcutaneous tissue and nylon mattress sutures for the skin.

POSTOPERATIVE MANAGEMENT

Postoperative management is similar to that used for the surgically treated acute calcaneal fracture. The patient is initially placed in a bulky dressing and the cryo-cuff. After about 3 days, a short leg non–weight-bearing cast for a period of 8 to

12 weeks is applied. When casting is discontinued, graduated weight bearing and range of motion exercises are begun.

With this realignment and arthrodesis of the calcaneus, the result depends to a large degree on obtaining a solid subtalar arthrodesis with the calcaneus narrowed and the tuberosity in an improved position. As with a subtalar arthrodesis alone, the subtalar motion is lost and compensation of the hindfoot to uneven ground surfaces is difficult. Pain relief is emphasized as the primary goal of treatment. Restoration of heel height and possible improvement in shoe use are secondary goals.

COMPLICATIONS

All the complications of a realignment with arthrodesis—infection, loss of correction, incomplete correction, and nonunion—may occur.

Infection is avoided by use of antibiotics during the operative procedure and 24 hours postoperative. Operative technique to prevent tissue ischemia and use of a compressive dressing with cryotherapy have all helped to decrease the incidence of possible infection.

Pseudarthrosis has not been a problem probably because of the large area of arthrodesis site in the subtalar joint and the use of bone graft along with stable fixation.

Inadequate realignment is probably the most common postoperative problem. A thorough understanding of the fracture position by preoperative radiographs and CT scanning allows proper planning of the appropriate tuberosity displacement. Where secondary fracture lines were present, the realignment will not be ideal but should be improved.

Breakage of fixation devices that occurred with bone block procedures and early weight bearing have not happened. I believe this is because the final construct is not dependent upon a graft bone block for stability or correction.

Neurologic injury has not been a problem with either this procedure or that for treating an acute calcaneal fracture.

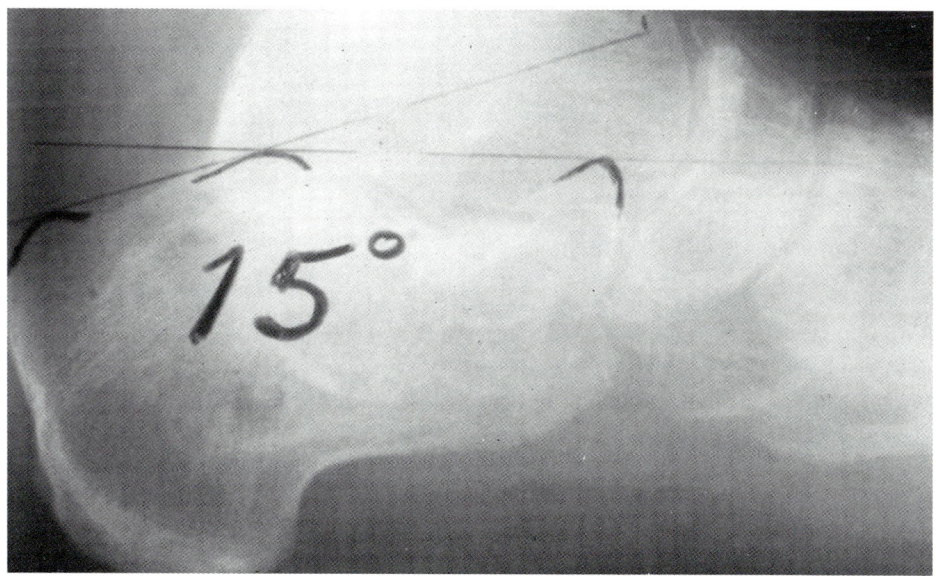

Figure 25. Preoperative radiograph with loss of calcaneal height and subtalar degenerative arthritis.

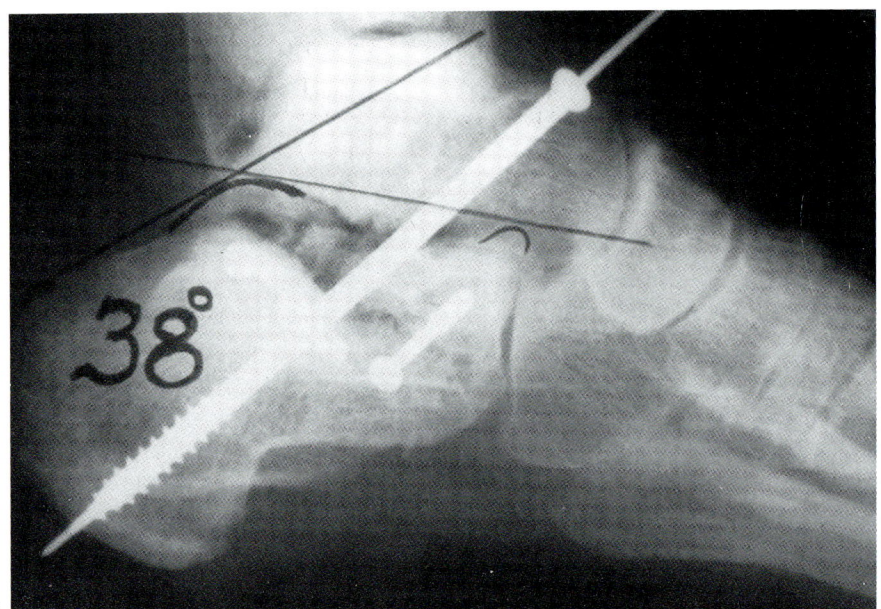 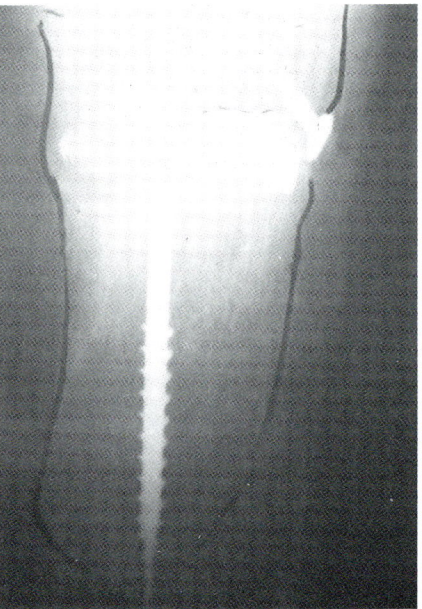

Figure 26. A: Postoperative radiograph corrective osteotomy and arthrodesis. Note cannula to aid in screw positioning. **B:** Postoperative axial view shows corrective osteotomy and arthrodesis.

ILLUSTRATIVE CASE FOR TECHNIQUE

A 32-year-old man fell from a ladder and incurred a fracture of his calcaneus. Two years later he was unable to work as a laborer because of incapacitating pain in his hindfoot with weight bearing. The lateral radiograph demonstrates the decrease in Böhler's angle to only 15° (Fig. 25).

The intraoperative view shows the repositioning of the tuberosity fragment and an increase in Böhler's angle to 38° (Fig. 26A). An axial view confirms the narrowing of the heel and the appropriate position of the cannulated screw (Fig. 26B).

The patient achieved excellent relief of his pain symptoms and was able to return to his work duties. He continued to have difficulty with climbing and walking on uneven ground.

RECOMMENDED READING

1. Bradley, S. A., and Davies, A. M.: Computerized tomographic assessment of old calcaneal fractures. *Br. J. Radiol.*, 63: 926–933, 1990.
2. Carr, J. B., Hansen, S. T., and Benirshke, S. K.: Subtalar distraction bone block fusion for late complications of the os calcis fractures. *Foot Ankle*, 9: 81–86, 1988.
3. Gallie, W. E.: Substragalr arthrodesis in fractures of the os calcis. *J. Bone Joint Surg.*, 25: 731–736, 1943.
4. Leung, K., Chan, W., Shen, W., et al.: Operative treatment of intra articular fractures of the os calcis. The role of rigid internal fixation and primary bone grafting: preliminary results. *J. Trauma*, 3: 232–240, 1989.
5. Romash, M. M.: Calcaneal fractures: three dimensional treatment. *Foot Ankle*, 8: 180–197, 1988.
6. Romash, M. M.: Reconstructive osteotomy of the calcaneus with subtalar arthrodesis for malunited calcaneal fractures. *Clin. Orthop.*, 228: 157–167, 1993

33

Ankle Instability Repair
The Bröstrom-Gould Procedure

William G. Hamilton

INDICATIONS/CONTRAINDICATIONS

In 1964 to 1966, Lennart Bröstrom wrote a series of six articles on ankle sprains in the *Acta Chirurgica Scandinavica* (1–6). In the last of these, he reported a success rate of 58 out of 60 patients, using a new operation for the correction of "chronic" ankle instability. In one of the earlier articles, he discussed the use of a similar operation for the acute ankle sprain (3).

His procedure involved tightening the stretched-out lateral ligaments to restore their normal anatomy without the use of supplemental tissues or "weaving" procedures. It was based upon the fact that the anterior talofibular (ATF) ligament lies within the anterolateral ankle capsule (similar to the anterior glenohumeral ligaments of the shoulder), and when the ATF ligament is torn it heals within the capsule in an elongated form. The operation shortened the stretched-out ATF and calcaneofibular (CF) ligaments to their normal lengths and sutured them to their anatomical locations.

In 1980, Nathaniel Gould reported his modification of the Bröstrom repair (7). It consisted of Bröstrom's operation followed by mobilizing the lateral portion of the extensor retinaculum and suturing it to the distal fibula over the ligament repair. This accomplishes three things: it reinforces the repair; it limits inversion, the position of reinjury; and it helps correct the subtalar component of the instability. The last of these factors is important, because the CF ligament is one of the main stabilizers of the subtalar joint (9). When it is torn, as in third-degree lateral sprains, a combined instability is usually present in both the tibiotalar and subtalar

---

W. G. Hamilton, M.D.: Department of Orthopaedic Surgery, Columbia University College of Physicians and Surgeons, New York, NY 10032; Department of Orthopaedic Surgery, St. Luke's-Roosevelt Hospital Center, New York, NY 10019; and *private practice*, 343 West 58th Street, New York, NY 10019.

joints. The retinacular reinforcement helps correct this combined instability because it runs parallel to the CF ligament and inserts in the lateral calcaneus.

There are several advantages to the modified Bröstrom procedure: it is a relatively easy procedure; it uses a small cosmetic incision; the sural nerve should not be in any danger; it does not require the sacrifice of a peroneal tendon; it is anatomic, and maintains a full range of motion in the ankle and subtalar joints; and, contrary to the various "weaving" procedures, it is difficult to make the repair so tight that the subtalar joint is locked in eversion.

Because of these factors, it is an ideal procedure for the athlete who needs ankle stability with a full range of motion and no loss of peroneal function, such as the ballet dancer, gymnast, ice skater, etc. We now use it routinely on all our patients.

Both Bröstrom and Gould described the use of their procedures for acute third-degree sprains in selected cases as well.

The indications for this procedure include chronic symptomatic lateral ankle instability that has not responded to physical therapy and rehabilitation (especially proprioceptive and peroneal strengthening), and selected cases of acute third-degree ankle sprains (usually professional level athletes).

This procedure is not recommended for the patient with a fixed heel varus. In this instance, a valgus osteotomy of the os calcis should be performed along with the repair. The procedure is also not recommended for patients of increased body weight, that is, athletes over 225 to 250 pounds. In these individuals, I recommend doing the modified Bröstrom and then adding an Evans type repair using half of the peroneus brevis. Peroneal weakness, palsy, and dysfunction are additional relative contraindications (e.g., Charcot-Marie-Tooth disease).

PREOPERATIVE PLANNING

The patient that is being considered for this surgical procedure will have a history of multiple sprains involving the lateral aspect of the ankle, which limits the functional ability to a significant degree. This type of surgical repair is particularly thought to be appropriate for the athlete since it does not tether subtalar motion to the degree that some of the procedures involving tendon weaving on the lateral aspect of the ankle will limit subtalar motion. During the physical examination it is particularly important to be aware that a fixed heel varus deformity in itself may cause lateral ankle stress and instability. If this fixed heel varus deformity is present, then a concomitant procedure with the lateral ankle repair would be an osteotomy of the os calcis to place the tuberosity of the calcaneus in a normal slight valgus position. Also at the time of physical examination, the strength of the peroneal muscles should be assessed. Weakness in the peroneal strength should be corrected prior to contemplation of any surgical care. At times, just strengthening of the peroneal muscles will obviate the need for surgical treatment.

Instability of the hindfoot can be evaluated by an inversion stress test and manual assessment of the amount of talar tilt. Probably the best instability sign that can be elicited is an anterior drawer of the ankle. This test is done by palpating with one hand the anterior lateral aspect of the ankle and then stressing the talus anterior on the tibia with the ankle in about 20° of plantar flexion. In my experience, this is the best predictor of instability of the ankle and needs to be compared with joint laxity present in the other ankle. It is also important to assess subtalar motion, which should be normal. If it is decreased, then the other diagnoses such as a coalition should be considered.

Routine radiographs are taken to be certain osteochondral fractures, anterior process fractures of the calcaneus, or other bone abnormalities are not present. Inversion stress views of the ankle are frequently done to look for a talar tilt. Since this test primarily stresses the calcaneofibular ligament, the talar tilt may not be increased and yet ankle instability still present. For this reason, stress views of the ankle are evaluated only in association with the history and physical findings and are not an absolute contraindication to surgical treatment if they do not show talar tilt instability.

SURGERY

The operation is usually performed as an outpatient procedure with the patient supine and a sandbag under the patient's hip so that the foot is in a vertical or slightly internally rotated position (Fig. 1). A thigh tourniquet is used over cast padding, so general, spinal, or epidural anesthesia is needed.

Technique. After exsanguination of the limb, a curvilinear incision is made along the anterior border of the distal fibula stopping at the peroneal tendons (Figs. 2 and 3). The sural nerve is just below this area, lying directly upon the peroneal tendons (Fig. 4). The lesser saphenous vein usually crosses the distal fibula at this level and will have to be ligated. In one case, the sural nerve also came across this area, so the surgeon should always be prepared for anatomical variations in this area.

The dissection is carried down to the joint capsule along the anterior border of the lateral malleolus. Laxity of the ATF and frequently the CF ligaments will be present (Fig. 5). The capsule is divided along the anterior border of the fibula down to the peroneal tendons, leaving a 2 to 3 mm cuff. The anterior talofibular ligament lies within this capsule, similar to the anterior glenohumeral ligaments of the shoulder. It frequently can be identified as a thickening in the capsule. It is best to leave a small cuff of tissue on the fibula rather than take the capsule off the bone by sharp dissection.

The calcaneofibular ligament must now be identified (Fig. 6). It lies deep to the peroneal tendons running obliquely downward and posteriorly to the calcaneus (Fig. 7) It will often be stretched out and attenuated, or it may be dislodged so that it lies outside the peroneals. On rare occasions it can be found avulsed from its calcaneal origin with a bone fragment. If it is in continuity, it is divided, leaving a cuff at its insertion on the fibula. By leaving a cuff of tissue at the insertion of the ligaments, the surgeon will be able to repair the ligaments in their exact anatomical locations, thus preserving isometry and an unrestricted range of motion [analogous to an anterior cruciate ligament (ACL) reconstruction in the knee].

The ligaments must now be shortened and repaired. The ankle should be placed in the fully reduced position in neutral dorsiflexion and slight eversion. The stumps

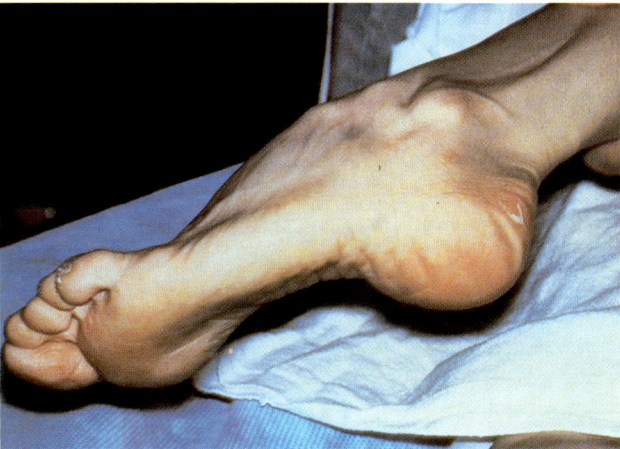

Figure 1. Positioning of the patient with a sandbag under the affected side allows excellent access to the anterolateral aspect of the ankle.

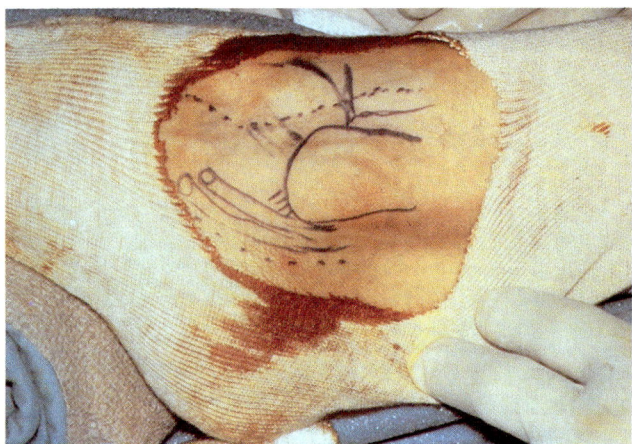

Figure 2. With the skin marking pen, the structures of the lateral aspect of the ankle are drawn. Starting inferior, the *dotted line* shows the usual location of the sural nerve. Next, the peroneal tendons and the calcaneofibular ligament coming off the tip of the fibula are marked. More anterior, the dome of the talus along with a *dotted line*, the lateral branch of the superficial peroneal nerve, is shown.

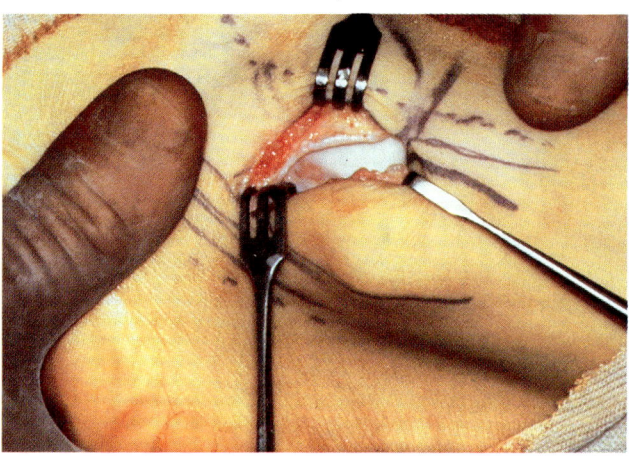

Figure 3. An oblique skin incision down through the capsule anterior to the fibula is made.

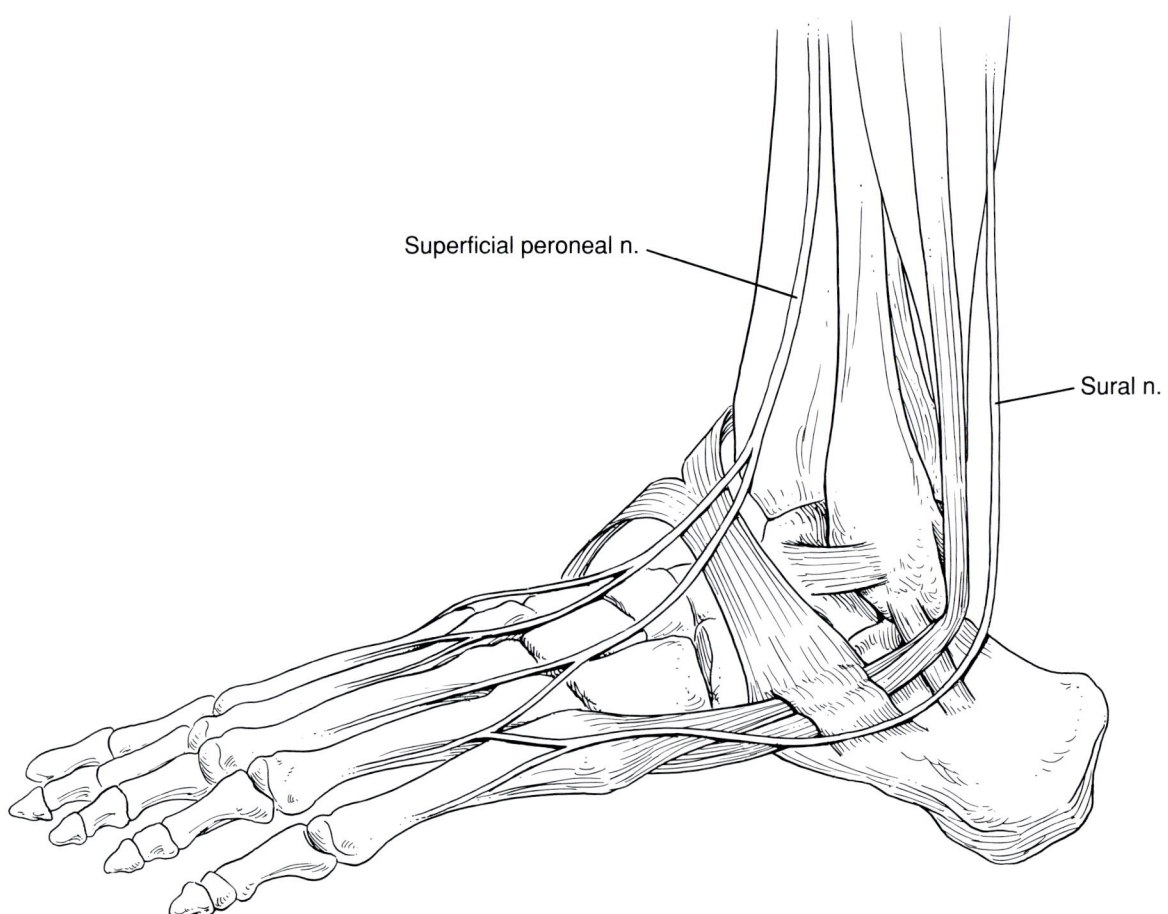

Figure 4. The relative positions of the sural nerve and the lateral branch of the superficial peroneal nerve, along with the inferior extensor retinaculum.

33 THE BRÖSTROM-GOULD PROCEDURE

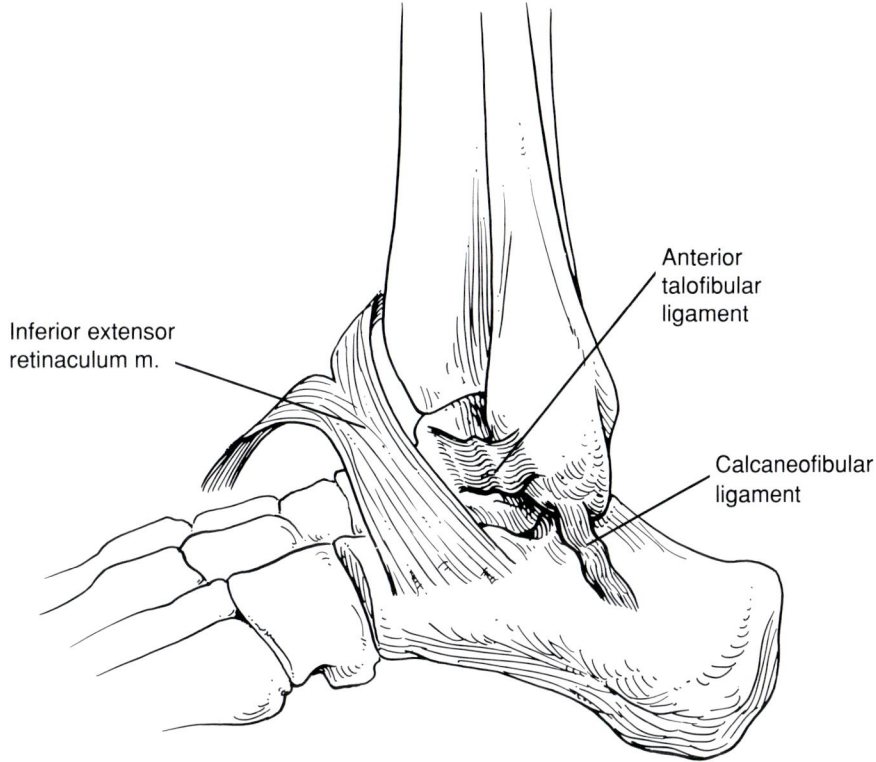

Figure 5. The position of the elongated anterior talofibular ligament and the calcaneal fibular ligament.

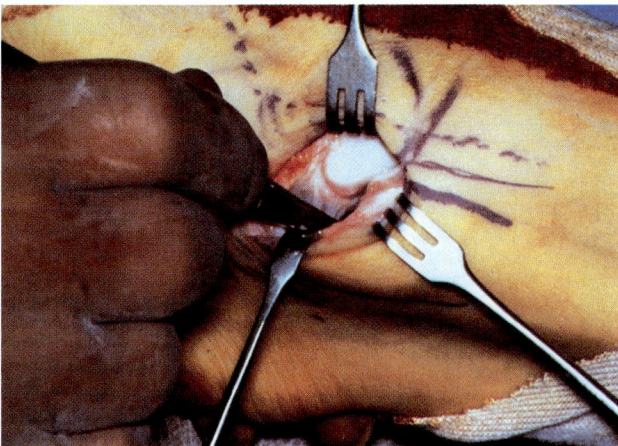

Figure 6. Deep to the tip of the fibula in the plane of the joint capsule, the tear of the calcaneofibular ligament is identified.

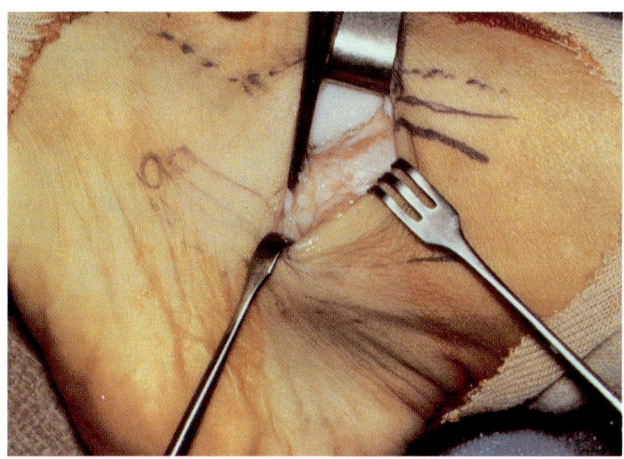

Figure 7. This torn distal portion of the calcaneofibular ligament is brought up in the wound and the ends freshened by removing the scar tissue.

of the ligaments are pulled up and the redundancy is trimmed. The ligaments are then sutured to their anatomical locations with 2-0 nonabsorbable sutures, starting with the CF ligament (Fig. 8) (because it is the most difficult to visualize) and then proceeding to the ATF ligament within the capsule (Figs. 9 and 10). This repair can be done by end to end suture, "pants over vest," or into drill holes (Figs. 11 and 12). On occasion, the capsular insertion on the fibula will be completely torn away or missing and it will be impossible to leave a cuff for repair. In this instance, the capsule and ATF ligament will need to be attached where the cuff should be. It will be necessary to make a small trough in the fibula with drill holes so that the capsule can be pulled into the trough for reattachment. I like to use a small bolster behind the distal tibia when performing this procedure. The bolster lifts the heel off the table so that the talus is not pushed forward in the anterior drawer position when the ligaments are repaired.

At this point the ankle should be examined for stability and a full range of dorsiflexion and plantar flexion. The lateral portion of the extensor retinaculum is then identified. It is dissected off the capsule and mobilized so that it can be pulled over the repair at the end of the procedure (Figs. 13 and 14). Care should be taken when working anterior to the malleolus because the lateral branch of the superficial peroneal nerve often lies in the subcutaneous tissues in this area and can be damaged by dissection or a sharp retractor. At times the extensor retinacu-

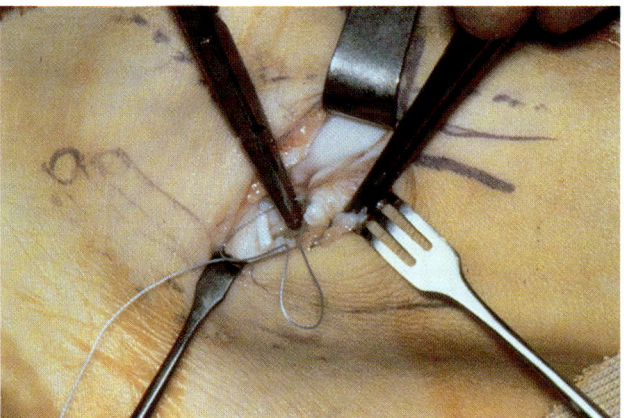

Figure 8. The two ends of the calcaneofibular ligament are then sutured, reestablishing its continuity.

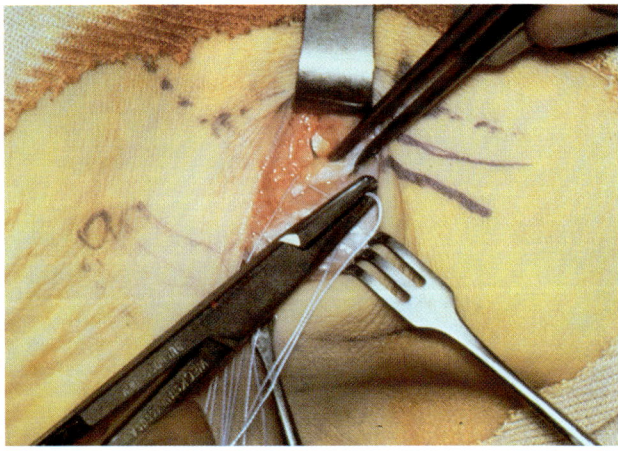

Figure 9. The anterior talofibular ligament represented as a thickening of the anterior joint capsule is also sutured to reestablish its proper length.

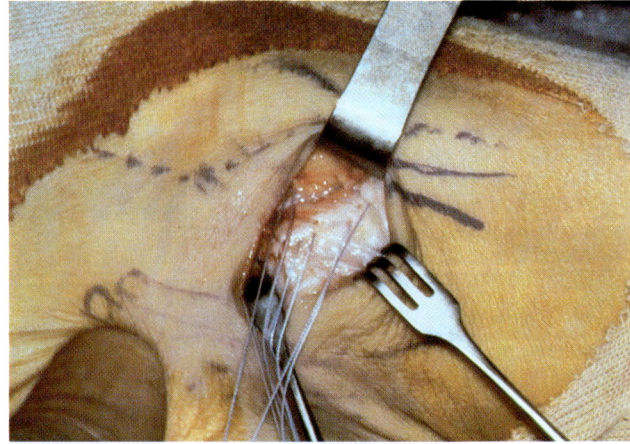

Figure 10. Multiple sutures closing up the anterior talofibular ligament and anterior lateral joint capsule.

33 THE BRÖSTROM-GOULD PROCEDURE

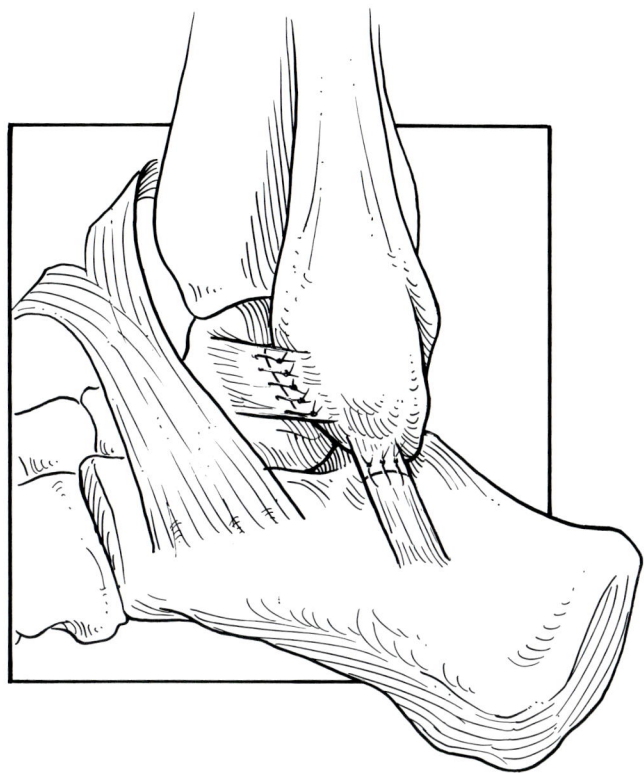

Figure 11. After suturing of the calcaneofibular and anterior talofibular ligaments, the ankle is ready for inferior extensor retinaculum translocation.

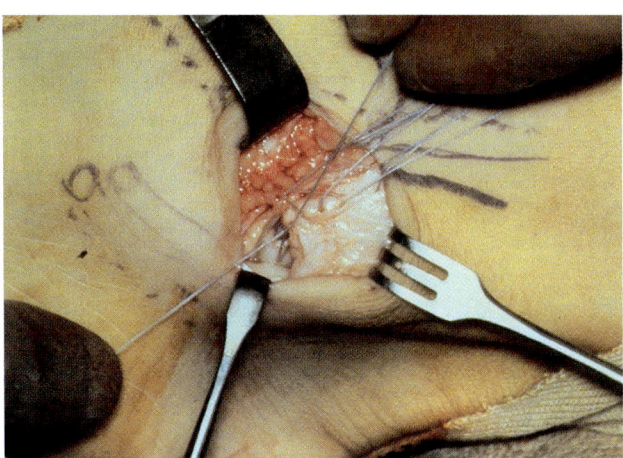

Figure 12. The inferior extensor retinaculum is seen just beneath the wide, more distal retractor.

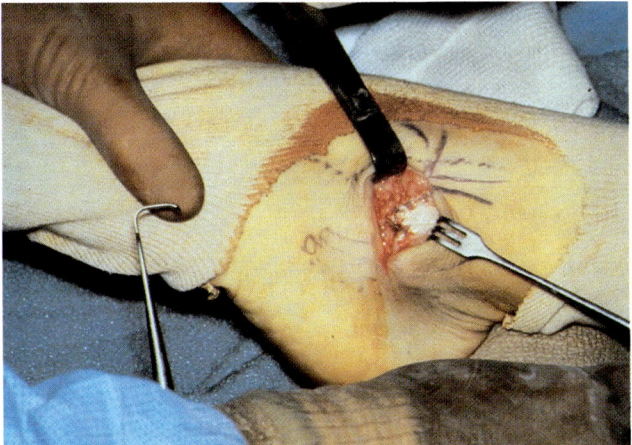

Figure 13. This larger view shows the exposure of the inferior extensor retinaculum superficial to the anterolateral joint capsule.

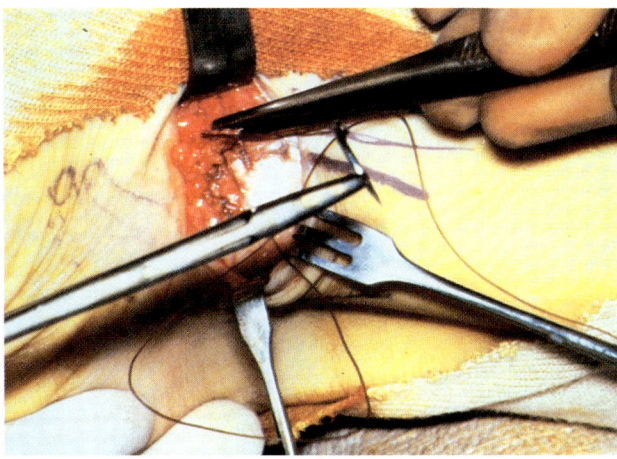

Figure 14. The retinaculum is mobilized and sutured to the anterior aspect of the fibula.

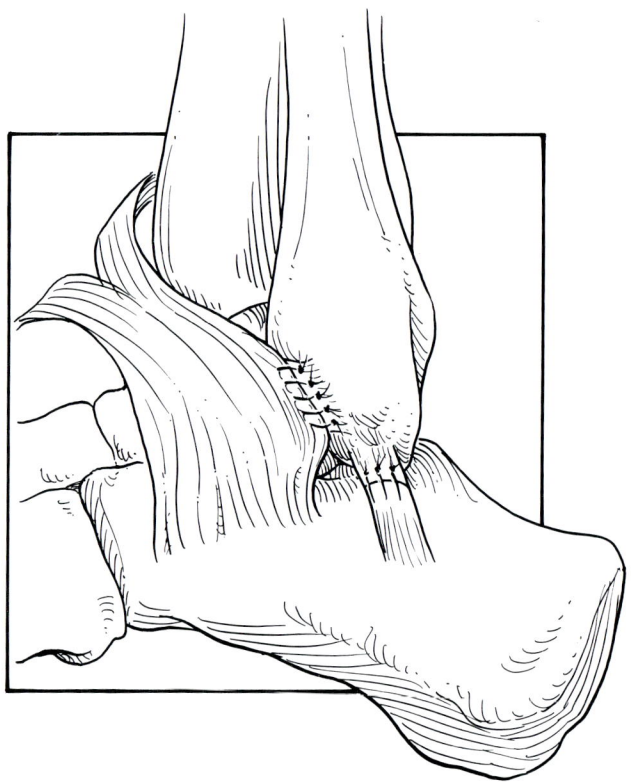

Figure 15. Suturing of the inferior extensor retinaculum to the anterior aspect of the fibula.

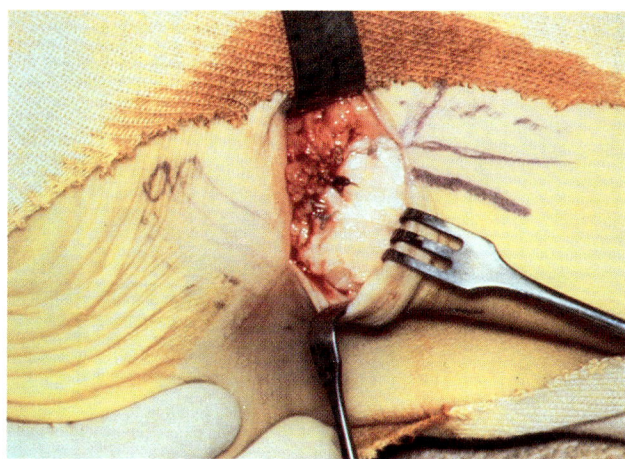

Figure 16. With completion of the procedure, both the lateral capsular ligaments and the inferior extensor retinaculum are in an appropriate position and allow full motion of the ankle.

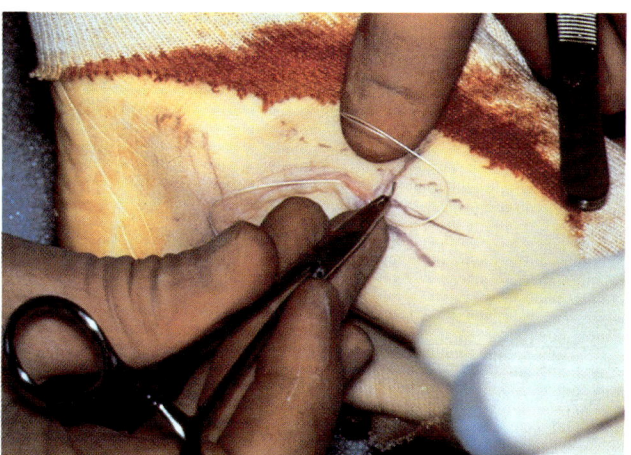

Figure 17. Skin closure is completed.

lum can be somewhat difficult to identify. Its fibers run at right angles to the joint capsule. If it cannot be identified, a larger incision will help. The mobilization of the extensor retinaculum can be performed either before or after the capsular incision.

The previously identified lateral extensor mechanism is then pulled over the repair and sutured to the tip of the fibula with 2-0 chromic catgut (Figs. 15 and 16). This accomplishes three things: it reinforces the repair, it limits inversion (the position of injury), and it helps correct the subtalar component of the instability. (As noted above, if the CF ligament is attenuated, there will be some degree of subtalar instability). The ankle is once again checked for stability and taken through a full range of motion.

A layered closure is then performed with an absorbable subcutaneous suture and Steri-strips (Fig. 17). The patient is placed in anterior-posterior plaster splints and discharged non–weight bearing with crutches.

POSTOPERATIVE MANAGEMENT

When the swelling has subsided, in 3 to 5 days, a short leg walking cast, or, if the patient is reliable, a removable short leg walker is applied for 3 to 4 weeks. The cast is removed 1 month postoperative and the ankle is protected with an air splint for another month. Swimming, range of motion, and isometric peroneal exercises are begun. Unrestricted activities are allowed at 10 to 12 weeks if full peroneal strength is present.

We started using this procedure in ballet dancers in 1980 and had such good results with it that we began to use it on all of our ligament repairs. As of 1992 we have over 40 cases, 55% of which are high level professional ballet dancers. The rest are recreational athletes and nonathletes. Average follow-up is 7 years. Of the 28 operations reviewed and reported (8), there were 26 "excellent," 1 "good," and 1 "fair" result. All the professional dancers have obtained excellent results and returned to their careers. As of this writing, there has been one failure (due to significant reinjury), but no long-term stretch-outs, "redos," or complications.

This operation is felt to be an excellent choice for the dancer, athlete, and nonathlete who needs a stable ankle with a full range of motion, and normal peroneal function.

COMPLICATIONS

Complications as a result of this procedure have been minimal.

It is possible when doing the repair of the capsule and anterior talofibular ligament structures to make the capsule too tight. If this is done, plantar flexion at the ankle may be limited. To avoid this, testing at the time of surgery to be certain the ankle can go into full plantar flexion while the hindfoot is in a neutral position is important. It is felt that the essence of this procedure is not only the static support to the ankle, but also the replacement of proprioception to the soft tissues about the ankle and subtalar joints.

The other complication that may occur involves the injury to the superficial sensory nerves about the lateral aspect of the ankle. If the incision is taken too far dorsal on the top of the foot, injury to the lateral branch of the superficial peroneal nerve can occur. Being aware of this as a possibility and protecting it from excessive stretching at the time of surgery is important. The other nerve is the sural nerve, which is less apt to be injured at the time of surgical care. Limiting the incision down to the level of the peroneal tendon, but not below that area, decreases the possibility of sural nerve damage. Also looking for that nerve on the inferior aspect of the wound should avoid transection of the nerve and result in hypesthesia in the lateral aspect of the foot distally.

ILLUSTRATIVE CASE FOR TECHNIQUE

An 18-year-old gymnast complained of instability in the lateral aspect of her ankle while doing exercises that tended to turn her hindfoot into inversion. The

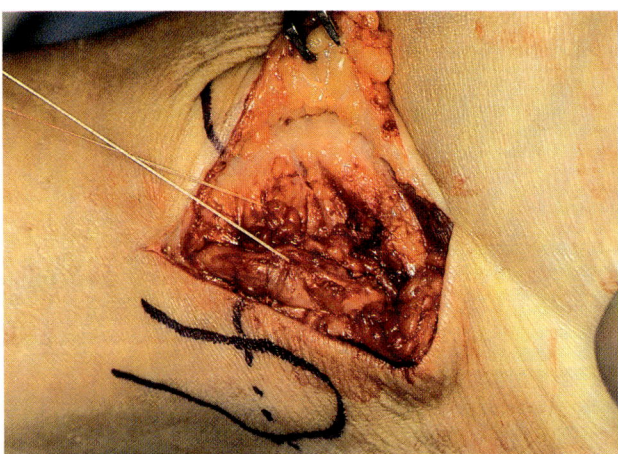

Figure 18. This is the right foot with the fibula drawn in on the lateral aspect of the ankle. The anterior talofibular ligament region is sutured in a "pants-over-vest" manner.

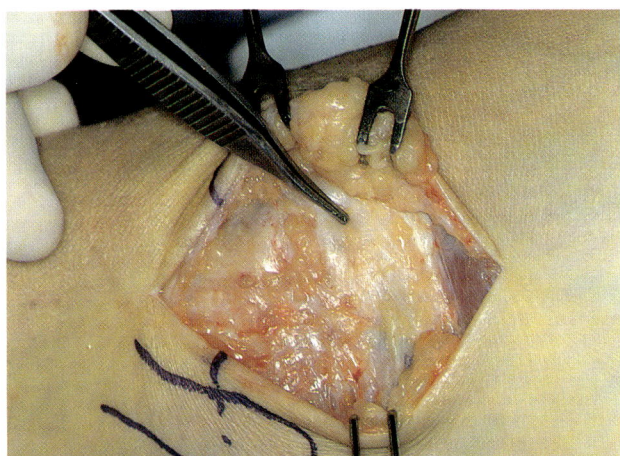

Figure 19. The inferior extensor retinaculum is seen with its transverse, white, thick fibers about 2 cm distal to the anterior margin of the fibula.

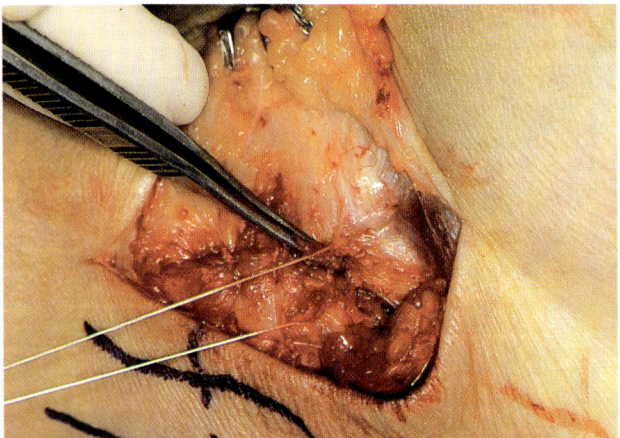

Figure 20. The mobilized inferior extensor retinaculum border is brought up to the anterior aspect of the fibula and sutured into its new position, providing stability and proprioception to the lateral aspect of the ankle and subtalar joint.

ankle would suddenly give way and she would fall with resultant swelling in the lateral aspect of her ankle. She had excellent strength in her peroneal muscle group and did not have any fixed heel varus and her subtalar motion was normal. Radiographs of her foot and ankle region did not show any abnormalities. Because of the chronicity of her ankle instability, it was felt that a surgical approach would be appropriate.

At the time of surgical treatment, the elongation of the anterior talofibular ligament was evident. These were resutured in a "pants over vest" manner (Fig. 18) and then the posterior border of the inferior extensor retinaculum (Fig. 19) was brought up to the anterior aspect of the fibula and sutured (Fig. 20). In this particular patient, a longitudinal incision was used in the skin, although a transverse incision is also felt to provide adequate exposure.

At 2 years following her ankle reconstruction, she has returned to gymnastics and has not had any recurrent episodes of instability involving that ankle.

RECOMMENDED READING

1. Bröstrom, L.: Sprained ankles. I. Anatomic lesions in recent sprains. *Acta Chir. Scand.*, 128: 483–495, 1964.
2. Bröstrom, L., Liljedahl, S., and Lindvall, N.: Sprained ankles. II. Arthrographic diagnosis of recent ligament ruptures. *Acta Chir. Scand.*, 129: 485–499, 1965.
3. Bröstrom, L.: Sprained ankles. III. Clinical observations in recent ligament ruptures. *Acta Chir. Scand.*, 130: 560–569, 1965.
4. Bröstrom, L., and Sundelin, P.: Sprained ankles. IV. Histological changes in recent and "chronic" ligament ruptures. *Acta Chir. Scand.*, 131: 483–490, 1966.
5. Bröstrom, L.: Sprained ankles. V. Treatment and prognosis in recent ligament ruptures. *Acta. Chir. Scand.*, 132: 537–550, 1966.
6. Bröstrom, L.: Sprained ankles. VI. Surgical treatment of "chronic" ligament ruptures. *Acta. Chir. Scand.*, 132: 551–565, 1966.
7. Gould, N., Seligson, D., and Gassman, J.: Early and late repair of lateral ligament of the ankle. *Foot Ankle*, 1: 84–89, 1980.
8. Hamilton, W., Thompson, F. M., and Snow, S. W.: The modified Bröstrom procedure for lateral ankle instability. *Foot Ankle*, 14: 1–7, 1993.
9. Kleiger, B.: Mechanisms of ankle injury. *Orthop. Clin. North Am.*, 5: 127, 1974.

PART VII

Ankle Joint

34
Malunited Ankle Fracture Realignment

Marion C. Harper

INDICATIONS/CONTRAINDICATIONS

The primary indication for realignment of an ankle malunion is some distortion of the normal tibiofibular-talar alignment associated with pain, which can be attributed to this malalignment. With increasing understanding of the primary role of the lateral malleolus in the reduction and stabilization of ankle injuries, attention has justifiably usually focused on the fibula as the key anatomic structure in most malunions. Based on the concept that the talus goes with and stays with the lateral malleolus, any malalignment of the talus beneath the tibial plafond must be linked directly to malalignment of the distal fibula.

Abnormality of the ankle mortise and talar position in some instances is clearly evident on plain radiographs. An example would be angular deformity of the fibula with shortening accompanied by lateral talar shift and widening of the medial joint space. In other instances, an abnormality may be quite subtle as in the case of rotational malalignment of the distal fibula associated with minimal, if any, medial joint space change. The latter occult deformity may only be fully evident on computed tomography (CT) scanning and indeed even the more obvious malalignments will usually be best defined by this technique, particularly as regards the rotational status of the fibula.

Assuming that a malalignment has been well defined and pain and disability are present or anticipated, the next major issue is the degree of degenerative joint disease. If only mild to moderate, it is reasonable to proceed with realignment based on the experience that symptoms will often improve and the progression of posttraumatic arthritis can be slowed or stopped. If, however, degenerative

---

M. C. Harper, M.D.: Department of Orthopaedic Surgery and Rehabilitation, Vanderbilt University, Nashville, TN 37203; and Centennial Medical Center, The Atrium, Nashville, TN 37203.

change is advanced, it is probably better to proceed with an ankle arthrodesis. In the absence of advanced arthritis, experience indicates that the interval from the original injury to the date of realignment is not a significant factor in the eventual outcome.

The status of the extremity must be considered with acceptable vascularity and reasonable health of the soft tissues being necessary. In addition, one should assess the neurologic status in terms of sensation, guarding against realignment surgery on an early Charcot joint. The latter must always be suspected in a patient with diabetes mellitus.

Finally, the patient must be of appropriate age, in reasonable general health, and understand that complete relief of symptoms may not ensue. Concomitant with the latter, the possible need for an eventual ankle arthrodesis must be understood.

PREOPERATIVE PLANNING

Preoperative planning should begin with the history and physical examination, attempting to confirm the ankle as the source of symptoms and eliminating other causes of lower extremity pain. One may be able to localize pain and tenderness to the specific area of abnormality, i.e., anterolateral tenderness with rotational deformities of the distal fibula. In some cases of widening of the ankle mortise, instability may be a major complaint and excessive medial-lateral excursion of the talus may be evident on examination.

Plain radiographs including anteroposterior (AP), lateral, and mortise views should be scrutinized carefully in several areas. The first is the medial aspect where the reduction of any medial malleolar fracture as well as the width of the medial joint space are noted. Any increase, even subtle, as compared to the joint

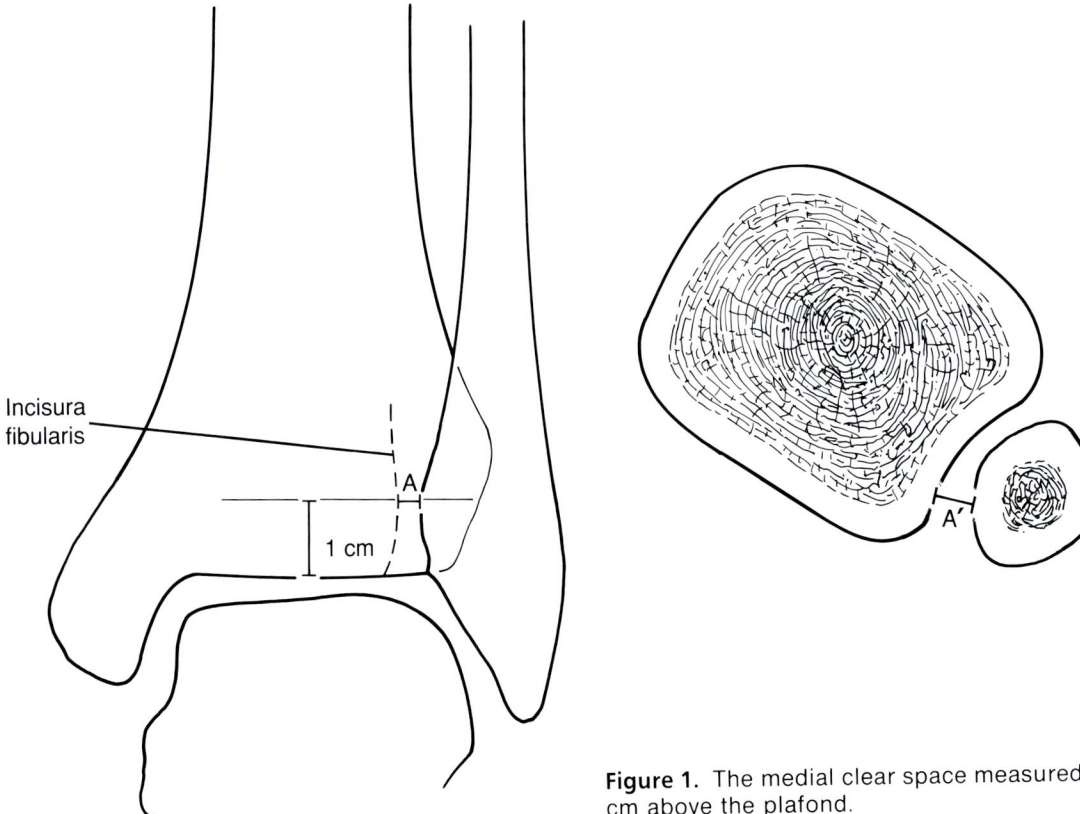

Figure 1. The medial clear space measured 1 cm above the plafond.

space beneath the tibial plafond should be considered abnormal. The second is the tibiofibular or syndesmotic interval where evidence of abnormal seating of the fibula in the incisura fibularis of the tibia should be looked for. The most common abnormal finding here will be some evidence of widening of this interval with the two parameters most often cited being diminished overlap of the distal fibula and anterior tibial tubercle and an increase in the tibiofibular clear space. Of these, the latter appears to be more reliable, with the normal width being less than 6 mm as measured 1 cm above the plafond (Fig. 1). Because the clear space represents the posterior aspect of the tibiofibular interval, its width can also vary with rotational deformity of the fibula. Internal fibular rotation, for instance, may contribute to an increase in this distance and external fibular rotation is possible in association with this interval appearing either normal or diminished. The final parameter to be evaluated on plain radiographs is fibular shortening. Several methods of measurement have been proposed to assess this important and commonly present element of malalignment, with none being totally reliable but all being of some value. The first two, as proposed by Weber, are seen on the mortise view: the integrity of "Shenton's line" as representing subchondral bone of the distal tibia and fibula (Fig. 2), and an unbroken curve between the lateral process of the talus and the distal fibular recess (Fig. 2). The final method is the talocrural angle representing the longitudinal axis of the tibia relative to a line across the tips of the malleoli (Fig. 3). This angle normally is within several degrees of that measured on radiographs of the contralateral ankle.

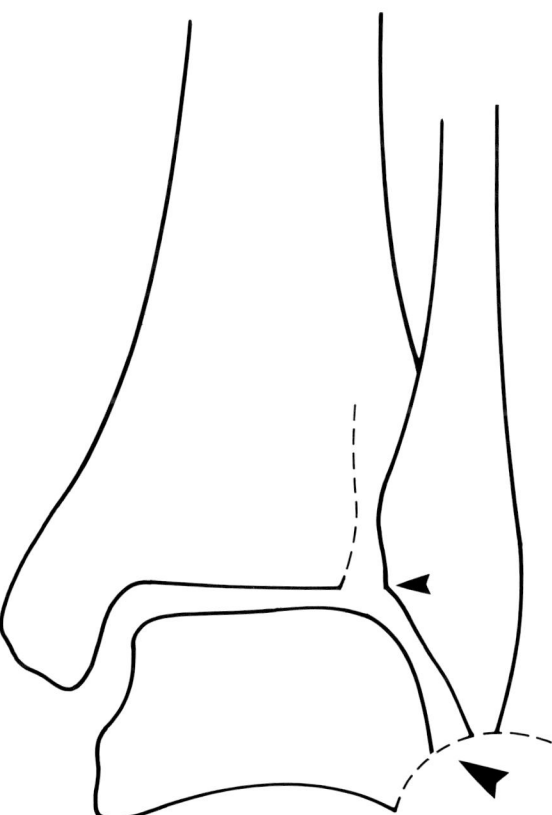

Figure 2. "Shenton's line" of the ankle *(small arrow)* reflecting the subchondral bone contour of the tibial plafond as it meets the subchondral bone of the fibula at the "fibular spike." Unbroken curve *(large arrow)* between lateral process of the talar surface and recess of the distal fibula.

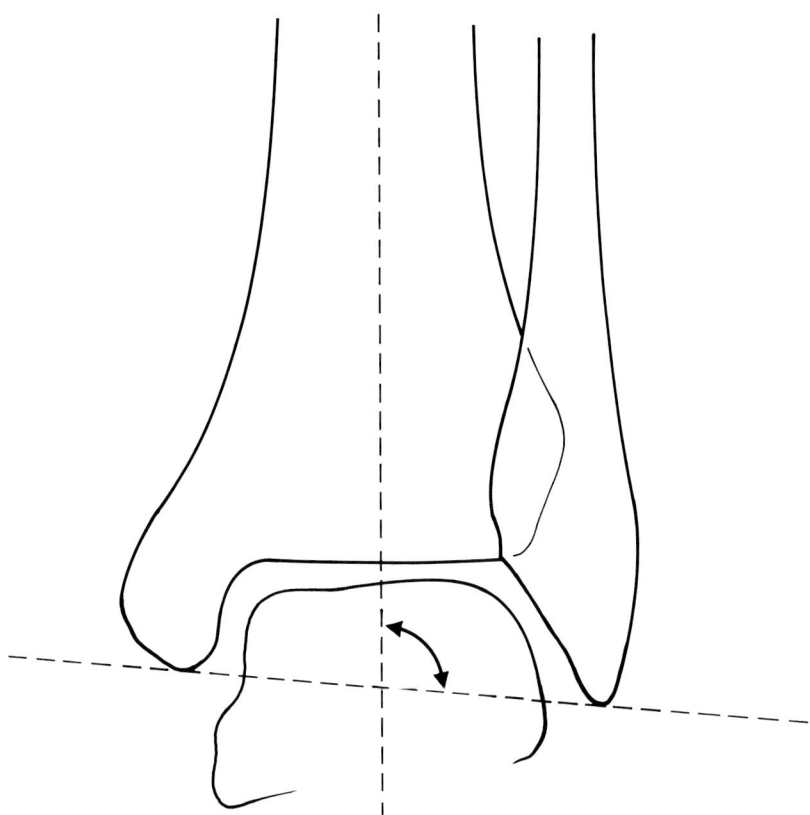

Figure 3. Talocrural angle reflecting the longitudinal axis of the tibia relative to a line across the tips of the malleoli.

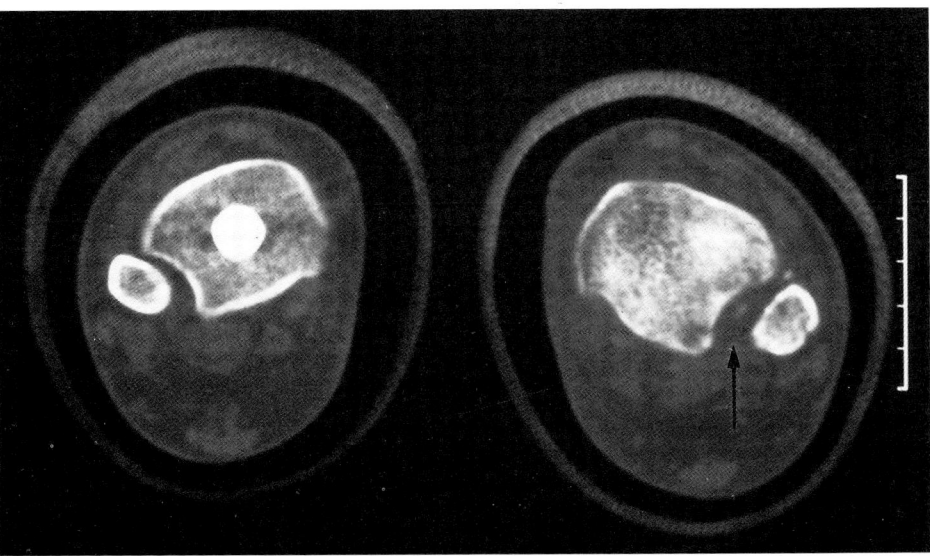

Figure 4. CT scan of the lower legs of an individual following open reduction and internal fixation of a pronation–external rotation ankle fracture on the left. Axial cuts across the distal tibiofibular interval reveal residual lateral translation and internal rotation of the distal fibula as indicated by more widening of the tibiofibular interval posteriorly *(arrow)* than anteriorly.

Although plain radiographs will usually provide useful information as to the nature of the malunion, the definitive study is the CT scan. Axial cuts across the tibiofibular interval and ankle mortise with comparison views of the normal ankle will accurately determine the amount of talar shift as well as the position of the fibula relative to the tibia. Malrotation of the fibula with both internal and external rotation being encountered can be assessed by noting the width of the tibiofibular interval at both the anterior and posterior aspects of the syndesmosis. External rotation of the relatively oval fibula will be manifested by asymmetrical widening anteriorly as versus internal rotation, which will appear as asymmetrical widening posteriorly (Fig. 4). Sagittal or coronal cuts will help determine the size and position of posterior malleolar fragments.

SURGERY

The patient is positioned supine with support beneath the buttock or in a half-lateral position if a posterolateral dissection is anticipated in order to correct a posterior malleolar malunion (Fig. 5). Under tourniquet control the distal fibula is exposed subperiosteally through a lateral longitudinal approach (Fig. 6).

Technique. The incision can be shifted anteriorly or posteriorly as desired to expose pertinent abnormalities, e.g., fractures of the anterior tibial tubercle or posterior malleolus. Usually the fibula will be malpositioned in the incisura fibularis of the tibia with some degree of widening of the syndesmosis. It is quite important to address and remove all interposed scar in this area in order to obtain and maintain a good reduction. When there has been either a proximal fibula fracture with little displacement, e.g., a Maisonneuve injury, or a diastasis without fracture, one may expose the syndesmosis anteriorly, progressively removing scar from anterior to posterior throughout the length of the syndesmotic interval.

In cases of distal fibula fracture with displacement and shortening, a fibular osteotomy will be necessary. This may be done in an oblique fashion through the fracture site or as a transverse osteotomy at or slightly above this area. The latter

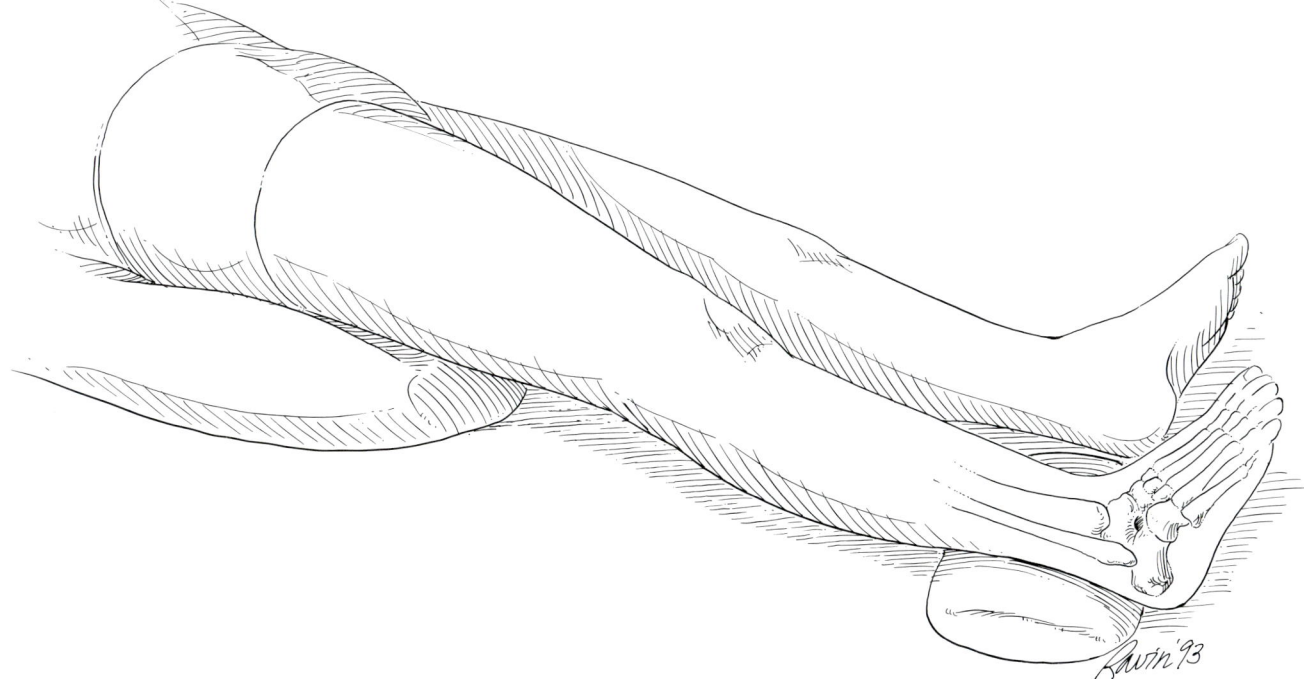

Figure 5. Semilateral patient positioning to facilitate fibular exposure.

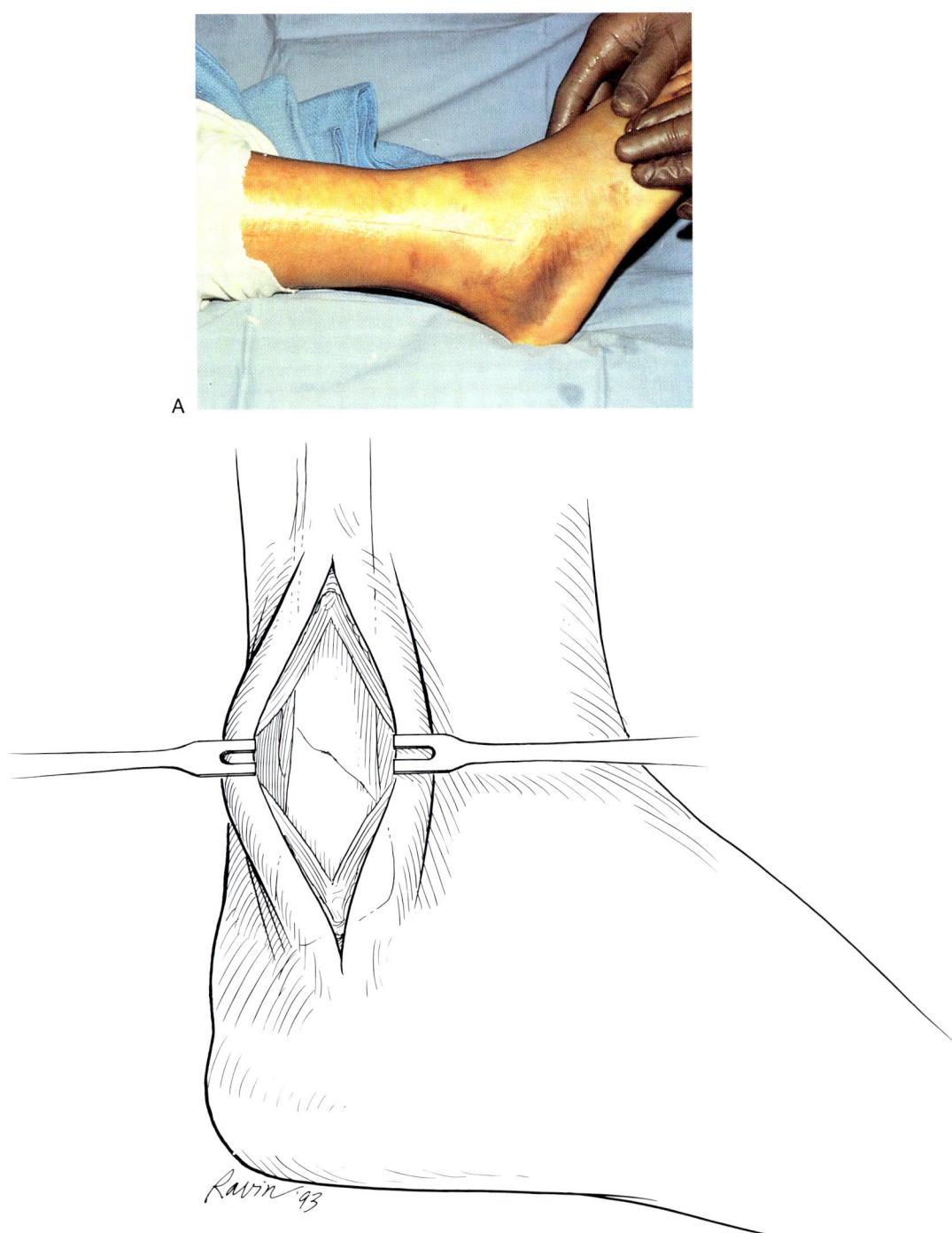

Figure 6. A: The skin incision is marked. **B:** Exposure of distal fibula and malunion site.

is often easier. The distal fibula is then progressively reflected either posteriorly or distally as in the approach of Gatellier and Chatang with concomitant division of the syndesmotic ligaments (Fig. 7). The former technique may be sufficient when the syndesmosis is only mildly widened primarily anteriorly, with the latter being helpful in cases of more severe widening both anteriorly and posteriorly. In either case, fairly extensive stripping of the distal fibula is often necessary in order to correct deformity and regain length. In my experience, this has not resulted in a clinical problem in terms of healing or avascular necrosis. Following

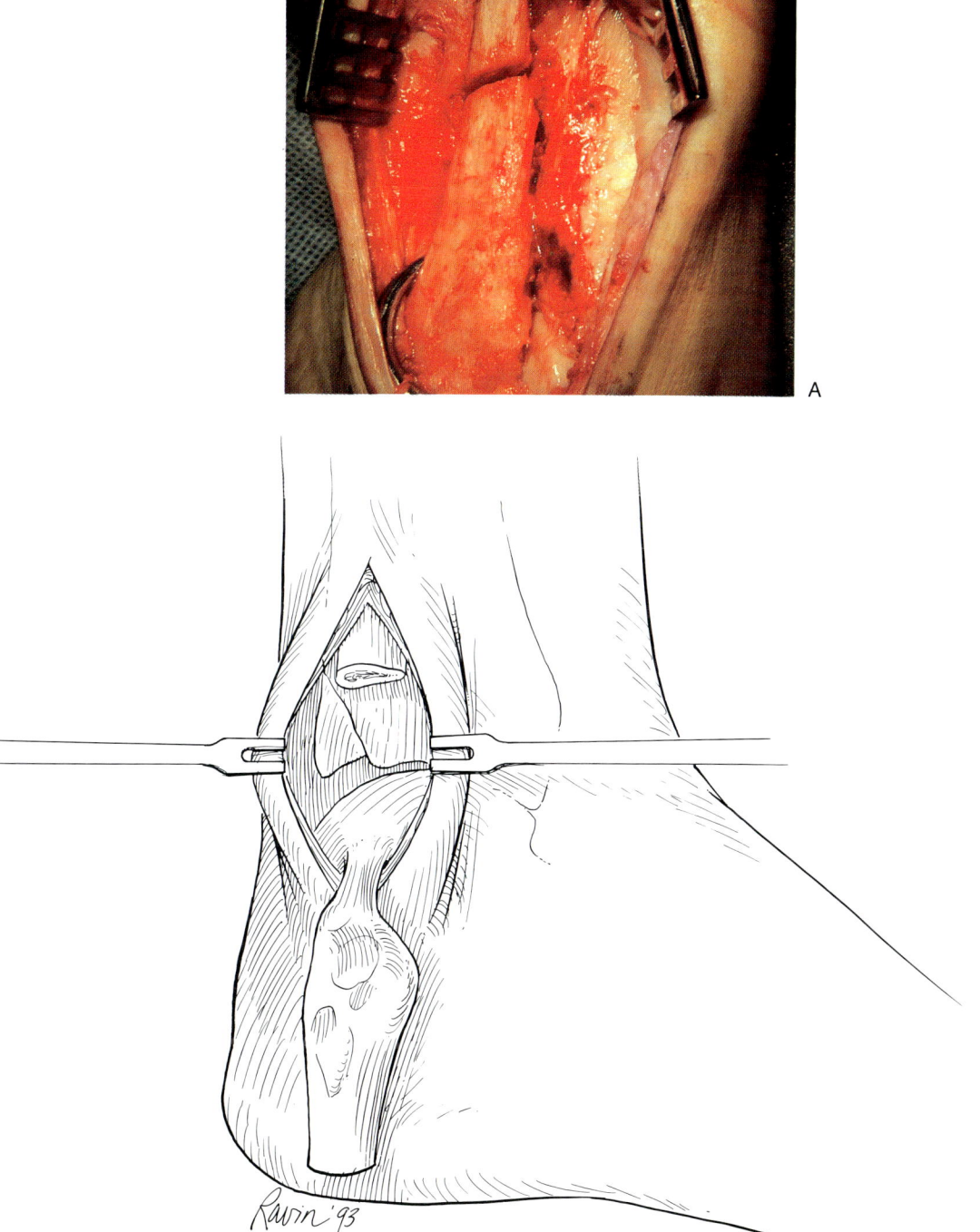

Figure 7. A: The fibula is osteotomized transversely. **B:** Reflection of fibula distally following fibular osteotomy with exposure of posterior malleolar fragment malunion. (**A**, from ref. 5.)

osteotomy and mobilization of the fibula, the posterior distal tibia can be well visualized laterally and any malunion of a posterior malleolar fracture addressed. Usually the fracture site can be "taken down" using osteotomes and the posterior fragment freed so as to be brought distally and anteriorly if necessary. Temporary stabilization with a large bone clamp or K-wires will allow subsequent screw fixation. A 4.0 cannulated screw proves helpful with placement either from posterior to anterior or anterior to posterior through a separate stab wound (Fig. 8).

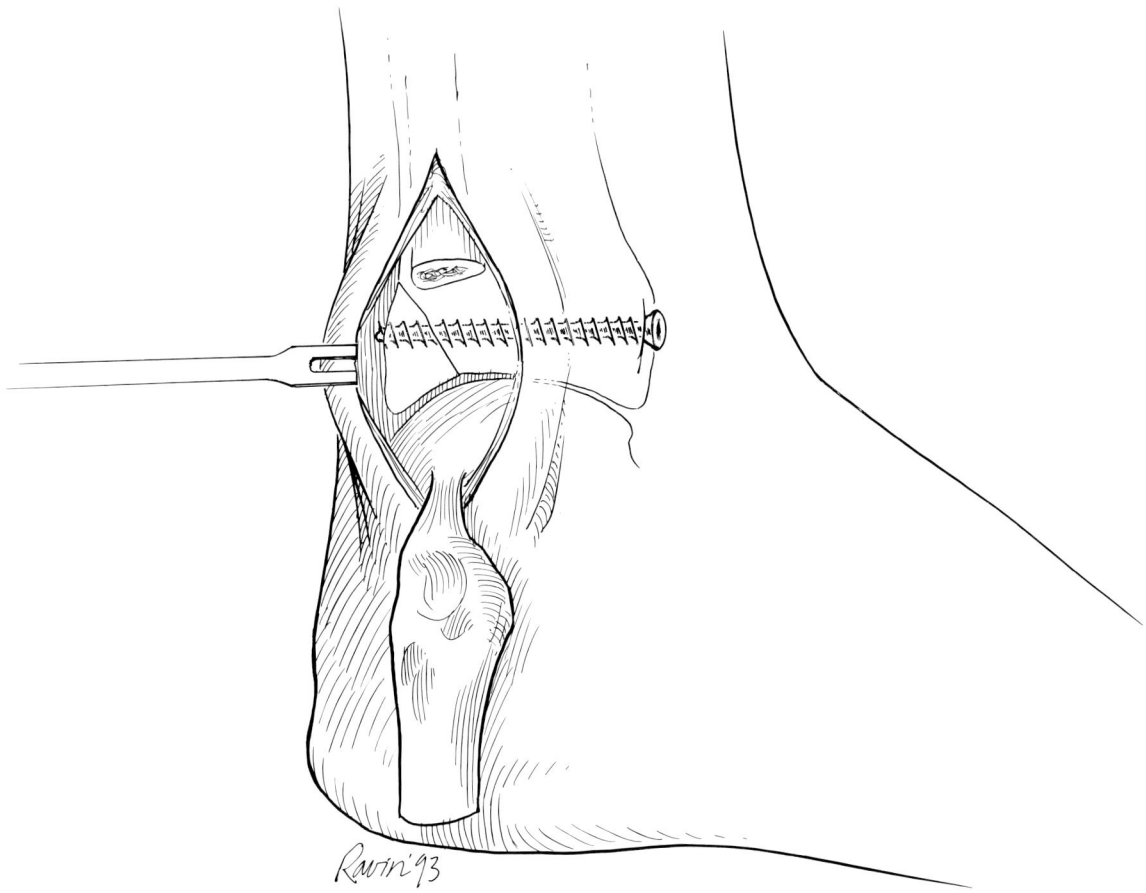

Figure 8. Internal fixation of reduced posterior malleolar fragment via cannulated 4.0-mm cancellous screw being placed from anterior to posterior over guide wire through a separate stab wound.

Prior to repositioning the distal fibula relative to the tibia and proximal fibula, any obstacle medially to anatomic positioning of the talus beneath the tibial plafond must be addressed. Usually this involves either interposed scar tissue in the medial joint space or a malunion or nonunion with lateral displacement of the medial malleolus. With the former, an anteromedial arthrotomy is necessary in order to completely debride scar, including a portion of the deep deltoid ligament if necessary. In the latter instance, a longitudinal medial incision curved anteriorly is used to expose and take down the malunion or nonunion. If the anatomic landmarks at the fracture margins are sufficiently clear so as to make an anatomic reduction apparent and feasible, stabilization of a medial malleolar fragment prior to reduction and stabilization of the fibula may be advantageous in terms of defining a buttress against which the talus may be reduced. Two 4.0-mm cancellous screws afford good fixation and compression for larger fragments, with K-wires often being better for small fragments. A small cancellous bone graft is indicated for any significant osseous defect. If anatomic repositioning of a medial malleolar fragment is not obvious, it may be better to initially reduce and stabilize the fibula, realizing that the common error is to not adequately seat the fibula in the incisura fibularis and thus not adequately reduce the talus from a position of lateral shift and tilt. If the incisura fibularis has been well debrided and correct fibula position and length have been regained, the talus should be correctly positioned beneath the plafond and can then be used as a buttress against which to reduce a medial malleolar fragment.

On the lateral side, the priorities are adequate seating of the fibula in the incisura fibularis, restoration of fibula length, and correction of any fibular rotational abnormality. These in turn depend initially upon adequate debridement of the syndesmosis, adequate mobilization of the distal fibula, and an appropriate preoperative analysis of the rotational status of the fibula. After the above plus fibular osteotomy have been accomplished, some method for applying forceful traction to the distal fibula with distraction at the osteotomy site is needed. With only mild shortening, manual traction via a bone clamp may be satisfactory. When greater length needs to be regained, a distraction device is very helpful. Options include the small AO distraction device utilizing threaded K-wires or Schanz pins placed anteriorly in the fibula, the AO articulating tension device attached to bone off the end of a plate (Fig. 9), and the AO femoral distractor. The latter utilizes Schanz pins placed in the anterolateral tibia and the calcaneus. Defining normal length intraoperatively may be difficult. Temporary K-wire fixation of the distal fibular fragment to the distal tibia or talus followed by an analysis of intraoperative radiographs using the criteria mentioned previously may be helpful. The more common error is to underestimate rather than overestimate the amount of lengthening necessary.

Next the need for a bone graft in the fibular defect created should be assessed. Small gaps, i.e., of several millimeters, can be grafted with cancellous bone, whereas larger defects require a structural corticocancellous graft (Fig. 10). Although small grafts may be harvested from the distal tibia, larger grafts are best obtained from the iliac crest. After the distal fibula has been reduced into the incisura fibularis with appropriate length and rotation being maintained, it is secured in this position with a plate, either a 3.5-mm dynamic compression plate (DCP) or a one-third semitubular. Securing the distal fragment to the plate with two or more screws prior to definitive positioning and stabilization may be helpful and in fact is necessary if the AO articulating tension device is used. Relatively little valgus bending of the plate is advisable in an effort to accentuate medial shift of the distal fibula and talus. Prior to definitive fixation, compression across the bone graft site may be obtained by simply releasing the previously applied distraction force or directly via the AO articulating tension device.

When a significant portion of the syndesmotic ligaments has been disrupted and this interval debrided of scar, a transsyndesmotic screw is indicated, placed either through or adjacent to the plate (Fig. 11). I use a 4.5-mm cortical screw, if possible, engaging both the fibular and the lateral tibial cortices. Ideally this should be a position screw placed in a nonlagged fashion, although occasionally a lag effect with overdrilling of the fibula is necessary in order to make the fibula seat well in the incisura fibularis and reposition the talus well beneath the tibial plafond. If compression is used across the syndesmosis, the ankle should be held in neutral flexion while the screw is tightened in order to avoid excessive narrowing of this interval and thus some loss of dorsiflexion. No repair of the syndesmotic or deltoid ligaments is necessary, as both heal well with correct repositioning of the talus and stabilization of the syndesmosis.

The subcutaneous tissue and skin are closed with interrupted sutures. Use of a small suction drain is advisable if there is excessive bleeding at the time of surgery. A compressive dressing with plaster splint immobilization is advisable.

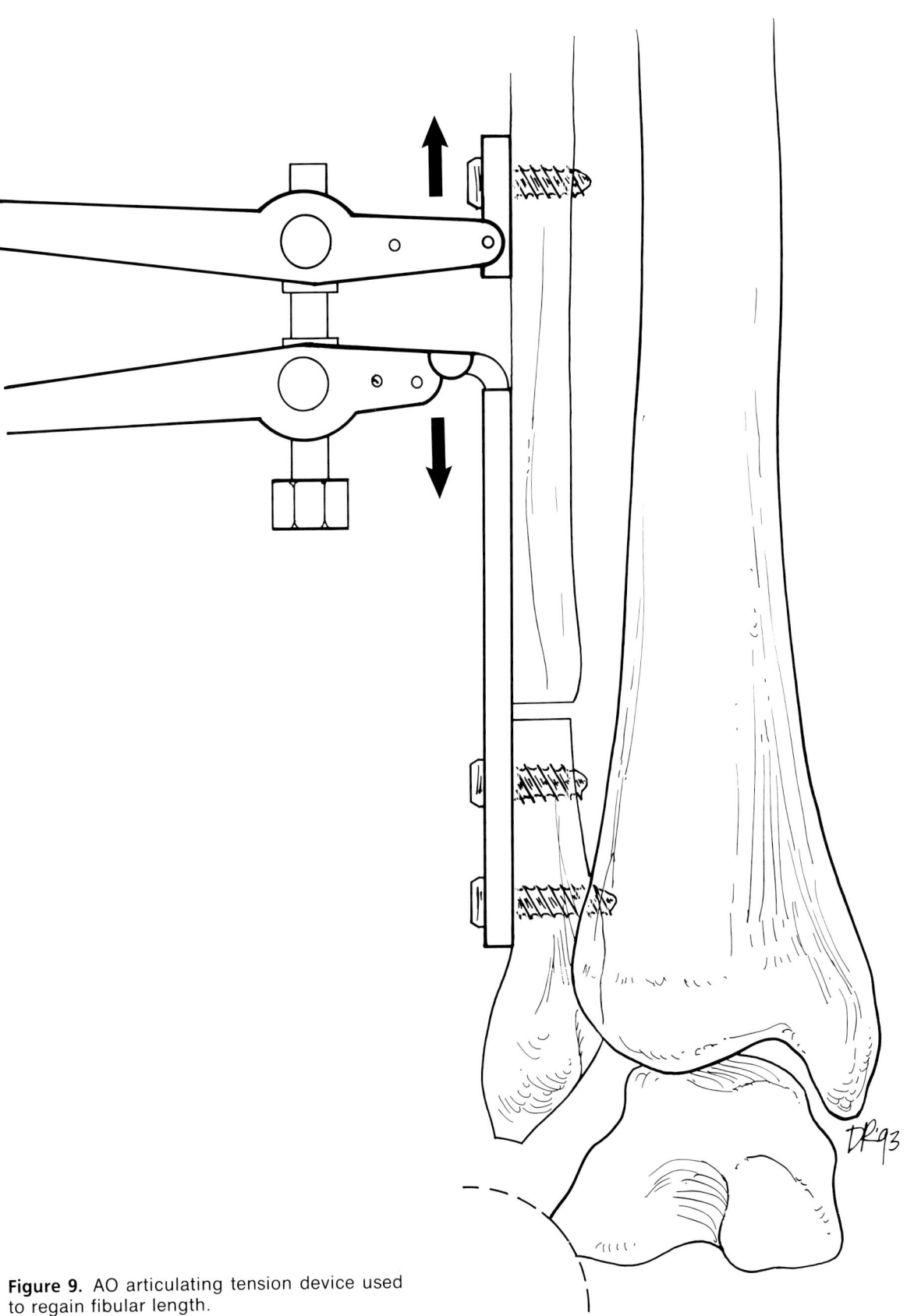

Figure 9. AO articulating tension device used to regain fibular length.

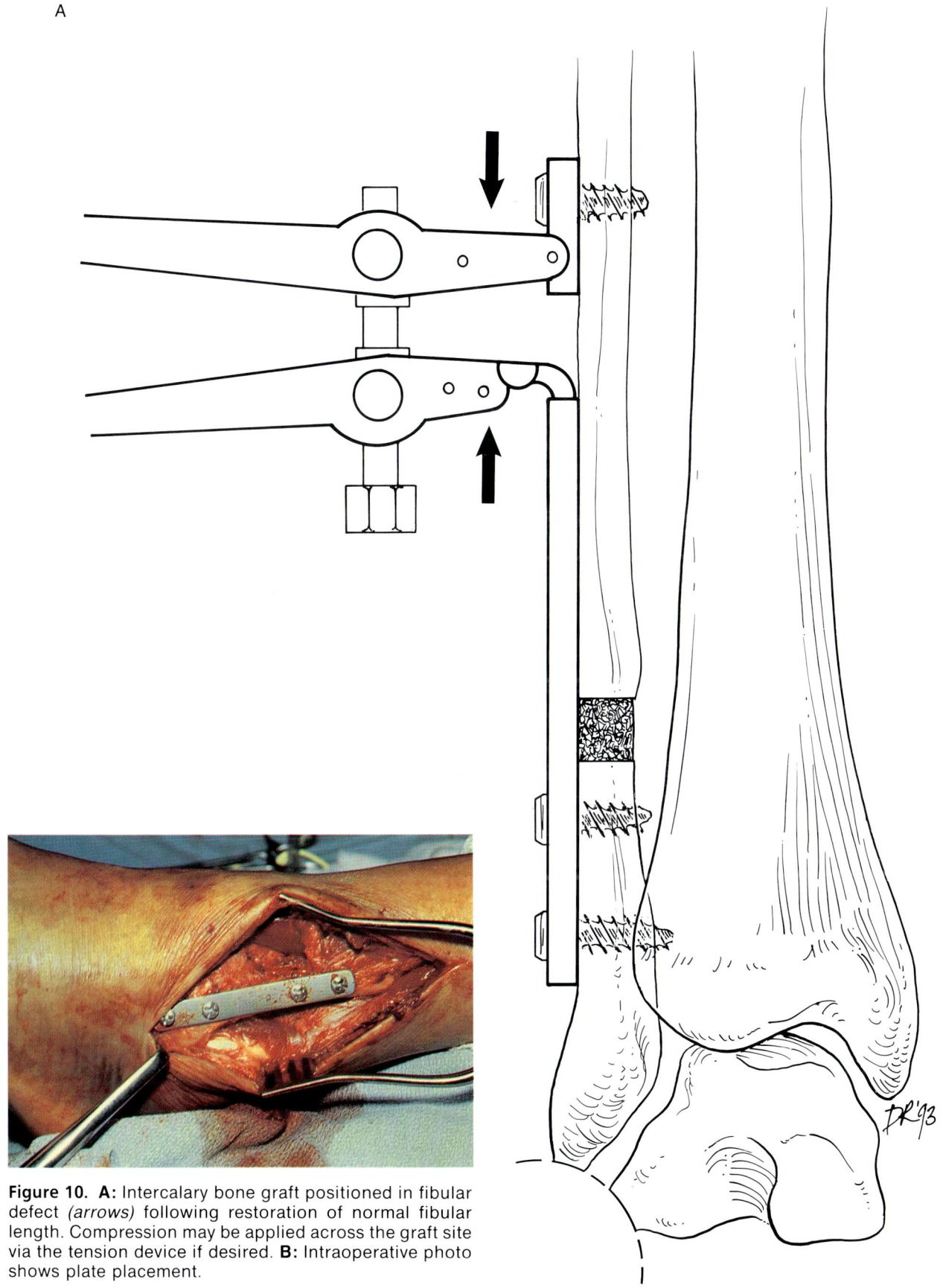

Figure 10. A: Intercalary bone graft positioned in fibular defect *(arrows)* following restoration of normal fibular length. Compression may be applied across the graft site via the tension device if desired. **B:** Intraoperative photo shows plate placement.

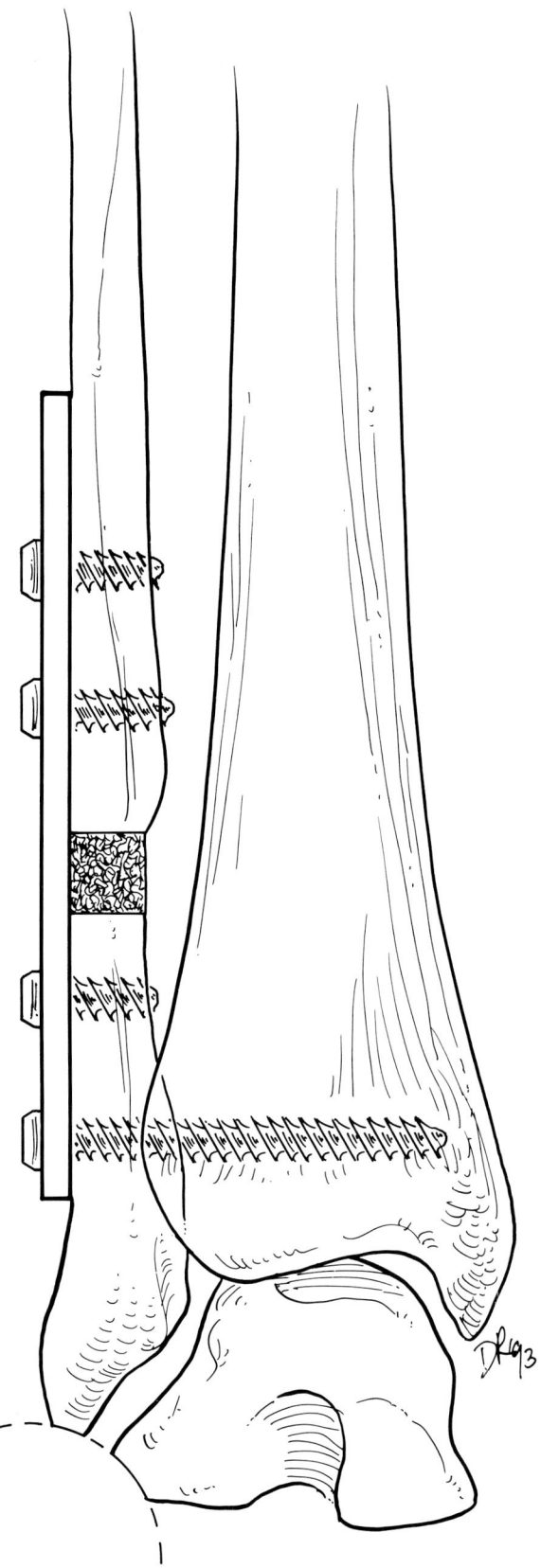

Figure 11. Placement of a transsyndesmotic screw through the plate.

POSTOPERATIVE MANAGEMENT

About 2 days after surgery, the compression dressing is removed. From then on, postoperative care is somewhat discretionary and dependent upon the experience of the surgeon, the reliability of the patient, and the stability of the fixation. Initial splinting with early motion is generally advantageous if feasible, followed typically by cast immobilization for 6 to 8 weeks. A removable fracture brace may be helpful thereafter, especially if significant bone grafting has been necessary. Early weight bearing is often permissible if fixation is secure and the transsyndesmotic screw is left in place for 3 to 4 months. If only one tibial cortex has been engaged, the screw will usually begin to loosen or toggle slightly but usually remain effective in terms of preventing recurrent diastasis during this period. Screw removal in the office or clinic under local anesthesia is often possible. Rehabilitation involves a standard physical therapy regimen for ankle and hindfoot motion plus lower leg strengthening.

A review of published results indicates that approximately 75% of patients undergoing realignment of an ankle malunion will obtain a satisfactory or good result. This appears to be valid despite the length of time from injury to realignment or the age of the patient, assuming that advanced posttraumatic arthritis is not present. There is evidence that the progression of mild to moderate arthritis may be slowed or stopped and ankle function often improved. Patients with severe arthritis and loss of motion should be counseled as to the advisability of an ankle arthrodesis.

COMPLICATIONS

Complications of this procedure include nonunion of the osteotomy site in the fibula. This can be prevented by using bone graft from the iliac crest and having the surfaces of the bone graft tightly apposed to the patient's own well-vascularized fibula. If necessary, the fibula can be resected back to bleeding bone to enhance later bone graft incorporation.

Loss of initial bone position may occur as a result of inadequate fixation of the syndesmosis. Placement of the screws through the fibula as described should prevent this complication.

Failure of anatomic reduction of the talus under the tibial plafond may be the result of an inadequate debridement of the medial joint space or the syndesmosis. Inadequate lengthening of the fibula will allow persistent inadvisable lateral displacement of the talus on the tibial plafond.

ILLUSTRATIVE CASE FOR TECHNIQUE

A 77-year-old woman sustained a trimalleolar ankle fracture that was treated with open reduction and internal fixation of the medial malleolus, with the lateral malleolus being reduced closed. Postoperatively she was maintained in a cast for 6 weeks. Unfortunately but somewhat predictably, she went on to exhibit progressive lateral and posterior displacement of the talus associated with early malunion of the fibula and posterior malleolus (Fig. 12). Two and one-half months postfracture, it was elected to proceed with surgical realignment.

A lateral incision shifted slightly posteriorly was used to subperiosteally expose the fibula. The fibula fracture site was identified and taken down using an osteotome. An AO femoral distractor was then applied to the lateral aspect of the lower leg using Schanz pins placed in the tibia and calcaneus. As traction was applied, the distal fibula was mobilized and reflected distally in association with division of the distal syndesmotic ligaments. The talofibular and calcaneofibular ligaments

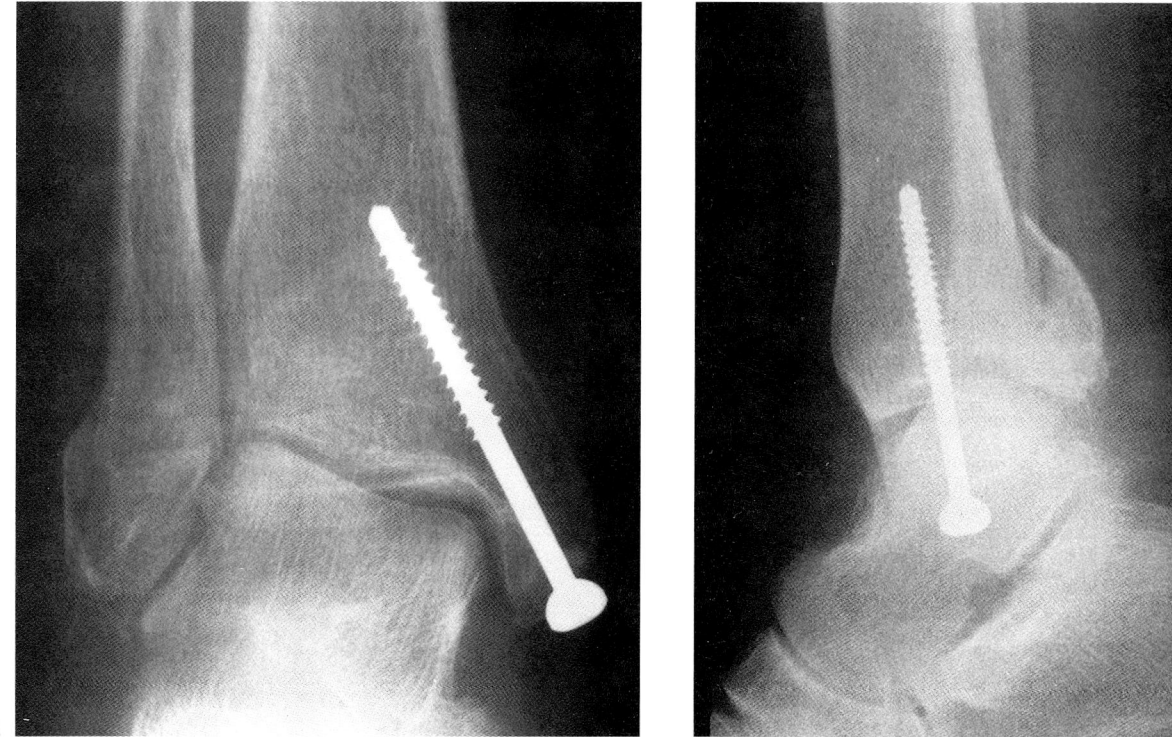

Figure 12. A and **B:** AP and lateral views of trimalleolar fracture malunion.

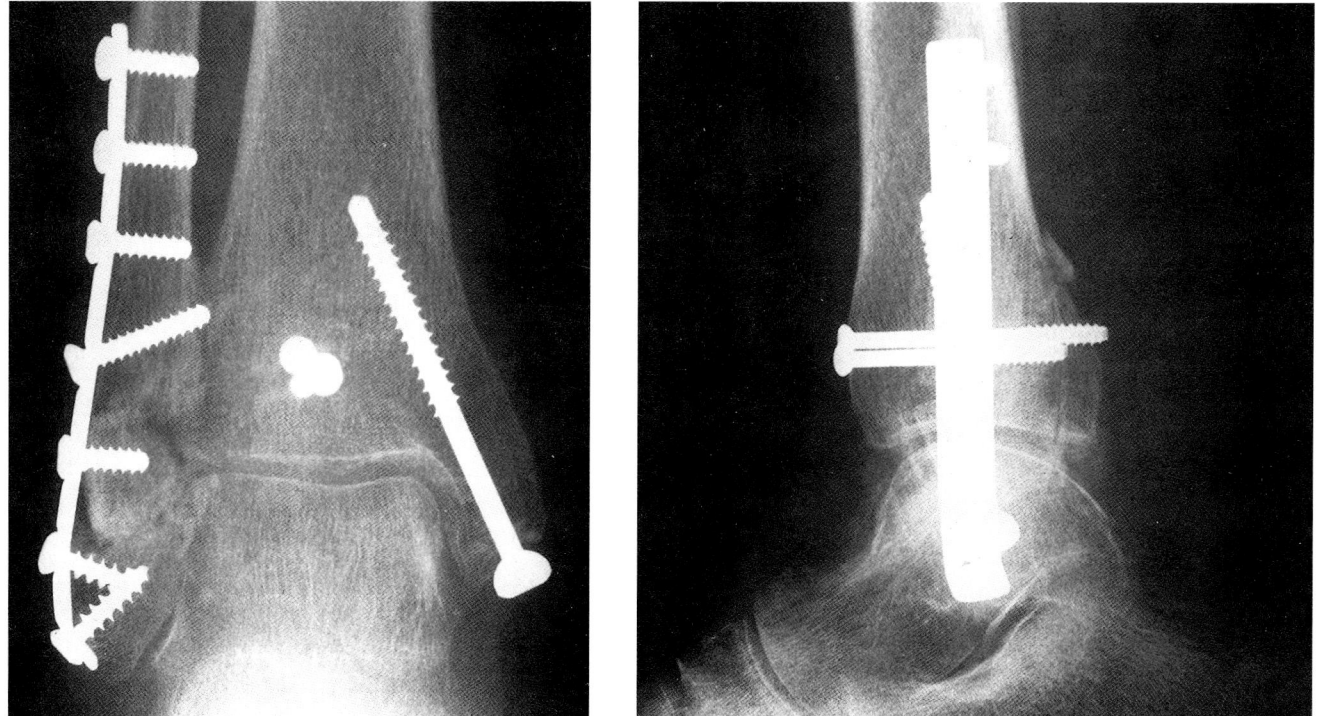

Figure 13. A and **B:** AP and lateral views following realignment.

distally were maintained largely intact. The distal aspect of the incisura fibularis was cleared of scar tissue and the lateral plafond and posterior malleolar fragment well visualized. An osteotome was used to free this fragment from the tibial metaphysis and allow accurate repositioning distally. Two 4.0-mm cannulated screws were then placed from anterior to posterior over guide wires through separate stab wounds into this fragment.

Traction was continued via the femoral distractor and a bone clamp until appropriate fibular length had been regained as confirmed on the image intensifier. The distal fibular fragment was then temporarily pinned to the talus using a small smooth K-wire placed across the talofibular articulation. A gap of approximately 1.5 cm was then apparent at the fracture site and thus a tricortical iliac crest bone graft of this length was harvested and placed in this interval. Next, a seven-hole one-third tubular plate was contoured appropriately and secured to the fibula using 3.5-mm cortical screws proximally and 4.0-mm cancellous screws distally. The intercalary graft was stabilized with one screw. Additional cancellous bone was packed around the fracture site followed by routine closure. Initially a plaster splint was applied, followed by a short leg cast that was maintained for approximately 3 months. Progressive weight bearing was begun at 6 weeks postoperatively. Follow-up radiographs 5 months postoperatively (Fig. 13) revealed progressive healing of the fibula with maintenance of a satisfactory reduction of the talus beneath the tibial plafond. Some joint space narrowing laterally over the talar dome as had been present preoperatively persisted. Ankle function was rated as good and pain was described as minimal. This apparently good result has been maintained with a total follow-up of 12 months.

RECOMMENDED READING

1. Marti, R. K., Raaymakers, E. L. F. B., and Nolte, P. A.: Malunited ankle fractures. The late results of reconstruction. *J. Bone Joint Surg.*, 72B: 709–713, 1990.
2. Offierski, C. M., Graham, J. D., Hall, J. H., Harris, W. R., and Schatzker, J. L.: Late revision of fibular malunion in ankle fractures. *Clin. Orthop.*, 171: 145–149, 1982.
3. Ward, A. J., Ackroyd, C. E., and Baker, A. S.: Late lengthening of the fibula for malaligned ankle fractures. *J. Bone Joint Surg.*, 72B: 714–717, 1990.
4. Weber, B. G., and Simpson, L. A.: Corrective lengthening osteotomy of the fibula. *Clin. Orthop.*, 199: 61–67, 1985.
5. Yablon, I. G., and Leach, R. E.: Reconstruction of malunited fractures of the lateral malleolus. *J. Bone Joint Surg.*, 71A: 521–527, 1989.

35

Ankle Arthrodesis

Ronald W. Smith

INDICATIONS/CONTRAINDICATIONS

The primary indication for ankle arthrodesis is arthritic pain that limits activities of daily living. Degenerative arthritis of the ankle may be caused by ankle fracture or, in rare cases, may result from chronic instability. Rheumatoid arthritis is a less common indication for ankle arthrodesis than the degenerative type, and often a rheumatoid patient's complaint of arthritis in the ankle is due to subtalar arthritis.

The radiographic appearance of arthritis is usually advanced when the arthritic process is severe enough to warrant arthrodesis. At least a portion of the joint has a complete loss of the cartilage space in most cases. Surprisingly, some patients who have severe radiographic arthritic findings do not have enough pain to significantly limit their daily activities, and postponement of arthrodesis is recommended.

Deformity is a relative indication for ankle arthrodesis. Occasionally equinus, varus, or valgus deformity may interfere with functional activities more than pain. The deformity may result from trauma or paralysis. Arthrodesis in such cases may lead to significant improvement in walking.

Failure of nonoperative care for the arthritic or paralyzed ankle is usually a prerequisite for recommending arthrodesis. The nonoperative regimen may include antiinflammatory medication, soft laced ankle gauntlet, or a motion-limiting brace.

The ankle arthrodesis technique described in this chapter involves a transverse resection of the distal articular surface of the tibia and is particularly useful in patients with deformity, whether varus-valgus, equinus, or rotational. The bimalleolar approach facilitates full correction of even severe deformities as well as allowing posterior displacement of the talus to improve the smoothness of gait. An attribute of this fusion technique is the orientation of the screws, which allows

---

R. W. Smith, M.D.: Division of Orthopaedic Surgery, Department of Surgery, University of California at Los Angeles School of Medicine, Los Angeles, CA 90024; Balance Orthopaedic Foot and Ankle Center, Long Beach, CA 90806.

relatively easy placement of *three* screws (instead of the commonly used two screws) without impingement between the screws. The use of screws as an alternative to external fixation obviates the occurrence of superficial pin track infections, which are common with the external fixator devices.

A simpler method of arthrodesis than the one described above may be appropriate in arthritic cases without significant deformity or bone loss: An arthrodesis in situ can be done without making a cross-sectional excision of the distal tibia and dome of the talus. In these cases, double screw fixation may be sufficient. Arthroscopic ankle arthrodesis is also applicable when there is no significant deformity or bone loss.

Avascular necrosis involving a "significant portion" of the talar body may be better treated with a Blair fusion than with the technique described in this chapter. In the Blair technique, the avascular body of the talus is removed and the tibia is fused to the talar neck. The term "significant portion" is not well defined in the literature, but if more than one-half of the talar body radiographically appears avascular, the Blair technique should probably be used.

Peripheral neuropathy, for example in diabetes, may be a contraindication to arthrodesis because of an increased likelihood of nonunion compared to arthrodesis in patients with normal sensory function. Neuropathy patients should be treated to the extent possible in immobilizing braces designed for sensory impaired patients. However, patients with severe deformity may be refractory to brace treatment due to skin breakdown. It has been shown that ankle arthrodesis in such patients is a reasonable alternative to amputation.

Severe osteoporosis is a relative contraindication to ankle arthrodesis with screw fixation. However, it is not clear from the literature that fixation with an external compression fixator is clearly better in these patients.

A failed total ankle arthroplasty may be a contraindication to screw fixation when there is insufficient talus remaining to effectively engage the threads of the screws. An external fixator may be a better fixation device under those conditions.

PREOPERATIVE PLANNING

The patient with ankle arthritis is carefully evaluated preoperatively for subtalar arthritis findings. Sinus tarsi tenderness and "ankle" pain with forced passive flexion are indicators of subtalar irritability. Computed tomography (CT) studies with coronal sections of the hindfoot may be helpful in assessing subtalar arthritis. If there is evidence of early subtalar arthritis, alert the patient to the possibility of persistent "ankle" pain that may require further surgery. When significant radiographic changes are present in the subtalar joint, plan to arthrodese the subtalar joint by making a small extension of the ankle arthrodesis exposure, adding bone graft, and using a talocalcaneal screw.

The presence of osteoporosis may lead to an intraoperative change in plans for fixation and immobilization. An external fixator such as the Calandruccio frame, a compression device designed for ankle fusions, should be available in the event that screw fixation is not satisfactory due to soft bone. Threaded $3/16''$ diameter Steinmann pins may be used axially from the calcaneus into the tibia as a last resort in rheumatoid patients if the bone is too soft for conventional fixation.

In planning for ankle arthrodesis to correct a valgus or varus deformity, the severity of the deformity influences the amount of bone to be resected in order to gain correction. This in turn influences the amount of limb shortening that will occur.

In postfracture cases, bone grafting of the distal tibia may be necessary if there are significant areas of bone loss. The resected malleoli usually provide enough bone in such circumstances. In contrast, arthrodesis of a failed total ankle arthroplasty usually requires a major bone graft such as from the iliac crest.

Scars from previous surgery may require modifications from the recommended incisions. One avoids making a parallel incision within 5 cm of a surgical scar or other incision. When necessary to incise across a linear scar, try to cross at right angles rather than at an acute angle.

The proper timing of arthrodesis following ankle fracture varies with the fracture's severity. In severe pilon fractures, waiting 1 to 2 years before arthrodesing may allow sufficient revascularization of the bone fragments and greater likelihood of successful arthrodesis. However, the presence of severe pain may prompt earlier arthrodesis.

Significant sclerosis, such as that seen on the tibial side of the ankle following severe pilon fractures, may require intramedullary drilling and more prolonged immobilization to avoid nonunion.

Preoperative counseling prepares the patient for realistic expectations. Items of information include general infection, nonunion, and neurovascular complications, and in addition, possibilities of

- shortening,
- prolonged casting,
- need for external fixator,
- need for bone graft, and/or
- need for shoe modifications postoperatively.

SURGERY

The patient is operated with a spinal or general anesthetic and positioned in a semilateral decubitus position with the operative side up (Fig. 1). The proper partial side-lying position is such that at rest the lateral side of the ankle is almost parallel to the floor, but with gentle external rotation the toes can be directed to the ceiling and the medial ankle is made accessible for the surgical exposure. A beanbag is used to hold the position. A radiograph table facilitates the use of an image intensifier.

A pneumatic tourniquet is used on the proximal thigh. Before the surgical scrub and draping, the surgeon repeats the evaluation of *rotational* alignment of the operative and *nonoperative* lower extremities by flexing the knee 90° and extending the ankle to neutral or as close to neutral as possible. A mental note is made of the rotational position by lining up the tibial tubercle with a landmark of the

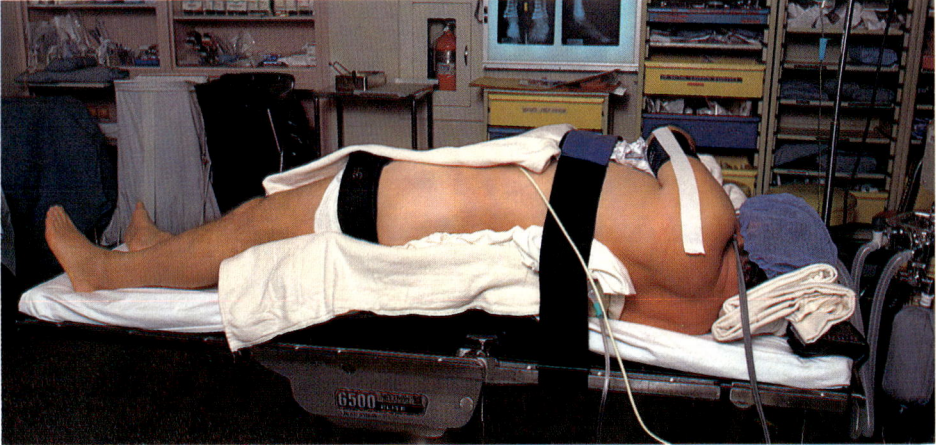

Figure 1. The patient is placed in a semilateral position. Hip external rotation allows toes to be directed toward the ceiling and gives access to the medial side of the ankle. Internal rotation allows easy access to the lateral side of the ankle.

forefoot such as the web space between the first and second toes. Surgical drapes are applied, leaving the foot, leg, and knee exposed in the surgical field (Fig. 2). This allows flexion of the knee to 90° and comparison of the rotational alignment of the foot to the knee during surgery (Fig. 3). If the patient has a previously fused ankle on the other extremity, it is helpful to scrub and drape the other leg in the surgical field to provide close symmetry in ankle position, if the other ankle is satisfactorily aligned.

Technique. The lateral incision begins over the distal fibula about 10 cm above the tip of the lateral malleolus (Fig. 4). The incision extends distally to the tip of the lateral malleolus and angles toward the fourth toe across the sinus tarsi, terminating near the dorsum of the cuboid. The soft tissue in the sinus tarsi is *not* excised, but the incision extends distally to allow easy exposure of the anterolateral surface of the talar body.

The lateral malleolus is osteotomized with an oscillating saw using a blade that is 0.5 to 1.0 cm in width (Fig. 5). The osteotomy begins about 4 cm proximal to the joint line and is directed distally and medially to make a beveled cut. The distal fragment is grasped with a Lewin bone clamp (a heavy towel clip-like tenaculum) and the soft tissue detached with scalpel, 1.2 cm Key elevator, and rongeurs. In proliferative osteoarthritis, bone spurs and dense soft tissue at the tibiofibular syndesmosis may require aggressive technique. Visualizing the peroneal tendons prevents injury to them when freeing up and excising the lateral malleolus.

Alignment reference guide pins are placed in the tibia prior to making the medial exposure (Fig. 6). Two 0.062" smooth wires are placed in the tibia about 12 cm proximal to the ankle joint. One pin is placed in the anterior cortex in an anterior to posterior direction. It is placed perpendicular to the tibia as one looks at the lateral surface of the leg. This pin serves to orient for the calcaneus-equinus position as the distal tibial cut is made. The second pin is placed in the lateral cortex in a lateral to medial direction, placing the pin perpendicular to the axis of the anterior surface of the tibia. This pin serves to orient for the varus-valgus position as the distal tibial osteotomy is made.

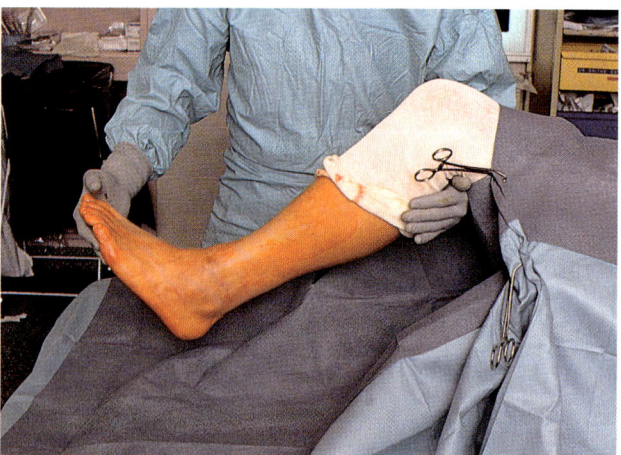

Figure 2. The lower extremity is draped to expose the knee and allow 90° of knee flexion for rotational alignment assessment.

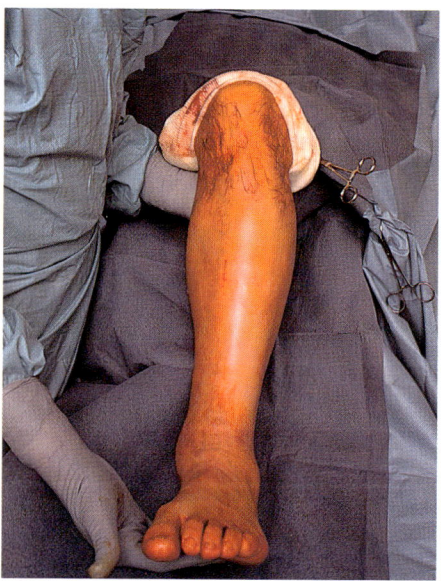

Figure 3. The frontal view allows assessment of rotational alignment. A mental note is made of which toe or interdigital space lines up with the tibial tubercle. A similar assessment is made of the other leg before surgery.

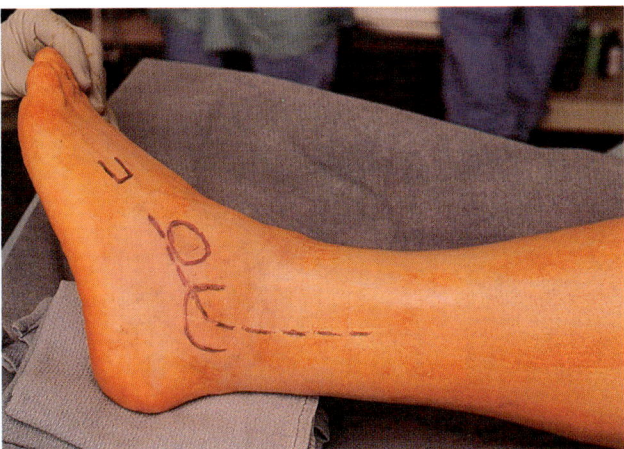

Figure 4. The lateral landmarks and planned incision are drawn on the skin. The *circle* depicts the sinus tarsi, and the *partial rectangle* marks the base of the fourth metatarsal.

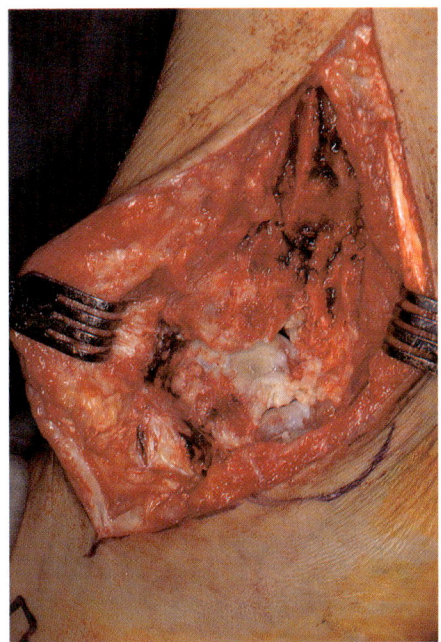

Figure 5. The lateral malleolus has been resected exposing the lateral talus. The *central white area* is the lateral surface of the talus.

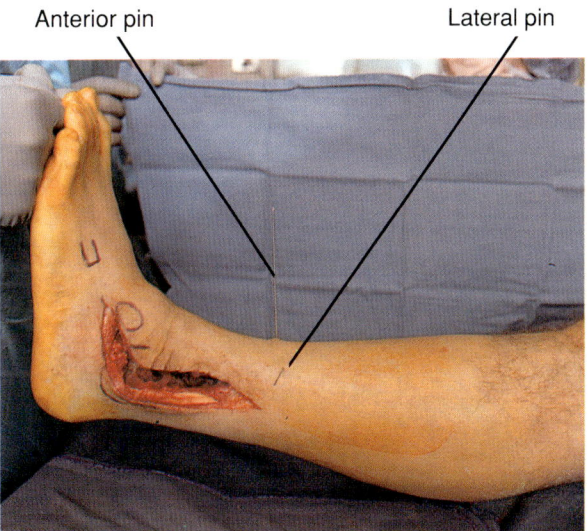

Figure 6. Guide pins are placed in orthogonal planes.

The leg is externally rotated to access the medial ankle, and incision is made beginning on the bone about 8 cm above the tip of the malleolus (Fig. 7). The incision is extended distally and at the tip of the malleolus is angled anteriorly to parallel the axis of the talar neck. The incision is continued to the level of the navicular to allow easy visualization of the ankle and medial talar neck.

With sharp dissection, free the tibialis posterior and flexor hallucis longus tendons from the posterior surface of the distal tibia. They may be adherent to the bone and can be injured as the articular surface of the tibia is osteotomized (Fig. 8).

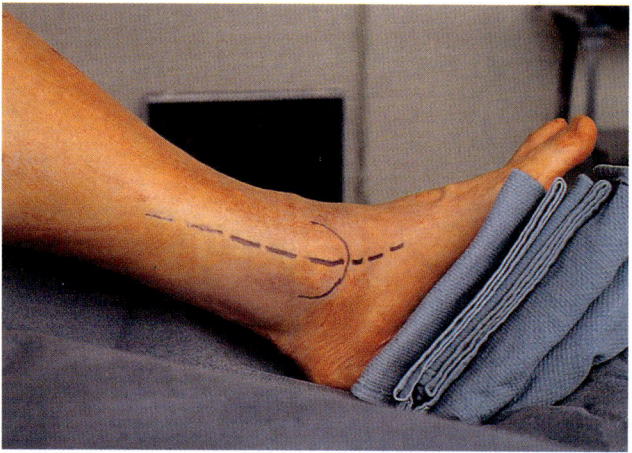

Figure 7. The planned medial incision is drawn. A smaller incision may be sufficient in cases not requiring extensive hardware removal.

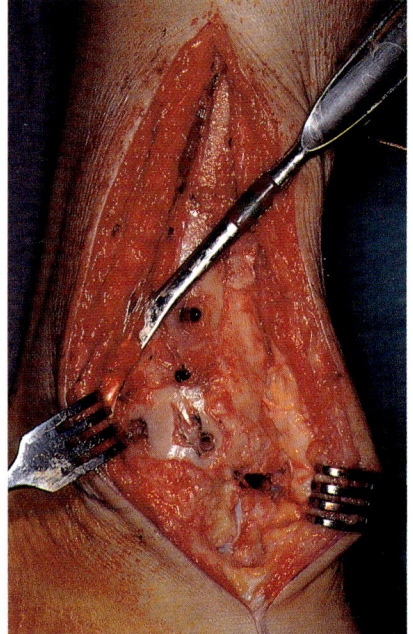

Figure 8. A fracture fixation plate has been removed from the medial tibia. A periosteal elevator is used to free up the tibialis posterior tendon that is scarred down on the posterior tibia.

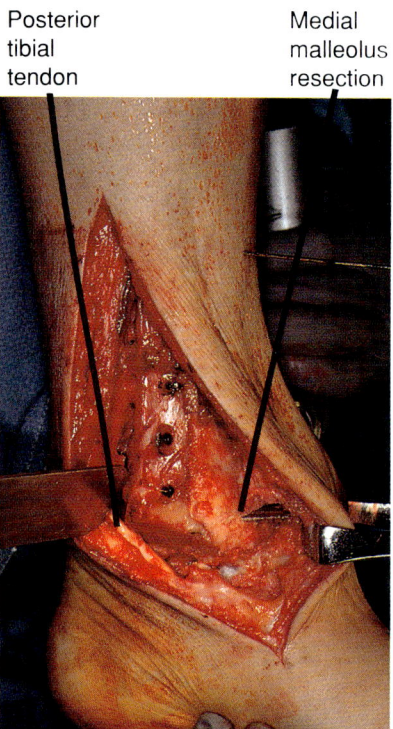

Figure 9. The medial malleolus has been resected at about a 45° angle.

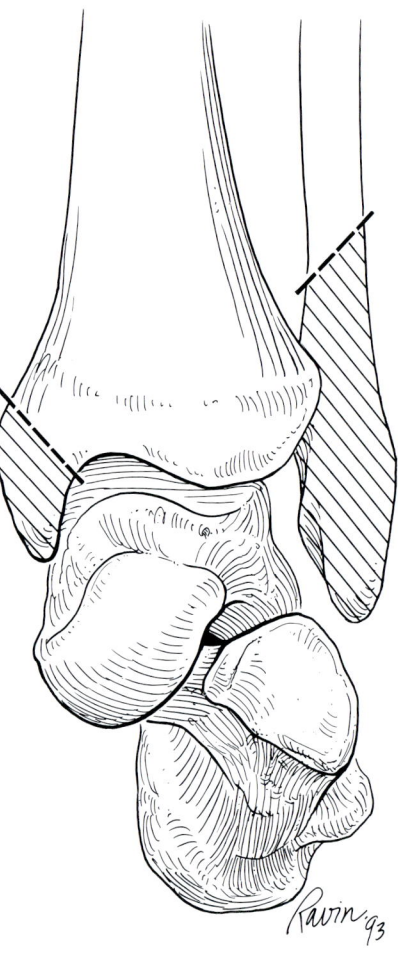

Figure 10. Anterior view drawing showing resection of malleoli.

Osteotomize the medial malleolus with about a 45° angle at the level of the plafond (Fig. 9). Doing this before osteotomizing the major articular surface of the tibia facilitates visualization of the vulnerable medial tendons. No further resection of the medial flare of the tibia should be needed at the end of the procedure. The small residual medial flare serves as a solid buttress for the medial screw (Fig. 10). Before osteotomizing the tibial articular surface, the anterior and posterior ankle capsule is well elevated or excised

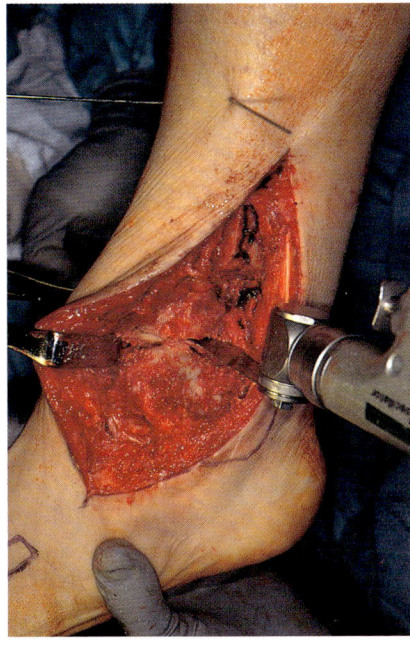

Figure 11. Resection of distal tibia from lateral to medial with oscillating saw. Army-navy retraction of anterior skin through medial and lateral incisions augments the views.

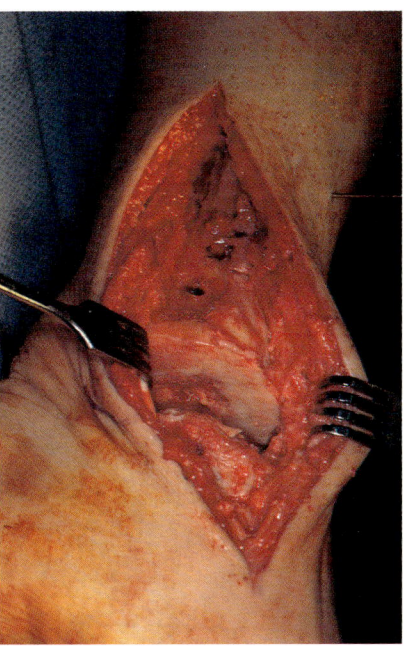

Figure 12. Cut surface of the distal tibia from medial view. Central bone defect is visible.

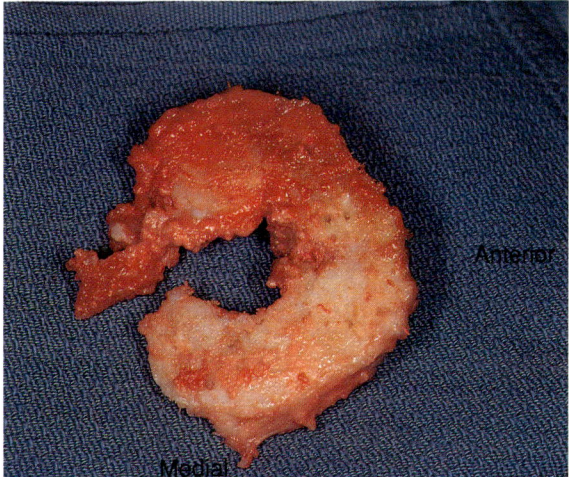

Figure 13. Resected surface of the distal tibia. Medial side is thicker to compensate for valgus deformity.

Excision of the tibial articular surface is made from lateral to medial using a large oscillating saw with a blade about 3 cm wide (Fig. 11). Visualization and protection of soft tissue is accomplished by placing blade-like retractors such as Chandler or Giannestras retractors posteriorly, both medially and laterally, interposed between bone and tendons. Anteriorly, army-navy retractors are placed medially and laterally and are lifted toward the ceiling with one hand of the assistant. The assistant surgeon and scrub assistant are involved in retraction at this point.

The surgeon resects the tibial articular surface, removing about 3 to 4 mm of bone (Figs. 12 and 13). Using the guide pins for orientation, the articular surface is cut perpendicular to the axis of the leg. Err toward valgus if necessary to avoid varus in making the osteotomy. Regardless of the deformity, the distal articular surface is osteotomized perpendicular to the axis of the leg. The resected fragment of bone may be wedge shaped, for example, thicker on the medial side if there

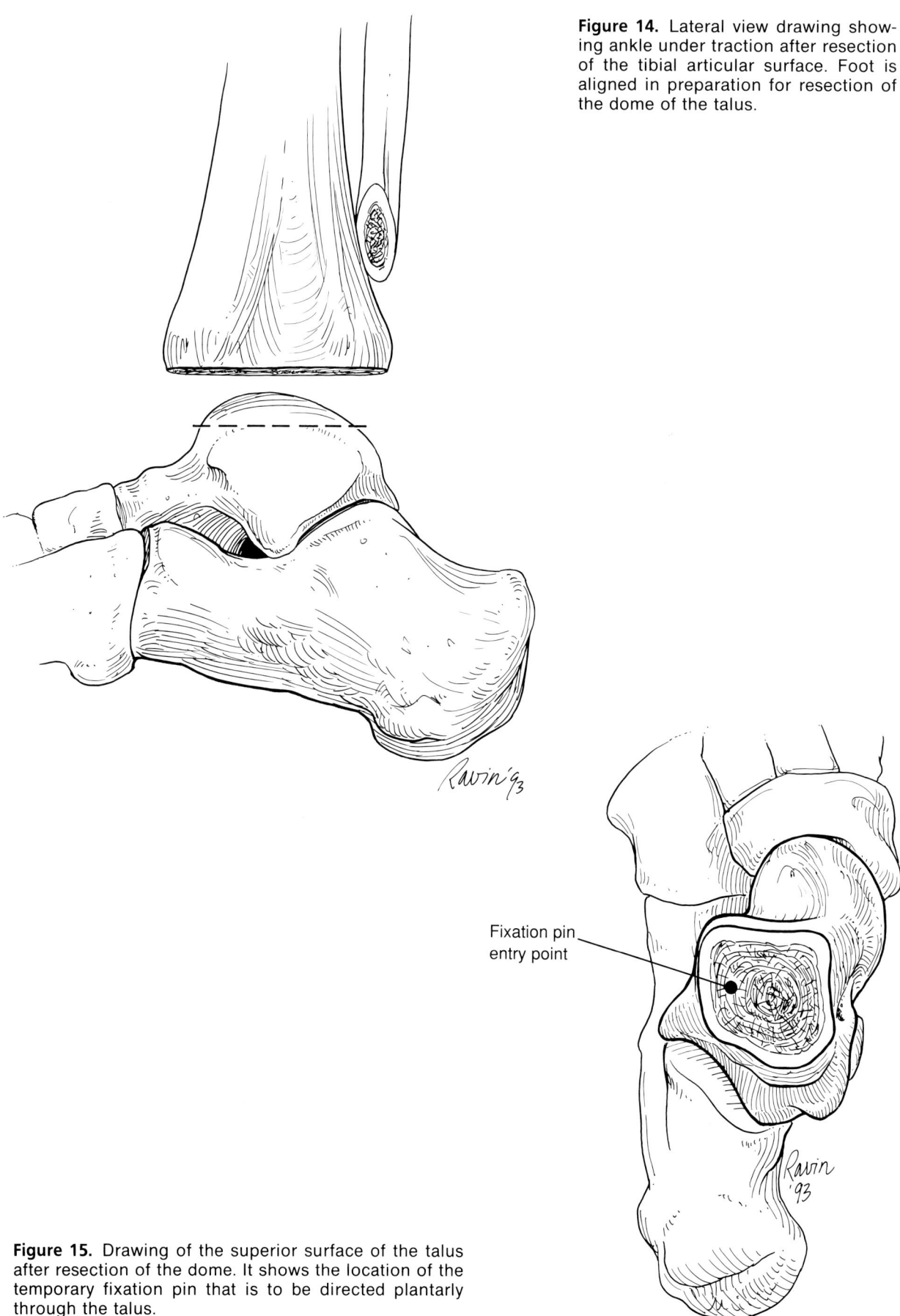

Figure 14. Lateral view drawing showing ankle under traction after resection of the tibial articular surface. Foot is aligned in preparation for resection of the dome of the talus.

Figure 15. Drawing of the superior surface of the talus after resection of the dome. It shows the location of the temporary fixation pin that is to be directed plantarly through the talus.

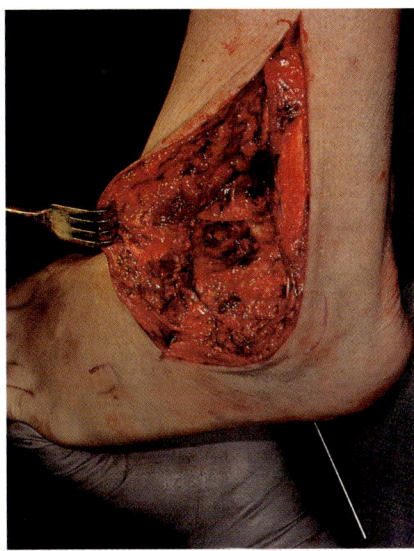

Figure 16. A ⅛" smooth Steinmann pin is driven plantarly to exit the plantar surface of the calcaneus. In the process, the ankle is adducted and the foot displaced laterally to expose the dorsal surface of the talus. However, care is taken to neutralize the hindfoot and avoid inversion when the pin crosses the subtalar joint.

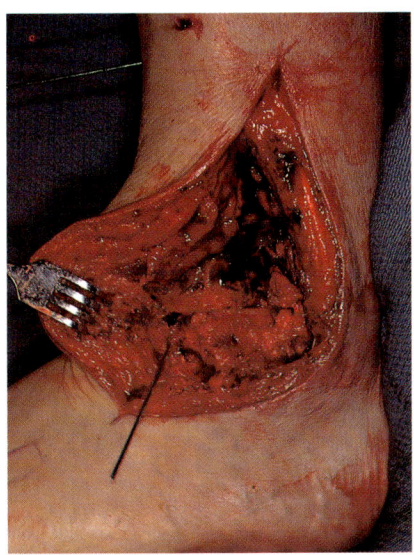

Figure 17. Lateral view. Arthrodesis surfaces have been reduced, the talus displaced posteriorly 5 to 8 mm, and the tibiocalcaneal pin advanced into the tibia while applying axial compression. A 0.062" K-wire has been added across the talotibial interval as temporary fixation to control rotation. The pin enters the talar body adjacent to the talar neck, sufficiently medial to allow entry of the first screw at the lateral face of the talar body.

was a preoperative valgus deformity. It may be a consideration to build in slight equinus if the female patient insists on wearing an elevated heel or if the leg length is already short preoperatively. However, it is this surgeon's feeling that the most consistent satisfaction in walking with a fused ankle comes with a neutral calcaneus-equinus position.

After removal of the articular surface of the tibia, the foot is lined up neutral to the leg with respect to calcaneus-equinus, varus-valgus, and rotation. The assistant surgeon holds the alignment, and the scrub assistant retracts the anterior skin with the medial and lateral retractors while the surgeon resects the dome of the talus, removing about 3 mm of dorsal surface (Fig. 14). A 2- to 2.5-cm blade width is used for the talar dome resection.

Temporary fixation is attained with an axial tibiotalocalcaneal ⅛" smooth Steinmann pin supplemented with a 0.062" smooth K-wire placed obliquely across the fusion site from the lateral talus to the medial tibia. The Steinmann pin is placed in the lateral surface of the cut dorsal surface of the talus and directed plantarly (Fig. 15). The lateral location for the axial pin avoids obstruction with the first two screws, which will be directed from anterolaterally to posteromedially. If the Steinmann pin is too posterior in the talus, it will cut out posteriorly when the pin is advanced proximally into the tibia after posteriorly displacing the talus on the tibia. Be sure to place the subtalar joint in neutral as the pin crosses the subtalar joint. The tendency is to leave the subtalar joint slightly inverted as the pin is advanced plantarly (Fig. 16). The Steinmann pin is retracted plantarly and the talus is displaced posteriorly. With the posterior displacement of the talus, the anterior flare of the distal tibia lines up near the junction of the head and neck of the talus or over a portion of the head of the talus. The posterior displacement

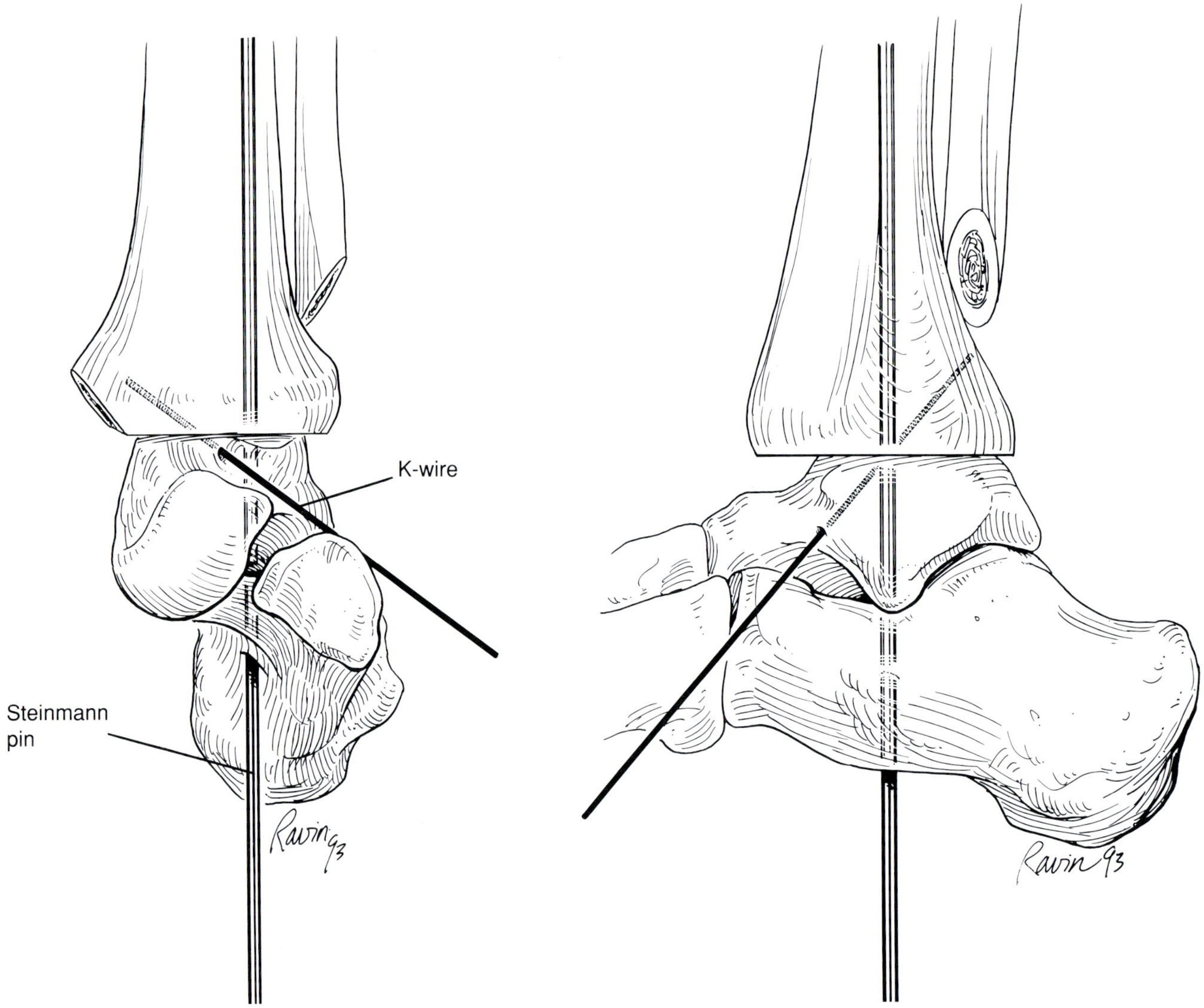

Figure 18. Anterior and lateral view drawings of pin placement for temporary fixation.

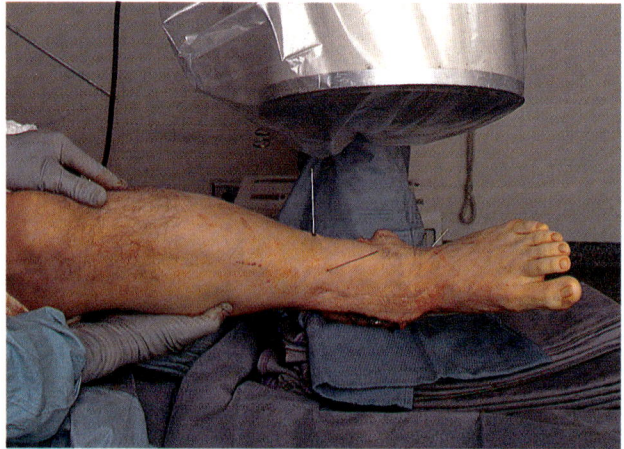

Figure 19. The leg is internally rotated to place the axis of the foot parallel to the floor for a lateral view using the image intensifier. If internal rotation is incomplete, the image X-ray beam is adjusted short of vertical to accomplish a true lateral view.

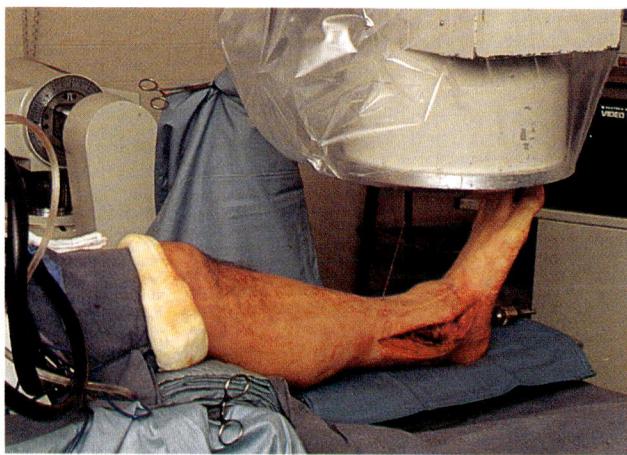

Figure 20. The leg is externally rotated and positioned for the anterior-posterior view.

of the talus reduces the length of the anterior lever arm of the ankle, allowing a smoother terminal stance phase of gait.

The tibiotalar joint surfaces are apposed, and the Steinmann pin is drilled into the tibia. Next, rotational alignment is rechecked and a K-wire is inserted to control the rotational alignment. The K-wire is inserted just lateral to the base of the talar neck on the anterior surface of the talar body and directed into the medial tibia (Figs. 17 and 18). If the pin is started too lateral, it will interfere with the first cannulated screw, which is started in the center of the anterior surface of the lateral talar body. One can use 7.0 mm cannulated stainless steel screws or 6.5 mm cannulated titanium screws. The strength of titanium allows a larger diameter hole in the screw and therefore a larger guide pin. The larger guide pin is easier to direct because it does not "bounce off" the far cortex but seems to penetrate the cortex better than smaller diameter guide pins.

The first cannulated screw is started on the anterior surface of the lateral talar body and is directed into the posteromedial tibia. At this point the image intensifier is used to evaluate the position of the arthrodesis and the location of the initial guide pin (Figs. 19 and 20). The standard technique of measuring for and inserting the cannulated screws is used. The opposite cortex is engaged if feasible. The first screw is not tightened until the second screw is inserted and the temporary fixation pins are removed.

The pin for the second screw is inserted on the anterolateral surface of the tibia about 2 to 2.5 cm proximal to the arthrodesis site. The pin and subsequent screw are directed into the posteromedial talus with the aid of the image intensifier (Fig. 21). After the second screw is placed, the temporary fixation pins are removed and both lateral screws are tightened.

The pin for the third screw is started in the medial surface of the tibia at about the midcoronal plane (Fig. 22). The pin is directed anteriorly toward the lateral talar neck. The screw may be quite oblique to the cortical surface and require some countersinking for the head of the screw. Countersinking is done with a 4-mm power bur on the proximal side of the drill hole after temporarily removing the guide pin. The use of a bur rather than the countersink cutter appears to maintain a better cortical shoulder distal to the drill hole. Inserting and tightening the third screw usually adds visibly to the solidness of the fusion site (Fig. 23).

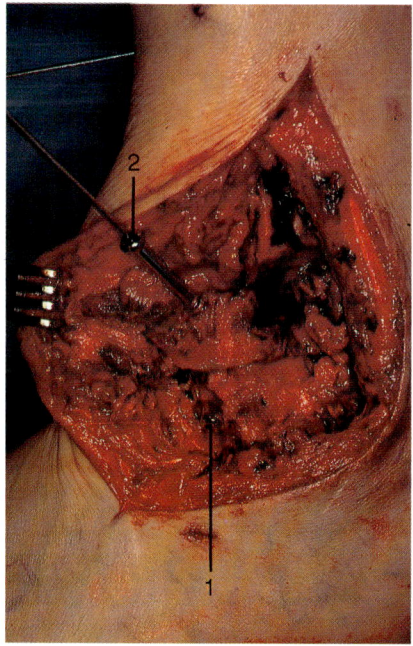

◀ **Figure 21.** Lateral view. The second cannulated screw (2) enters the anterolateral surface of the distal tibia and is directed into the posteromedial talus. The first screw (1) has already been placed and the screw head is seated on the anterior surface of the talar body and is directed into the posterior medial tibia.

▶ **Figure 22.** The third cannulated screw enters the medial tibia and is directed toward the anterolateral body or neck of the talus.

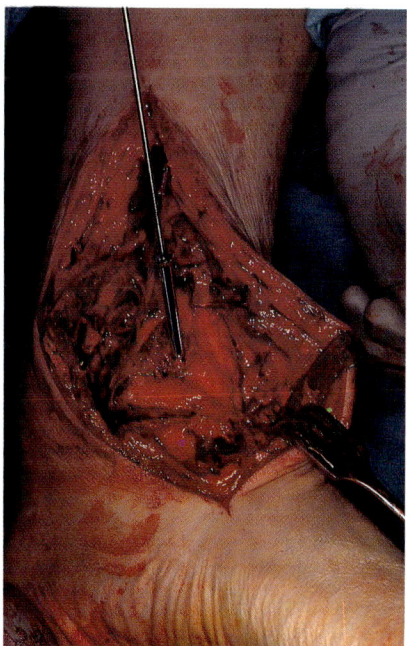

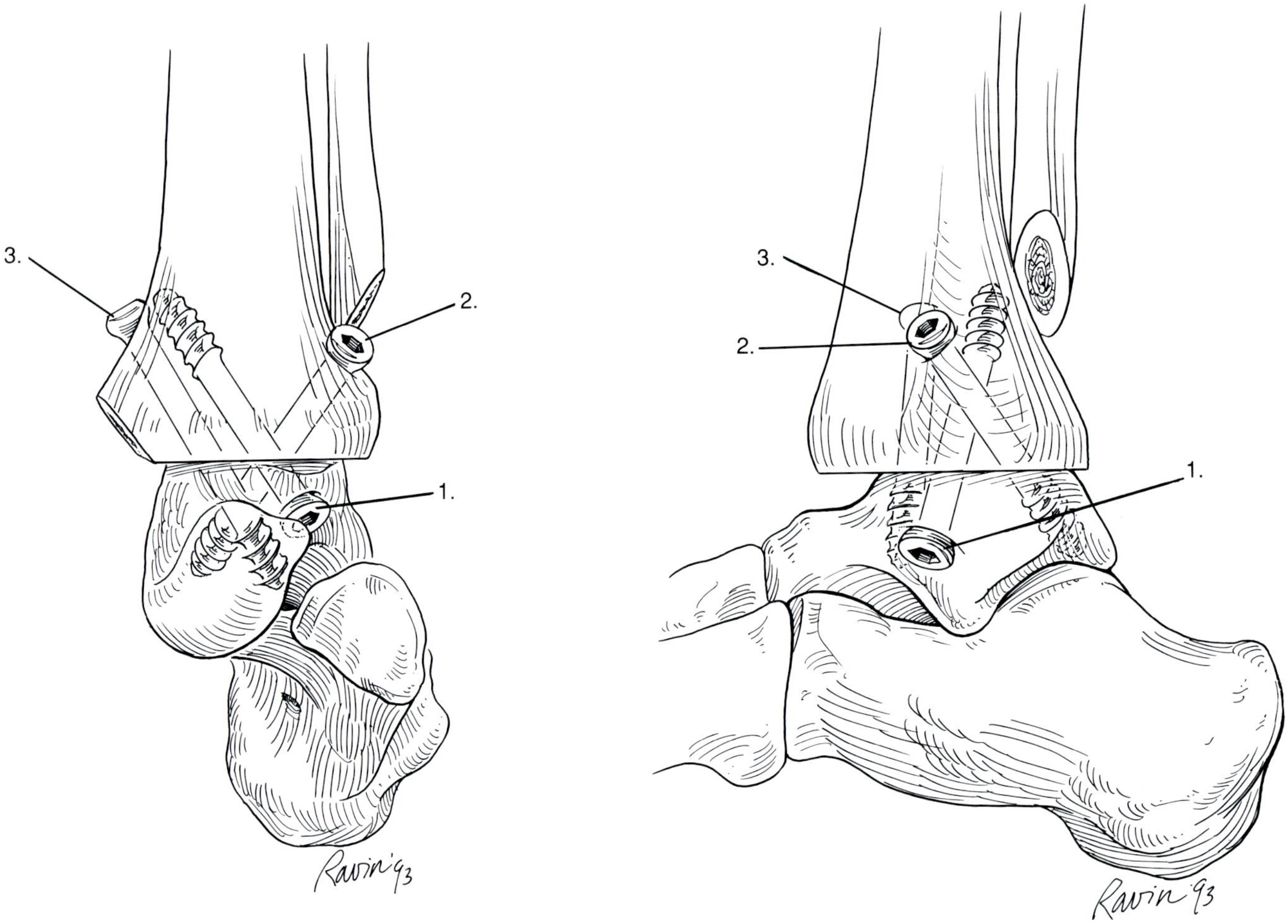

Figure 23. Anterior and lateral view drawings showing screw placement.

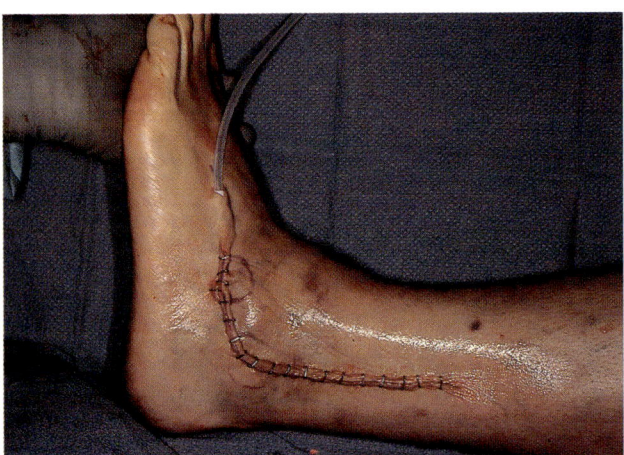

Figure 24. Lateral view after wound closure.

At any of the screw sites, a washer may be necessary if cortical softness allows penetration of the head of the screw. The utmost care is taken to avoid penetrating the subtalar joint with the second and third screws (proximal-to-distal screws). Radiographic imaging and checking subtalar motion help identify inadvertent screw extension into the subtalar joint.

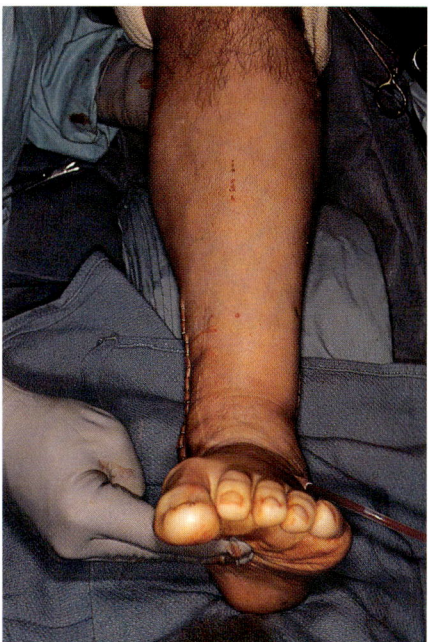

Figure 25. Frontal view after wound closure.

A soft suction drain is brought out from the lateral ankle at the dorsum of the foot, just proximal to the base of the fourth metatarsal.

The wound is closed with absorbable subcutaneous sutures and nylon sutures or stainless steel staples on the skin (Figs. 24–25).

POSTOPERATIVE MANAGEMENT

A well-padded short leg cast is applied with two rolls of 6″ plaster and no splints. This lightweight cast is easily univalved and spread if required because of pain following surgery. The drain is usually pulled on the first postoperative day and the cast closed and reinforced with a layer of fiberglass on the second day. The patient usually starts brief non–weight-bearing ambulation on the second day and goes home on the second or third postoperative day. Bed rest with elevation of the ankle at least 12 inches above the heart is emphasized for the first 3 days. Thereafter, the patient progresses with sitting, using another chair for elevation.

The cast is changed about 2 weeks after surgery, sutures or staples are removed, and a short leg fiberglass cast is reapplied. Non–weight bearing or toe touch ambulation is prescribed for 3 months, and calf isometric exercises are instructed. Cast changes are made at 4- to 6-week intervals, and weight bearing is initiated at 3 months postoperatively. The patient is advised to gradually progress with weight bearing as long as there is no pain.

Four months postoperatively, the patient is expected to be ambulating at full weight bearing in a short leg cast without pain at that time. The cast is converted to a "bivalve," anterior and posterior shells of the fiberglass cast that can be used as a removable cast. This device allows a gradual weaning from immobilization. In the security of the home, the patient can walk cast-free for an hour or so three to four times the first day and progress with cast-free walking on subsequent days as long as there is no pain. An elastic stocking is worn with and without the bivalve cast for at least 3 months to prevent or minimize swelling.

Physical therapy is started when the "bivalve program" (weaning from the cast) is started. Subtalar range of motion and foot and leg strengthening are emphasized. The surgeon or physical therapist may suggest footwear modifications. An elevated heel or rocker bottom sole may aid in developing a maximally smooth gait. In this surgeon's experience, ankle fusion patients improve the smoothness of their walking for at least 9 to 12 months following surgery. Patients usually walk better with shoes than barefooted. Contrary to popular belief, transverse tarsal motion does not increase with time.

Conservative guidelines for patient expectations include playing golf at 9 to 12 months and doubles tennis at 1 to 2 years. Stationary bicycle riding is encouraged as a form of aerobic exercise but not jogging, even after the arthrodesis is well healed. There is concern that the repetitive impact loading of jogging may accelerate arthritic problems in the subtalar joint or knee.

It is reasonable to expect a 10% nonunion rate, higher in extenuating circumstances (see Complications). Malalignment complaints may occur in about 15% of patients.

COMPLICATIONS

1. *Pseudarthrosis*. Pseudarthrosis occurs in about 10% of cases (range 0–30%) of reported ankle fusions. An increased rate of pseudarthrosis is associated with the severity of the initial trauma in cases caused by fracture and in cases of neuropathy.

    Several points may help prevent pseudarthrosis. An adequate area of cancellous bone apposition promotes arthrodesis. Removal of only 1 or 2 mm off the dome of the talus in order to minimize shortening may not provide a large enough surface area of cancellous bone to assure arthrodesis. The cross-sectional area of the talus is larger 3 to 4 mm below the dorsal surface.

    If the distal tibia is sclerotic, as may be seen with arthritis following pilon fractures, make multiple intramedullary drill holes in the tibial surface. Fill bone defects with morcellized bone from the malleoli.

    Additional protection with a flexed knee long leg cast may be necessary in patients who are prone to pseudarthrosis. Such patients include those who had a high-energy ankle fracture and patients who may be noncompliant in avoiding weight bearing postoperatively. Be suspicious of a delay in healing if a patient has significant pain, swelling, or warmth at the ankle 3 months after surgery. A long leg cast and an electrical stimulator may be considerations at that point *even* if the radiographs look satisfactory.

    Bone grafting and revision of the internal fixation is a consideration as early as 6 months after initial fusion if there is a delayed union. Often there is fibrous tissue stability, and the arthrodesis does not have to be completely taken down.

2. *Malalignment*. The most common malalignment problems associated with ankle arthrodesis are equinus, varus, and internal rotation. Equinus deformity causes a knee hyperextension gait deformity and makes barefoot walking difficult. Prevention requires carefully aligning the lateral border of the plantar surface of the foot with the axis of the fibula at the time temporary fixation is accomplished. Resecting the distal articular surface of the tibia perpendicular to the long axis of the tibia is imperative.

    A postoperative varus deformity causes the patient to walk on the lateral border of the foot. Prevention requires resecting the distal articular surface of the tibia with a minimal valgus angle.

    Avoidance of rotational deformity is aided by the use of guide pins and by flexing the knee 90° when judging rotational alignment.

The occurrence of malalignment is treated with footwear modifications if the deformity is mild. An osteotomy just proximal to the fusion site may be necessary in more severe circumstances.

Occasionally, a slowly developing internal rotation/varus deformity may result from progressive subtalar arthritis.

3. *Persistent postoperative pain despite a solid fusion.* This is most likely due to subtalar arthritis. Occasionally subtalar irritability will be caused by penetration of the screws into the talocalcaneal joint. Use of the image intensifier while placing the guide pins and screws, as well as checking the subtalar motion after removing the temporary fixation, helps to avoid this problem.
4. *Tendon lacerations.* The tibialis posterior and the long flexor of the hallux are vulnerable during the resection of the distal tibial articular surface. Carefully resecting a portion of the medial malleolus exposes the tendons and allows their further mobilization. The tendons are often adherent to the medial tibia in cases of previous fracture.

ILLUSTRATIVE CASE FOR TECHNIQUE

The case of a 51-year-old machine operator is used to illustrate this technique of ankle arthrodesis.

The man suffered an intraarticular fracture of the ankle 3 years prior to his arthrodesis while cross-country skiing. The fracture was treated surgically, but progressive pain and valgus deformity developed (Fig. 26).

The prefusion examination revealed a moderate limp and moderate heel valgus. There was a mild lateral translation of the foot relative to the longitudinal axis of the leg. Examination showed a mild loss of ankle extension and moderate loss of flexion. Subtalar motion was almost absent. Well-healed surgical scars were present over the anteromedial distal tibia and distal aspect of the fibula. There was a significant loss of active flexion of the great toe.

At surgery, sclerotic bone and a bone defect were encountered in the distal tibia. The flexor hallucis longus was incarcerated in scar at the posterior surface

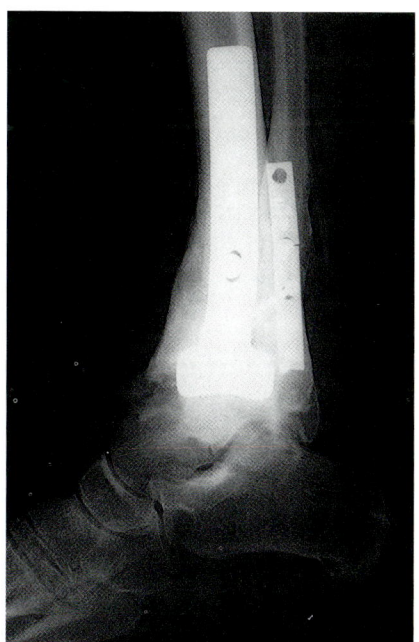
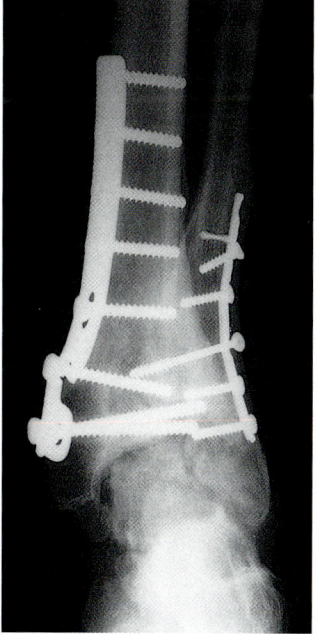

Figure 26. **A** and **B**: Radiographs preoperative.

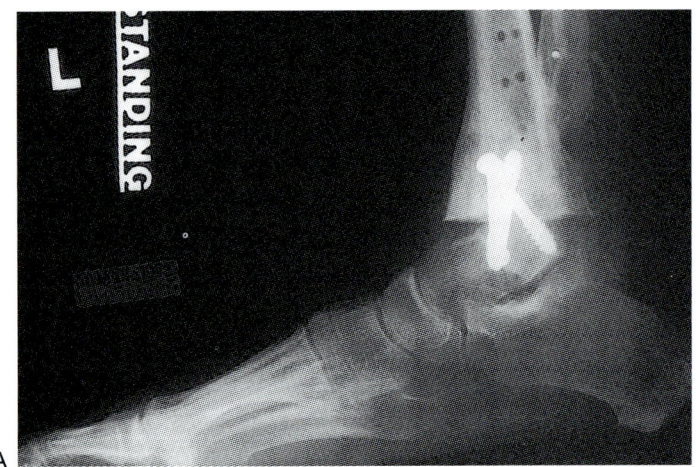
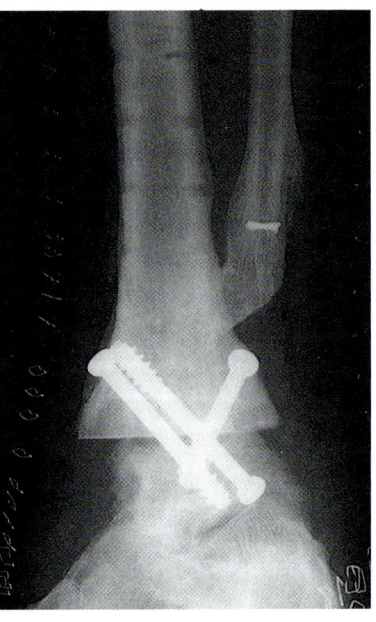

Figure 27. A and **B**: Radiographs 2 weeks postoperative.

of the distal tibia, and tenolysis was performed. At the completion of operation, ankle position was approximately neutral with regard to dorsiflexion-flexion and valgus-varus. The foot was externally rotated about 15° (Fig. 27).

The patient was discharged from the hospital on the third postoperative day. He is early in his postoperative course and will be kept non–weight bearing for at least 3 months, with the expectation of slow bone union due to sclerosis.

RECOMMENDED READING

1. Buck, P., Morrey, B. F., and Chao, E. Y. S. The optimum position of arthrodesis of the ankle—a gait study of the knee and ankle. *J. Bone Joint Surg.*, 69A: 1052–1062, 1987.
2. Cracchiolo, A., guest editor. Symposium on methods and follow-up statistics on ankle arthrodeses. *Clin. Orthop.*, 1991.
3. Johnson, K. A. *Surgery of the Foot and Ankle*. Raven Press, New York, pp. 151–177, 1989.
4. Kenzora, J. E., Simmons, S. C., Burgess, A. R., Edwards, C. C. External fixation arthrodesis of the ankle following trauma. *Foot Ankle*, 7: 49–61, 1986.
5. Morgan, C. D., Henke, J. A., Bailey, R. W., Kaufer, H. Long term results of tibiotalar arthrodesis. *J. Bone Joint Surg.*, 67A: 546–550, 1985.
6. Morris, H. D., Hand, W. L., Dunn, A. W. The modified Blair fusion for fractures of the talus. *J. Bone Joint Surg.*, 53A: 1289–1297, 1971.
7. Myerson, M., Quill, G. Ankle arthrodesis. A comparison of an arthroscopic and an open method of treatment. *Clin. Orthop.*, 268: 56–64, 1991.
8. Ouzounian, T. J., Kleiger, B. Arthrodesis in the foot and ankle. In: *Disorders of the Foot and Ankle*, 2nd ed, edited by M. H. Jahss, W.B. Saunders, Philadelphia, pp. 2614–2623, 1991.
9. Waters, R. L., Barnes, G., Husserl, T., Silver, L., Liss, R. Comparable energy expenditure after arthrodesis of the hip and ankle. *J. Bone Joint Surg.*, 70: 1032–1037, 1988.

36

Tibiocalcaneal Arthrodesis

Kenneth A. Johnson

INDICATIONS/CONTRAINDICATIONS

When degeneration and/or deformity involves both the tibiotalar and talocalcaneal articulations of the hindfoot, the appropriate treatment may be an arthrodesis from the tibia to the calcaneus. There are a variety of reasons for a tibiocalcaneal (TC) arthrodesis, such as avascular necrosis of the talus following trauma, failed total ankle placement with subtalar intrusion, failed ankle arthrodesis, rheumatoid arthritis, severe deformity secondary to untreated talipes equinovarus or neuromuscular disease, and posttraumatic arthrosis. The posterior approach for this procedure avoids the medial and lateral aspects of the ankle. Not infrequently prior surgical procedures or trauma will have injured skin in these areas and the only approach available through healthy skin will be posteriorly. A posterior TC arthrodesis is a versatile procedure that allows for a large correction of deformity and accurate repositioning of the foot in a plantigrade position.

Contraindications for this procedure would be impaired circulation or a history of infection that may be dormant or active.

PREOPERATIVE PLANNING

Factors that need to be considered in preoperative planning include the extent of hindfoot joint involvement, skin condition at the operative site, bone vascularity, and deformity.

If there are degenerative changes in the calcaneocuboid and talonavicular articulations, these may also need to be treated with an arthrodesis procedure. Plain radiographs of the foot and ankle should be sufficient to evaluate these joints.

K. A. Johnson, M.D.: Division of Foot and Ankle Surgery, Mayo Clinic Scottsdale, Scottsdale, AZ 85259.

Skin condition is important since delayed healing or necrosis can occur. Prior surgical posterior approaches or injury may make the posterior incision inadvisable.

The vascularity, particularly of the talus body, should be assessed if trauma is the inciting incident. When in doubt, magnetic resonance imaging should be done to demonstrate the extent of avascular bone.

Deformity is largely evident by physical examination. The goal of the procedure is to place the foot in a plantigrade position. With a large hindfoot varus or valgus, an osteotomy of the fibula is necessary. Flexion deformity is largely corrected by resecting wedges from the talar dome and distal tibial plafond.

A proper physical examination along with plain radiographs of the foot and ankle, and an occasional magnetic resonance imaging study, should allow proper surgical planning for the tibiocalcaneal arthrodesis. With stress testing of the ankle separately from stress testing of the subtalar joint, the origin of pain can be determined. Crepitus and stiffness with swelling are indicators of degeneration. When there is doubt, a technetium scan with delayed views will highlight the pattern of joint degeneration.

SURGERY

After induction of general or spinal anesthesia, the patient is placed on the operating room table in a prone position on chest rolls. With the knee flexed to a right angle, the involved extremity is sterilely prepared and draped. An adhesive surgical drape is placed about the forefoot to seal off the toes from the surgical wound. The posterior iliac crest on the same side as the involved extremity is also sterilely prepared for bone graft harvesting.

Technique. To limit tourniquet time, bone graft from the posterior iliac crest is taken first. By removing the upper aspect of the posterior iliac crest (Fig. 1) as well as the outer table of the posterior ilium, copious bone graft is available (Fig. 2). If two surgeons are available, the iliac crest bone can be removed while the second surgeon is exposing the hindfoot through the posterior approach. The bone graft is meticulously cleaned of soft tissue with a large rongeur and then morcellated with a bone mill, which mixes the cortical and cancellous bone fragments (Fig. 3). A hand-operated bone mill (Kirschner Co.) provides the desired 2 to 4

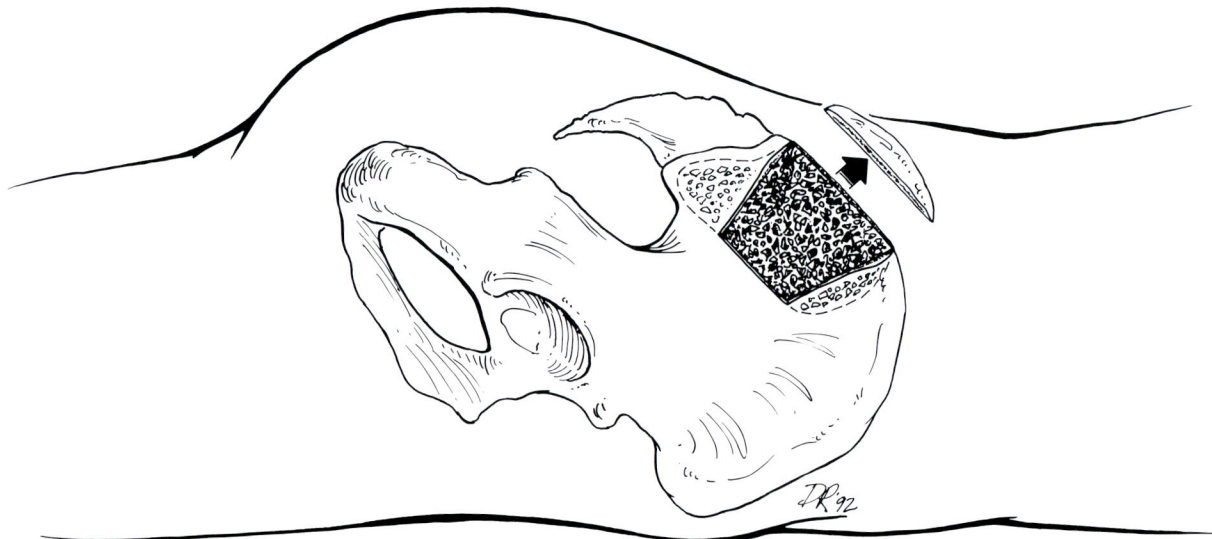

Figure 1. Diagrammatic representation of bone graft harvesting from the posterior iliac crest.

mm in diameter bone particles. The posterior iliac crest wound is closed in layers over a small suction drain after a large Gelfoam saturated with thrombin is placed in the wound.

For the posterior ankle area, hemostasis is provided by rubber bandage exsanguination and thigh tourniquet (Fig. 4). A posterolateral slightly curved incision about 20 cm long is made along the lateral border of the Achilles tendon (Fig. 5).

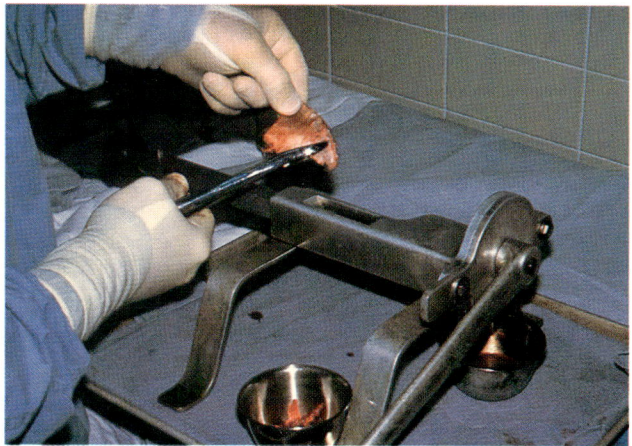

Figure 2. Bone graft is removed from the outer aspect of the posterior iliac crest and cut into strips before being placed in the bone mill.

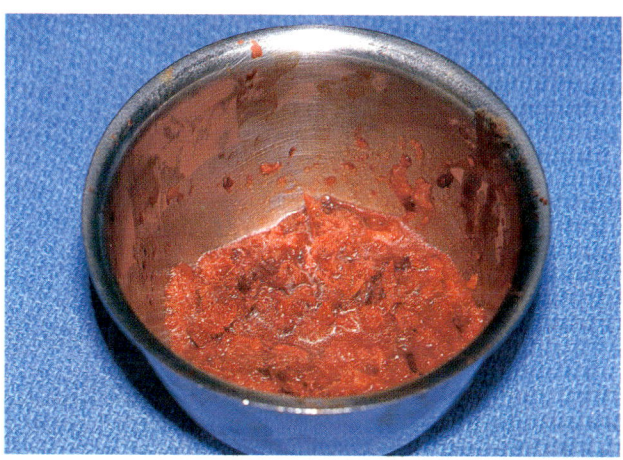

Figure 3. After the bone graft has been run through the bone mill, it forms a slurry of small bone chips that will mold to the arthrodesis site.

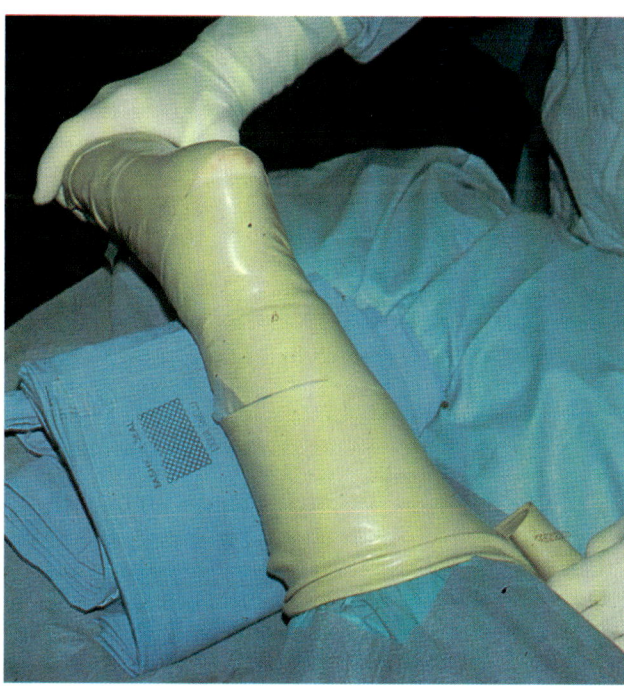

Figure 4. The patient is placed prone on the operating room table and the procedure is done under thigh tourniquet hemostasis.

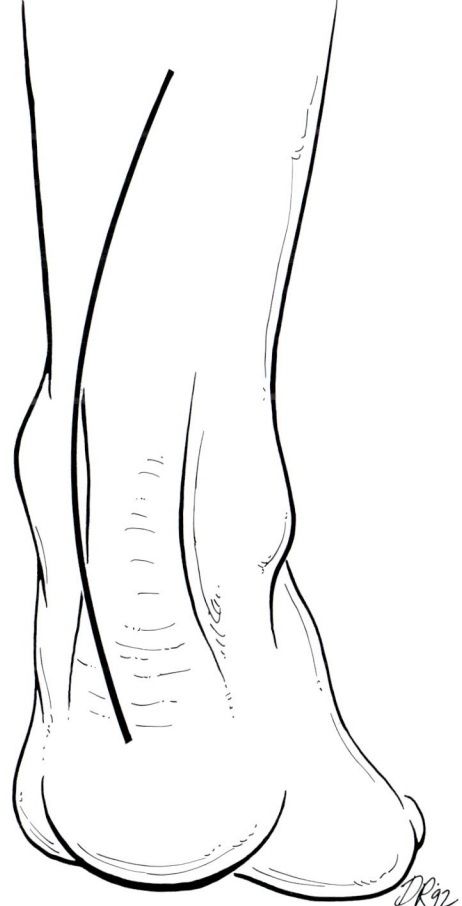

Figure 5. Location of the incision just lateral to the Achilles tendon.

Special attention is given to preserving thickness and gentle handling of the skin and subcutaneous tissue flap from over the tendon. The Achilles tendon is split in a coronal plane at its distal third (Fig. 6). The anterior half of the tendon is transected at its distal level and the posterior half at the proximal extent of the coronal split (Fig. 7). The tendon is then kept moist with two short lengths of

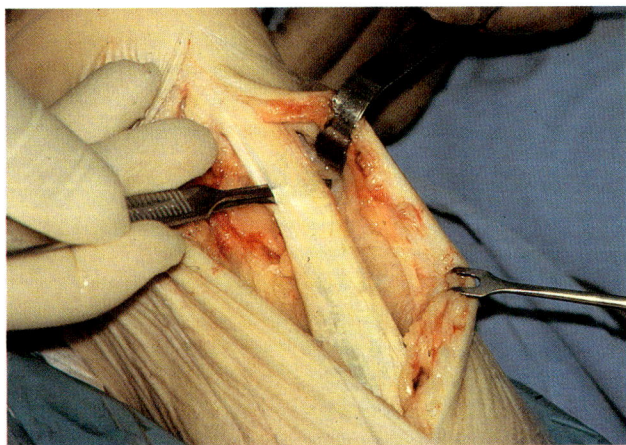

Figure 6. Transverse splitting of the Achilles tendon.

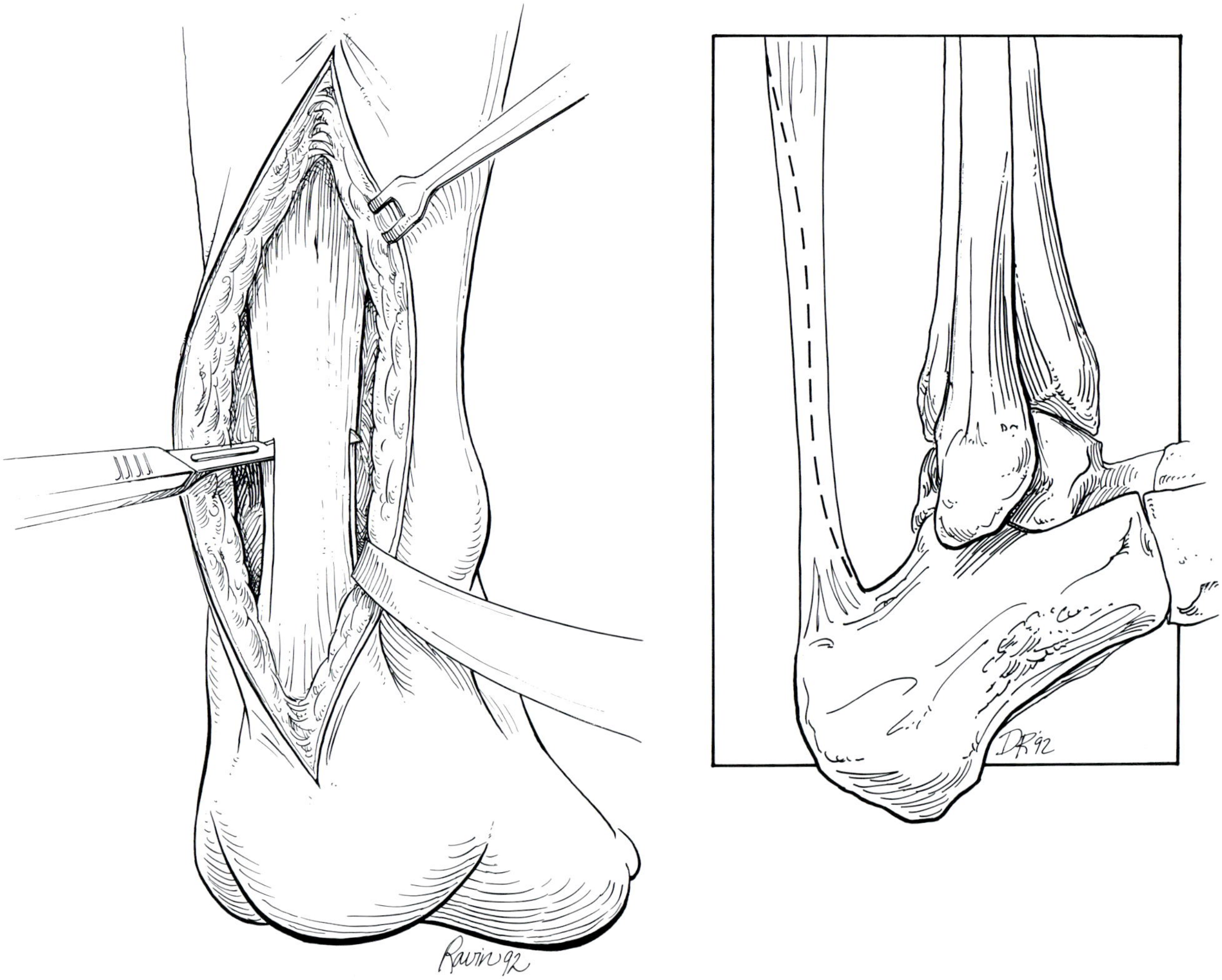

Figure 7. Diagrammatic illustration showing plane of resection of the Achilles tendon.

moistened finger tube gauze and the tendon halves retracted. The investing fascia of the deep posterior compartment is uncovered by dividing in the midline the fatty tissue just anterior to the Achilles tendon (Fig. 8). This fascia of the deep posterior compartment is split in the midline from the level of the ankle joint to well up into the leg. Beneath the fascia, the muscle belly of the flexor hallucis longus (FHL), is uncovered (Fig. 9). The origin of the FHL from the posterior aspect of the fibula and interosseous membrane is released and reflected medially to protect the tibial nerve and artery. The posterior aspect of the tibia and talus and posterosuperior tuberosity of the calcaneus are thus exposed (Fig. 10).

The arthrodesis recipient site is prepared by first removing the superior aspect of the calcaneal tuberosity, the posterior prominence (Stieda's process) of the talus, and the posterior margin and cortex of the tibia (Fig. 11). A trough is then made from the tibia to the calcaneus across the body of the talus. The medial and lateral cortices of the talar body are left intact. The trough is developed anteriorly to the anterior margin of the tibia and to the neck region of the talus and down

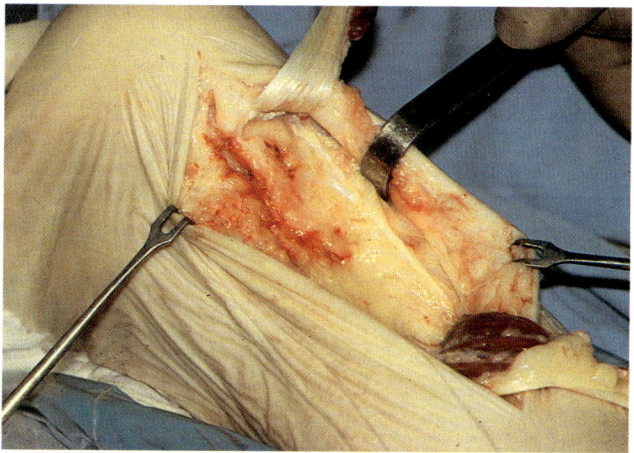

Figure 8. Retraction of the Achilles tendon proximally and distally allows access to the deep fascia of the posterior compartment.

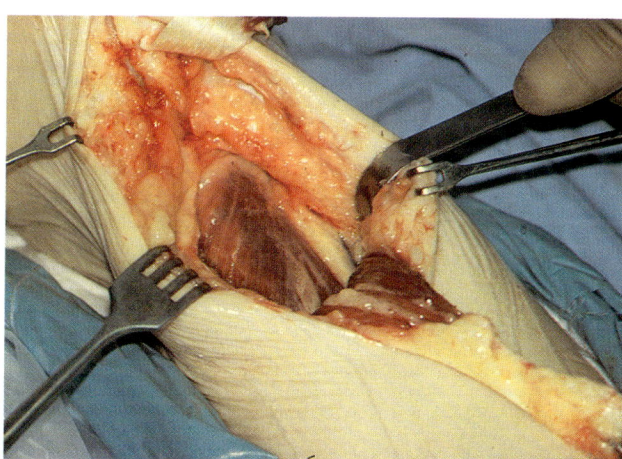

Figure 9. After the deep fascia is incised, the muscle belly of the flexor hallucis longus is seen with its tendon along the medial aspect of the muscle belly.

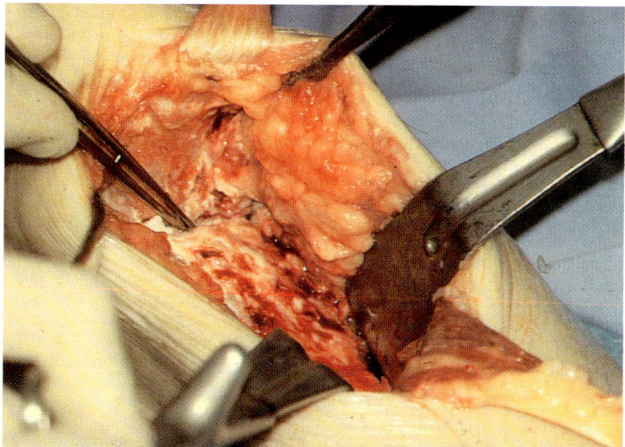

Figure 10. Exposure of the posterior aspect of the tibia down to the superior aspect of the calcaneal tuberosity is shown. The tip of the forceps is in the ankle joint at its posterior aspect.

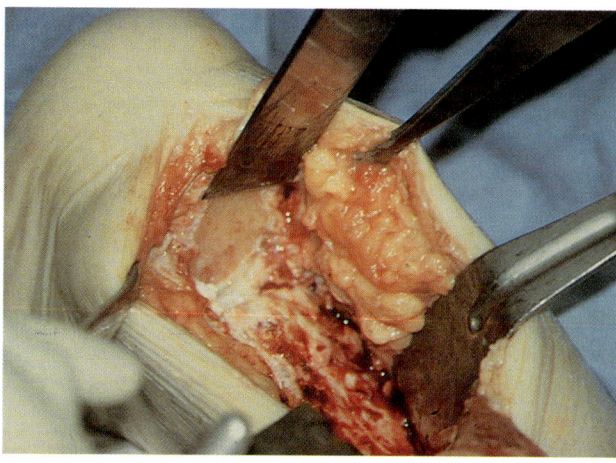

Figure 11. An osteotome removes the cortical surface from the superior aspect of the calcaneal tuberosity.

into the calcaneus in the region of the middle subtalar facet and sustentaculum tali (Fig. 12). Articular cartilage of the ankle and subtalar joints is removed medially and laterally with bone rongeur and osteotomes (Fig. 13).

If deformity is present, realignment of the hindfoot can be obtained by excessive resection of the talus dome and distal tibial. Sometimes the fibula will hold the hindfoot in an abnormal position. Osteotomy of the fibula through the posterior incision or through a separate short lateral incision will allow proper positioning of the hindfoot into a valgus orientation of about 5°, neutral dorsiflexion–plantar flexion and external rotation to match the contralateral foot, which usually is about the midportion of the patella with the first web space (Fig. 14).

When the foot is in an appropriate position, a large Steinmann pin is inserted from the inferior surface of the heel, transfixing the calcaneus and talus to the tibia in the desired position. The short transverse stab incision is made in line with the tibia about 2 cm posterior from the anterior margin of the thickened heel pad skin.

Stabilization of the arthrodesis site may be achieved with an external fixator or more recently an intramedullary rod. The usual external fixator is a modified Calandruccio device (Smith and Nephew Richards, Inc., Memphis, TN) (Fig. 15).

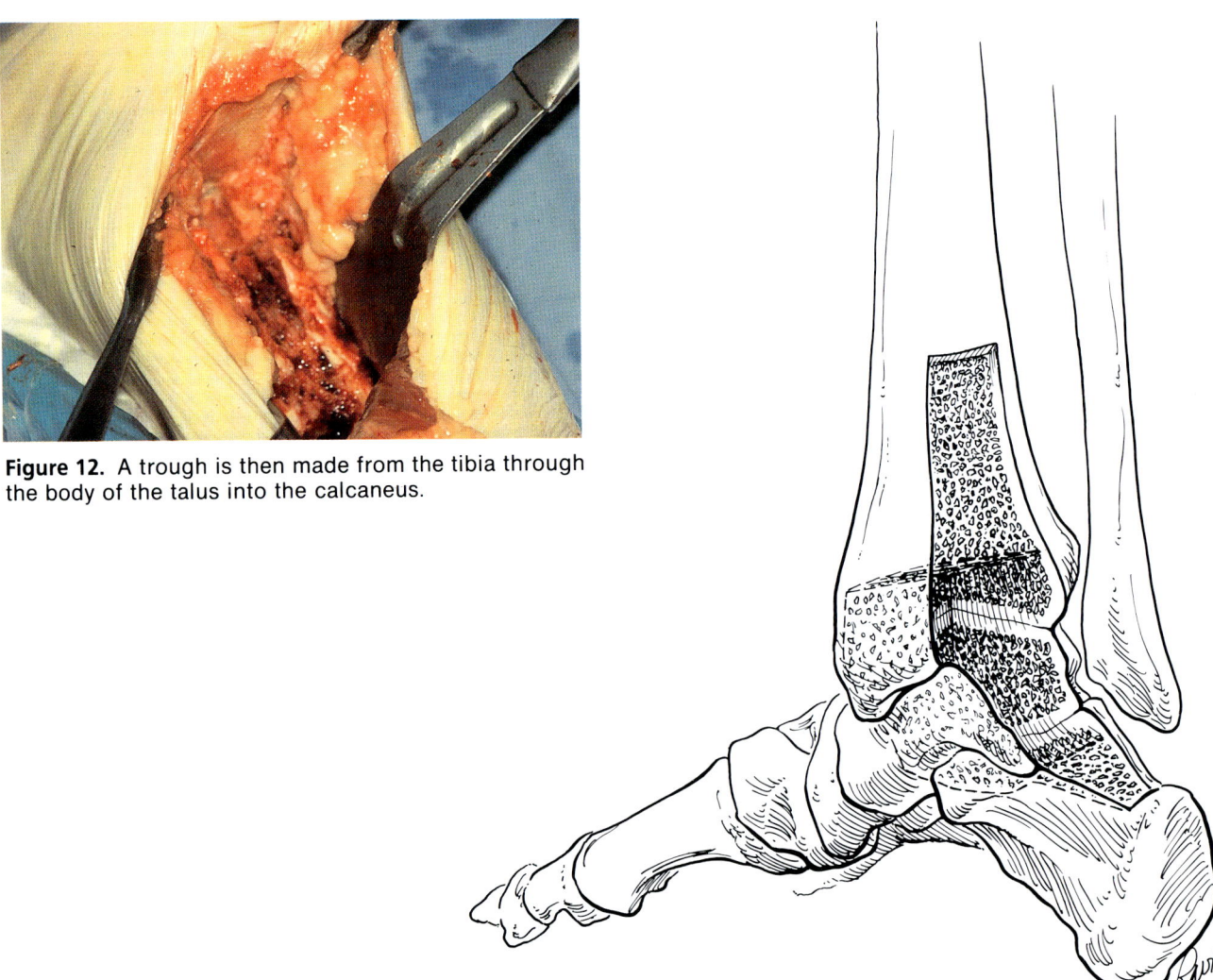

Figure 12. A trough is then made from the tibia through the body of the talus into the calcaneus.

Figure 13. The usual extent of the cancellous bone exposed at the posterior aspect of the tibia and the superior aspect of the calcaneus, as well as the trough from the tibia through the talar body into the calcaneus.

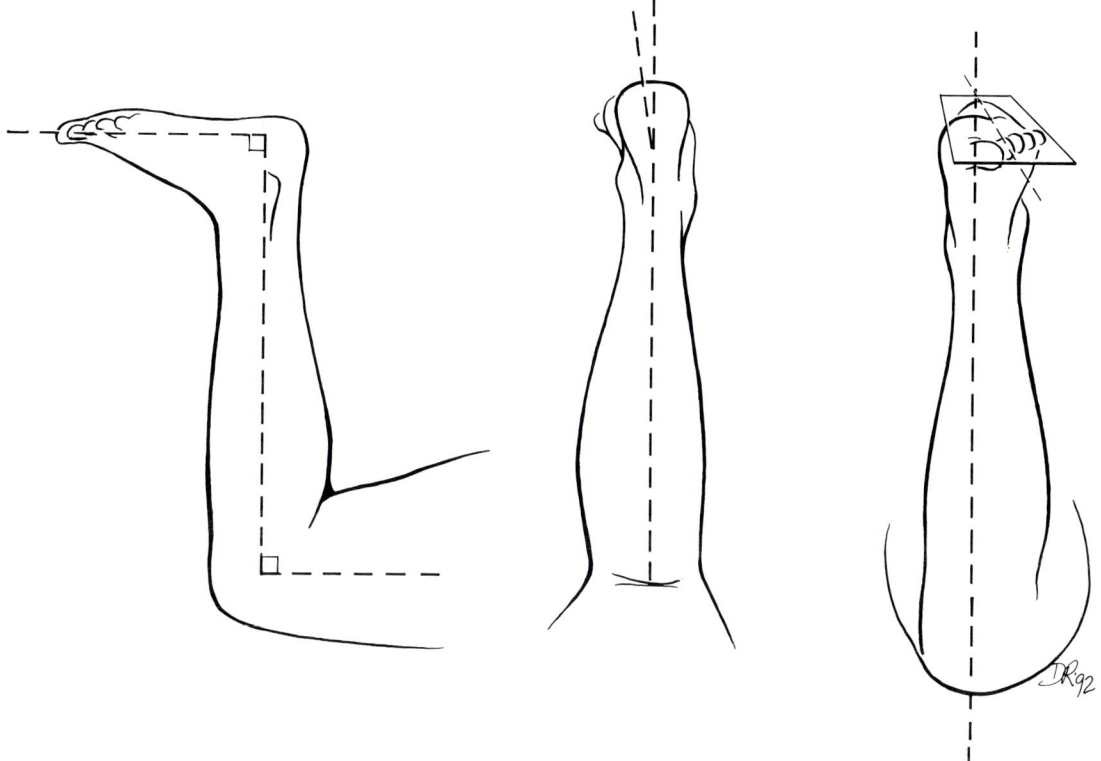

Figure 14. With the patient in the prone position, positioning of the foot can be quite accurate since the relationship of the foot to the tibia in flexion is readily seen. The hindfoot varus-valgus position is evident and rotation with the knee flexed is also accurately assessed.

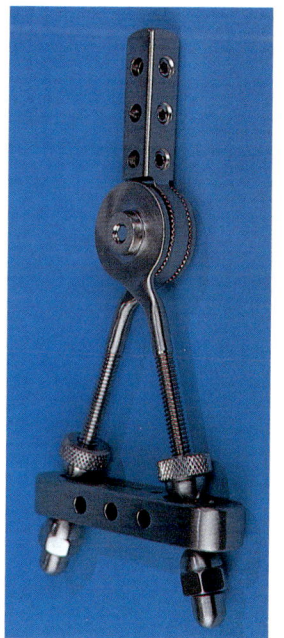
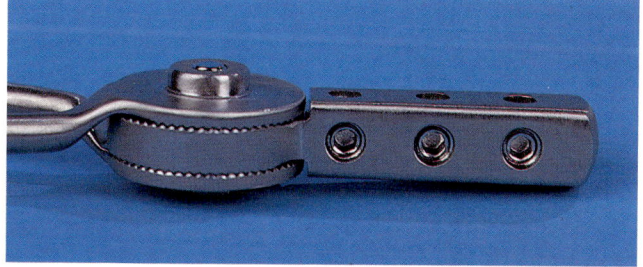

Figure 15. A: The Calandruccio device. **B:** A close-up view shows the mechanism to secure the hinge of the Y-shaped device.

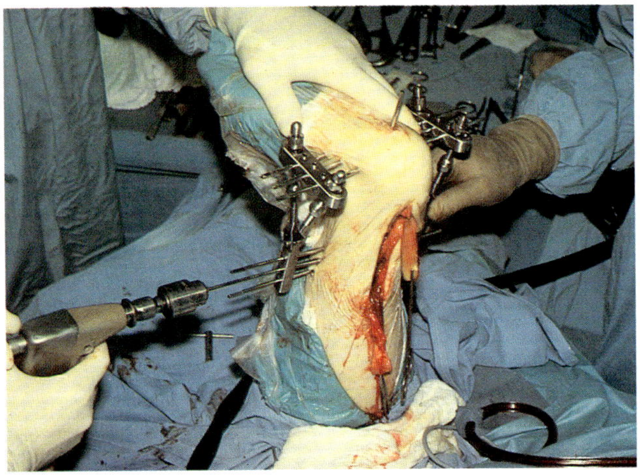

Figure 16. After the longitudinal Steinmann pin has been inserted the Calandruccio device is applied.

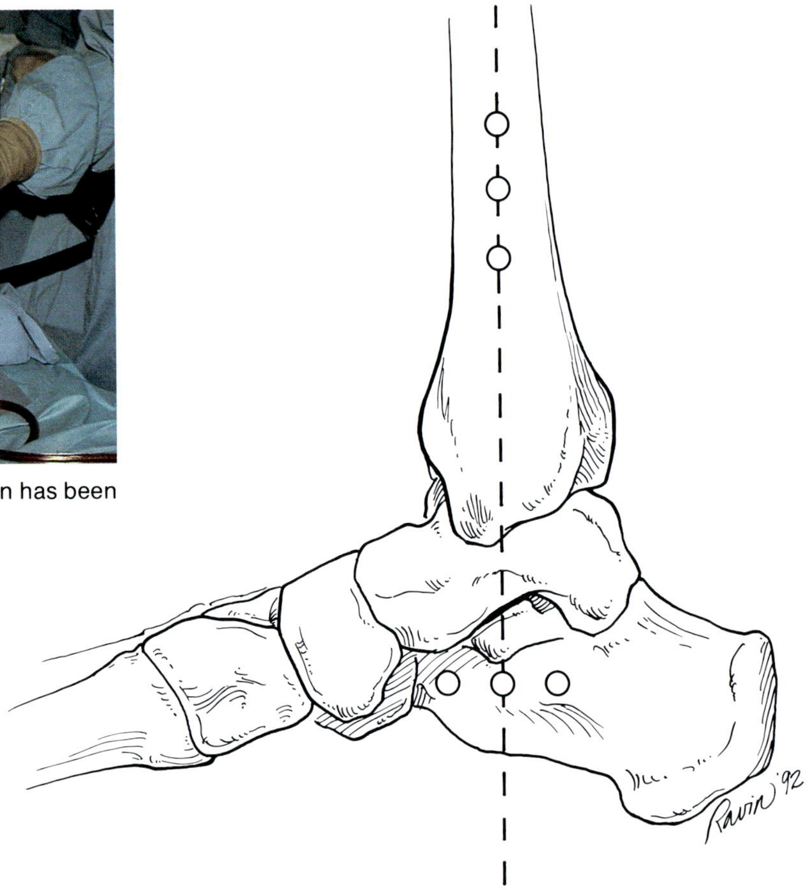

Figure 17. Positioning of the transfixing pins for application of the Calandruccio apparatus.

The modification involves a locking bolt at the Y hinge of the device. This bolt secures the external fixator in a sagittal plane and prevents inadvertent flexion. Three transfixion pins are placed through the calcaneus from lateral to medial using the external fixator as a template (Fig. 16). The skin incisions are made in a longitudinal orientation sparing the subcutaneous tissue where injury to a nerve such as the sural may occur. Pushing the self-drilling transfixation pin through the subcutaneous and deep tissues to the surface of the calcaneus before drilling

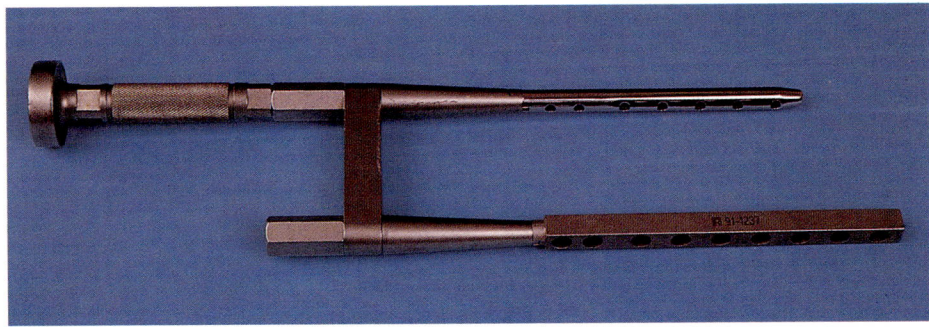

Figure 18. Intramedullary rod with attached external hole localizing device. This allows for an interlocking screw stabilization of the rod through the tibia and calcaneus.

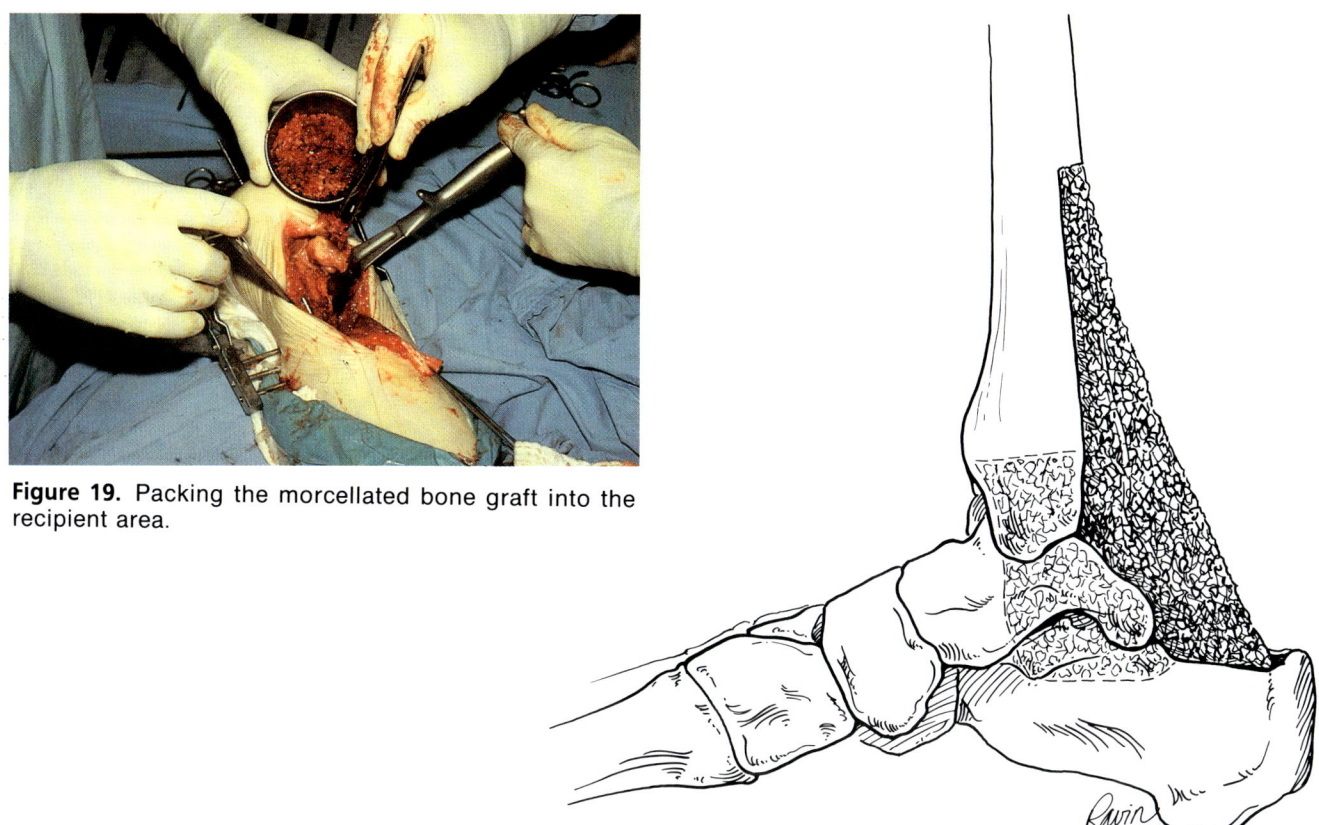

Figure 19. Packing the morcellated bone graft into the recipient area.

Figure 20. Diagrammatic representation of the final arthrodesis site.

the pin through the bone mill obviates neurovascular injury with insertion. Likewise after the appropriate surface of the calcaneus is broadened, the soft tissues are pushed gently over the pin end with minimal drilling and then tented skin only is incised. The middle pin in the calcaneus is placed close to the longitudinal Steinmann pin so that approximately straight longitudinal compression is provided when the external fixator is tightened. Three pins are placed through the tibia from lateral to medial and the external fixator applied (Fig. 17). By making the skin incisions for the tibial pins at an obliquity of about 30° from vertical, avoidance of one long skin incision is possible. *By tightening the external fixator, the arthrodesis site is compressed.* If flexion-extension control is not provided by the external fixator, then the longitudinal Steinmann pin should be left in place.

Recently an intramedullary rod (Richards, Inc.) has been used to provide arthrodesis site stability and save the patient the discomfort and inconvenience of an external fixator. This rod utilizes an attached external hole-centering device (Fig. 18). Two or three interlocking screws through the calcaneus-talus region and two or three through the tibia provide excellent fixation. An image intensifier is necessary for accurate rod placement.

The morcellated autogenous bone graft is tightly packed in the recipient trough and along the posterior aspect of the tibia and superior aspect of the calcaneus (Fig. 19) to create both an intraarticular and extraarticular arthrodesis (Fig. 20).

The flexor hallucis longus muscle belly is returned to its normal position over the bone graft and sutured into place providing a vascular supply to the arthrodesis site (Fig. 21). A suction drain is inserted and the Achilles tendon sutured loosely into place (Fig. 22). The posterior wound is very, very carefully closed with ab-

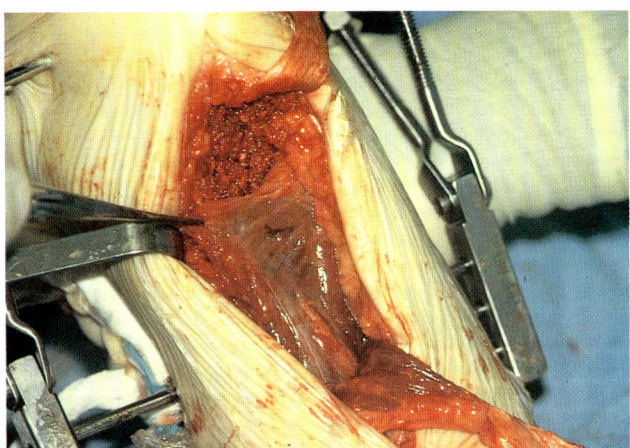

Figure 21. The muscle belly of the flexor hallucis longus is pulled across the graft to provide vascular supply.

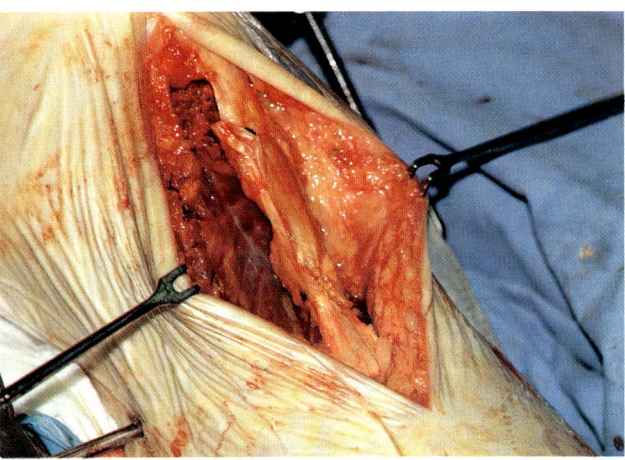

Figure 22. Loose closure of the now nonfunctional Achilles tendon.

sorbable subcutaneous sutures and 2-0 nylon mattress sutures just coapting but not strangulating the skin. A bulky compression dressing and plaster stirrup splint are applied distal to the knee.

As a result of prior experience, there are three aspects of this procedure that have become evident. First, the ability to realign severe deformity is present. Osteotomy of the fibula along with resection of the talar dome and distal tibia plafond and sometimes resection of the medial malleolus will allow realignment of a severely deformed hindfoot into a plantar-grade position prior to bone grafting and fixation.

Second, the fixation with an external fixator that allows a hinge motion at the arthrodesis site is not satisfactory in all cases. Even though a longitudinal Steinmann pin was left in place, the windshield wiper motion of the pin in the tibia medullary canal or pin bending in a few instances allowed late flexion of the ankle and a resultant malpositioned hindfoot in about 10° of flexion. Modifying the otherwise very satisfactory Calandruccio apparatus to have a hinge that can be stabilized eliminated the need for the long-term longitudinal Steinmann pin and prevented a late flexion deformity. More recently a longitudinal interlocking intramedullary rod has provided excellent stability. Technically it is more involved and long-term results are not known as yet for this type of rod fixation.

Third, it is important that the trough through the talar body be extended to viable bone at the head and neck position of the talus if avascular necrosis of the talus is the indication for operative treatment. This arthrodesis should be envisioned as the tibia to talus arthrodesis coupled with a talus to calcaneus arthrodesis. It is not a tibia to calcaneus arthrodesis that bypasses the talus.

POSTOPERATIVE MANAGEMENT

The patient initially is placed in a bulky Jones type of compressive dressing. The following day crutch or walker training is begun in the hospital. At 3 to 5 days postoperative, the dressing is removed. For the external fixator type of stabilization, daily soaking of the foot up to above the fixator is done. Lukewarm soapy water is placed in fresh appropriate-sized refuse container for soaking. After about 30 minutes, the foot is dried and the pin tracts are cleansed of any crusting that may occur. An iodine-based ointment is placed on each pin tract site and gauze dressings are split and placed about the pins to stabilize the skin. Usually only once a day soaking is necessary but if pin tract infection occurs it is increased to two times each day and oral antibiotics are started. Such daily soaking is continued until the fixator is removed. No cast is necessary with the external fixator. If an internal intramedullary rod is used, a cast is applied at about 3 to 5 days, and soakings are not necessary.

The posterior nylon sutures are removed at about 3 weeks postoperative along with the iliac crest donor site staples.

Return visits occur at about 6-week intervals. At 12 weeks, the radiograph should show early consolidation and the external fixator is removed and a walking cast applied for an additional 6 weeks. It takes a total of about 18 weeks postoperative for the final cast to be removed and the patient allowed to bear weight without fixation. If there is any doubt about the arthrodesis site stability, an additional 6 weeks in a removable cast/brace can be utilized. When the final cast has been removed, the patient is instructed to use a compression stocking for a few months only during the day to control swelling. A postoperative stiff-soled shoe is provided and gradually the patient progresses back toward normal footwear such as athletic shoes or a soft leather lace-up type shoe.

Although the report of 1988 (5) indicated 75% satisfactory results, that is probably higher now with further experience and improved fixation. Osseous union was radiographically evident in 18 of 21 patients. With normal walking after a tibiocalcaneal arthrodesis, there will be a slight limp with a shorter step and increased flexion in the arthrodesis extremity. Pain relief should be very good. No formal rehabilitation is prescribed. Sometimes a shoe with a cushioned heel and rocker bottom sole is helpful. In fact, however, the patient soon tires of having the shoes modified and usually opts for a conservative soft lace-up type of off-the-shelf shoe.

COMPLICATIONS

Complications may occur during the treatment of a tibiocalcaneal arthrodesis and will be considered.

A nonunion may develop. This complication can be avoided by using copious autogenous bone graft, secure fixation, and a well-vascularized recipient site. Bone graft from the posterior iliac crest is abundant. Fixation is with the rigid modified Calandruccio or the intramedullary rod. Taking the recipient trough all the way anterior to the neck of the talus will enhance union. If a nonunion is evident at about 6 months, reapplication of an external fixator with non–weight bearing and an electrical stimulator would be all that is necessary. Repeat bone grafting across the nonunion with stabilization is the usual treatment, however.

Malunion can be a problem if the type of fixation permits the ankle to plantarflex during the healing period. If such a deformity inadvertently occurs, a single appropriately sized heel lift may be all that is necessary. Surgically such a deformity can be corrected if necessary by a dome osteotomy in the distal tibia metaphysis just above the arthrodesis site along with a fibula osteotomy and appropriate fixation.

Late fracture of the tibia at a pin tract site of the external fixator has occurred. This is indicated by pain in the distal tibia a few months after the patient has become pain free and normally active. The pin tract, particularly if close to the bone cortex, will act as a stress riser and allow fracture. Simple cast immobilization is all that is necessary to let such a completed stress fracture heal.

As with all external fixator devices, a pin tract infection can occur. Maintaining adequate pin care technique, with skin stabilization with a dressing between the skin and external fixator frame, along with oral antibiotics should heal the pin tract infection. The most susceptible pin site location for infection seems to be at the calcaneal area.

Finally, wound dehiscence and necrosis may occur. It usually will be at the most distalward aspect of the incision. Keeping the skin flap thick, avoiding surgi-

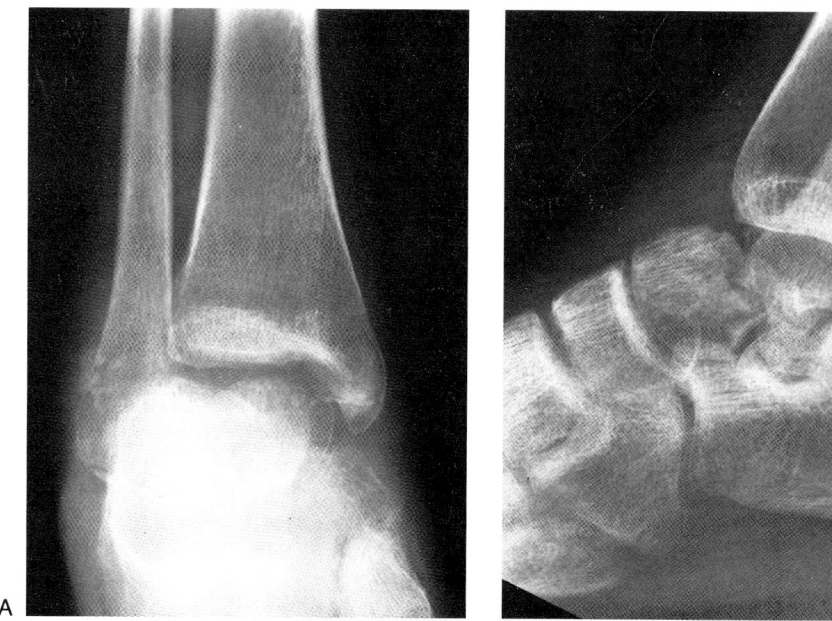

Figure 23. A: AP radiograph shows loss of the talar dome. **B:** Lateral radiograph demonstrates the absence of the body of the talus.

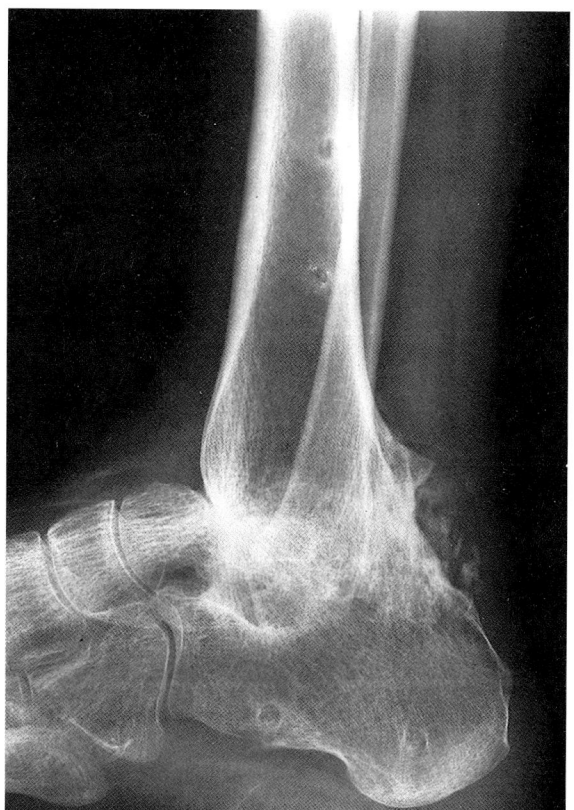

Figure 24. Lateral radiograph shows the arthrodesis of the tibia to the calcaneus with maintenance of the hindfoot height. For this patient only two pins in the tibia and two pins in the calcaneus were felt to be necessary.

ILLUSTRATIVE CASES FOR TECHNIQUE

Case 1. An 18-year-old woman was involved in a motor vehicle accident 4 months previously. Along with multiple other injuries, she had an open fracture of her left hindfoot. Apparently the body of the talus was extruded through the medial ankle wound and not recovered. All wounds healed, but she was left with a very painful shortened distal lower extremity (Fig. 23).

She underwent a tibia to calcaneal arthrodesis as a salvage procedure. The bone grafting was extended to the viable neck of the talus and restoration of hindfoot height was achieved with relief of her pain symptoms (Fig. 24).

Case 2. A 57-year-old man gave a history of a severe injury to his left hindfoot 4 years ago. This was a Hawkins type III talar neck fracture dislocation. Unfortunately, he developed avascular necrosis of the body of the talus and a nonunited talar neck fracture (Fig. 25). Because of severe pain he sought further care.

The radiographs show direct involvement of both the tibiotalar and talocalcaneal joints so a posterior tibia to calcaneal arthrodesis was done through a posterior approach.

The unique aspect of his treatment was the use of an interlocking intramedullary rod for fixation along with bone grafting from the posterior iliac crest (Figs. 26 and 27). He went on to hindfoot bony union and excellent pain relief.

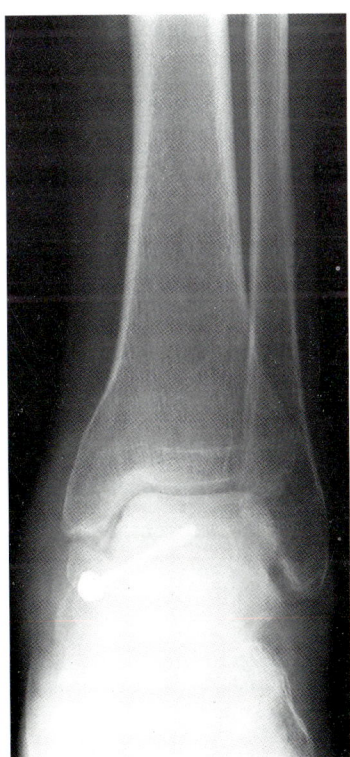 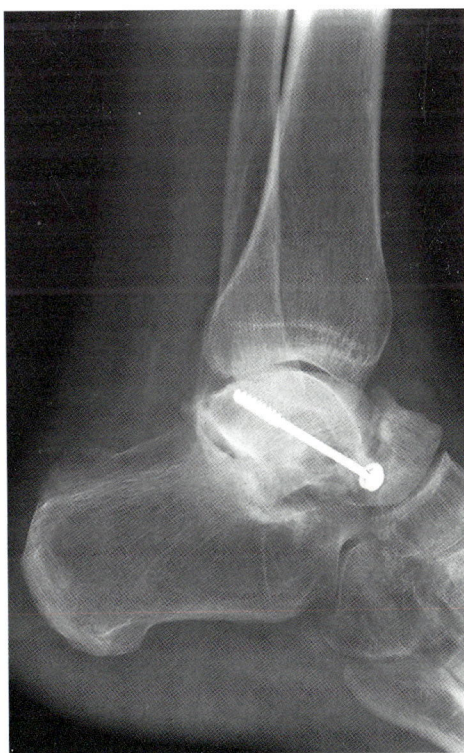

Figure 25. A: AP radiograph shows maintenance of cartilage space, but with loss of vascularity to the body of the talus. **B:** Lateral radiograph shows the nonunion of the talar neck fracture as well as a malposition.

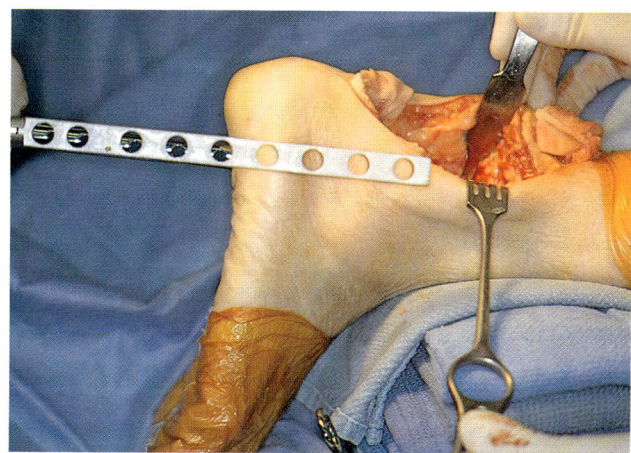

Figure 26. The intramedullary rod is being inserted through the heel with the external transfixing screw localizing device outside of the foot.

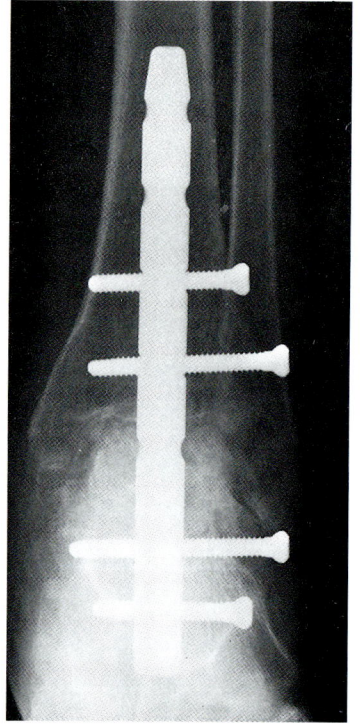
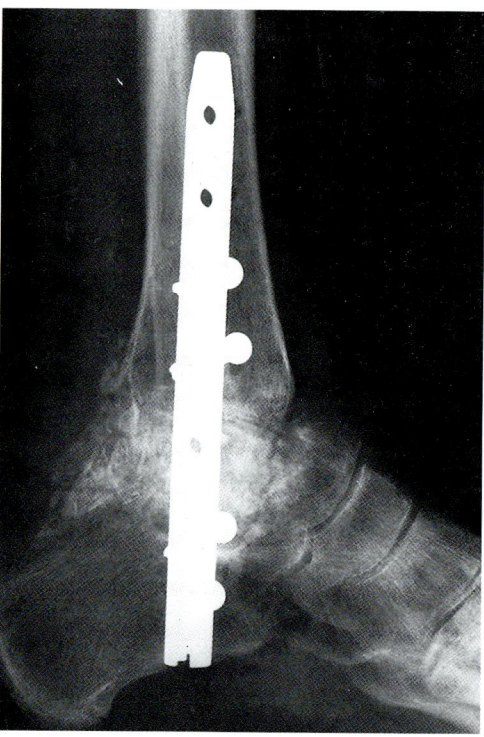

Figure 27. A: AP radiograph shows the position of the rod with transfixing screws. One screw went through the fibula before entering the tibia and the intramedullary rod. **B:** Lateral radiograph shows the bone graft in the talar body area along with the intramedullary rod.

RECOMMENDED READING

1. Blair, H. Z.: Comminuted fractures and fracture dislocations of the body of the talus. Operative treatment. *Am. J. Surg.*, 59: 37–43, 1943.
2. Canale, S. T., and Kelly, F. B.: Fractures of the neck of the talus. Long-term evaluation of seventy-one cases. *J. Bone Joint Surg.*, 60A: 143–156, 1978.
3. Papa, J. A., and Myerson, M. S.: Plantar and tibiotalocalcaneal arthrodesis for post-traumatic osteoarthrosis of the ankle and hindfoot. *J. Bone Joint Surg.*, 74A(7): 1042–1049, 1992.
4. Reckling, F. W.: Early tibiocalcaneal fusion in the treatment of severe injuries of the talus. *J. Trauma*, 12: 390–396, 1972.
5. Russotti, G. M., Johnson, K. A., and Cass, J. R.: Tibiocalcaneal arthrodesis for arthritis and deformity of the hind part of the foot. *J. Bone Joint Surg.*, 70A: 1304–1307, 1988.

37

Syme Amputation

James W. Brodsky

INDICATIONS/CONTRAINDICATIONS

The Syme amputation is indicated for the patient who requires amputation of most of the foot because of loss of viability due to infection, gangrene, or trauma. This is the patient for whom a partial foot amputation is no longer possible, and yet who still has a viable heel pad. The advantages of the Syme amputation over the next amputation alternative in a patient with a nonviable foot, viz., a below-knee amputation are enormous: they are manifested in its mechanical, physiological, and functional superiority. The mechanical advantage of the Syme amputation is the tremendously longer lever given to the function of the quadriceps muscles and to the knee joint. Physiologically, this results in a lower energy expenditure in walking than in patients with a more proximal amputation, an important factor in all patients, but especially in patients with underlying debilitating chronic disease such as diabetes or chronic peripheral vascular disease (5).

Functionally, the patient with a Syme amputation requires only a fraction of the rehabilitation and training to become ambulatory required by a below-knee amputee. Not only is the extensive training in donning and doffing the prosthesis not necessary, but almost none of the Syme amputees require admission to a rehabilitation facility for gait training. In addition, the Syme amputation has the advantage that the distal stump is covered with plantar skin and the pad of the heel, and is therefore thicker and better able to withstand the pressure of weight bearing. The Syme stump is partially end-bearing on this specialized tissue, with the remaining pressure distributed through the proximal tibial metaphysis, where all of the pressure is borne in a below-knee amputation. Some patients (while not advised to do so by their surgeons) nonetheless report weight bearing directly on the stump when getting up in the night to go to the bathroom.

The Syme amputation has also been widely and successfully utilized in various congenital deformities and deficiencies of the lower limb, including proximal focal

---

J. W. Brodsky, M.D.: Department of Orthopaedic Surgery, University of Texas Southwestern Medical School, Dallas, TX; Department of Orthopaedic Surgery, Baylor University Medical Center, Dallas, TX 75246; and *private practice*, Orthopaedic Associates of Dallas, 411 N. Washington #7000, Dallas, TX 75246.

femoral deficiency, fibular hemimelia, and congenital pseudarthrosis of the tibia. As in amputations at other levels, the most common underlying disease is diabetes, followed by arteriosclerotic peripheral vascular disease, and trauma.

The primary and absolute contraindication to a Syme ankle disarticulation is the absence of an intact and viable heel pad. This means that the patient needs to have completely intact skin over the posterior, medial and lateral, and plantar aspect of the heel. Posterior skin compromise in particular, especially over the Achilles tendon, will doom the procedure to failure. The only exception would be in the unusual case of a Syme amputation to be performed for trauma in an otherwise healthy individual, in which superficial injury to the heel soft tissue might rapidly heal, particularly with normal vascularity of the limb.

The Syme amputation is likewise contraindicated in patients for whom the procedure is contemplated due to severe infection of the foot, but in whom the infection has extended too far proximally, and involves the area of the heel itself. Because the primary advantages of this procedure are focused on the enhancement of the patient's walking ability, there is no indication to perform this procedure rather than a below-knee amputation in a wheelchair bound or otherwise nonambulatory patient. Partial foot amputations are still generally preferable to a Syme procedure whenever a viable outcome is possible, because partial foot amputations can usually be fitted with shoe modifications in order to ambulate, whereas the Syme amputation is the lowest level amputation that requires a prosthesis. A properly performed Chopart amputation (which must *always* include Achilles tenotomy) usually requires the use of a polypropylene ankle foot orthosis, which also extends to just below the knee. Although this is also somewhat cumbersome, it is still more cosmetic, and lighter than a Syme prosthesis, and can fit into a limited range of shoe-wear, all of which are preferable to a prosthesis.

PREOPERATIVE PLANNING

The most important determinant of a successful outcome in the Syme amputation, as in many surgeries, is proper patient selection. The purpose of the preoperative planning is to identify those patients with sufficient vascularity and the appropriate problem that warrant Syme amputation. Radiographs should be taken to make certain that there is not osteomyelitis of the distal tibia or fibula. Osteomyelitis of the talus would also be a likely contraindication.

The role of magnetic resonance imaging (MRI) is not as clearly defined. This technique is so sensitive as to be difficult to interpret. The marrow edema (change from adipose to water density) of infection is nonspecific, and trauma or even reaction to nearby infection may elicit this indistinct change. On the other hand, if the MRI shows a plantar abscess that extends into the heel pad, this information is clearly most helpful in the decision-making.

Most important to the preoperative planning is evaluation of the vascular status of the patient's lower limbs. This is particularly true since the majority of patients who require this procedure are either diabetic or dysvascular, or both. The arterial Doppler ultrasound is still the most widely available and most readily applied test of limb perfusion. However, it is to be considered a screening test and not a definitive measure of perfusion. Other technologies, including transcutaneous oxygen measurement and arteriography, are more authoritative with regard to the amount of tissue perfusion (see chapter by Brodsky, "Transmetatarsal Amputation"). A vascular surgery consultation is frequently required prior to proceeding with this operation. The key issue is that there be adequate perfusion of the heel pad, which is supplied by branches of the posterior tibial artery. Although the adipose tissue of the heel pad is a relatively avascular tissue, the absence of sufficient perfusion to this area is the primary cause of failure of the Syme amputation.

SURGERY

Although there are points of technical finesse to be elucidated in any operative procedure, much amputation surgery is relatively straightforward. However, the Syme amputation is not only the least commonly performed, but unquestionably the most technically difficult of lower extremity amputations. Its functional superiority makes worthwhile the effort expended by the surgeon to obtain a good result with this operation.

Although the "two-stage" Syme amputation has been much discussed and written about, most Syme amputations are now done at a single sitting ("one-stage"). The second stage, which is usually performed 6 or more weeks after the initial procedure, refers to delayed resection of the malleoli. This has been recommended in the past for severely infected cases in which the surgeon does not wish to expose the medullary cavities of the tibia and fibula to likely infection. The number of Syme amputations that currently are considered to require a second stage are few.

The patient is placed in the supine position. If there is much external rotation of the hip in this position, a pad, made of two to three folded sheets is placed beneath the ipsilateral buttock to compensate by internally rotating the limb. If there is an open, draining wound (Fig. 1), it can be covered and sealed off prior

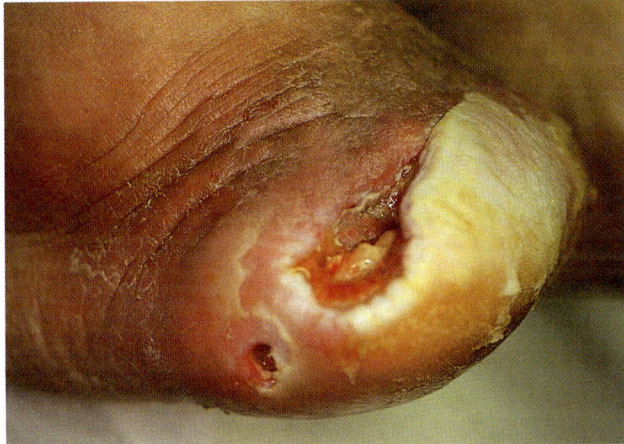

Figure 1. Infected, failed transmetatarsal amputation with deep plantar abscess that does not extend to the heel pad. Revision to Syme amputation was elected.

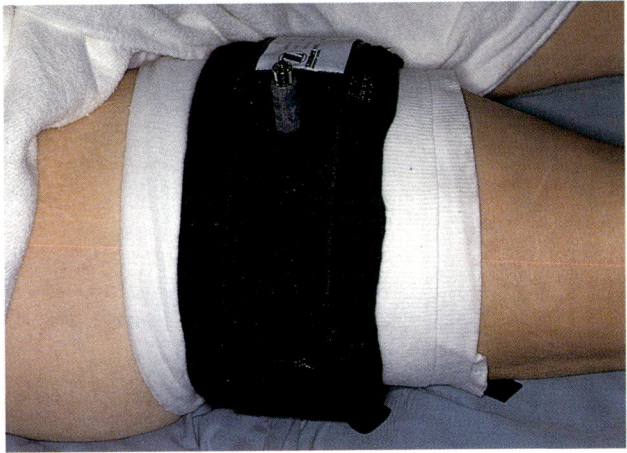

Figure 2. The pneumatic tourniquet is applied on the proximal thigh over cast padding.

to the prep using an adhesive plastic incise drape. The draped off area is included in the prep, and any drainage is blocked from the area of the incisions. If a tourniquet is used, which is frequently the case, it is a pneumatic cuff placed high on the thigh over several layers of cast padding (Fig. 2). If there has been a previous vascular bypass in the thigh, the tourniquet is usually foregone. An Esmarch bandage can still be considered for use as a tourniquet at the ankle level. Preoperative antibiotics are usually given, but can be withheld until the deep wound cultures are taken, so as not to confuse the culture results.

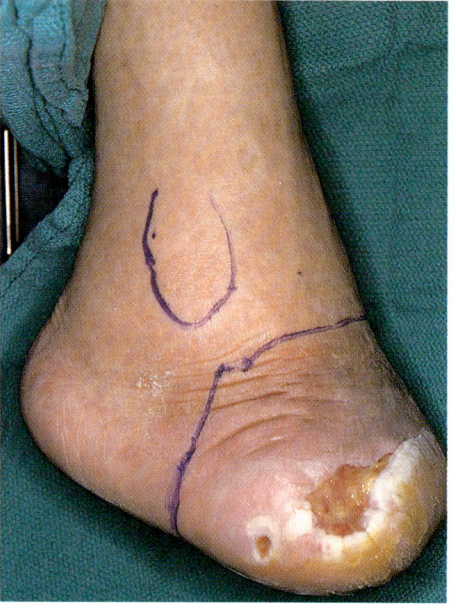

Figure 3. The anterior skin incision is marked out. The line connects two points which are placed at or 1 cm distal to the tips of the malleoli.

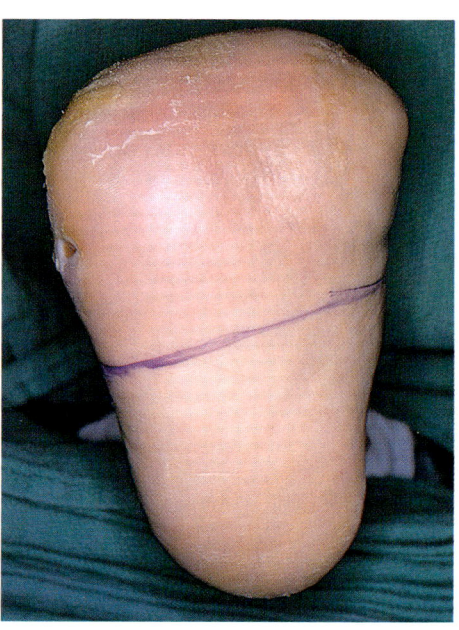

Figure 4. The plantar incision is marked out.

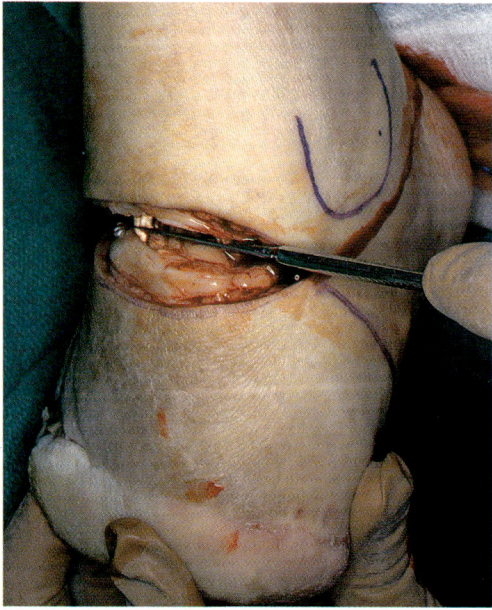

Figure 5. Using a #10 blade, the dorsal incision is made full thickness down to the dome of the talus.

37 SYME AMPUTATION

Technique. First, the skin incisions are marked out (Figs. 3 and 4). In a two-stage procedure, the anterior incision is along a line that connects two points that are placed 1 to 1.5 cm below and 1 to 1.5 cm anterior to the midpoint of the tip of each malleolus. In the one-stage procedure, especially if done for trauma, the points from which the incisions originate can be more proximal, either on the tips of the malleoli or on the midpoints of the two malleoli. The two malleolar points are then connected by a second incision across the sole, which will delineate the plantar side of the closure.

Using a #10 scalpel, the dorsal incision is made down to the dome of the talus (Fig. 5). The plantar incision is then made all the way down to bone, i.e., down to the calcaneus (Figs. 6 and 7). The collateral ligaments of the talus are released, working back and forth from lateral to medial while pulling the talus forward and down (Figs. 8 and 9). A large bone hook in the talus is extremely helpful, if not essential, to obtain the forward and downward traction to keep the soft tissue dissection under tension (Fig. 10).

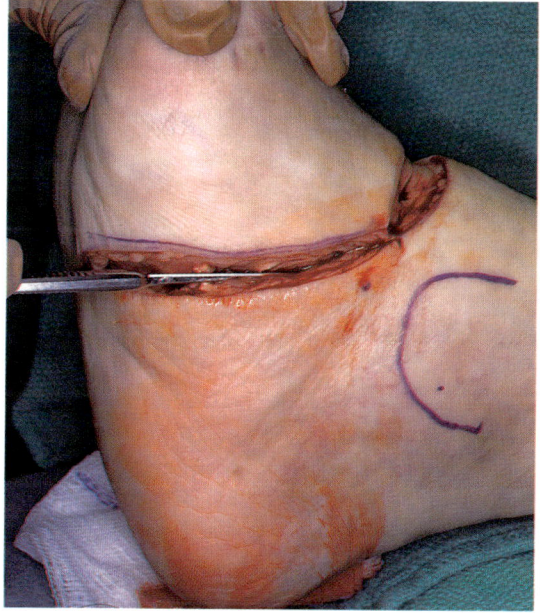

Figure 6. The plantar incision is then made down to the calcaneus (side view).

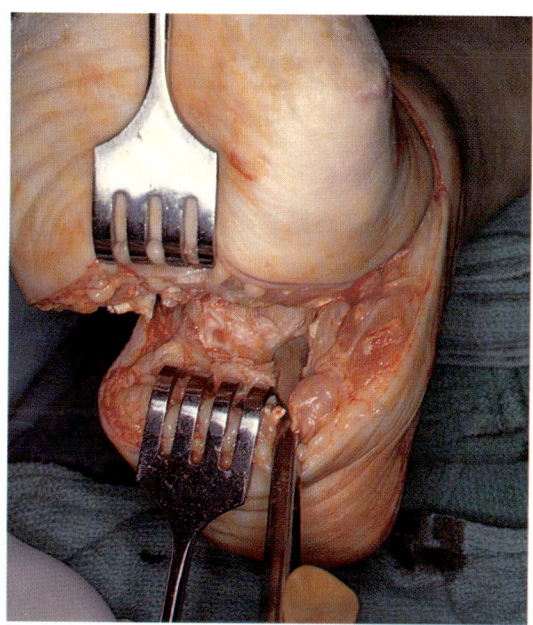

Figure 7. Plantar view of figure 6, with retraction in place.

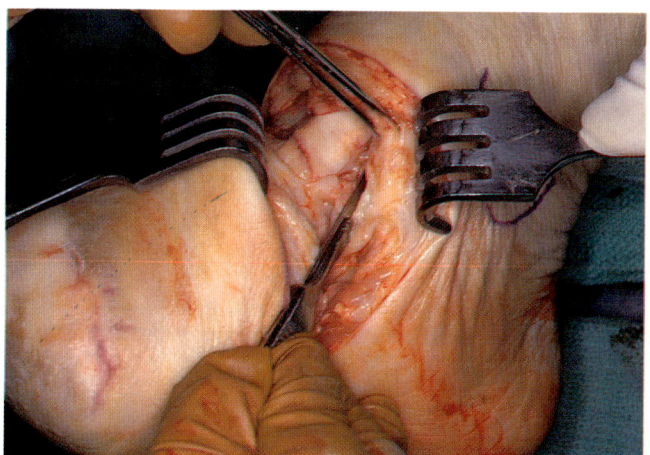
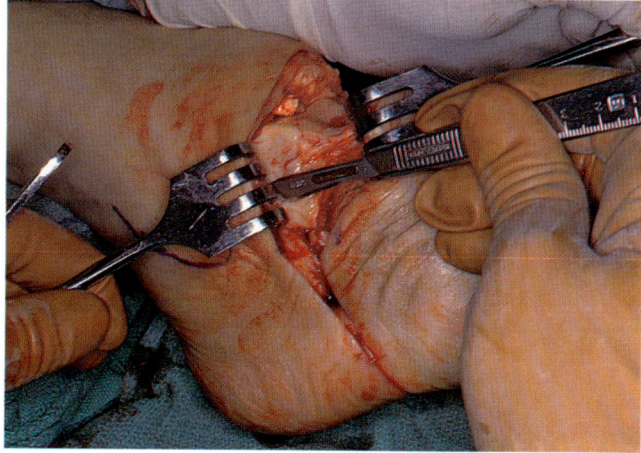

Figures 8 and 9. The collateral ligaments of the talus are then released working alternatively on medial (**left**) and lateral (**right**) sides while pulling the talus downward and forward.

Great care is taken to circumvent the neurovascular bundle, one of the two most critical points of the operation, as was even described by Syme himself. The bundle lies between the flexor hallucis longus and the flexor digitorum longus, and can be accidentally injured if care is not taken (Fig. 11). The flexor hallucis longus tendon is the primary landmark, as the bundle lies just behind it. Once it is identified, a blunt dissection is done, e.g., with a broad Key elevator, to separate the bone from the entire soft tissue envelope (Fig. 12).

The dissection of the calcaneus, and its neat separation from the soft tissue is the second major danger point in the operation, viz., the subcutaneous attachment of the Achilles tendon. Penetrating or "buttonholing" through the skin at this

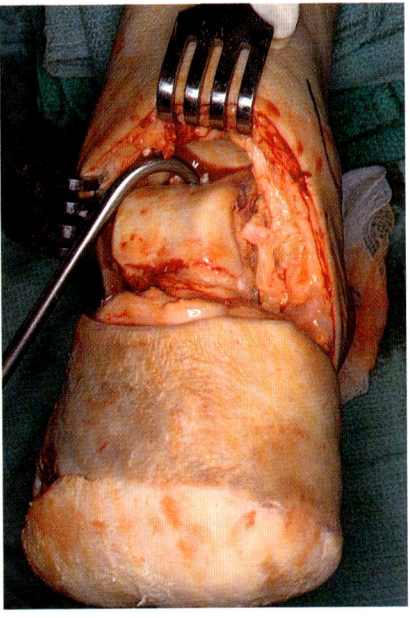

Figure 10. A large bone hook placed into the dome of the talus is essential to apply the traction needed to keep the dissection under tension. This is essential in order to "peel" the calcaneus out of its soft tissue envelope.

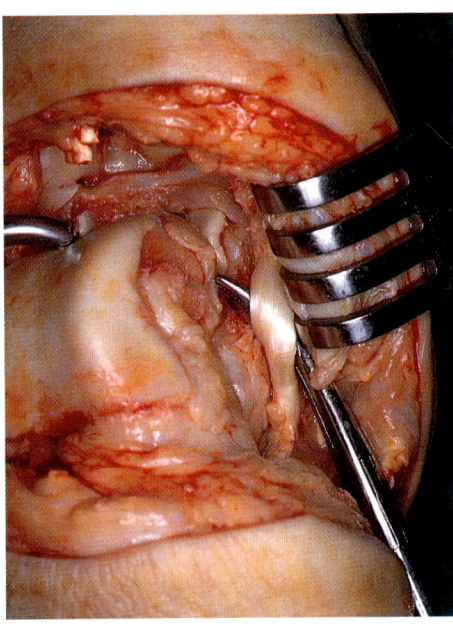

Figure 11. Care is taken to protect and avoid the neurovascular bundle between the flexor digitorum (on the clamp) and flexor hallucis tendons (at the point of clamp).

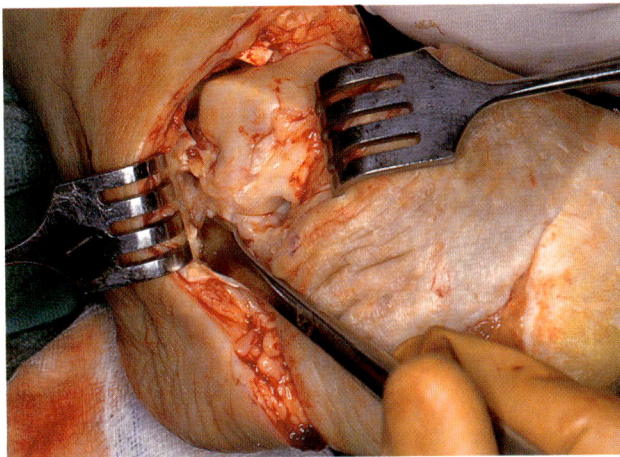

Figure 12. Blunt dissection with a broad elevator is done to separate the calcaneus from the full-thickness flap of soft tissue.

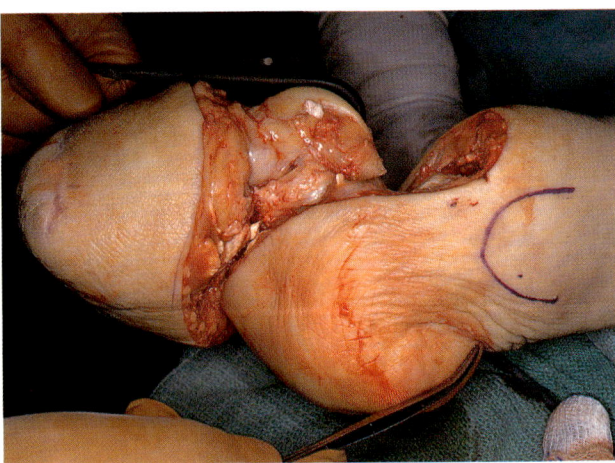

Figure 13. The clamp points to a dimple in the posterior skin where the attachment of the calcaneus is closest to the surface. This is the point of greatest danger in the operation. Penetration of the skin while dissecting out the calcaneus will cause failure.

point will usually condemn the procedure to failure since the Syme stump will not heal after this type of injury to the heel pad. Note in Fig. 13 how close the attachment of the Achilles tendon is to the skin posteriorly. This is the point at which penetration of the skin is the greatest danger.

Alternating use of sharp and blunt dissection with scalpel and periosteal elevator works best (Figs. 14 and 15). It is this portion of the procedure that is responsible for making the Syme amputation the most technically difficult foot amputation. At this point in the operation it is important to work methodically and patiently, exercising vigilance to avoid a penetrating stroke to the posterior soft tissue.

The subperiosteal dissection alternates from above at the Achilles tendon and from the undersurface and sides of the calcaneus until the bone is free from the soft tissue. This then leaves the hollow of the stump ready for final shaping and closure. Note the appearance of the specimen once the dissection has been completed (Fig. 16).

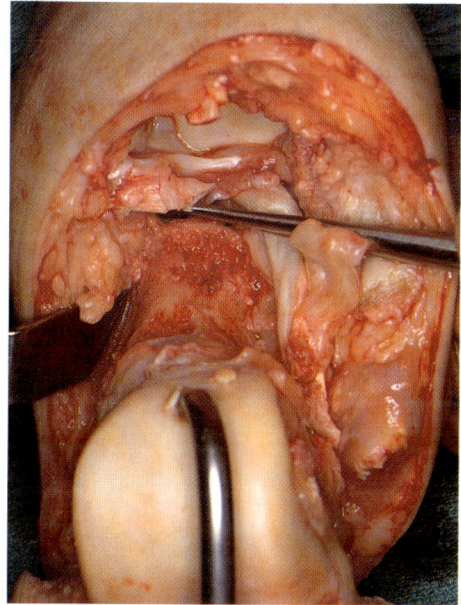 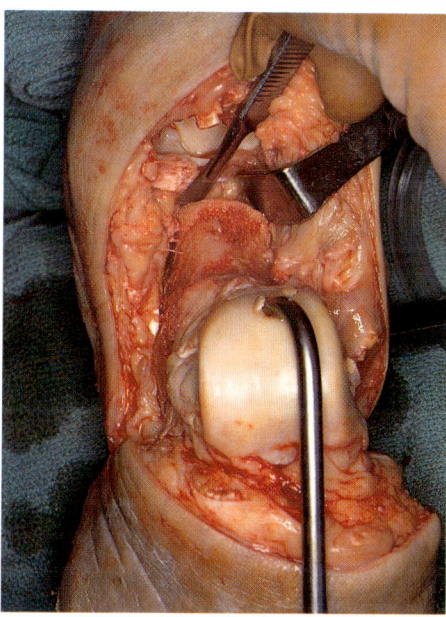

Figures 14 and 15. Alternating sharp and blunt dissection on the calcaneus works best for the difficult task of dissecting the bone from the thin layer of soft tissue.

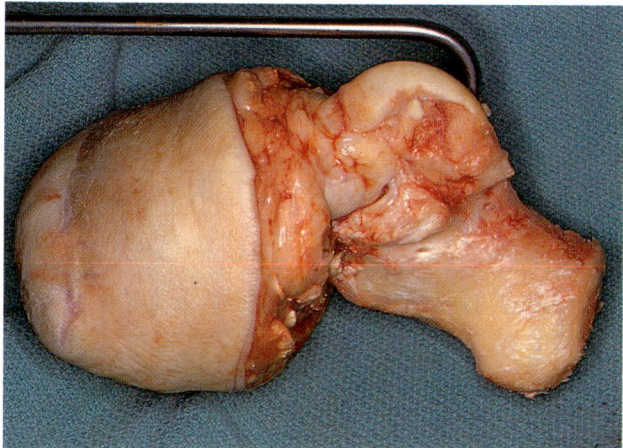

Figure 16. The appearance of the specimen once the dissection is completed.

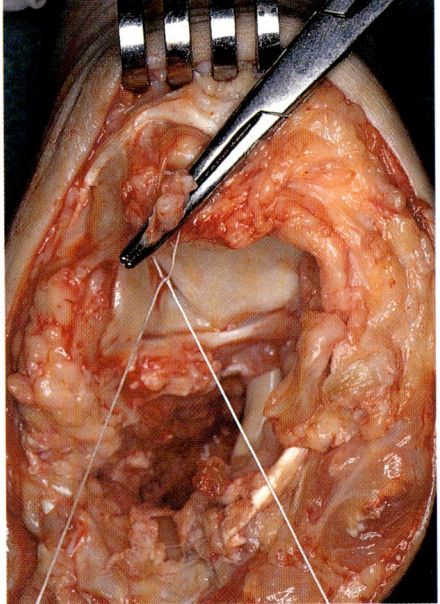

Figure 17. The anterior vascular bundle is ligated.

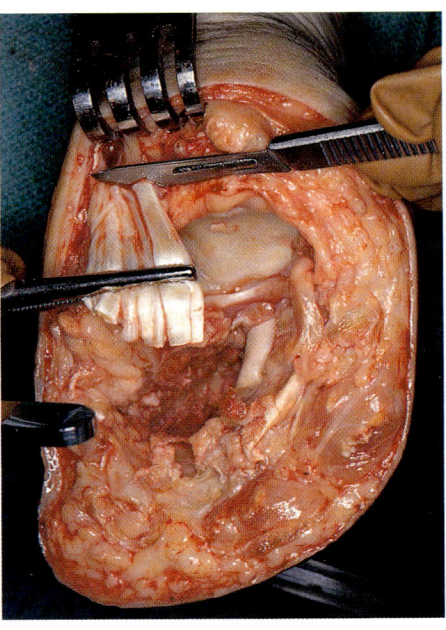

Figure 18. The extensor tendons are divided under tension.

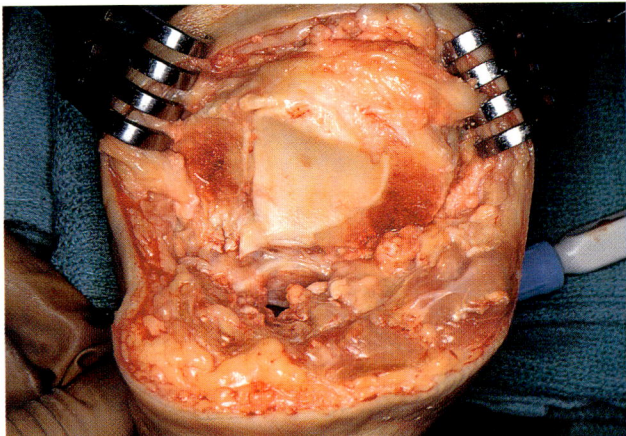

Figure 20. The appearance after resection of both malleoli.

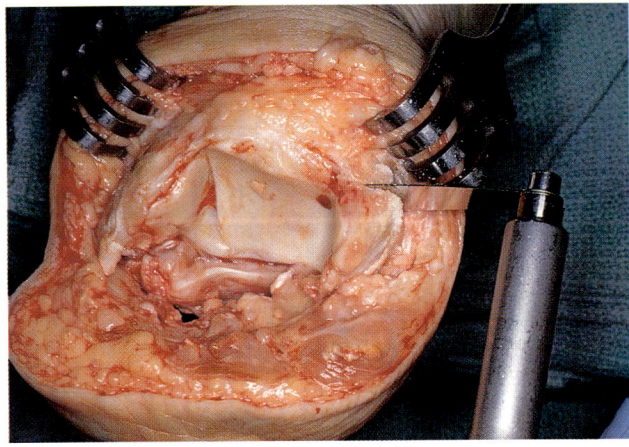

Figure 19. The malleoli are resected at the level of the tibial plafond using the small oscillating saw.

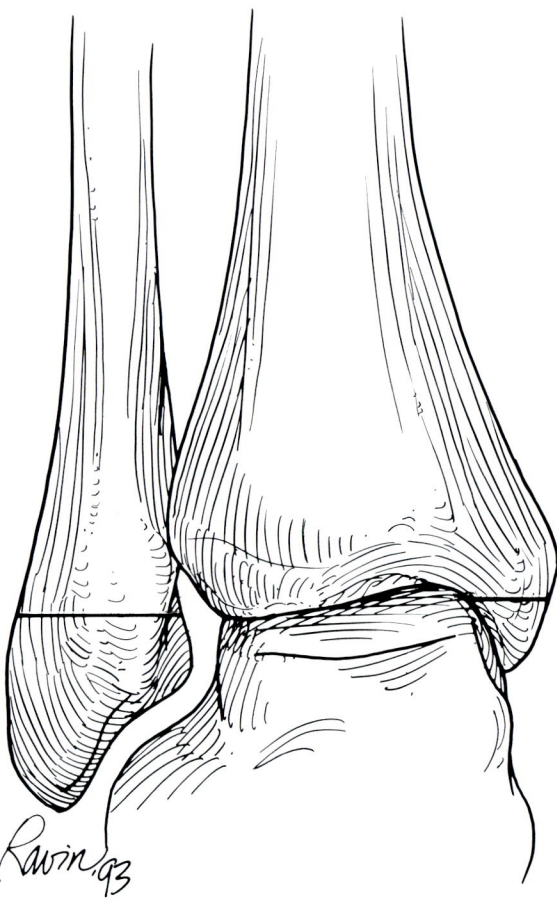

Figure 21. The level of bone resection of the malleoli.

The anterior tibial artery and accompanying veins are then ligated (Fig. 17). The extensor and flexor tendons are then pulled distally with a large clamp and divided so that they retract proximally (Fig. 18). Avoid the bundle within the posterior flap as described in order not to damage the blood supply to the heel pad.

Prior to performing the closure the malleoli are cut off flush with the level of the tibial plafond (Figs. 19 and 20). Although some authors have advised narrowing the medial-lateral flare of the tibial metaphysis, it is desirable to conserve the flare because it gives wider internal support to the bulbous Syme stump. It is specifically important because the tibial flare is the main structure that holds the prosthesis on and keeps it from slipping up and down (Fig. 21). It is not necessary to remove the cartilage from the distal tibia.

The pad is then gently held up and the closure is tested with digital pressure (Fig. 22). If the pad appears to be too mobile at the time of closure, additional tissue should be resected from the distal (plantar) edge of the heel pad, and the pad sutured to the bone. If the soft tissue is too thick to allow easy apposition of the two skin edges, it is usually due to the thick plantar fat pad on the inferior side. It is often necessary to carefully thin or "plane" down this fat pad so that it does not distract the edges of the wound. Prudence must be applied to prevent excessive thinning, and thus devascularization of the flap.

The closure is done over a suction drain that is brought out through a separate tiny stab wound proximally (Figs. 23 and 24).

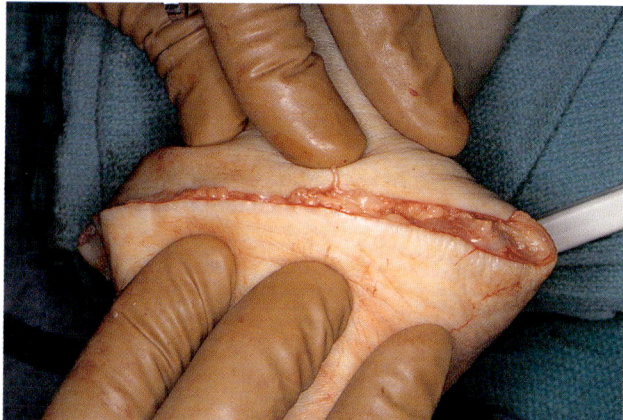

Figure 22. The final shape of the stump is checked with gentle manual approximation to verify the easy apposition of the flaps.

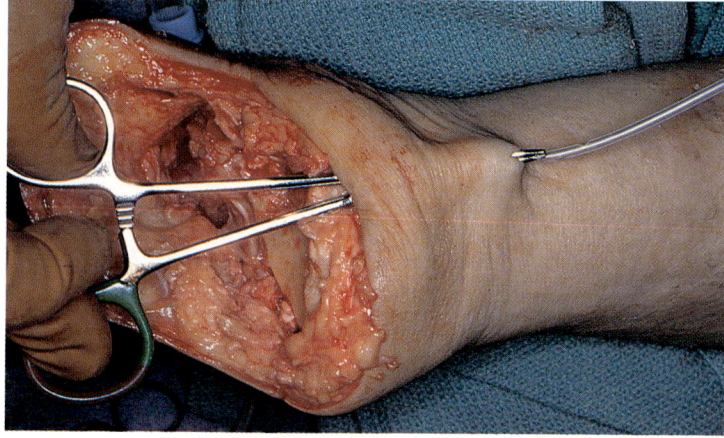

Figure 23. Closure is done over a ⅛-inch suction drain brought through a separate, proximal stab incision.

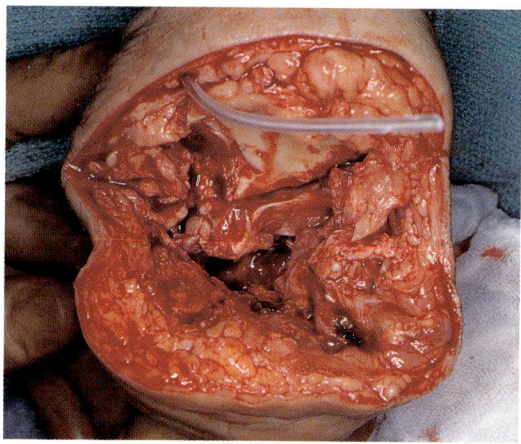

Figure 24. The drain is placed in the wound.

Drill holes are made in the anterior lip of the tibial plafond (Fig. 25) in order to anchor the plantar fascia. Alternatively, the plantar fascia can be sutured to the deep fascia anteriorly.

The closure is done in three layers. First, the plantar fascia is sutured either through the drill holes in the distal tibia or to the fascia as described (Figs. 26 and 27). This is followed by a subcutaneous closure with inverted interrupted absorbable sutures (Fig. 28). The skin is closed with nylon sutures or staples (Fig. 29). A soft dressing is applied.

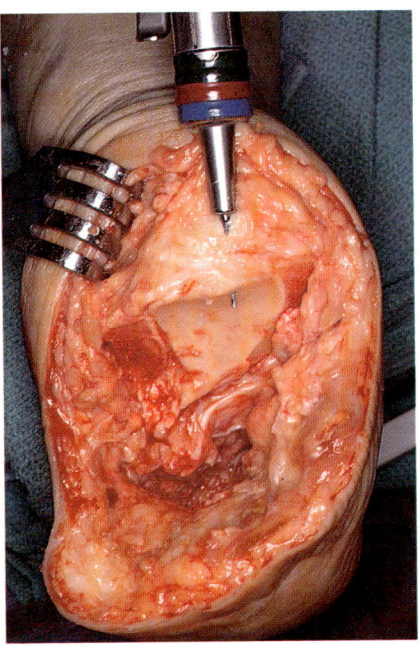

Figure 25. Drill holes are made in the anterior lip of the distal tibial plafond to anchor sutures to the plantar fascia.

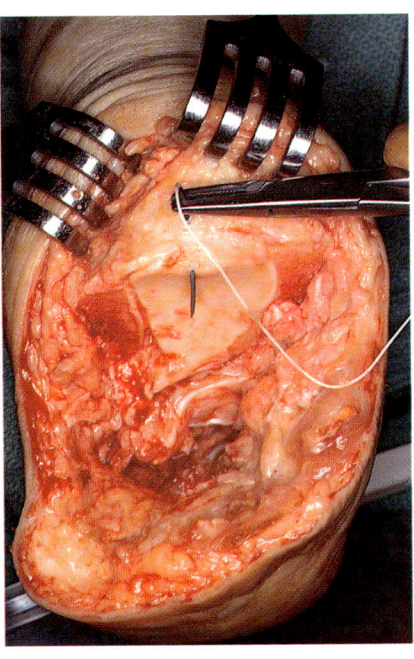

Figure 26. The suture is placed through the drill holes in the anterior margin of the tibia.

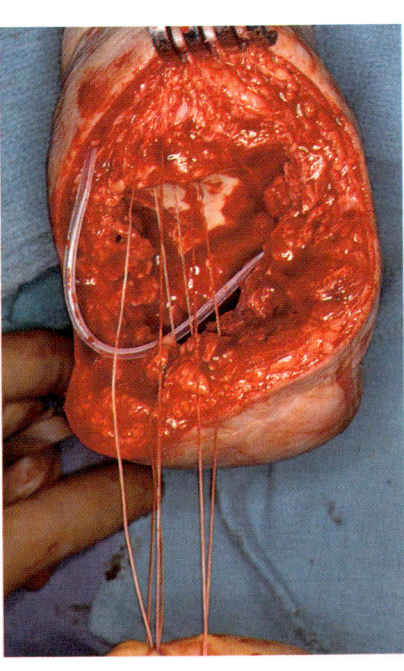

Figure 27. The sutures are then passed through the plantar fascia, taking care to avoid entrapping the drain.

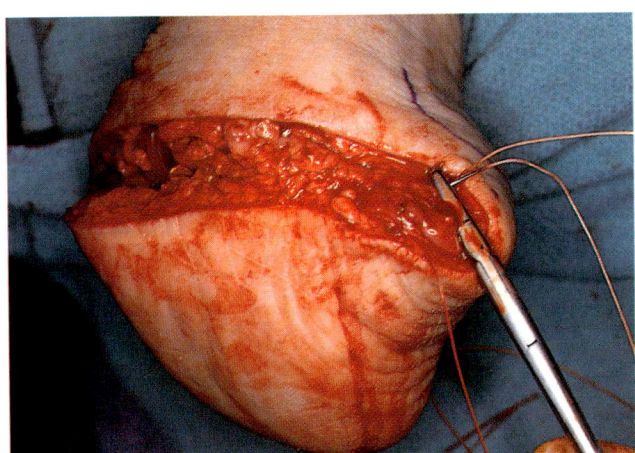

Figure 28. A subcutaneous closure is done with interrupted, inverted absorbable sutures.

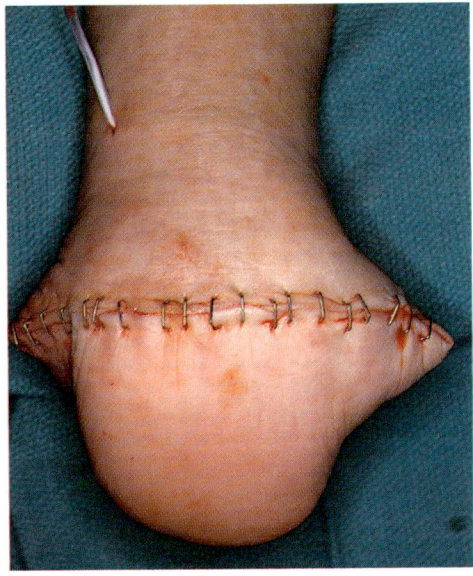

Figure 29. The skin is closed with staples or interrupted sutures.

In the two-stage Syme procedure, done for infected cases, the resection of the malleoli is deferred at the time of the initial operation. At the second stage, the "dog ears" of soft tissue on the medial and lateral sides are excised. The malleoli are then resected through the elliptical openings thus created on either side, prior to closure. If the pad is excessively mobile at this stage, correction is obtained by removing larger ellipses of skin and subcutaneous tissue.

POSTOPERATIVE MANAGEMENT

Initially, either a soft dressing or a plaster shell over the dressing can be used. The suction drain is usually removed after 24 hours. The patient is instructed in proper technique for non–weight-bearing gait using crutches or walker. After the first week, a cast is usually applied to protect the stump. If the patient is diabetic or dysvascular, non–weight bearing is maintained for at least 4 to 6 weeks. Earlier ambulation on the cast can sometimes be allowed in amputations done for trauma, depending on the advancement of wound healing.

The removal of the skin sutures or staples may be delayed until 6 to 8 weeks after surgery, or even more. Sutures are generally left in place a minimum of 4 weeks. It is not unusual to see a small amount of serous drainage after closure, as occurs in most foot amputations, but this usually resolves over the first 1 to 2 weeks.

Prosthetic fitting, especially in the diabetic and dysvascular patients is done once complete healing of the stump has occurred. Weight bearing is not permitted if areas of delayed soft tissue healing persist. Most patients with a successful outcome will be able to be fitted with a prosthesis and ambulate at least on a limited basis, within 10 to 12 weeks.

The success rate of Syme amputations varies from 50% to 90%. At this time, most authors report about a 70% to 75% success rate for healing of Syme amputations in diabetic and dysvascular patients.

The vast majority of failures in this population occur early as the result of failure to achieve primary wound healing, usually due to ischemia of the heel pad, which, as noted above, is supplied by branches of the posterior tibial artery.

Late failure of the Syme amputation is usually due to progressive peripheral vascular occlusion, which results in gangrene through a wider area of the lower limb, rather than complications inherent within the Syme stump.

REHABILITATION

Good prosthetic fitting of the Syme stump is vital, and usually requires a prosthetist with experience. The difficulty lies in the fact that a secure fit is required but the broad, bulbous end of the stump must pass through a narrow portion of the prosthesis corresponding to the narrow width of the distal tibia just above the metaphysis. This challenge has been handled with a number of different techniques including placing a hinged window in the prosthesis, placing a wraparound filler above the bulb, or using an elastic double-wall construction for the distal part of the prosthesis. Many prostheses are equipped with a solid ankle cushion heel (SACH) that enhances the patient's gait.

A minor, and, in fact, the only significant disadvantage of the Syme amputation compared to a below-knee amputation is that the Syme prosthesis is less cosmetic because of the wide "ankle" portion of the prosthesis, which is required to allow passage of the stump, as described above.

However, in virtually every other way, the Syme prosthesis is preferable to a below-knee amputation. The Syme stump is partially end-bearing, as described previously, and even diabetic patients have fewer problems with skin breakdown over the proximal leg that would occur with a below-knee amputation. Suprapatellar suspension straps are not needed. The mechanical advantage of a full lower leg segment is immense. Even more important, most patients with Syme amputations need minimal prosthetic training, and require much less extensive physical therapy because the Syme amputation functions like a partial foot amputation. Prosthetic walking is similar to the use of a cast, which most of the patients have used previously. The lower energy "cost" (oxygen consumption per meter) of the Syme amputation when compared to more proximal amputations was noted in the introduction to this chapter. The Syme amputee also has a higher velocity of gait and a longer stride length (5).

COMPLICATIONS

The Syme amputation is an excellent procedure with potentially excellent function for the patient. Because this is often used as a "salvage" type of procedure, in an attempt to avert performing a below-knee amputation, there will be a certain number of failures and complications, and the numbers will be related to the individual surgeon's threshold criteria for doing this procedure. Although the morbidity of a second, more proximal amputation is not negligible, the ultimate result for the patient is not significantly prejudiced by the need to revise to a below-knee amputation if the Syme amputation fails.

There are five major complications of the Syme amputation:

1. *Early (dysvascular) failure of the wound to heal:* The most common complication of the Syme procedure is primary failure of the soft tissue to heal. Some occurrences of this complication cannot be precluded if the surgeon strives for the goal of maximal limb salvage. However, proper preoperative vascular evaluation is the solution in order to keep the frequency of this complication to a reasonable level. At the time of surgery, if the wound edges do not demonstrate adequate bleeding once the disarticulation is completed, it is advisable to proceed to a more proximal amputation.
2. *Hypermobility or migration of the stump:* Some mobility of the stump is normal, and a few patients can even dorsiflex and plantar flex the stump through the action of the residual tendons. Stump mobility becomes problematic when the stump moves or migrates side to side, because this can interfere with or compromise the fitting and function of the prosthesis. If modification of the prosthesis is unsuccessful, excision of full-thickness wedges of tissue from the medial and lateral sides of the stump is the solution. Suturing the fascia of the distal pad to the tibia through drill holes is rarely required as well.
3. *Late ulceration of the stump:* Infrequently, late ulceration around the stump can occur. This occurs primarily in diabetics. While this may be due to an isolated incident of trauma to the tissue, it is usually caused by pressure from the distal edge of the fibula. Stump mobility, and shrinkage of the tissue can exacerbate the problem. Initial treatment is with local wound care and total contact casts. If the problem persists, the treatment is excision of a portion of the distal fibula to relieve the underlying bony pressure on the skin. The ulcer can be debrided or excised as well.
4. *Poor cosmesis:* The cosmetic appearance of the prosthesis in the Syme amputee is occasionally a problem, particularly for women who would like to wear dresses instead of pants. It is important to discuss this with the patient preoperatively, and if necessary, even show photos of the prosthesis so that the patient understands what to expect of the appearance. Most patients will opt for function over image.
5. *Painful stump:* Painful stumps occur very infrequently, and usually in Syme amputations that have been done for trauma. The most common cause of pain

is neuroma formation in one of the major nerves or anterior superficial sensory nerves near the level of the ankle joint where they have been transected. The treatment is surgical excision or burying the nerve. Diagnosis is aided by selective injection with small amounts of local anesthetic.

Rarely, the entire pad of the stump will be persistently painful in a patient who has had the amputation done for a crushing injury to the hindfoot. Most of these are industrial accidents. Treatment is by revision to a long below-knee amputation.

ILLUSTRATIVE CASE FOR TECHNIQUE

This patient is a 23-year-old construction worker who sustained a severe crushing injury on the job while working with a paving machine. The forefoot was mangled and the midfoot was contaminated and degloved. The patient underwent initial aggressive debridement, followed by redebridement and a partial foot amputation that was left open (Figs. 30 and 31). The patient was then treated with appropriate intravenous antibiotics and vigorous local wound care. The open amputation was converted to a Syme amputation 1 week after injury.

Initially, the patient was kept non–weight bearing until all the skin sutures were removed. He was then placed in a temporary prosthesis made of synthetic cast material with a rubber heel and started on a vigorous physical therapy program.

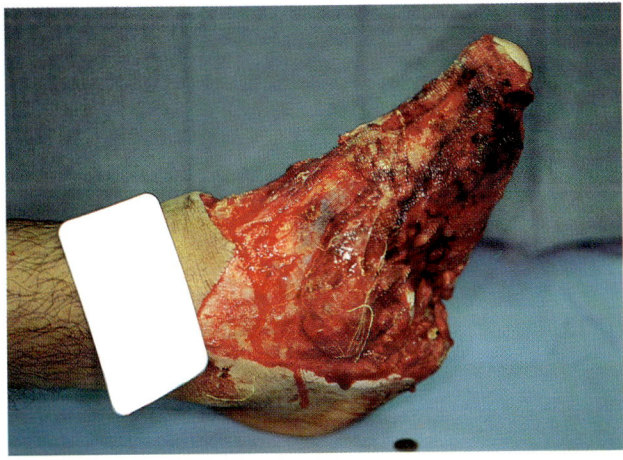

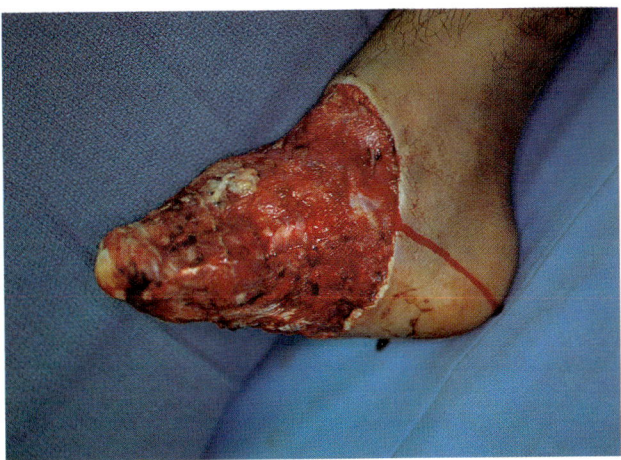

Figures 30 and 31. Appearance of the foot after primary debridements, local wound care and antibiotics, and prior to performing the Syme procedure.

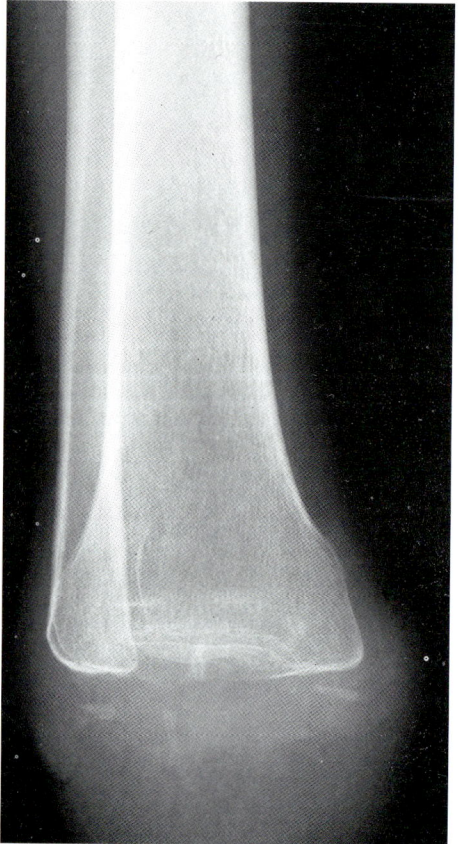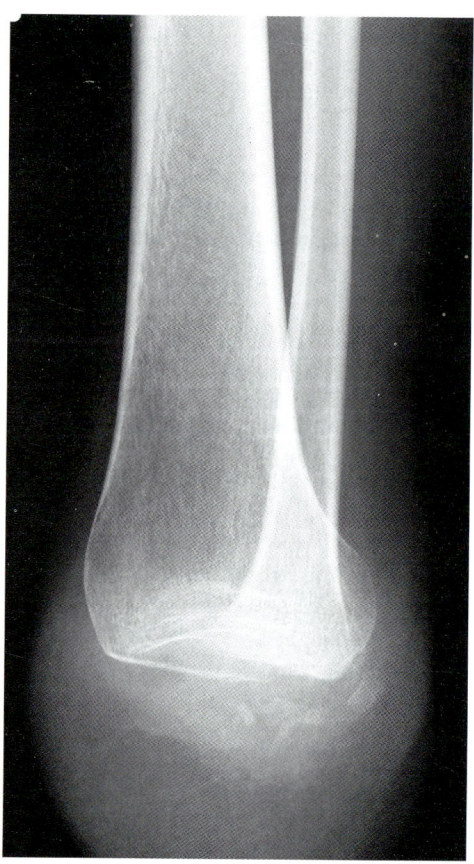

Figure 32. Radiographs of the Syme stump 6 months postoperatively.

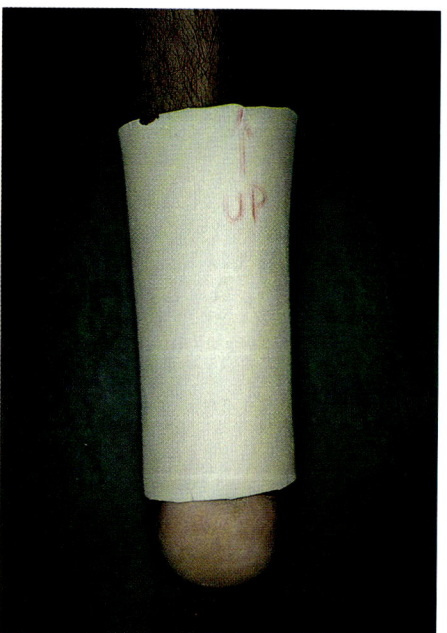

Figure 33. The Syme limb with a Plastazote molded filler applied just above the bulb. This "converts" the limb to a cylinder, facilitating early prosthetic fitting.

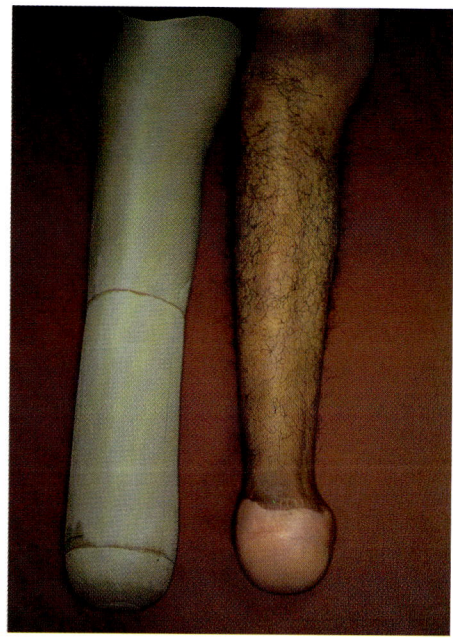

Figure 34. The appearance of the limb and the liner for the prosthesis 9 months postoperatively.

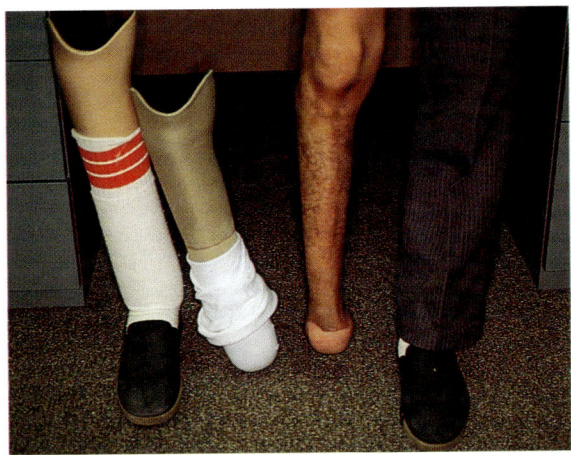

Figure 35. From **left** to **right:** the Syme prosthesis, the liner of the prosthesis, the Syme limb, and normal limb 9 months postoperatively.

He was fitted with a Syme prosthesis at about 2½ months postoperatively. The patient had significant persistent pain for many months, presumably due to the crushing nature of the injury. The patient required another 3 months of physical therapy because of his stump pain and slow progress. There were no problems with healing of the wound, and no specific point tenderness could be found that might indicate neuroma formation. The radiographic appearance of the limb is seen in (Fig. 32). Eventually the patient became independent in his ambulation and virtually pain free, and returned to a sedentary type of job at about 9 months postinjury. The limb and the patient's prosthesis at the time of completion of his treatment are pictured in Figs. 33–35.

RECOMMENDED READING

1. Anderson, L., Westin, G. W., and Oppenheim, W. L.: Syme amputation in children: indications, results, and long-term follow-up. *J. Pediatr. Orthop.*, 4: 550–554, 1984.
2. Francis, H. III, Roberts, Jr., et al.: The Syme amputation: success in elderly diabetic patients with palpable ankle pulses. *J. Vasc. Surg.*, 12: 237–240, 1990.
3. Herring, J.. A., Barnhill, B., and Gaffney, C.: Syme amputation. *J. Bone Joint Surg.*, 68A: 573–578, 1986.
4. Jany, R. S., and Burkus, J. K.: Long-term follow-up of Syme amputations for peripheral vascular disease associated with diabetes mellitus. *Foot Ankle*, 9: 107–110, 1988.
5. Waters, R. L., Perry, J., Antonelli, D., et al.: Energy cost of walking of amputees: the influence of level of amputation. *J. Bone Joint Surg.*, 56A: 42–46, 1976.

Subject Index

A

Abductor digiti quinti nerve release, 333–340
  ankle block, 334
  closure, 335
  complications, 339
  contraindications, 333
  heel pain, 334
  illustrative case, 339–340
  incision, 334
  indications, 333
  medial calcaneal nerve branch, 339
  postoperative management, 339
  preoperative planning, 333–334
  prognosis, 339
  surgical procedure, 334–338
Achilles tendon. *See also* Achilles tendon acute repair; Achilles tendon delayed repair
  anatomy, 301–302
  avulsion, calcaneal prominence resection, 348
  rupture, 299
    diagnosis, 299–300
    Thompson test, 299–300
  tendinosis, 343
Achilles tendon acute repair, 299–308
  closure, 304–305
  complications, 306–307
  contraindications, 300
  illustrative case, 307–308
  incision, 301
  indications, 299–300
  postoperative management, 305–306
  preoperative planning, 300
  rehabilitation, 306
  surgical procedure, 301–305
Achilles tendon delayed repair, 311–321
  closure, 319
  complications, 319
  contraindications, 311
  flexor digitorum longus, 316, 317
  illustrative case, 319, 320, 321
  incision, 313
  indications, 311
  postoperative management, 319
  preoperative planning, 312–313
  sural nerve neuroma, 319
  surgical procedure, 313–319
  V-Y sliding tendinous flap, 317, 318
Adolescent bunion
  cuneiform-metatarsal arthrodesis, 107
  metatarsocuneiform arthrodesis, 107
Age
  bunion, 31, 107
  chevron osteotomy, 31
  cuneiform-metatarsal arthrodesis, 107
  metatarsocuneiform arthrodesis, 107
Akin procedure, 65–72
  ankle block, 66
  apex plantar, 70
  bone apposition, 70
  closing, 69
  complications, 71
  contraindications, 65
  deformity recurrence, 71
  great toe valgus deformity, 65
  hallux valgus, 65
  hallux valgus interphalangeus, 65
  illustrative case, 71–72
  indications, 65
  Kirschner wire, 68, 69
  nonunion, 70
  pitfalls, 70
  plantar angulation, 70
  postoperative management, 70
  preoperative planning, 66
  surgical procedure, 66–70
Anesthesia
  ankle instability repair, 439
  Bröstrom-Gould procedure, 439
  calcaneal tuberosity osteotomy, 353
  chevron osteotomy, 33
  chevron type fifth metatarsal osteotomy, 190–191

Anesthesia (*contd.*)
  distal fifth chevron metatarsal
    osteotomy, 190–191
  fifth metatarsal osteotomy, 190–191
  hallux metatarsophalangeal
    arthrodesis, 55
  marginal toenail ablation, 4
  peroneal tendon repair-reconstruction,
    288
  phenol matrixectomy, 17
  plantar fascia release, 325
  proximal first metatarsal osteotomy,
    89–90
  second toe resection arthroplasty, 152
  secondary interdigital neuroma
    resection, 183–184
  subtalar arthrodesis, 359–368
  talocalcaneal arthrodesis, 359–368
  talonavicular arthrodesis, 250
  third toe resection arthroplasty, 152
Ankle arthrodesis, 467–482
  closure, 479
  complications, 480–481
  contraindications, 468
  diabetes, 468
  fixation, 475–478
  illustrative case, 481–482
  incision, 470
  indications, 468
  Kirschner wire, 475, 477
  malalignment, 480–481
  osteoporosis, 468
  patient position, 469
  peripheral neuropathy, 468
  persistent postoperative pain, 481
  postoperative management, 479–480
  preoperative planning, 468–469
  pseudarthrosis, 480
  Steinmann pin, 475, 476, 477
  surgical procedure, 469
  tendon laceration, 481
Ankle block
  abductor digiti quinti nerve release,
    334
  Akin procedure, 66
  cheilectomy, 123
  hallux metatarsophalangeal
    arthrodesis, 55
  hallux proximal phalanx osteotomy, 66
  marginal toenail ablation, 4
  Mitchell osteotomy, 74
  Morton's neuroma resection, 168
  plantar fascia release, 325
  primary interdigital neuroma resection,
    168
  proximal first metatarsal osteotomy,
    89–90
Ankle fracture realignment
  degenerative joint disease, 451–452
  diabetes, 452
  malunion
    closure, 459
    complications, 463
    contraindications, 451–452
    fixation, 457–459
    illustrative case, 463–465
    incision, 455

  indications, 451–452
  postoperative management, 463
  preoperative planning, 452–455
  surgical procedure, 455
  patient education, 452
Ankle instability repair, 437–447
  advantages, 438
  anesthesia, 439
  ankle sprain, 437
  anterior talofibular ligament, 437,
    441–443
  calcaneal fibular ligament, 437,
    441–443
  closure, 444–445
  complications, 445
  contraindications, 438
  extensor retinaculum, 437
  illustrative case, 445–447
  incision, 439, 440
  indications, 438
  postoperative management, 445
  preoperative planning, 438–439
  surgical procedure, 439–445
Ankle inversion injury, peroneal tendon
  repair-reconstruction, 285
Ankle joint, 451–511
Ankle pain, lateral, 165
Ankle sprain
  ankle instability repair, 437
  Bröstrom-Gould procedure, 437
Ankle valgus, 372
Anterior talofibular ligament
  ankle instability repair, 437, 441–443
  Bröstrom-Gould procedure, 437,
    441–443
Anteromedial heel pad field block,
  plantar fascia release, 325
Apex plantar
  Akin procedure, 70
  hallux proximal phalanx osteotomy, 70
Arteriosclerotic peripheral vascular
  disease, Syme amputation,
  497–498
Arthritis, interphalangeal joint, 21
Arthrosis, posttraumatic, 483
Avascular necrosis
  chevron osteotomy, 45
  talar body, 468
  talus, 483

B
Böhler's angle, 403, 404, 411, 412
Biplanar metatarsal neck osteotomy,
  Mitchell osteotomy, 83
Blair fusion, talar body, 468
Bone apposition
  Akin procedure, 70
  hallux proximal phalanx osteotomy, 70
Bone graft
  hallux metatarsophalangeal
    arthrodesis, 58, 59, 60, 61, 62, 63
  posterior iliac crest, 484–485
Bröstrom-Gould procedure, 437–447
  advantages, 438
  anesthesia, 439
  ankle sprain, 437

anterior talofibular ligament, 437, 441–443
calcaneal fibular ligament, 441–443
calcaneal fibular ligaments, 437
closure, 444–445
complications, 445
contraindications, 438
extensor retinaculum, 437
illustrative case, 445–447
incision, 439, 440
indications, 438
postoperative management, 445
preoperative planning, 438–439
surgical procedure, 439–445
Bunionectomy, 21, 107
  Mitchell's. *See* Mitchell osteotomy

C

Calandruccio device, tibiocalcaneal arthrodesis, 488, 489, 490
Calcaneal fibular ligament
  anatomy, 286
  ankle instability repair, 437, 441–443
  Bröstrom-Gould procedure, 437, 441–443
Calcaneal fracture
  calcaneal arthrodesis
    calcaneocuboid joint, 428
    complications, 435
    contraindications, 427–428
    illustrative case, 436
    incision, 429–430
    indications, 427–428
    instrumentation, 428–429
    malunion, 425–436
    postoperative management, 434–435
    preoperative planning, 428
    screw fixation, 432–434
    surgical procedure, 428–434
    sustentacular fragment, 431–433
  calcaneal osteotomy
    calcaneocuboid joint, 428
    complications, 435
    contraindications, 427–428
    illustrative case, 436
    incision, 429–430
    indications, 427–428
    instrumentation, 428–429
    malunion, 425–436
    postoperative management, 434–435
    preoperative planning, 428
    screw fixation, 432–434
    surgical procedure, 428–434
    sustentacular fragment, 431–433
  compartment release, 257
  fracture blister, 406, 407
  functional losses, 426–427
  Kirschner wire, 413
  open reduction and fixation, 401–422
    closure, 413–414
    complications, 416
    contraindications, 401
    illustrative case, 417–422
    indications, 401
    postoperative management, 415–416
    preoperative planning, 402–408
    surgical procedure, 409–414, 415
  pathomechanics, 425, 426
  staple fixation, 410–411
  Steinmann pin, 410–411
  sural nerve, 416
  sustentaculum tali, 425, 431
  tibial nerve, 416
  wound necrosis, 416
Calcaneal prominence resection, 341–349
  Achilles tendon avulsion, 348
  complications, 348
  contraindications, 342
  Haglund's syndrome, 341
  illustrative case, 348, 349
  incision, 343, 344
  indications, 342
  postoperative management, 348
  preoperative planning, 342–343
  retrocalcaneal bursitis, 341
  surgical procedure, 343–347
Calcaneal tuberosity displacement, 426–427
Calcaneal tuberosity osteotomy, 351–357
  anesthesia, 353
  complications, 356
  contraindications, 351–353
  illustrative case, 356–357
  incision, 353–354
  indications, 351–353
  patient education, 355
  postoperative management, 355
  preoperative planning, 353
  Steinmann pin, 355
  surgical procedure, 353–355
Calcaneocuboid joint, 428
Calcaneal arthrodesis
  calcaneal fracture
    calcaneocuboid joint, 428
    complications, 435
    contraindications, 427–428
    illustrative case, 436
    incision, 429–430
    indications, 427–428
    instrumentation, 428–429
    malunion, 425–436
    postoperative management, 434–435
    preoperative planning, 428
    screw fixation, 432–434
    surgical procedure, 428–434
    sustentacular fragment, 431–433
  nonunion, 435
  Steinmann pin, 430, 431, 432
Calcaneal osteotomy
  calcaneal fracture
    calcaneocuboid joint, 428
    complications, 435
    illustrative case, 436
    incision, 429–430
    indications, 427–428
    instrumentation, 428–429
    malunion, 425–436
    postoperative management, 434–435
    preoperative planning, 428
    screw fixation, 432–434
    surgical procedure, 428–434
    sustentacular fragment, 431–433
  nonunion, 435
  Steinmann pin, 430, 431, 432

Calcaneus
  displacement after fracture, 426
  function, 425–426
  normal, 402, 426
  relationships, 402
Callus
  groove, 15, 16
  rheumatoid forefoot reconstruction, 208
Charcot-Marie-Tooth disease, 21
  talus-calcaneus-cuboid arthrodesis, 369
Cheilectomy, 119–132
  ankle block, 123
  closure, 127–128
  complications, 129–130
  contraindications, 120
  extensor hallucis longus tendon, 130
  hallux rigidus, 119
  illustrative case, 130, 131, 132
  incision, 123
  indications, 119–120
  joint arthrodesis, 129
  Keller resection arthroplasty, 129
  metatarsal head resection, 126, 127, 128
  metatarsal prominence excision, 125–126
  osteophyte excision, 126–127
  postoperative management, 128
  preoperative planning, 120–121
  prognosis, 129
  rehabilitation, 129
  sesamoid metatarsal complex, 127
  surgical procedure, 123–128
  variations, 128
Chevron osteotomy, 31–48
  age, 31
  anesthesia, 33
  avascular necrosis, 45
  closing, 42–43
  complications, 45–46
  contraindications, 31–33
  drill orientation, 37–39
  forefoot, insufficient narrowing, 45
  hallux valgus deformity, 31
  hallux valgus night splint, 44
  illustrative case, 46–48
  incision, 34, 35
  indications, 31–33
  medial eminence pain, 31
  metaphysis resection, 41–42
  metatarsal head, 36, 37, 38
  metatarsophalangeal joint, incongruity, 45–46
  metatarsophalangeal joint arthritis, 32–33
  metatarsophalangeal valgus, recurrent, 45
  modified osteotomy arms correct location, 36, 37
  outpatient vs. inpatient, 33
  patient expectations, 44–45
  postoperative management, 44–45
  potential pitfalls, 36
  preoperative planning, 40–41
  previous hallux valgus surgery, 33
  radiology, 33
  screw fixation, 33→34, 39–41
  soft tissue reconstruction, 42
  spica soft tissue dressing, 44
  surgical procedure, 34–43
  varus-valgus stress, 32
  walking cast, 44
Chevron type fifth metatarsal osteotomy
  anesthesia, 190–191
  closure, 194
  complications, 195
  contraindications, 189–190
  illustrative case, 195, 196
  incision, 191
  indications, 189
  postoperative management, 194–195
  preoperative planning, 190
  prognosis, 195
  surgical procedure, 190–194
Chronic synovitis, 135
Claw hallux, 21
Claw toe
  second toe resection arthroplasty, 149
  third toe resection arthroplasty, 149
Compartment release, 257–267
  calcaneal fracture, 257
  compartment syndrome, 257
  complications, 266
  contraindications, 257
  fasciotomy, 261–265
  foot compartment syndrome, 257
  illustrative case, 267
  incision, 261–265, 266
  indications, 257
  postoperative management, 265–266
  preoperative planning, 258–261
  surgical procedure, 260, 261–265
  trauma, 257
Compartment syndrome, 257
Congenital pseudarthrosis of tibia, Syme amputation, 497–498
Cross-over toe deformity, 135–148
Crural fascia, 301–302
Cuneiform-metatarsal arthrodesis, 107–116, 231–246
  adolescent bunion, 107
  age, 107
  complications, 115, 242–244
  contraindications, 108, 231–233
  hallux valgus, 107
  hypermobility, 107
  illustrative case, 115–116, 244–246
  incision, 110, 111–112, 234–235
  indications, 107–108, 231–233
  malunion, 244
  metatarsocuneiform arthritis, 107
  metatarsus adductus, 108
  metatarsus primus varus, 107
  nonunion, 244
  patient education, 110
  postoperative management, 115, 241–242
  preoperative planning, 108–110, 233–234
  resection, 111–112
  screw fixation, 112, 114
  surgical procedure, 110–115, 234–240, 241
Cuneiform-metatarsal joint, 230–246

SUBJECT INDEX

D

Degenerative arthritis, proximal first metatarsal osteotomy, 86
Degenerative joint disease, ankle fracture realignment, 451–452
Degenerative osteophyte, first metatarsal head, 119, 120
Delayed union, proximal first metatarsal osteotomy, 102
Diabetes
    ankle arthrodesis, 468
    ankle fracture realignment, 452
    phalanges, 3, 10
    phenol matrixectomy, 15
    transmetatarsal amputation, 213
Diffuse peripheral neuritis, 180
Digital block
    marginal toenail ablation, 4
    phenol matrixectomy, 17
Distal fifth chevron metatarsal osteotomy
    anesthesia, 190–191
    closure, 194
    complications, 195
    contraindications, 189–190
    illustrative case, 195, 196
    incision, 191
    indications, 189
    postoperative management, 194–195
    preoperative planning, 190
    prognosis, 195
    surgical procedure, 190–194
Distal soft tissue realignment, proximal first metatarsal osteotomy, 85
Dorsal proper digital nerve, hallux metatarsophalangeal arthrodesis, 59–60
DuVries arthroplasty, second toe realignment, 145

E

Electromyography, 334
Enchondroma, 3
Epinychium, phenol matrixectomy, 17, 19, 20
Erythema, phalanges, 10
Extension contracture
    second toe resection arthroplasty, 149
    third toe resection arthroplasty, 149
Extensor digitorum brevis, second toe realignment, 142–145
Extensor digitorum longus, second toe realignment, 142–145
Extensor hallucis brevis, 22
Extensor hallucis longus, 22
    cheilectomy, 130
Extensor retinaculum
    ankle instability repair, 437
    Bröstrom-Gould procedure, 437

F

Fasciotomy, compartment release, 261–265
Fibular hemimelia, Syme amputation, 497–498
Fibular sesamoid, 88

Fifth metatarsal osteotomy, 189–196
    anesthesia, 190–191
    closure, 194
    complications, 195
    contraindications, 189–190
    illustrative case, 195, 196
    incision, 191
    indications, 189
    postoperative management, 194–195
    preoperative planning, 190
    prognosis, 195
    surgical procedure, 190–194
First metatarsal head
    degenerative osteophyte, 119, 120
    lateral displacement osteotomy, 81
First metatarsophalangeal joint, congruency, 87–88
Fixed hindfoot deformity, talus-calcaneus-cuboid arthrodesis, 369
Flatfoot, plantar fascia release, 331
Flexor digitorum longus
    Achilles tendon delayed repair, 316, 317
    posterior tibial tendon release-substitution, 271–280
    second toe realignment, 140–142
    tibialis posterior tendon release-substitution, 271–280
Flexor hallucis brevis, 22
    detachment, 21
Flexor hallucis longus, 22
Foot
    compartments, 258
    dorsal view, 232–233
Foot compartment syndrome, compartment release, 257
Forefoot, chevron osteotomy, insufficient narrowing, 45
Fracture blister, calcaneal fracture, 406, 407
Fungal infection
    diagnosis, 16
    marginal toenail ablation, 3, 9–10
    phenol matrixectomy, 16

G

Gait instability, rheumatoid forefoot reconstruction, 208
Gangrene, transmetatarsal amputation, 213
Great toe valgus deformity
    Akin procedure, 65
    hallux proximal phalanx osteotomy, 65
Groove, callus, 15, 16

H

Haglund's syndrome
    calcaneal prominence resection, 341
    conservative treatment, 341, 342
Hallux, motion, 108, 109
Hallux interphalangeal arthrodesis, 21–27
    closure, 25
    complications, 26
    contraindications, 21
    fixation, 24, 25, 26

Hallux interphalangeal arthrodesis
(*contd.*)
  illustrative case, 27
  incision, 22–24
  indications, 21
  Kirschner wire, 24, 26
  nonunion, 26
  postoperative management, 26
  preoperative planning, 21–22
  screw length, 22
  screw removal, 26
  surgical procedure, 22–26
Hallux metatarsophalangeal arthrodesis, 49–64
  anesthesia, 55
  ankle block, 55
  apposition of existing bone, 56–57
  bone graft, 58, 59, 60, 61, 62, 63
  closing, 56–57
  complications, 59–60
  conical technique, 53
  contraindications, 49
  dorsal proper digital nerve, 59–60
  hallux position, 50
    axial (varus-valgus) plane, 51–52, 53
    coronal plane rotation, 52–53
    sagittal (flexion-extension) plane, 50–51, 52
  illustrative cases, 60–64
  implant arthroplasty, 49–50
  incision, 55
  indications, 49
  malposition, 59
    salvage, 59
  Marin reamer, 54–55
  nonunion, 59
    salvage, 59
  postoperative management, 59
  preoperative planning, 50–55
  resection arthroplasty, 49–50
  rongeur, 54
  screw fixation, 53, 56
  silastic implant, 50
  surgical procedure, 55–59
  tricortical graft, 58, 59, 62, 63
Hallux position, hallux metatarsophalangeal arthrodesis, 50
  axial (varus-valgus) plane, 51–52, 53
  coronal plane rotation, 52–53
  sagittal (flexion-extension) plane, 50–51, 52
Hallux proximal phalanx osteotomy, 65–72
  ankle block, 66
  apex plantar, 70
  bone apposition, 70
  closing, 69
  complications, 71
  contraindications, 65
  deformity recurrence, 71
  great toe valgus deformity, 65
  hallux valgus, 65
  hallux valgus interphalangeus, 65
  illustrative case, 71–72
  indications, 65
  Kirschner wire, 68, 69
  nonunion, 70
  pitfalls, 70
  plantar angulation, 70
  postoperative management, 70
  preoperative planning, 66
  surgical procedure, 66–70
Hallux rigidus
  advanced, 121, 122
  cheilectomy, 119
  clinical features, 119
  conservative treatment, 119
  grading, 121, 122
  mild, 121
  Mitchell osteotomy, 81
  moderate, 121, 122, 130
  physical examination, 120
  proximal first metatarsal osteotomy, 86
Hallux valgus
  Akin procedure, 65
  angle, 86, 87
  chevron osteotomy, 31
  cuneiform-metatarsal arthrodesis, 107
  hallux proximal phalanx osteotomy, 65
  metatarsocuneiform arthrodesis, 107
  Mitchell osteotomy, 73
  proximal first metatarsal osteotomy, 85
  recurrence, 101
  second toe realignment, 137–139
Hallux valgus interphalangeus
  Akin procedure, 65
  hallux proximal phalanx osteotomy, 65
Hallux varus, 21
  proximal first metatarsal osteotomy, 102
Hammer toe
  second toe resection arthroplasty, 149
  third toe resection arthroplasty, 149
Heel pad, Syme amputation, 498
Heel pain, 323, 324
  abductor digiti quinti nerve release, 334
  conservative treatment, 323
  plantar fascia release, 323
Heel spur
  conservative treatment, 323
  plantar fascia release, 323
  surgical removal, 326, 327–329
Herbert screw
  lateral displacement osteotomy, 81
  Mitchell osteotomy, 79
Hindfoot, 271–447
Hindfoot valgus, 370
Hindfoot varus, 370
Hypermobility
  cuneiform-metatarsal arthrodesis, 107
  evaluation, 108
  medial ray, 108, 109
  metatarsocuneiform arthrodesis, 107
  second metatarsal base, 108, 109

I

Implant arthroplasty, hallux metatarsophalangeal arthrodesis, 49–50
Inferior peroneal retinaculum, anatomy, 286

SUBJECT INDEX

Ingrown toenail
  nail bed, 15
  nail plate, 15
  recurrent, 15
  surgical management, 3–12
Interdigital neuroma
  diagnosis, 163–167
  resection. *See* Primary interdigital neuroma resection; Secondary interdigital neuroma resection
Intermetatarsal ligament, primary interdigital neuroma resection, 169
Intermetatarsal nerve, primary interdigital neuroma resection, 169–174
Interphalangeal joint, arthritis, 21
Intramedullary rod, tibiocalcaneal arthrodesis, 488, 490 491

J
Joint arthrodesis, cheilectomy, 129
Joker retractor, Mitchell osteotomy, 75

K
Keller resection arthroplasty, cheilectomy, 129
Kirschner wire
  Akin procedure, 68, 69
  ankle arthrodesis, 475, 477
  calcaneal fracture, 413
  hallux interphalangeal arthrodesis, 24, 26
  hallux proximal phalanx osteotomy, 68, 69
  proximal first metatarsal osteotomy, 97
  rheumatoid forefoot reconstruction, 205
  talus-calcaneus-cuboid arthrodesis, 387, 389, 392
Knee replacement, 375

L
Lateral displacement first metatarsal neck osteotomy, medial sesamoid, 82
Lateral displacement osteotomy
  first metatarsal head, 81
  Herbert screw fixation, 81
Lateral plantar nerve, first branch, 333–340
Lisfranc arthrodesis, 231–246
  complications, 242–244
  contraindications, 231–233
  illustrative case, 244–246
  incision, 234–235
  indications, 231–233
  malunion, 244
  nonunion, 244
  postoperative management, 241–242
  preoperative planning, 233–234
  surgical procedure, 234–240, 241
Loupe magnification, marginal toenail ablation, 5, 10

M
Malposition
  ankle arthrodesis, 480–481
  hallux metatarsophalangeal arthrodesis, 59
    salvage, 59
  talus-calcaneus-cuboid arthrodesis, 395
Malunion
  ankle fracture realignment
    closure, 459
    complications, 463
    contraindications, 451–452
    fixation, 457–459
    illustrative case, 463–465
    incision, 455
    indications, 451–452
    postoperative management, 463
    preoperative planning, 452–455
    surgical procedure, 455
  calcaneal fracture, 425–436
  calcaneus arthrodesis, 425–436
  calcaneus osteotomy, 425–436
  proximal first metatarsal osteotomy, 102–103
  talonavicular arthrodesis, 254
  tibiocalcaneal arthrodesis, 493
Marginal toenail ablation, 3–12
  anesthesia, 4
  ankle block, 4
  closing, 7–8, 12
  complications, 9–10
  contraindications, 3
  digital block, 4
  fungal infection, 3, 9–10
  illustrative case, 10–13
  indications, 3
  loupe magnification, 5, 10
  matricectomy, 6–7, 10, 11, 12
    complete, 7
    partial, 6–7
  nail splitter, 5
  postoperative management, 8–9, 13
  preoperative planning, 3–4
  surgical procedure, 4–8, 10–13
Marin reamer, hallux metatarsophalangeal arthrodesis, 54–55
Matricectomy, marginal toenail ablation, 6–7, 10, 11, 12
  complete, 7
  partial, 6–7
Medial calcaneal nerve branch, abductor digiti quinti nerve release, 339
Medial capsule, elevation, 34, 35
Medial eminence
  removal, 32, 35–36
  sagittal sulcus, 88, 89
  size, 88
Medial eminence pain
  chevron osteotomy, 31
  proximal first metatarsal osteotomy, 86
Medial longitudinal arch, weight bearing, 108
Medial ray, hypermobility, 108, 109
Medial sesamoid, lateral displacement first metatarsal neck osteotomy, 82

Metatarsal, 163–227
  osteotomy, 36
Metatarsal head
  cartilage pathologic changes, 124–125
  chevron osteotomy, 36, 37, 38
Metatarsocuneiform arthritis
  cuneiform-metatarsal arthrodesis, 107
  metatarsocuneiform arthrodesis, 107
Metatarsocuneiform arthrodesis, 107–116
  adolescent bunion, 107
  age, 107
  complications, 115
  contraindications, 108
  hallux valgus, 107
  hypermobility, 107
  illustrative case, 115–116
  incision, 110, 111–112
  indications, 107–108
  metatarsocuneiform arthritis, 107
  metatarsus adductus, 108
  metatarsus primus varus, 107
  patient education, 110
  postoperative management, 115
  preoperative planning, 108–110
  resection, 111–112
  screw fixation, 112, 114
  surgical procedure, 110–115
Metatarsophalangeal joint, 31–159
  chevron osteotomy, incongruity, 45–46
  collateral ligament rupture, 150
  proximal first metatarsal osteotomy
    noncongruent, 86, 88
    subluxated, 86, 88
  testing for instability, 151
Metatarsophalangeal joint arthritis
  chevron osteotomy, 32–33
  proximal first metatarsal osteotomy, 86
Metatarsophalangeal joint capsule,
    medial exposure, 34, 35
Metatarsophalangeal joint dorsiflexion
  second toe resection arthroplasty, 157
  third toe resection arthroplasty, 157
Metatarsophalangeal resection
    arthroplasty, second toe
    realignment, 145
Metatarsophalangeal valgus, chevron
    osteotomy, recurrent, 45
Metatarsus adductus
  cuneiform-metatarsal arthrodesis, 108
  proximal first metatarsal osteotomy, 86
Metatarsus primus varus, cuneiform-
    metatarsal arthrodesis 107
Midtarsal, 249–267
Mitchell osteotomy, 73–84
  ankle block, 74
  biplanar metatarsal neck osteotomy, 83
  closure, 79, 82
  complications, 80–82, 83
  contraindications, 73
  hallux rigidus, 81
  hallux valgus, 73
  Herbert screw arthrodesis, 79
  illustrative case, 83, 84
  incision, 74–75
  indications, 73
  Joker retractor, 75
  lateral correction, 75–79
  postoperative management, 82–83
  preoperative planning, 73–74
  prognosis, 93
  resection of medial eminence, 75
  surgical technique, 74–82
Mitchell's bunionectomy. *See* Mitchell
    osteotomy
Morton's neuroma
  diagnosis, 163–167
  second web space, 163, 164
  third web space, 163, 164
Morton's neuroma resection, 163–177
  ankle block, 168
  contraindications, 163–164
  incision, 168
  indications, 163–164
  patient education, 175
  preoperative planning, 164–167
  recurrence, 174, 175, 179–188
  surgical procedure, 167–168
Mulder's click, 166
Myotendinous junction, 301–302, 303

N
Nail bed, ingrown toenail, 15
Nail plate, ingrown toenail, 15
Nail spike, 9
Nail splitter, marginal toenail ablation, 5
Nerve conduction study, 334
Neuroma, talonavicular arthrodesis, 254
Nonunion
  Akin procedure, 70
  calcaneus arthrodesis, 435
  calcaneus osteotomy, 435
  hallux interphalangeal arthrodesis, 26
  hallux metatarsophalangeal
      arthrodesis, 59
    salvage, 59
  hallux proximal phalanx osteotomy, 70
  rheumatoid forefoot reconstruction,
      208
  subtalar arthrodesis, 366
  talocalcaneal arthrodesis, 366
  talonavicular arthrodesis, 254
  talus-calcaneus-cuboid arthrodesis,
      395–396

O
Os calcis abnormality, 351
Osteoarthritis, talus-calcaneus-cuboid
    arthrodesis, 369 396
Osteoporosis, ankle arthrodesis, 468

P
Paratenon, 301, 302
Patient education
  ankle fracture realignment, 452
  calcaneal tuberosity osteotomy, 355
  cuneiform-metatarsal arthrodesis, 110
  metatarsocuneiform arthrodesis, 110
  Morton's neuroma resection, 175
  primary interdigital neuroma resection,
      175

talus-calcaneus-cuboid arthrodesis, 369–370, 377
Peripheral neuropathy, ankle arthrodesis, 468
Peroneal tendon, course, 287
Peroneal tendon repair-reconstruction, 285–297
   anesthesia, 288
   ankle inversion injury, 285
   complications, 296
   contraindications, 285–286
   illustrative case, 297
   incision, 288
   indications, 285
   postoperative management, 296
   preoperative planning, 286–288
   surgical procedure, 288–296
Phalanges, 1–27
   diabetes, 3, 10
   erythema, 10
Phenol
   storage, 20
   technique, 20
Phenol matrixectomy, 15–20
   advantages, 15
   anesthesia, 17
   closing, 18, 19
   complications, 19–20
   contraindications, 15–16
   diabetes, 15
   digital block, 17
   epinychium, 17, 19, 20
   fungal infection, 16
   illustrative case, 20
   indications, 15–16
   postoperative management, 19
   preoperative planning, 16, 17
   serous drainage, 19
   surgical procedure, 17–19
Plantar angulation
   Akin procedure, 70
   hallux proximal phalanx osteotomy, 70
Plantar condylectomy, 74
Plantar fascia release, 323–332
   anesthesia, 325
   ankle block, 325
   anteromedial heel pad field block, 325
   closure, 329
   complications, 330–331
   contraindications, 324
   flatfoot, 331
   heel pain, 323
   heel spur, 323
   illustrative case, 331–332
   incision, 326
   indications, 324
   nerve damage, 331
   plantar fasciitis, 323
   plantar intrinsic muscle damage, 331
   postoperative management, 329–330
   preoperative planning, 324–325
   rehabilitation, 330
   surgical procedure, 325–329
Plantar fasciitis, 324
   conservative treatment, 323
   plantar fascia release, 323
Plantar nerve, anatomy, 181

Plantar scar, secondary interdigital neuroma resection, 187
Plantaris tendon, 302, 303
Plantaris tendon repair, 313, 315
Posterior iliac crest, bone graft, 484–485
Posterior tibial tendon release-substitution
   complications, 280
   contraindications, 272
   flexor digitorum longus, 271–280
   illustrative case, 280–282
   incision, 273
   indications, 271–272
   postoperative management, 279–280
   preoperative planning, 272–273
   surgical procedure, 273–278, 279
Primary interdigital neuroma resection, 163–177
   ankle block, 168
   closure, 174
   complications, 175–176
   contraindications, 163–164
   incision, 168
   indications, 163–164
   intermetatarsal ligament, 169
   intermetatarsal nerve, 169–174
   patient education, 175
   postoperative management, 175
   preoperative planning, 164–167
   prognosis, 175
   recurrence, 174, 175, 179–188. *See also* Secondary interdigital neuroma resection
   surgical procedure, 167–168
Proximal first metatarsal osteotomy, 85–105
   advantages, 85
   alignment, 98–100
   anesthesia, 89–90
   ankle block, 89–90
   closure, 100
   complications, 101–103
   contraindications, 85–86
   correct angle, 94, 95–96
   degenerative arthritis, 86
   delayed union, 102
   distal soft tissue realignment, 85
   hallux rigidus, 86
   hallux valgus, 85
      recurrence, 101
   hallux varus, 102
   illustrative case, 103–105
   incision, 90–93
   indications, 85–86
   Kirschner wire, 97
   malunion, 102–103
   medial eminence pain, 86
   metatarsophalangeal joint
      noncongruent, 86, 88
      subluxated, 86, 88
   metatarsophalangeal joint arthritis, 86
   metatarsus adductus, 86
   postoperative management, 100–101
   preoperative planning, 86–89
   saw position, 93, 94–96
   surgical procedures, 89–99

Proximal focal femoral deficiency, Syme amputation, 497–498
Pseudarthrosis, ankle arthrodesis, 480

R

Reflex sympathetic dystrophy syndrome, 180
Rehabilitation
   Achilles tendon acute repair, 306
   cheilectomy, 129
   plantar fascia release, 330
   Syme amputation, 507–508
   transmetatarsal amputation, 222–224
Resection arthroplasty, hallux metatarsophalangeal arthrodesis, 49–50
Retrocalcaneal bursa, anatomy, 342, 343
Retrocalcaneal bursitis
   calcaneal prominence resection, 341
   conservative treatment, 341, 342
Rheumatoid arthritis, 483
   metatarsophalangeal joint involvement, 197
   talus-calcaneus-cuboid arthrodesis, 369
Rheumatoid forefoot reconstruction, 197–211
   callus formation, 208
   closure, 201, 203, 206
   complications, 207–208
   contraindications, 197
   gait instability, 208
   illustrative case, 208–211
   incisions, 199–200
   indications, 197
   Kirschner wire, 205
   nonunion, 208
   osteoporotic forefoot, 200
   postoperative management, 207
   preoperative planning, 198
   screw fixation, 205
   surgical procedure, 198–206

S

Sagittal sulcus
   location, 35
   medial eminence, 88, 89
Second metatarsal base, hypermobility, 108, 109
Second metatarsal head pain, 80
Second metatarsophalangeal joint
   dorsofibular capsular rupture, 136
   synovitis, 143
Second metatarsophalangeal joint pain, 135
Second metatarsophalangeal joint subluxation
   second toe resection arthroplasty, 149
   third toe resection arthroplasty, 149
Second toe
   overlapping, 135–148
      pathophysiology, 135, 136
      spreading between, 149, 150
Second toe realignment, 135–148
   complications, 147–148
   contraindications, 137
   deformity recurrence, 147
   delayed wound healing, 147
   DuVries arthroplasty, 145
   extensor digitorum brevis, 142–145
   extensor digitorum longus, 142–145
   flexor digitorum longus, 140–142
   hallux valgus, 137–139
   illustrative case, 146, 147, 148
   indications, 135, 136
   metatarsophalangeal resection arthroplasty, 145
   postoperative management, 146–147
   preoperative planning, 137–140
   reduced voluntary control, 147
   surgical procedure, 140–146
Second toe resection arthroplasty, 149–159
   anesthesia, 152
   claw toe, 149
   closure, 155, 156
   complications, 157–158
   contraindications, 150
   extension contracture, 149
   hammer toe, 149
   illustrative case, 158–159
   incision, 154
   indications, 149–150
   metatarsophalangeal joint dorsiflexion, 157
   postoperative management, 156–157
   preoperative planning, 150, 151
   principle, 150, 151
   prognosis, 157
   second metatarsophalangeal joint subluxation, 149
   surgical procedure, 152–155, 156
   third metatarsophalangeal joint subluxation, 149
   toe shortening, 157
   toe stability loss, 157
Second web space, Morton's neuroma, 163, 164
Secondary interdigital neuroma resection, 174, 175, 179–188
   anesthesia, 183–184
   closure, 185, 186
   complications, 187
   contraindications, 179–180
   dorsal approach, 183
   illustrative case, 187–188
   incision, 184
   indications, 179–180
   plantar approach, 182, 183
   plantar scar, 187
   postoperative management, 185–186
   preoperative planning, 180–183
   prognosis, 186
   surgical procedure, 183–185, 186
Sensation testing, 167
Serous drainage, phenol matrixectomy, 19
Sesamoid, 88
Sesamoidectomy, 21
Shenton's line, 453
Shoe, transmetatarsal amputation, 223
Silastic implant, hallux metatarsophalangeal arthrodesis, 50

SUBJECT INDEX

Steinmann pin
  ankle arthrodesis, 475, 476, 477
  calcaneal fracture, 410–411
  calcaneal tuberosity osteotomy, 355
  calcaneus arthrodesis, 430, 431, 432
  calcaneus osteotomy, 430, 431, 432
  subtalar arthrodesis, 359–368
  talocalcaneal arthrodesis, 359–368
Subtalar arthrodesis
  anesthesia, 359–368
  complications, 365–366
  contraindications, 360
  illustrative case, 366–368
  incision, 360
  indications, 359–360
  nonunion, 366
  postoperative management, 365
  preoperative planning, 360
  Steinmann pin fixation, 359–368
  surgical procedure, 360
Subtalar intrusion, 483
Subtalar joint
  comminution, 401
  decreased range of motion, 416
  posterior facet, 401
Superficial peroneal nerve, injury, 242
Superior peroneal retinaculum, anatomy, 286
Sural nerve, 301–302
  calcaneus fracture, 416
Sural nerve neuroma, Achilles tendon delayed repair, 319
Sustentacular fragment, 407
Syme amputation, 497–511
  advantages, 497
  arteriosclerotic peripheral vascular disease, 497–498
  closure, 505–506
  complications, 508–509
  congenital pseudarthrosis of tibia, 497–498
  fibular hemimelia, 497–498
  heel pad, 498
  illustrative case, 509–511
  incision, 501
  neurovascular bundle, 502
  one-stage, 499
  postoperative management, 507
  preoperative planning, 498
  proximal focal femoral deficiency, 497–498
  rehabilitation, 507–508
  surgical procedure, 499–507
  trauma, 497–498
  two-stage, 499, 507
  ulceration, 508
  vascular status evaluation, 498
Synovitis
  chronic, 135
  second metatarsophalangeal joint, 143

T

Talar body
  avascular necrosis, 468
  Blair fusion, 468
Talipes equinovarus, 483
Talocalcaneal arthrodesis
  anesthesia, 359–368
  complications, 365–366
  contraindications, 360
  illustrative case, 366–368
  incision, 360
  indications, 359–360
  nonunion, 366
  postoperative management, 365
  preoperative planning, 360
  Steinmann pin fixation, 359–368
  surgical procedure, 360
Talocrural angle, 453, 454
Talonavicular arthrodesis, 249–256
  anesthesia, 250
  closure, 252
  complications, 254
  contraindications, 249
  illustrative case, 254–256
  indications, 249
  malunion, 254
  neuroma, 254
  nonunion, 254
  postoperative management, 252
  preoperative planning, 249–250
  surgical procedure, 250–252, 253
Talonavicular joint, 249
Talus
  anatomic reduction, 463
  avascular necrosis, 483
Talus-calcaneus-cuboid arthrodesis, 369–399
  Achilles tendon lengthening, 385
  Charcot-Marie-Tooth disease, 369
  closure, 393–394
  complications, 395–396
  contraindications, 369
  debridement, 383–385
  fixation, 387–392
  fixed hindfoot deformity, 369
  illustrative case, 396–399
  indications, 369
  Kirschner wire, 387, 389, 392
  malposition, 395
  nonunion, 395–396
  osteoarthritis, 369, 396
  patient education, 369–370, 377
  postoperative management, 394–395
  preoperative planning, 369–377
  recovery period, 370, 377
  rheumatoid arthritis, 369
  in situ, 377
  surgical procedure, 377
Third metatarsophalangeal joint subluxation
  second toe resection arthroplasty, 149
  third toe resection arthroplasty, 149
Third toe, spreading between, 149, 150
Third toe resection arthroplasty, 149–159
  anesthesia, 152
  claw toe, 149
  closure, 155, 156
  complications, 157–158
  contraindications, 150
  extension contracture, 149
  hammer toe, 149

Third toe resection arthroplasty (*contd.*)
  illustrative case, 158–159
  incision, 154
  indications, 149–150
  metatarsophalangeal joint dorsiflexion, 157
  postoperative management, 156–157
  preoperative planning, 150, 151
  principle, 150, 151
  prognosis, 157
  second metatarsophalangeal joint subluxation, 149
  surgical procedure, 152–155, 156
  third metatarsophalangeal joint subluxation, 149
  toe shortening, 157
  toe stability loss, 157
Third web space, Morton's neuroma, 163, 164
Thompson test, Achilles tendon rupture, 299–300
Tibial mechanical axis, 373
Tibial nerve
  anatomy, 181
  calcaneal fracture, 416
Tibial plafond, 463
Tibialis posterior tendon
  abnormalities, 271
    stages, 271, 272
  preoperative situation, 278
Tibialis posterior tendon release-substitution
  complications, 280
  contraindications, 272
  flexor digitorum longus, 271–280
  illustrative case, 280–282
  incision, 273
  indications, 271–272
  postoperative management, 279–280
  preoperative planning, 272–273
  surgical procedure, 273–278, 279
Tibiocalcaneal arthrodesis, 483–496
  bone graft, 484–485, 491
  Calandruccio device, 488, 489, 490
  closure, 491–492
  complications, 493–495
  contraindications, 483
  fixation, 488–492
  illustrative cases, 495, 496
  incision, 485, 486
  indications, 483
  intramedullary rod, 488, 490, 491
  malunion, 493
  nonunion, 493
  postoperative management, 492–493
  preoperative planning, 483–484
  surgical procedure, 484–492
Tibiofibular-talar alignment, 451
Toe box impingement, 135, 136
Toe shortening
  second toe resection arthroplasty, 157
  third toe resection arthroplasty, 157
Toe stability loss
  second toe resection arthroplasty, 157
  third toe resection arthroplasty, 157
Toenail. *See* Marginal toenail ablation
Transmetatarsal amputation, 213–227
  advantages, 213–215
  closure, 220–222
  complications, 224
  contraindications, 213–215
  diabetes, 213
  gangrene, 213
  healing, 224
  illustrative case, 225, 226–227
  indications, 213–215
  pitfall, 222
  postoperative management, 222
  preoperative planning, 215
  rehabilitation, 222–224
  as salvage procedure, 214
  shoe, 223
  surgical procedure, 215–222
  trauma, 213
  ulceration, 224
Trauma
  compartment release, 257
  Syme amputation, 497–498
  transmetatarsal amputation, 213
Tricortical graft, hallux metatarsophalangeal arthrodesis 58, 59, 62, 63
Triple arthrodesis, 369–399, 427, 428
  Achilles tendon lengthening, 385
  Charcot-Marie-Tooth, 369
  closure, 393–394
  complications, 395–396
  contraindications, 369
  debridement, 383–385
  fixation, 387–392
  fixed hindfoot deformity, 369
  illustrative case, 396–399
  indications, 369
  Kirschner wire, 387, 389, 392
  malposition, 395
  nonunion, 395–396
  osteoarthritis, 369, 396
  patient education, 369–370, 377
  postoperative management, 394–395
  preoperative planning, 369–377
  recovery period, 370, 377
  rheumatoid arthritis, 369
  in situ, 377
  surgical procedure, 377
Tubular nail, 4, 15

U
Ulceration
  Syme amputation, 508
  transmetatarsal amputation, 224

V
Varus-valgus stress, chevron osteotomy, 32
Vascular compromise of digit, 148

W
Walking cast, chevron osteotomy, 44
Weight bearing, medial longitudinal arch, 108